Traditional and Alternative Medicine

Traditional and Alternative Medicine

Edited by Brendon Gould

SYRAWOOD
PUBLISHING HOUSE
New York

Published by Syrawood Publishing House,
750 Third Avenue, 9th Floor,
New York, NY 10017, USA
www.syrawoodpublishinghouse.com

Traditional and Alternative Medicine
Edited by Brendon Gould

International Standard Book Number: 978-1-68286-478-4 (Hardback)

Cataloging-in-Publication Data

Traditional and alternative medicine / edited by Brendon Gould.
p. cm.
Includes bibliographical references and index.
ISBN 978-1-68286-478-4
1. Traditional medicine. 2. Alternative medicine. 3. Medicine, Chinese. I. Gould, Brendon.
R733 .T73 2017
615.5--dc23

Printed in China.

TABLE OF CONTENTS

PREFACE

Medicinal practices that were developed and practiced before the invention of modern medicine is termed as traditional medicine. This book on traditional and alternative medicine discusses topics that are concerned with therapeutic practices and its effects relating to long-term health and nutritional patterns. These medicinal practices rely on harnessing the body's energy for therapeutic aid. The topics included in this book on traditional and alternative medicine are of utmost significance and bound to provide incredible insights to readers. While understanding the long-term perspectives of the topics, the book makes an effort in highlighting their impact as a modern tool for the growth of the discipline. This book will be helpful for students and researchers in the field of physiotherapy traditional and alternative medicinal practices.

This book unites the global concepts and researches in an organized manner for a comprehensive understanding of the subject. It is a ripe text for all researchers, students, scientists or anyone else who is interested in acquiring a better knowledge of this dynamic field.

I extend my sincere thanks to the contributors for such eloquent research chapters. Finally, I thank my family for being a source of support and help.

Editor

GABA-A Receptor Modulation and Anticonvulsant, Anxiolytic, and Antidepressant Activities of Constituents from *Artemisia indica* Linn

Imran Khan,[1] Nasiara Karim,[2] Waqar Ahmad,[2] Abeer Abdelhalim,[3] and Mary Chebib[4]

[1]*Department of Pharmacy, University of Swabi, Khyber Pakhtunkhwa 23340, Pakistan*
[2]*Department of Pharmacy, University of Malakand, Khyber Pakhtunkhwa 18800, Pakistan*
[3]*Faculty of Science, Taibah University, Medina 30001, Saudi Arabia*
[4]*Faculty of Pharmacy, University of Sydney, Sydney, NSW 2006, Australia*

Correspondence should be addressed to Nasiara Karim; nasiara.karim@hotmail.com

Academic Editor: Carmen Mannucci

Artemisia indica, also known as "Mugwort," has been widely used in traditional medicines. However, few studies have investigated the effects of nonvolatile components of *Artemisia indica* on central nervous system's function. Fractionation of *Artemisia indica* led to the isolation of carnosol, ursolic acid, and oleanolic acid which were evaluated for their effects on GABA-A receptors in electrophysiological studies in *Xenopus* oocytes and were subsequently investigated in mouse models of acute toxicity, convulsions (pentylenetetrazole induced seizures), depression (tail suspension and forced swim tests), and anxiety (elevated plus maze and light/dark box paradigms). Carnosol, ursolic acid, and oleanolic acid were found to be positive modulators of $\alpha 1\beta 2\gamma 2L$ GABA-A receptors and the modulation was antagonized by flumazenil. Carnosol, ursolic acid, and oleanolic acid were found to be devoid of any signs of acute toxicity (50–200 mg/kg) but elicited anticonvulsant, antidepressant, and anxiolytic activities. Thus carnosol, ursolic acid, and oleanolic acid demonstrated CNS activity in mouse models of anticonvulsant, antidepressant, and anxiolysis. The anxiolytic activity of all three compounds was ameliorated by flumazenil suggesting a mode of action via the benzodiazepine binding site of GABA-A receptors.

1. Introduction

Artemisia indica is known as "Mugwort" in the local community in South Asia and belongs to the family "Asteraceae." The plant is perennial shrub with height of 2–8 meters tall, found in Northern area of Pakistan as well as in Asia and Europe at high altitude of cold temperate zone [1]. *Artemisia* species possesses antiplasmodial [2], antispasmodic and bronchodilator [3], antihypertensive [4], antiallergic [5], hepatoprotective [3], and antibacterial activities [6]. Furthermore, various species of this plant have been reported to possess antihyperglycemic effects as well [1]. Several species of *Artemisia* have been reported to possess CNS activities. For example, *Artemisia absinthium* has been shown to possess antidepressant activity in mouse models of tail suspension and forced swimming tests [7]. Also, *Artemisia dracunculus* has been reported to possess central antinociceptive effect [8].

Phytochemical studies have featured the presence of various classes of substances including essential oils, flavonoids, amino acids, triterpenes, coumarins, phenolic compounds, and carotenoids [9, 10]. The flavonoids isolated from various species of Asteraceae include apigenin-4-O-methyl ether, isoscutellarein-8-O-methyl ether, isoscutellarein-8,4-dimethyl ether, 8-methoxyluteolin, 5,3,4-trihydroxy-6,7,8-trimethoxyflavone, 5,7,3,4-tetrahydroxy-3,6,8-trimethoxyflavone, and 5,3,4-trihydroxy-3,6,7,8-tetramethoxyflavone [11]. Terpenes isolated from various species of Asteraceae include monoterpenoids, triterpenoids, and sesquiterpenoids such as dihydroartemisinic acid, artemisinic acid, artemisinin, and arteannuin B [12]. Various phenolic compounds isolated from Asteraceae family include caffeoyl derivatives, that is, chlorogenic acid, cichoric acid, 1,5-, 3,5-, and 4,5-di-*O*-caffeoylquinic acids, and 3-caffeoylquinic acid [13]. Chlorogenic

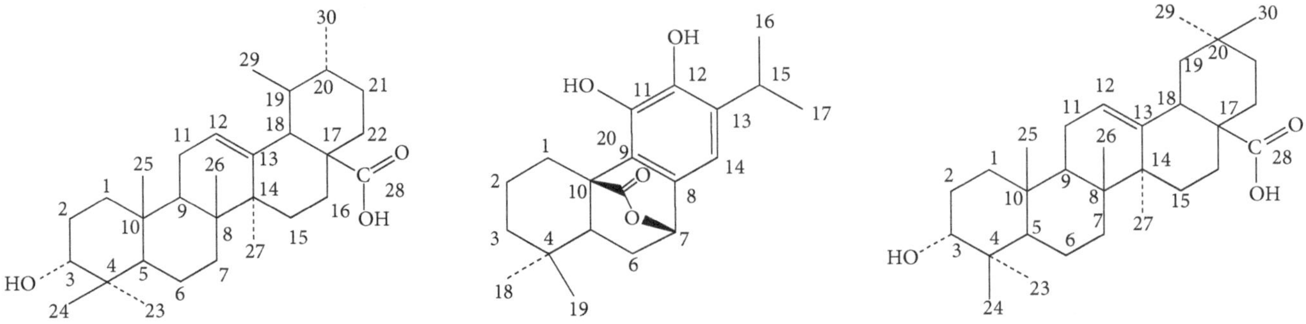

Ursolic acid Carnosol Oleanolic acid

FIGURE 1: Chemical structure of the compounds isolated from *Artemisia indica* Linn.

acid isolated from *Artemisia capillaris* has been shown to possess antidepressant activity [14]. Flavonoids from *Artemisia herba-alba* have been shown to possess in vitro GABA-A benzodiazepine receptor activity [15].

γ-Aminobutyric acid (GABA) is the major inhibitory neurotransmitter in the mammalian central nervous system (CNS) activating neurons through a number of pharmacologically and structurally different receptor subtypes: ionotropic GABA-A and GABA-C and metabotropic GABA-B receptors. GABA-A receptor plays an important role in the overall balance between neuronal inhibition and excitation [16]. The GABA-A receptor is possibly the most complex member of the ligand-gated ion channel and is a pharmacological target not only for GABA but also for general anaesthetics, barbiturates, picrotoxin, and neurosteroids and a number of flavonoids modulate GABA-A receptors in CNS [17, 18].

Although the phytochemical profile of various *Artemisia* species has been extensively studied, this is the first study reporting the phytochemical and CNS pharmacological profile of *Artemisia indica*. Carnosol, ursolic acid, and oleanolic acid (Figure 1) isolated from *Artemisia indica* were evaluated for their positive modulatory effects on GABA-A receptors expressed in *Xenopus* oocytes and were subsequently investigated in mouse models of toxicity and anticonvulsant, antidepressant, and anxiolytic activity to correlate the in vitro and in vivo findings.

2. Materials and Methods

2.1. Chemicals, Materials, Instrumentation, and Drugs. All chemicals used were purchased from Aldrich Chemical Co., Ltd. (St. Louis, MO, USA), and were of highest commercially available purity. Silica gel for column chromatography (CC) was performed on silica gel (Merck silica gel 60H, particle size 5–40 μm) and Sephadex LH-20 gel. Thin layer chromatography (TLC) was performed on Merck aluminium backed plates, precoated with silica (0.2 mm, 60F254). UV spectra were recorded on Hitachi's U-2000 Double-Beam UV/Vis Spectrophotometer. Mass spectra were carried out on a Thermo Finnigan PolarisQ Ion Trap system (Waltham, MA, USA) using a direct exposure probe. Nuclear magnetic resonance ^{1}H NMR and ^{13}C NMR spectra were recorded at 400 and 100 MHz, respectively, on a Varian Gemini spectrometer (Palo Alto, CA, USA). Melting points were determined using a Stuart SMP10 melting point apparatus (Stone, Staffordshire, UK).

Diazepam was kindly donated by the Department of Pharmacy, University of Peshawar. Imipramine, DMSO, Tween solution (TWEEN® 80), flumazenil (Sigma-Aldrich, USA), and pentylenetetrazol (Tokyo Chemical Industries Co., Ltd.) were purchased for the study. All chemicals and solvents used in this research were of analytical grade.

2.2. Plant Material and Extraction. The whole part of the plant was dried in the shade at room temperature and crushed into fine powder. 5 kg of dried powdered sample was extracted with 100% methanol. The methanol extract was filtered and three sample replicates were extracted under the same conditions with new solvent. The methanol extract was filtered and evaporated under reduced pressure using a vacuum rotary evaporator at 45°C which yields 700 g of semisolid crude methanolic extract of *Artemisia indica*. The crude methanolic extract was then suspended in deionized water and partitioned sequentially with n-hexane, chloroform, ethyl acetate (EtOAc), and butanol (water saturated BuOH) fractions and was then evaporated using a vacuum rotary evaporator to get different extracts.

2.3. Purification. In the preliminary assay of the crude methanolic extract of *Artemisia indica* Linn, the chloroform fraction was found to be the most active one and possessed various important pharmacological activities. The chloroform fraction 250 g was subjected to column chromatography (Φ28 × 4.5 cm) on silica gel (70–230 mesh size) for further isolation and purification which yielded the three new compounds from *Artemisia indica* Linn for the first time. These included ursolic acid, carnosol, and oleanolic acid.

The chloroform fraction (250 g) was subjected to column chromatography (Φ28 × 4.5 cm) which was initially eluted with pure hexane and then the polarity gradually increased using ethyl acetate affording three subfractions F1, F2, and F3. F1 (62 g) was further subjected to column chromatography (Φ24 × 3 cm) with 5% ethyl acetate/hexane as the solvent system which afforded carnosol (3 g). F2 (47.8 g) was subjected to column chromatography (Φ25 × 3 cm) (8% ethyl acetate/hexane as the solvent system) that gave the ursolic acid (3.8 g). F3 (obtained from the soluble fraction of 200 g of chloroform) was separated by column chromatography (Φ21 × 3.5 cm) to yield oleanolic acid (2 g) (15% ethyl acetate/hexane as the solvent system).

2.4. Spectroscopic Data of the Isolated Compounds

Ursolic Acid. Colorless needles; ESMS m/z (%): 479.4 (100), 457 (5), 439 (15), 425 (44), 413 (12). IR spectrum showed the presence of carbonyl at (1697 cm^{-1}), OH group at absorption (3510 cm^{-1}), and trisubstituted double bond at (1635 and 820 cm^{-1}). The ^{1}H NMR (DMSO-d_6) δ ppm: 2.99 (^{1}H, s, H-3), 5.11 (^{1}H, s, H-12), 2.08 (^{1}H, d, H-18), 0.89 (^{1}H, s, H-23), 0.73 (^{1}H, s, H-24), 0.65 (^{1}H, s, H-25), 0.87 (^{1}H, s, H-26), 1.02 (^{1}H, s, H-27), 0.79 (^{1}H, d, H-29), 0.84 (^{1}H, d, H-30), 2.08 (^{1}H, d, J = 11.6 Hz, H-28). ^{13}C NMR (DMSO-d_6) δ ppm: 38.7 (C-1), 27.4 (C-2), 77.3 (C-3), 38 (C-4), 55.2 (C-5), 18.4 (C-6), 33.2 (C-7), 39.5 (C-8), 47.5 (C-9), 37 (C-10), 23.3 (C-11), 125 (C-12), 138.6 (C-13), 42.1 (C-14), 28.7 (C-15), 24.3 (C-16), 47.3 (C-17), 52.8 (C-18), 38.9 (C-19), 38.8 (C-20), 30.6 (C-21), 36.8 (C-22), 28.7 (C-23), 16.5 (C-24), 15.70 (C-25), 17.4 (C-26), 23.7 (C-27), 178.7 (C-28), 17.5 (C-29), 21.5 (C-30).

Carnosol. White solid; UV λ_{max}: 209 and 285 nm; ESMS m/z (%): 683.4 (100), 331.0 (19); ^{1}H NMR (DMSO-d_6) δ ppm: 2.64dd, 2.43dd (H-α:β, H-1), 1.5 m (H-2), 1.42dd, 1.21dd (H-α:β, H-3), 1.59dd (H-5), 2.01ddd, 1.6 m (H-α:β, H-6), 5.44dd (H-7), 6.68s (H-14), 3.21s (H-15), 1.10d (H-16), 1.10d (H-17), 0.79s (H-18), 0.77s (H-19). ^{13}C NMR (DMSO-d_6) δ ppm: 29.2 (C-1), 19.0 (C-2), 41.0 (C-3), 34.6 (C-4), 45.4 (C-5), 29.7 (C-6), 77.4 (C-7), 132.0 (C-8), 122.3 (C-9), 48.3 (C-10), 143.7 (C-11), 143.5 (C-12), 134.7 (C-13), 111.7 (C-14), 26.6 (C-15), 23.1 (C-16), 23.2 (C-17), 31.2 (C-18), 19.8 (C-19), 175.9 (C-20).

Oleanolic Acid. White solid; ESMS m/z (%): 456 (100), 431 (15), 391 (8); ^{1}H NMR (DMSO-d_6) δ ppm: 2.98 (^{1}H, t, H-1), 5.14 (^{1}H, H-12), 2.78 (^{1}H, dd, H-18), 0.65 (^{1}H, s, H-23), 0.85 (^{1}H, s, H-24), 0.87 (^{1}H, s, H-15). ^{13}C NMR (DMSO-d_6) δ ppm: 38.5 (C-1), 27.4 (C-2), 77.3 (C-3), 38.9 (C-4), 55.5 (C-5), 55.5 (C-6), 32.5 (C-7), 38.8 (C-8), 47.5 (C-9), 37.0 (C-10), 23.1 (C-11), 122.0 (C-12), 144.3 (C-13), 41.8 (C-14), 27.6 (C-15), 23.3 (C-16), 45.9 (C-17), 41.3 (C-18), 46.1 (C-19), 30.8 (C-20), 33.8 (C-21), 32.9 (C-22), 28.7 (C-23), 16.5 (C-24), 15.5 (C-25).

2.5. Pharmacological Activities

2.5.1. Animals. Male Swiss mice with a weight range of 20 to 30 g were purchased from the National institute of health (NIH), Islamabad, Pakistan. Animals were housed in the Department of Pharmacy, University of Malakand's animal house, with fresh water and standard food available ad libitum. The animals were maintained at a 12-hour light and dark cycle and with room temperature of 22–25°C in the animal house. All animal procedures have been approved by the Departmental Animal Ethical Committee (DAEC/PHARM/2012/13) and were conducted according to the UK animal scientific procedure act, 1986.

2.6. GABA Receptor Subunit Constructs. Human GABA-A α1, β2, and γ2L cDNA subcloned in pCDM8 were linearized with the appropriate restriction endonucleases and capped transcripts were produced from linearized plasmids using the "mMessage mMachine" T7 transcript kit from Ambion (Austin, TX, USA). The quality of mRNA was determined by 0.5% agarose gel electrophoresis. mRNA concentrations were measured by *NanoDrop*® ND-1000 UV-Vis Spectrophotometer. mRNA was diluted with nuclease-free water and stored at −80°C.

2.7. Expression of Recombinant GABA Receptors in Xenopus Oocytes

2.7.1. Oocyte Preparation. Sexually mature female *Xenopus laevis* were kept under optimal conditions by authorized animal keepers at the University of Sydney Animal House and fed standard frog food. Stages V-VI oocytes were harvested under 0.1% tricaine (3-aminobenzoic acid ethyl ester) anesthesia. Oocytes were defolliculated by shaking for approximately 1 h at 18°C in collagenase (2 mg/mL) dissolved in OR2 solution containing (in mmol/L) NaCl 96, KCl 2, $CaCl_2$ 1, $MgCl_2$ 1, and HEPES 5, pH 7.4.

Stages V-VI oocytes were sorted and injected (Nanoject, Drummond Scientific Co., Broomall, PA) with cRNA reconstituted in nuclease-free water in a ratio of 1α (25 ng) : 1β (25 ng) : 5 (γ) (125 ng). Oocytes were incubated for up to 4–8 days in standard ND96, pH 7.4, supplemented with pyruvate (2.5 mM), theophylline (0.5 mM), gentamycin (50 μg/mL), and 2% horse serum at 18°C.

2.7.2. Electrophysiology. Currents were recorded using the two-electrode voltage clamp technique as described elsewhere [19]. Glass microelectrodes were filled with 3 M KCl (0.5–2 MΩ). Oocytes were clamped at −60 mV and continuously superfused with ND96 solution (96 mM NaCl, 2 mM KCl, 1 mM $MgCl_2$, 1.8 mM $CaCl_2$, and 5 mM HEPES, pH 7.5). Current amplitudes were calculated off-line using Chart software v3.6 (ADInstruments, NSW, Australia). Responses to GABA applications were normalized as $I\% = (I/I_{max}) \times 100$, where I is the peak amplitude of current response and I_{max} is the maximum current produced by GABA measured from individual cells.

Modulation of GABA-elicited currents was tested by coapplying increasing concentrations of the drugs with a concentration of GABA that produced 5% of maximal activation (EC_5, determined for each cell). Current responses were recorded and normalized as % potentiation = $((I_{drug+GABA} - I_{GABA})/I_{GABA}) \times 100$, where $I_{drug+GABA}$ is the control GABA current in the presence of a given concentration of drug and I_{GABA} is the amplitude of the control GABA current alone.

2.8. Acute Toxicity. The acute toxicity study was conducted according to the modified method described by Adebiyi and Abatan [20]. Swiss albino mice (25–30 g) were randomly divided into ten groups (n = 6). Animals were fasted overnight but had access to water ad libitum and then were treated intraperitoneally with carnosol, ursolic acid, or oleanolic acid (50, 150, and 200 mg/kg). Mice in the control group received 10 mL/kg i.p. of vehicle (0.9% w/v). Animals were keenly observed for any signs of toxic effects during the first 6 hours after the treatment and then carefully monitored for the subsequent 66 hours (3-day observation) for any changes in behaviors including grooming, hyperactivity, sedation, respiratory arrest, convulsion, increased or decreased motor activity, and mortality, if any.

2.9. Assessment of Anxiolytic Activity

2.9.1. Elevated Plus Maze (EPM). The apparatus consisted of two open arms (30 cm × 5 cm) and two closed arms (30 cm × 5 cm × 15 cm) made of black plexiglas connected by an open central platform (5 cm × 5 cm) and elevated 40 cm from ground level. A raised ledge (3 mm high and 1 mm thick) surrounded the perimeter of the open arms. Mice were injected with vehicle or drug and 20 min later placed in the center of the apparatus facing an open arm and allowed to explore the maze for 5 min. An arm entry was defined by having all four paws inside the arm. All sessions were videotaped by a camera positioned above the maze, and, at the end of the test, the number of arm entries and time spent in arms were recorded. To assess the involvement of the GABAergic system, animals were given vehicle or flumazenil (2.5 mg/kg) i.p. 20 minutes before treatment with carnosol, ursolic acid, or oleanolic acid. The % of open-arm entries and the % of time spent in the open arms were recorded as a measure of anxiety state [18].

2.9.2. Light/Dark Box Test (LDB). The light/dark apparatus consists of an acrylic box of dimensions 44 cm × 21 cm × 21 cm, divided into a small dark compartment (one-third) and a large illuminated compartment (two-thirds); the division between zones contains an opening of 6 cm × 3 cm. The box is equipped with 16 light beams, 11 in the lit area and 5 in the dark area, which detect the movement of the animal. The box is connected to a computer that records the number of transitions between areas, latency to the first transition, time and activity in each zone, and total activity in a 5 min session. An increase in the exploration of the lit area is associated with an anxiolytic effect; as such, two parameters were selected as a measure of anxiety: the time spent in the lit compartment and the total number of transitions [18].

2.10. Assessment of Anticonvulsant Activity

2.10.1. PTZ-Induced Seizures. PTZ-induced convulsions test was used to evaluate anticonvulsant activity of carnosol, ursolic acid, and oleanolic acid [18]. In this test, 48 mice were divided into eight groups of six animals each. Group I (control) was treated with vehicle (5% DMSO, 1% Tween 80, and 94% saline) i.p. Group II received standard drug diazepam i.p. in a dose of 1 mg/kg. Groups II, III, IV, and V were treated with carnosol; groups VI, VII, VIII, and IX were treated with ursolic acid, whereas groups X, XI, XII, and XIII were treated with oleanolic acid i.p. in a dose of 1, 10, 30, and 100 mg/kg, respectively. All the drugs were given thirty minutes before PTZ (70 mg/kg). Each animal was placed in a transparent chamber for observation lasting forty-five minutes after i.p. injection of PTZ. The onset of seizure, duration, and mortality in treated mice were recorded. Mice that did not convulse 60 min after PTZ administration were considered to be protected.

2.11. Assessment of Antidepressant Activity

2.11.1. The Tail Suspension Test. Mice were hung by their tail on the tail hanger using sticky tape for tail fixation, at approximately 1 cm from the end of the tail. The hanger was fixed in the black plastic box (20 × 20 × 45 cm) with the opening at the top front. The distance between the hanger and floor was approximately 40 cm. The mouse was suspended in the air by its tail and the immobility time was recorded over a period of 5 minutes. The duration of immobility was defined as the absence of all movements except for those required for respiration [21].

2.11.2. The Forced Swim Test. The forced swim test was carried out in a glass cylinder (diameter 20 cm, height 30 cm) filled with water to the height of 20 cm. The water temperature was approximately 25–28°C. Mice were gently placed into the water and the immobility time was recorded by an observer over a period of 5 minutes. Immobility was defined as absence of all movements and remaining floating passively in the water with the head just above the water surface [22].

2.12. Locomotor Activity. The locomotor activity arena measured 50 × 40 cm and the floor was divided by lines into 4 equal-sized rectangular zones. Mice ($n = 6$ per group) were habituated to laboratory conditions 90 min prior to testing. Doses of carnosol, ursolic acid, oleanolic acid, or vehicle were administered intraperitoneally and animals were placed in the recording apparatus 30 min later. Group mean line-crossing counts were subsequently recorded between 1 and 30 min following introduction to the arena by means of a Cat Eye camera, coupled to a remote personal computer [23].

2.13. Statistical Analysis. Data were expressed as mean ± SEM. When several treatments were compared, one-way ANOVA was used and post hoc comparisons between vehicle and drug treated groups were made using Dunnett's multiple comparison test using GraphPad Prism version 5. In all tests, the criterion for significance was $P < 0.05$.

3. Results

3.1. Positive Modulation of GABA-Induced Currents at $\alpha 1\beta 2\gamma 2L$ GABA-A Receptors. Carnosol, ursolic acid, and oleanolic acid enhanced the response to 5 μM GABA at $\alpha 1\beta 2\gamma 2L$ GABA-A receptors (Figure 2). Figures 2(a)–2(c) show the concentration dependent enhancement of GABA-EC5-evoked response by carnosol, ursolic acid, and oleanolic acid (1, 10, 30, 100, and 300 μM) at $\alpha 1\beta 2\gamma 2L$ receptors. Carnosol, ursolic acid, and oleanolic acid at 300 μM maximally potentiated GABA-EC5-induced currents by 250 ± 30%, 230 ± 25%, and 220 ± 20% at $\alpha 1\beta 2\gamma 2L$ receptors, respectively. We then studied the ability of neutralizing benzodiazepine antagonist flumazenil to block the potentiation of carnosol, ursolic

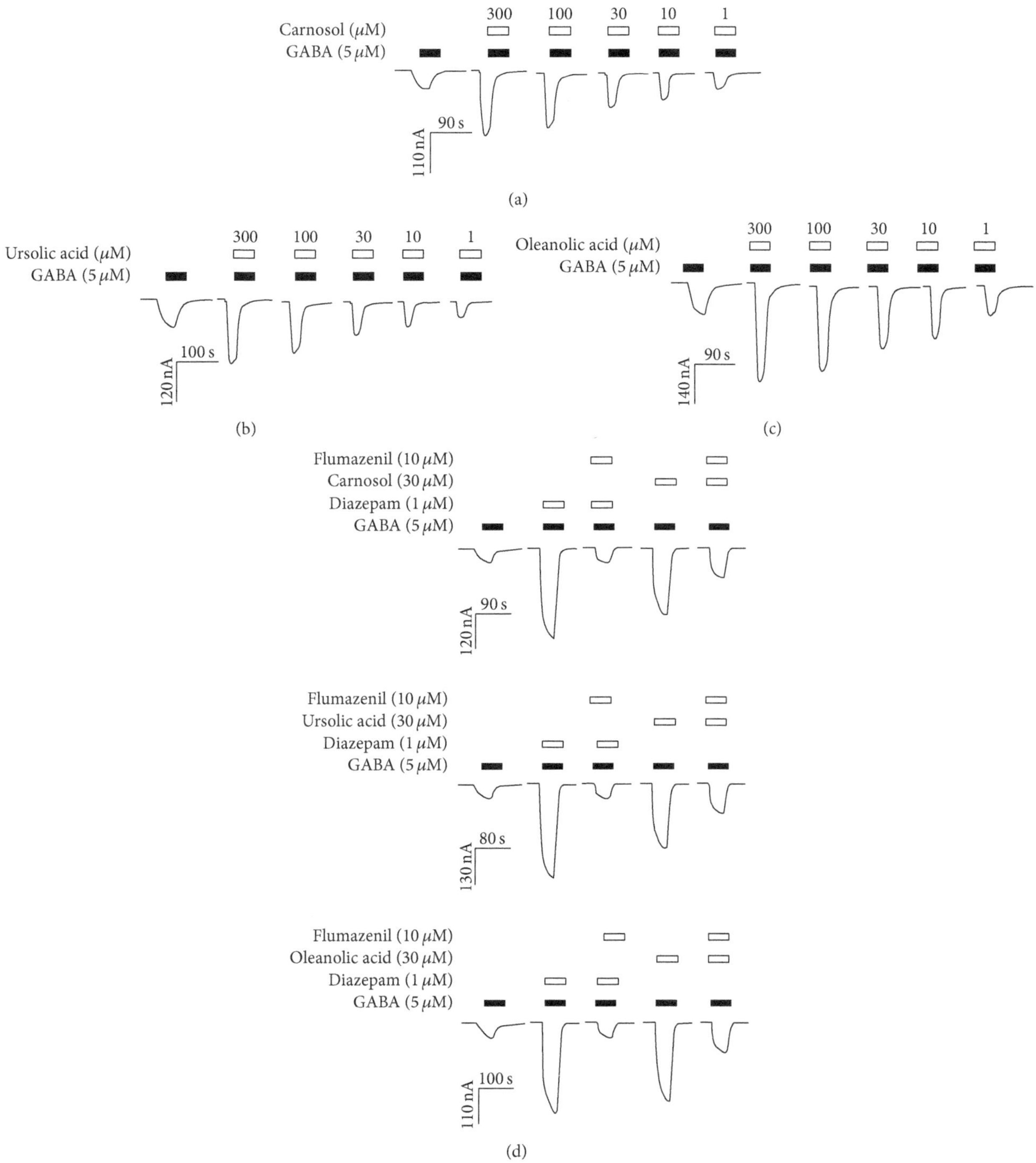

FIGURE 2: Carnosol, ursolic acid, and oleanolic acid are positive modulators of α1-containing GABA-A receptors expressed in *Xenopus* oocytes. Representative current trace showing the potentiation of GABA-EC5 by various concentrations of carnosol, ursolic acid, and oleanolic acid (1, 10, 30, 100, and 300 μM) at human recombinant $\alpha1\beta2\gamma2$L GABA-A receptors ((a)–(c)). The potentiating effect of carnosol, ursolic acid, and oleanolic acid was attenuated by flumazenil (10 μM) similar to that of diazepam (d). Horizontal bars show the duration of drug application.

acid, and oleanolic acid at $\alpha1\beta2\gamma2$L GABA-A receptors. The positive modulation by carnosol, ursolic acid, and oleanolic acid at $\alpha1\beta2\gamma2$L GABA-A receptors was mostly sensitive to antagonism by flumazenil (10 μM) (Figure 2(d)). This effect was similar to the antagonism of diazepam induced potentiation of GABA effects at $\alpha1\beta2\gamma2$L GABA-A receptors, indicating that these compounds bind to the benzodiazepine site of GABA-A receptors.

3.2. Acute Toxicity. Carnosol, ursolic acid, and oleanolic acid in the dose range of 50–200 mg/kg did not produce any noticeable effects on grooming, sedation, respiratory arrest, convulsions, or muscle activity. Furthermore, not a single case of lethality was found. Food and water consumption remained normal throughout the test period.

3.3. Assessment of Anxiolytic Activity in EPM. The anxiolytic effects of carnosol, ursolic acid, and oleanolic acid or diazepam in the elevated plus maze using diazepam as a positive control are summarized in Figure 3. Carnosol, ursolic acid, and oleanolic acid significantly reduced the anxiety in mice. All the three compounds at the doses of 10, 30, and 100 mg/kg i.p. significantly increased the % of open-arm entries ($^{*}P < 0.05$ and $^{**}P < 0.01$; $n = 6$, one-way ANOVA followed by Dunnett's test) and % of time spent in open arms of the elevated plus maze (EPM) ($^{*}P < 0.05$, $^{**}P < 0.01$, and $^{***}P < 0.001$; $n = 6$, one-way ANOVA followed by Dunnett's test).

Similarly, diazepam (1 mg/kg, i.p.) also increased % of open-arm entries ($^{**}P < 0.01$) and the % of time spent in open arms of the EPM ($^{***}P < 0.001$; $n = 6$, one-way ANOVA followed by Dunnett's test).

3.4. Effect of Flumazenil on the Anxiolytic Activity of Carnosol, Ursolic Acid, and Oleanolic Acid in the Elevated Plus Maze. The anxiolytic activity of carnosol, oleanolic acid, and ursolic acid was decreased by coadministration of flumazenil (2.5 mg/kg) with carnosol, oleanolic acid, and ursolic acid (30 mg/kg), indicating that the benzodiazepine binding site of GABA-A receptors is involved in the anxiolytic activity induced by these compounds (Figure 4).

3.5. Assessment of Anxiolytic Activity in Light Dark Test. The anxiolytic effects of carnosol, oleanolic acid, and ursolic acid in the light dark box test are shown in Figure 5. The results indicate that carnosol, oleanolic acid, and ursolic acid at the doses of 10, 30, and 100 mg/kg i.p. significantly increased the time spent in the light compartment ($^{*}P < 0.05$, $^{**}P < 0.01$, and $^{***}P < 0.001$; $n = 6$, one-way ANOVA followed by Dunnett's test) and the number of transitions between light and dark compartments ($^{*}P < 0.05$, $^{**}P < 0.01$, and $^{***}P < 0.001$; $n = 6$, one-way ANOVA followed by Dunnett's test).

The positive control drug diazepam (1 mg/kg, i.p.) also significantly ($^{***}P < 0.001$) increased the time spent in the light area of the light dark box, indicating antianxiety activity and confirming that the paradigm is valid.

3.6. Assessment of Antidepressant Activity in Tail Suspension Test. The effects of carnosol, ursolic acid, and oleanolic acid on active behavior in the tail suspension test (TST) are shown in Table 1. Intraperitoneal administration of the positive control, imipramine, at the dose of 60 mg/kg, caused a significant reduction in the immobility time as compared to the vehicle ($^{***}P < 0.001$). Carnosol, ursolic acid, and oleanolic acid at the doses of 10, 30, and 100 mg/kg caused a significant decrease in the immobility time as compared to the vehicle control group ($^{*}P < 0.05$; $^{**}P < 0.01$).

3.7. Assessment of Antidepressant Activity in Forced Swim Test. The effects of carnosol, ursolic acid, and oleanolic acid on active behavior in the forced swim test (FST) of mice are summarized in Table 2. Intraperitoneal administration of carnosol, ursolic acid, and oleanolic acid at doses of 10, 30, and 100 mg/kg significantly decreased the immobility time in the FST as compared to the vehicle control ($^{*}P < 0.05$; $^{**}P < 0.01$; $^{***}P < 0.001$; one-way ANOVA followed by Dunnett's test). The reference drug imipramine 60 mg/kg also caused a significant decrease in the immobility time as compared to vehicle control ($^{***}P < 0.001$; one-way ANOVA followed by Dunnett's test).

Table 1: Effect of carnosol, ursolic acid, and oleanolic acid on immobility period (sec) of mice using tail suspension test.

Group	Treatment	Dose (mg/kg)	Immobility time (sec)
1	Control	—	170 ± 10.5
2		10	139.4 ± 13.5*
3	Carnosol	30	115.7 ± 11.3**
4		100	100.5 ± 10.2**
5		10	135.4 ± 14.8*
6	Ursolic acid	30	115.3 ± 11.5**
7		100	105.1 ± 10.4**
8		10	125.8 ± 5.2*
9	Oleanolic acid	30	115.3 ± 10.3**
10		100	95.6 ± 15.1**
11	Imipramine	60	60.2 ± 11.6***

All values are expressed in mean ± SEM ($n = 6$). $^{*}P < 0.05$, $^{**}P < 0.01$, and $^{***}P < 0.001$ compared to the vehicle group. Differences between groups were analyzed by analysis of variance (one-way ANOVA) followed by Dunnett's test.

Table 2: Effect of carnosol, ursolic acid, and oleanolic acid on immobility period (sec) of mice using forced swimming test.

Group	Treatment	Dose (mg/kg)	Immobility time (sec)
1	Control	—	184.6 ± 13.5
2		10	149.4 ± 10.5*
3	Carnosol	30	125.7 ± 12.3**
4		100	80.5 ± 11.2***
5		10	135.4 ± 10.5*
6	Ursolic acid	30	120.3 ± 11.4**
7		100	74.9 ± 10.5***
8		10	148.8 ± 10.2*
9	Oleanolic acid	30	125.3 ± 11.3**
10		100	95.6 ± 14.1***
11	Imipramine	60	70.2 ± 12.6***

All values are expressed in mean ± SEM ($n = 6$). $^{*}P < 0.05$, $^{**}P < 0.01$, and $^{***}P < 0.001$ compared to the vehicle group. Differences between groups were analyzed by analysis of variance (one-way ANOVA) followed by Dunnett's test.

3.8. Locomotor Activity of Carnosol, Ursolic Acid, and Oleanolic Acid. Keeping in view the possible effect of exploration on antidepressant effect, the effects of carnosol, ursolic acid, and oleanolic acid on locomotor activity were evaluated. The results showed that carnosol, ursolic acid, and oleanolic acid, at the dose level of 1–100 mg/kg, i.p., did not have any significant effect on locomotor activity compared to the

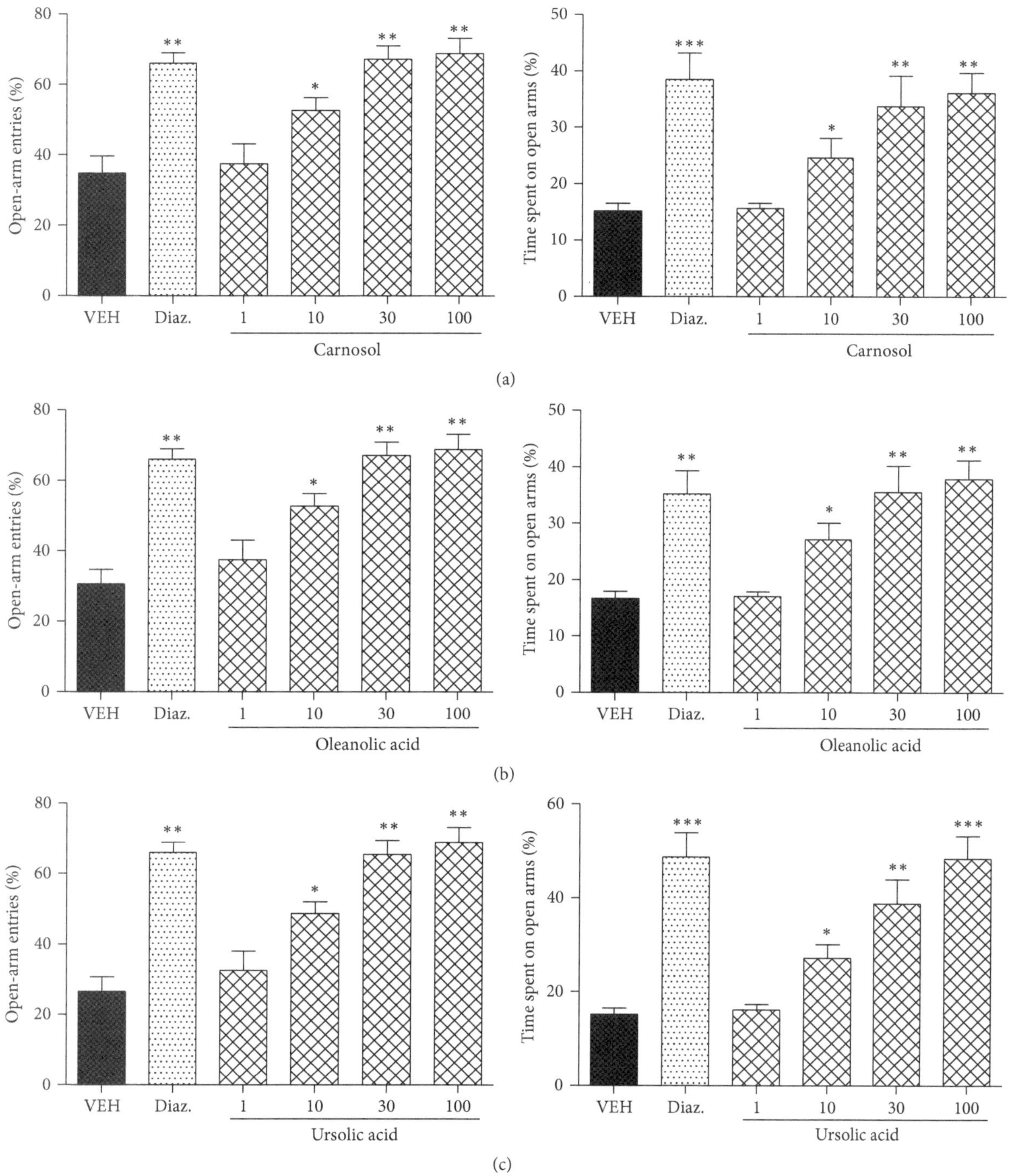

Figure 3: Effect of carnosol, oleanolic acid, ursolic acid, and diazepam on the behavior of mice in the elevated plus maze. (a) % of open-arm entries (left panel) and % of time spent in open arms (right panel) registered over a session of 5 min after 20 min of an i.p. injection of carnosol (1, 10, 30, and 100 mg/kg). (b) % of open-arm entries (left panel) and % of time spent in open arms (right panel) registered over a session of 5 min after 20 min of an i.p. injection of oleanolic acid (1, 10, 30, and 100 mg/kg), diazepam (1 mg/kg), or vehicle. (c) % of open-arm entries (left panel) and % of time spent in open arms (right panel) registered over a session of 5 min after 20 min of an i.p. injection of ursolic acid (1, 10, 30, and 100 mg/kg). Columns represent mean ± SEM (n = 6/group). $^{*}P < 0.05$, $^{**}P < 0.01$, and $^{***}P < 0.001$ compared with vehicle group using one-way ANOVA followed by Dunnett's test.

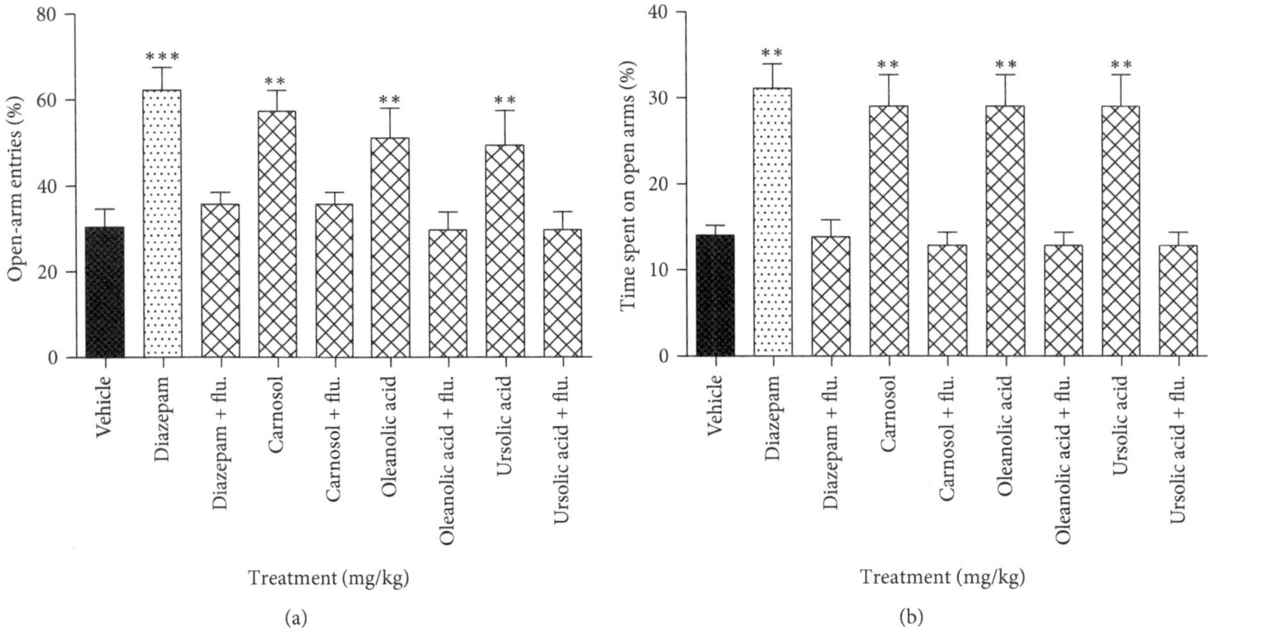

FIGURE 4: Effect of flumazenil on the anxiolytic activity of carnosol, oleanolic acid, and ursolic acid in the elevated plus maze. (a) % of open-arm entries and (b) % of time spent in open arms registered over a session of 5 min after 20 min of an i.p. injection of vehicle, diazepam (1 mg/kg), carnosol, oleanolic acid, and ursolic acid (10 mg/kg) in the presence of flumazenil (2.5 mg/kg). Columns express mean ± SEM (n = 6/group). $^{**}P < 0.01$ and $^{***}P < 0.001$ compared with vehicle control group using one-way ANOVA followed by Dunnett's test.

TABLE 3: Effect of carnosol, ursolic acid, and oleanolic acid in locomotor activity test.

Group	Treatment	Dose (mg/kg)	Line-crossing counts (mean ± SEM)
1	Control	—	44.6 ± 6.5
2		10	45.4 ± 3.5
3	Carnosol	30	43.7 ± 5.3
4		100	36.5 ± 3.2
5		10	45.4 ± 3.5
6	Ursolic acid	30	43.3 ± 2.4
7		100	35.9 ± 4.5
8		10	40.8 ± 2.2
9	Oleanolic acid	30	42.3 ± 3.3
10		100	34.6 ± 4.1
11	Imipramine	60	40.2 ± 2.6
12	Diazepam	1	35.5 ± 3.5

All values are expressed in mean ± SEM (n = 6). $P > 0.05$ compared to the vehicle group. Differences between groups were analyzed by analysis of variance (one-way ANOVA) followed by Dunnett's test.

vehicle (Table 3). At 100 mg/kg, all the three compounds caused a slight reduction in locomotor line crossing; however, this effect was statistically not significant.

3.9. Anticonvulsant Actions of Carnosol, Ursolic Acid, and Oleanolic Acid in PTZ Test. Carnosol, ursolic acid, and oleanolic acid showed significant anticonvulsant activity against PTZ-induced convulsions in mice. Carnosol, ursolic acid, and oleanolic acid caused a dose dependent increase in the duration of onset of tonic-clonic convulsions and decreased the duration of convulsions. Carnosol, ursolic acid, and oleanolic acid at doses of 10, 30, and 100 mg/kg caused a significant increase in the duration of onset ($^*P < 0.05$; $^{**}P < 0.01$; $^{***}P < 0.001$; ANOVA with Dunnett's post hoc test; $n = 6$) and decreased the duration of clonic-tonic seizures ($^*P < 0.05$; $^{**}P < 0.01$; ANOVA with Dunnett's post hoc test; $n = 6$). The reference anticonvulsant diazepam at doses of 1 mg/kg also significantly delayed the onset of clonic-tonic seizures and decreased the duration of clonic-tonic seizures ($^{***}P < 0.001$; ANOVA with Dunnett's post hoc test; $n = 8$). Carnosol, ursolic acid, and oleanolic acid caused a dose dependent reduction in PTZ-induced mortality and provided 100, 83.33, 66.7, and 33.34% protection at doses of 100, 30, 10, and 1 mg/kg, respectively (Table 4).

4. Discussion

In the present study, we have evaluated three constituents, carnosol, ursolic acid, and oleanolic acid, from *Artemisia indica* for their ability to modulate GABA-induced currents at GABA-A $\alpha 1\beta 2\gamma 2L$ receptor subtype expressed in *Xenopus* oocytes. Carnosol, ursolic acid, and oleanolic acid were subsequently evaluated for various neuropharmacological activities in mouse models. The results indicate that carnosol, ursolic acid, and oleanolic acid were positive modulators of $\alpha 1\beta 2\gamma 2L$ recombinant GABA-A receptor. Furthermore, the potentiation at $\alpha 1\beta 2\gamma 2L$ GABA-A receptor subtype was blocked by flumazenil under conditions, where flumazenil also inhibited diazepam induced enhancement, indicating

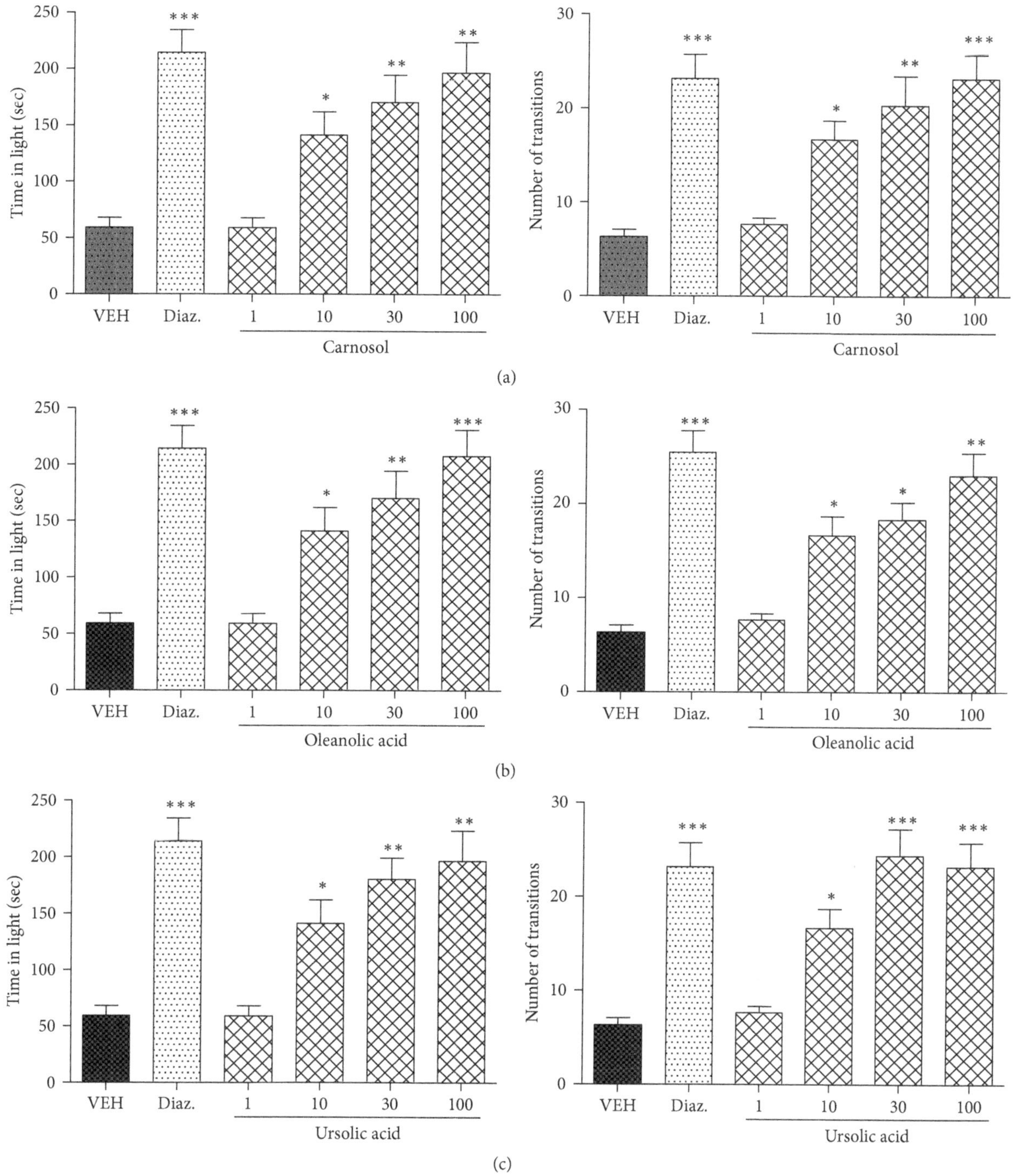

FIGURE 5: Effect of carnosol, oleanolic acid, ursolic acid, and diazepam on the behavior of mice in the light dark box test. (a) Time spent in lit area (left panel) and number of transitions (right panel), recorded over a session of 5 min, after 20 min of an i.p. injection of carnosol (1, 10, 30, and 100 mg/kg), diazepam (0.5, 1, and 3 mg/kg), or vehicle. (b) Time spent in lit area (left panel) and number of transitions (right panel), recorded over a session of 5 min, after 20 min of an i.p. injection of oleanolic acid (1, 10, 30, and 100 mg/kg), diazepam (0.5, 1, and 3 mg/kg), or vehicle. (c) Time spent in lit area (left panel) and number of transitions (right panel), recorded over a session of 5 min, after 20 min of an i.p. injection of ursolic acid (1, 10, 30, and 100 mg/kg), diazepam (0.5, 1, and 3 mg/kg), or vehicle. Values are expressed as mean ± SEM (n = 6/group). $^{*}P < 0.05$, $^{**}P < 0.01$, and $^{***}P < 0.001$ compared with vehicle group using one-way ANOVA followed by Dunnett's test.

TABLE 4: Effect of carnosol, ursolic acid, and oleanolic acid on PTZ-induced seizure.

Treatment	Dose (mg/kg)	Onset of clonic-tonic convulsions (sec)	Duration of clonic-tonic convulsions (sec)	% mortality	% protection against mortality
Control	—	72.5 ± 8.5	39 ± 4.5	100%	0
Diazepam	1	197 ± 10.6***	15.8 ± 2.6**	0.00	100
Carnosol	1	77.1 ± 12.9$^{\text{n.s.}}$	35 ± 3.5$^{\text{n.s.}}$	66.6	33.34
Carnosol	10	117.3 ± 6.8*	26 ± 2.6*	33.3	66.67
Carnosol	30	158.3 ± 11.6**	17.6 ± 1.8**	16.3	83.33
Carnosol	100	185.8 ± 8.8***	7.5 ± 1.1**	0.00	100
Ursolic acid	1	75.1 ± 13.5$^{\text{n.s.}}$	33 ± 3.5$^{\text{n.s.}}$	66.6	33.34
Ursolic acid	10	120.3 ± 7.5*	25 ± 3.6*	33.3	66.67
Ursolic acid	30	148.5 ± 11.5**	19.6 ± 2.8**	16.3	83.33
Ursolic acid	100	195.8 ± 8.8***	15.5 ± 2.5**	0.00	100
Oleanolic acid	1	78.1 ± 14.5$^{\text{n.s.}}$	34 ± 3.5$^{\text{n.s.}}$	66.6	33.34
Oleanolic acid	10	130.3 ± 9.5*	23 ± 2.6*	33.3	66.67
Oleanolic acid	30	150.8 ± 13.5**	18.5 ± 2.8**	16.3	83.33
Oleanolic acid	100	190.8 ± 8.8***	14.5 ± 2.5**	0.00	100

The data represent the mean ± SEM ($n = 6$). $^{*}P < 0.05$, $^{**}P < 0.01$, and $^{***}P < 0.001$ represent significant difference compared to PTZ-induced seizure control.
n.s.: not significant.

that carnosol, ursolic acid, and oleanolic acid elicit potentiation via the benzodiazepine binding site. A fraction of the positive modulation produced by carnosol, ursolic acid, and oleanolic acid remained flumazenil insensitive indicating that a component of GABA-A receptor potentiation might be mediated by nonbenzodiazepine sites. Such a flumazenil independent positive modulation of GABA-A receptors has previously been reported with flavonoids [17, 18].

Anxiolytics are known to exert their pharmacological action by causing an increase in GABAergic neurotransmission in the brain [18, 22]. The elevated plus maze and light dark tests are routinely used for the assessment of anxiolytic activity of substances in rodents [24–26]. GABA-A receptors are involved in the anxiolytics effects of benzodiazepines [27]. Flavonoids have also been shown to mediate their anxiolytic effects via modulation of GABA-A receptors [25, 28]. Recently, we have shown that synthetic flavones such as 2′-methoxy-6-methylflavone [24], 3-hydroxy-2′-methoxy-6-methylflavone [25], and viscosine [18] exert their anxiolytic effects via modulation of GABA-A receptors. In this study, carnosol, ursolic acid, and oleanolic acid exerted significant anxiolytic effects at the doses of 10–100 mg/kg in both the elevated plus maze and light dark tests. Furthermore, the anxiolytic effect exerted by carnosol, ursolic acid, and oleanolic acid was antagonized by flumazenil indicating that the effect is mediated through the benzodiazepine site of GABA-A receptors.

The anticonvulsant activity of carnosol, ursolic acid, and oleanolic acid was determined using chemically induced (PTZ test) convulsions in mice. The results of the current study indicate that carnosol, ursolic acid, and oleanolic acid at the dose level of 10–100 mg/kg possess significant anticonvulsant activity in mice in PTZ-induced seizures which may elicit seizures by inhibiting GABAergic mechanisms [18, 29, 30]. GABA is the major inhibitory neurotransmitter and glutamic acid is the excitatory neurotransmitter in the brain. The inhibition of GABA and enhancement of the action of glutamate neurotransmitters are believed to be the underlying factors in epilepsy [31]. GABA-A receptor agonists as well as drugs which allosterically modulate GABA-A receptors are useful in convulsive seizures [32, 33]. The standard antiepileptic drug diazepam is believed to be mediating its anticonvulsant action by enhancing the action of GABA at GABA-A receptors [34]. Thus it is possible that the anticonvulsant effects shown by carnosol, ursolic acid, and oleanolic acid against PTZ-induced seizures may be due to the activation of GABAergic neurotransmission.

The forced swimming and tail suspension tests are well known models of depression sensitive to all classes of antidepressant including monoamine oxidase inhibitors, tricyclic antidepressants, and selective serotonin reuptake inhibitors [20, 35]. Both tests are widely used screening methods for antidepressants in mice [20, 21]. Carnosol, ursolic acid, and oleanolic acid exerted significant antidepressant effect as evidenced by the reduction of immobility time in both the tail suspension test and the forced swimming test. To avoid the possibility of false positive effect, these compounds were evaluated for their effects on locomotor activity tests. Carnosol, ursolic acid, and oleanolic acid did not exert any significant effect on the locomotor activity indicating that the decrease in immobility in the forced swimming and tail suspension tests is caused by an antidepressant-like effect rather than a locomotor-enhancing effect. Studies have shown that GABA-A receptors are involved in the pathophysiology of depression [36]. Patients suffering from depression have been shown to have deficient GABA levels as well as decreased cortical GABA-A receptors. Thus those substances which mimic the GABAergic system may have potential effects on depression [36]. Since carnosol, ursolic acid, and oleanolic acid potentiated GABA-induced currents at $\alpha 1\beta 2\gamma 2L$ GABA-A receptor, it is possible that the antidepressant effects shown by carnosol, ursolic acid, and oleanolic acid may also be due to the activation of GABAergic mechanisms.

5. Conclusions

In conclusion, carnosol, ursolic acid, and oleanolic acid modulate $\alpha 1\beta 2\gamma 2L$ GABA-A receptors via the benzodiazepine binding site. Furthermore, carnosol, ursolic acid, and oleanolic acid demonstrated significant anticonvulsant, anxiolytic, and antidepressant activities in mouse models of anticonvulsant, antidepressant, and anxiolysis. We have also shown that the anxiolytic activity is mediated by the GABAergic system. However, further studies are required to investigate possible mechanisms of action of these compounds in epilepsy and depression and to investigate these compounds on other GABA-A receptor subtypes.

Competing Interests

The authors declare that there are no competing interests regarding the publication of this paper.

Acknowledgments

The authors acknowledge the Higher Education Commission of Pakistan for providing financial support to carry out this research work. The authors also acknowledge the International Center for Chemical and Biological Study (ICCBS), HEJ, Karachi University, for providing the opportunity to carry out the experimental part of this research work.

References

[1] W. Ahmad, I. Khan, M. A. Khan, M. Ahmad, F. Subhan, and N. Karim, "Evaluation of antidiabetic and antihyperlipidemic activity of *Artemisia indica* linn (aeriel parts) in Streptozotocin induced diabetic rats," *Journal of Ethnopharmacology*, vol. 151, no. 1, pp. 618–623, 2014.

[2] Q. L. Tran, Y. Tezuka, J.-Y. Ueda et al., "In vitro antiplasmodial activity of antimalarial medicinal plants used in Vietnamese traditional medicine," *Journal of Ethnopharmacology*, vol. 86, no. 2-3, pp. 249–252, 2003.

[3] A. H. Gilani, S. Yaeesh, Q. Jamal, and M. N. Ghayur, "Hepatoprotective activity of aqueous-methanol extract of Artemisia vulgaris," *Phytotherapy Research*, vol. 19, no. 2, pp. 170–172, 2005.

[4] X. T. Tigno, F. de Guzman, and A. M. T. V. Flora, "Phytochemical analysis and hemodynamic actions of Artemisia vulgaris L.," *Clinical Hemorheology and Microcirculation*, vol. 23, no. 2–4, pp. 167–175, 2000.

[5] R. Rodrigues-Alves, A. Pregal, M. C. Pereira-Santos et al., "Anaphylaxis to pine nut: cross-reactivity to *Artemisia vulgaris*?" *Allergologia et Immunopathologia*, vol. 36, no. 2, pp. 113–116, 2008.

[6] V. Chen and C. D. Ianuzzo, "Dosage effects of streptozotocin on rat tissue enzyme activities and glycogen concentration," *Canadian Journal of Physiology and Pharmacology*, vol. 60, no. 10, pp. 1251–1256, 1982.

[7] M. Mahmoudi, M. A. Ebrahimzadeh, F. Ansaroudi, S. F. Nabavi, and S. M. Nabavi, "Antidepressant and antioxidant activities of *Artemisia absinthium* L. at flowering stage," *African Journal of Biotechnology*, vol. 8, no. 24, pp. 7170–7175, 2009.

[8] A. Eidi, S. Oryan, J. Zaringhalam, and M. Rad, "Antinociceptive and anti-inflammatory effects of the aerial parts of Artemisia dracunculus in mice," *Pharmaceutical Biology*, vol. 54, no. 3, pp. 549–554, 2015.

[9] B. Zapata, C. Durán, E. Stashenko, L. Betancur-Galvis, and A. C. Mesa-Arango, "Antifungal activity, cytotoxicity and composition of essential oils from the Asteraceae plant family," *Revista Iberoamericana de Micologia*, vol. 27, no. 2, pp. 101–103, 2010.

[10] A. K. Mondal, S. Parui, and S. Mandal, "Analysis of the free amino acid content in pollen of nine *Asteraceae* species of known allergenic activity," *Annals of Agricultural and Environmental Medicine*, vol. 5, no. 1, pp. 17–20, 1998.

[11] Z. Šesták, "Bohm, B.A., Stuessy, T.F.: flavonoids of the sunflower family (Asteraceae)," *Biologia Plantarum*, vol. 45, no. 2, p. 226, 2002.

[12] T. Carbonara, R. Pascale, M. P. Argentieri et al., "Phytochemical analysis of a herbal tea from Artemisia annua L.," *Journal of Pharmaceutical and Biomedical Analysis*, vol. 62, pp. 79–86, 2012.

[13] D. Fraisse, C. Felgines, O. Texier, and L. J. Lamaison, "Caffeoyl derivatives: major antioxidant compounds of some wild herbs of the *Asteraceae* family," *Food and Nutrition Sciences*, vol. 2, no. 3, pp. 181–192, 2011.

[14] S.-H. Park, Y.-B. Sim, P.-L. Han, J.-K. Lee, and H.-W. Suh, "Antidepressant-like effect of chlorogenic acid isolated from *Artemisia capillaris* Thunb," *Animal Cells and Systems*, vol. 14, no. 4, pp. 253–259, 2010.

[15] S. M. Salah and A. K. Jäger, "Two flavonoids from Artemisia herba-alba Asso with in vitro GABA A-benzodiazepine receptor activity," *Journal of Ethnopharmacology*, vol. 99, no. 1, pp. 145–146, 2005.

[16] R. W. Olsen and A. J. Tobin, "Molecular biology of GABAA receptors," *The FASEB Journal*, vol. 4, no. 5, pp. 1469–1480, 1990.

[17] J. R. Hanrahan, M. Chebib, and G. A. R. Johnston, "Flavonoid modulation of GABAA receptors," *British Journal of Pharmacology*, vol. 163, no. 2, pp. 234–245, 2011.

[18] N. Karim, S. Irshad, I. Khan et al., "GABA(A) receptor modulation and neuropharmacological activities of viscosine isolated from Dodonaea viscosa (Linn)," *Pharmacology Biochemistry and Behavior*, vol. 136, pp. 64–72, 2015.

[19] N. Karim, J. Curmi, N. Gavande et al., "2′-Methoxy-6-methylflavone: a novel anxiolytic and sedative with subtype selective activating and modulating actions at GABA A receptors," *British Journal of Pharmacology*, vol. 165, no. 4, pp. 880–896, 2012.

[20] O. E. Adebiyi and M. O. Abatan, "Phytochemical and acute toxicity of ethanolic extract of Enantia chlorantha (oliv) stem bark in albino rats," *Interdisciplinary Toxicology*, vol. 6, no. 3, pp. 145–151, 2013.

[21] L. Steru, R. Chermat, B. Thierry, and P. Simon, "The tail suspension test: a new method for screening antidepressants in mice," *Psychopharmacology*, vol. 85, no. 3, pp. 367–370, 1985.

[22] R. D. Porsolt, G. Anton, N. Blavet, and M. Jalfre, "Behavioural despair in rats: a new model sensitive to antidepressant treatments," *European Journal of Pharmacology*, vol. 47, no. 4, pp. 379–391, 1978.

[23] F. Subhan, N. Karim, A. H. Gilani, and R. D. E. Sewell, "Terpenoid content of *Valeriana wallichii* extracts and antidepressant-like response profiles," *Phytotherapy Research*, vol. 24, no. 5, pp. 686–691, 2010.

[24] A. Abdelhalim, N. Karim, M. Chebib et al., "Anxiolytic and antinociceptive activities of constituents from rosmarinus officinalis," *Journal of Pharmacy & Pharmaceutical Sciences*, vol. 18, no. 4, pp. 448–459, 2015.

[25] T. Mennini, S. Caccia, and S. Garattini, "Mechanism of action of anxiolytic drugs," *Progress in Drug Research*, vol. 31, pp. 315–347, 1987.

[26] N. Karim, N. Gavande, P. Wellendorph, G. A. R. Johnston, J. R. Hanrahan, and M. Chebib, "3-Hydroxy-2ʹ-methoxy-6-methylflavone: a potent anxiolytic with a unique selectivity profile at GABA A receptor subtypes," *Biochemical Pharmacology*, vol. 82, no. 12, pp. 1971–1983, 2011.

[27] E. Poleszak, "Benzodiazepine/GABAA receptors are involved in magnesium-induced anxiolytic-like behavior in mice," *Pharmacological Reports*, vol. 60, no. 4, pp. 483–489, 2008.

[28] S. P. Fernandez, K. N. Mewett, J. R. Hanrahan, M. Chebib, and G. A. Johnston, "Flavan-3-ol derivatives are positive modulators of $GABA_A$ receptors with higher efficacy for the α_2 subtype and anxiolytic action in mice," *Neuropharmacology*, vol. 55, no. 5, pp. 900–907, 2008.

[29] M. G. Corda, O. Giorgi, B. Longoni, M. Orlandi, and G. Biggio, "Decrease in the function of the γ-aminobutyric acid-coupled chloride channel produced by the repeated administration of pentylenetetrazol to rats," *Journal of Neurochemistry*, vol. 55, no. 4, pp. 1216–1221, 1990.

[30] D. A. Golombek, E. Escolar, L. J. Burin, M. G. De Brito Sánchez, D. F. Duque, and D. P. Cardinali, "Chronopharmacology of melatonin: inhibition by benzodiazepine antagonism," *Chronobiology International*, vol. 9, no. 2, pp. 124–131, 1992.

[31] H. F. Bradford, "Glutamate, GABA and epilepsy," *Progress in Neurobiology*, vol. 47, no. 6, pp. 477–511, 1995.

[32] S. J. Enna and H. Mohler, *The GABA Receptors*, Humana Press, New York, NY, USA, 3rd edition, 2007.

[33] D. M. Treiman, "GABAergic mechanisms in epilepsy," *Epilepsia*, vol. 42, no. 3, pp. 8–12, 2001.

[34] H. S. White, M. D. Smith, and K. S. Wilcox, "Mechanisms of action of antiepileptic drugs," *International Review of Neurobiology*, vol. 81, pp. 85–110, 2007.

[35] J. F. Cryan, A. Markou, and I. Lucki, "Assessing antidepressant activity in rodents: recent developments and future needs," *Trends in Pharmacological Sciences*, vol. 23, no. 5, pp. 238–245, 2002.

[36] H. Möhler, "The GABA system in anxiety and depression and its therapeutic potential," *Neuropharmacology*, vol. 62, no. 1, pp. 42–53, 2012.

2

Study on the Mechanism Underlying the Regulation of the NMDA Receptor Pathway in Spinal Dorsal Horns of Visceral Hypersensitivity Rats by Moxibustion

L. D. Wang,[1] J. M. Zhao,[1] R. J. Huang,[1] L. Y. Tan,[1] Z. H. Hu,[2] Z. J. Weng,[1] K. Wang,[1] H. G. Wu,[1] and H. R. Liu[1]

[1]*Key Laboratory of Acupuncture and Immunological Effects, Shanghai Research Institute of Acupuncture and Meridian, 650 South Wanping Road, Shanghai 200030, China*
[2]*Shanghai TCM-Integrated Hospital, Shanghai University of TCM, Shanghai 200082, China*

Correspondence should be addressed to H. G. Wu; wuhuangan@126.com and H. R. Liu; lhr_tcm@139.com

Academic Editor: Thomas Lundeberg

Visceral hypersensitivity is enhanced in irritable bowel syndrome (IBS) patients. Treatment of IBS visceral pain by moxibustion methods has a long history and rich clinical experience. In the clinic, moxibustion on the Tianshu (ST25) and Shangjuxu (ST37) acupoints can effectively treat bowel disease with visceral pain and diarrhea symptoms. To investigate the regulatory function of moxibustion on the Tianshu (ST25) and Shangjuxu (ST37) acupoints on spinal cord NR1, NR2B, and PKCε protein and mRNA expression in irritable bowel syndrome (IBS) visceral hypersensitivity rats, we did some research. In the study, we found that moxibustion effectively relieved the IBS visceral hyperalgesia status of rats. Analgesic effect of moxibustion was similar to intrathecal injection of Ro 25-6981. The expression of NR1, NR2B, and PKCε in the spinal dorsal horns of IBS visceral hyperalgesia rats increased. Moxibustion on the Tianshu and Shangjuxu acupoints might inhibit the visceral hypersensitivity, simultaneously decreasing the expression of NR1, NR2B, and PKCε in spinal cord of IBS visceral hyperalgesia rats. Based on the above experimental results, we hypothesized NR1, NR2B, and PKCε of spinal cord could play an important role in moxibustion inhibiting the process of central sensitization and visceral hyperalgesia state.

1. Introduction

Visceral pain is one of the major symptoms in functional gastrointestinal disease patients. It usually causes inconvenience and massive economic burden to this group of patients. Visceral pain is the most common in irritable bowel syndrome (IBS) patients [1]; therefore, relief or elimination of the patient's pain becomes the main purpose of treatment. Active exploration and popularization of effective measures for treating visceral pain in IBS are important goals in the medical field. With visceral hypersensitivity (visceral pain), nonnociceptive stimulation and nociceptive stimulation both induce peripheral and central level changes. Central sensitization is a current research hotspot and is considered a key factor in the development and progression of visceral hypersensitivity and its visceral hyperalgesia [2]. Therefore, studying the mechanism underlying the treatment of IBS visceral hypersensitivity by moxibustion through the perspective of central sensitization will be important in elucidating the mechanism underlying the development and progression of conduction and transduction of analgesic signals by moxibustion.

Currently, the treatment of IBS visceral pain by western medicine is mainly limited to symptomatic treatment; there are too many drugs and severe side effects [3]. Treatment of IBS visceral pain by moxibustion methods has a long history and rich clinical experience. In the clinic, moxibustion can effectively treat bowel disease with visceral pain and diarrhea symptoms [4–6]. There are many records of "abdominal pain" (similar to IBS visceral pain) in ancient medical books. The Tianshu and Shangjuxu acupoints are the two commonly and frequently used acupoints for treatment of IBS [7–9].

The combinatorial use of these two acupoints belongs to the classic He-Mu combination acupoints for treating bowel diseases in the clinic. This combination acupoint method matches the Lower He-Sea point of six organs and the Front MU acupoint. However, modern science has few studies on the pathway underlying the transduction of the stimulation signal of moxibustion on the treatment of IBS visceral pain. Therefore, it is necessary to study the mechanism underlying the treatment of IBS visceral pain by moxibustion on these bases to determine the scientific basis of the analgesic effect of moxibustion. Such research will provide laboratory data and a theoretic basis for the popularization of moxibustion therapy in the treatment of IBS visceral pain.

The N-methyl-D-aspartate (NMDA) receptor is a heteromeric complex that includes three different subunits, NR1, NR2, and NR3. The NR2B subunit can form a functional NMDA receptor only when interacting with NR1. The NR2B subunit plays an important role in the transmission of nociceptive signals at the spinal cord level and in the production and maintenance of hyperalgesia [10–12]. The NMDA receptor channel composed of NR1/NR2B has high Ca^{2+}-selective permeability and temperature sensitivity. Tyrosine phosphorylation of NR2B can enhance the activity of the NMDA receptor channel and promote intracellular signal transduction. When the persistent nociceptive stimulation signals are transmitted to the spinal dorsal horn, the release of excitatory amino acids (mainly glutamate) will increase. Glutamate can bind to the NMDA receptor and activate ion channels to cause Ca^{2+} influx; after interaction with the protein kinase C (PKC) regulatory region, the catalytic region is turned on to activate PKC [13]. Activated PKC can phosphorylate various receptor proteins and ion channels (including the NMDA receptor). On the one hand, activated PKC relieves the blocking effect of Mg^{2+} on NMDA receptor ion channels to open NMDA receptor ion channels at a relatively low potential condition to promote Ca^{2+} influx. On the other hand, it promotes the increase of NOS expression and NO production. Through the complex function of NO, the excitation of spinal neurons is changed and maintained at an excitatory status for a long time thus causing central sensitization [14]. Using this positive feedback amplification effect, neurons further transmit nociceptive stimulation signals to central nervous system [15] to induce hyperalgesia. As a subtype of PKC, PKCε plays a certain regulatory role in the process of transduction of pain signals at the spinal cord level [16, 17]. The role of PKC in sensory afferents, especially the process of central pain transduction, has received much attention.

Therefore, blocking the spinal NR1, NR2B, and PKCε signals may become an important pathway to prevent or inhibit the central sensitization process of the development of visceral pain. Here, we observed the changes in spinal NR1, NR2B, and PKCε in IBS visceral hyperalgesia rats, and we compared the regulatory effects on spinal NR1, NR2B, and PKCε in IBS visceral hyperalgesia rats treated with moxibustion versus intrathecal injection of Ro 25-6981, a selective antagonist of the NMDA receptor channel composed of NR1/NR2B. This study will improve our understanding of the signal conduction and transduction mechanisms underlying the regulation of central sensitization by moxibustion, which can help us investigate the analgesic mechanism of moxibustion.

Table 1: Abdominal withdrawal reflex (AWR) scoring criteria.

Score 0	No behavioral response to colorectal distension (CRD)
Score 1	Immobility during distension of colorectum (CR) and occasional appearance of brief head motion after a pause at the onset of the stimulation
Score 2	A mild contraction of abdominal muscles, but no lifting of the abdomen off the platform
Score 3	A strong contraction of abdominal muscles and lifting of abdomen off the platform, no lifting of pelvic structure off the platform
Score 4	Arching body and lifting of pelvic structure and scrotum

2. Experimental Animals and Methods

2.1. Model Establishment. A total of 68 newborn male specific pathogen-free- (SPF-) grade SD rats (5 days old) were provided by the Experimental Animal Center of Shanghai University of Traditional Chinese Medicine. Lactating rats were given free access to food and water. The housing environment was 12 h light/12 h dark, 20 ± 2°C, and 50–70% humidity. After adaptive feeding for 3 days, the experiments began. During the experimental process, animal treatment conformed to the guidelines of the International Association for the Study of Pain (IASP).

Using the complete randomization method, the 68 8-day-old neonatal rats were divided into the normal control group ($n = 18$) and the model group ($n = 50$). Neonatal rats in the normal group only received genital scratching without other stimuli. For neonatal rats in the model group, colorectal stimulation balloons for IBS visceral hyperalgesia were prepared according to the method of Al-Chaer et al. [18]. Colorectal distension (CRD) was performed in awake animals. During the operation, liquid paraffin was applied to the surface of each balloon. The balloon was gently inserted anally along the physiological curvature of rectum to the descending colon at a depth of approximately 2 cm. At this point, the balloon began to inflate to 0.2 mL over 1 min. The injector was slowly withdrawn, and the balloon was removed. After 1 hour, the same stimulation was repeated once. The balloon stimulation was performed once every day at a fixed time for 14 days. The balloon stimulation was not performed for the next 21 days. Rats were continuously fed until week 6, when the experimental grouping and processing were performed.

The AWR scoring standards followed the method of Li et al. [19] (Table 1). CRD stimulation used homemade balloons that were connected to a desktop sphygmomanometer and an injector through a three-way valve. Before scoring, animals were fasted for food but not water for 8–12 h to reduce the formation of feces. Before distension stimulation, the head end of the balloon gently touched the anus to facilitate defecation by rats. The balloon was gently inserted anally along the physiological curvature of rectum to the descending colon. The injector was pushed to provide constant pressure for distension stimulation. The sphygmomanometer connected to the three-way valve was used to control the pressure of balloon dilation. Four different pressures, 20 mmHg, 40 mmHg, 60 mmHg, and 80 mmHg, were supplied to perform CRD stimulation. Three AWR scores were recorded for each rat. CRD stimulation was performed for 20 s each time at 5-minute intervals. The mean of the three AWR scores was used as the final score. Within 60 min of the last moxibustion treatment, CRD was performed to observe the AWR scores of rats in each group (Figure 2).

2.2. Animal Grouping. After the model was successfully established, rats in the model group were grouped using the complete randomization method into the model group, moxibustion group, and Ro 25-6981 group. (1) The normal group ($n = 16$) rats were normally treated without CRD stimulation. (2) The model group ($n = 16$) rats were not treated after the model was established successfully. (3) The moxibustion group ($n = 16$) received stimulation at the "Tianshu" (bilateral) and "Shangjuxu" (bilateral) acupoints (the position of the acupoints followed Experimental Acupuncture [20] and relevant literature [21, 22]). Rats were immobilized on a fixing frame. A moxa stick was lighted, and the lighted end was placed perpendicularly to the acupoint, approximately 2 cm above it. This was performed for 10 min once every day for 7 days [23] (Figure 1). The Tianshu point was approximately 5 mm away from the Shenque acupoint (the distance to subxiphoid area and pubic symphysis at a ratio of 8 : 5, i.e., 8 from the top and 5 from the bottom). The Shangjuxu acupoint was 1 mm from the line that connected the horizontal surface of the medial tibial condyle and external malleolus at 6 : 10 (6 from the top and 10 from the bottom). (4) The Ro 25-6981 group ($n = 16$) received intrathecal injection of 5 μg/μL Ro 25-6981 [11, 24–26]. The treatment was performed once every day for 7 days. Rats were anesthetized by intraperitoneal injection of 2% pentobarbital sodium at 0.25 mL/100 g. The fur at the waist was shaved, and disinfection was performed using 75% alcohol cotton balls. Rats were placed in the prone position. The left thumb and middle finger were placed at both sides of the interval between L5 and L6 of the spinal cord. The right hand held a microinjector to aspirate 20 μL Ro 25-6981. The needle was slowly inserted perpendicularly to the spinous process interval. The quiver or lateral swing of the rat tail was a marker of successful puncture. The drug was slowly injected.

2.3. Specimen Collection and Processing. After the treatment was finished, intraperitoneal injection of 2% pentobarbital sodium at 0.25 mg/100 g was performed immediately to anesthetize animals and collect specimens. Specimens were prefixed in 4% paraformaldehyde, and the descending colon at 10 cm above the anus was collected. The colon was cut at 3 cm from its end, the intestinal tube was cut open longitudinally, and other debris such as the mesenteric membrane and connective tissues were removed. Feces on the intestinal wall were washed using PBS, and specimens were fixed in preprepared 4% paraformaldehyde. The L6-S2 segment of the spinal cord was used for western blot and real-time quantitative polymerase chain reaction (PCR).

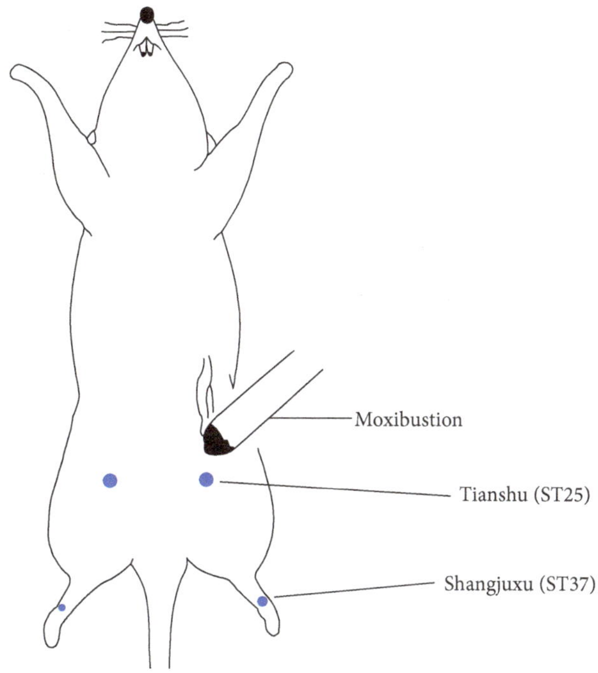

FIGURE 1: Diagram of moxibustion in rats. Rats were immobilized on a fixing frame. A moxa stick was lighted, and the lighted end was placed perpendicularly to the acupoint, approximately 2 cm above it. This was performed for 10 min once every day for 7 days.

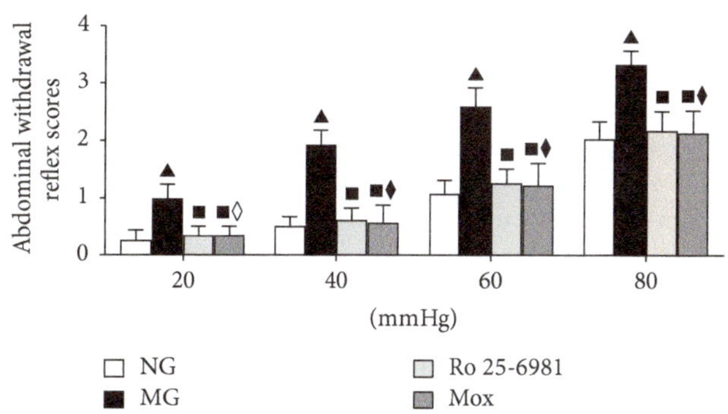

FIGURE 2: AWR scores of rats in each group after moxibustion intervention. Under the same intensity of CRD stimulation, compared to the normal group, ▲$P < 0.001$; compared to the model group, ■$P < 0.001$; compared to the Ro 25-6981 group, ♦$P < 0.05$, ◊$P > 0.05$.

2.4. Real-Time PCR. Total RNA was extracted from the L6-S2 segment of spinal dorsal horn tissues. cDNA was synthesized using the reverse transcriptase reaction system (Jrdun Biotechnology (Shanghai) Co., Ltd.). The relative gene expression level was controlled using the ΔΔCT method. Data were analyzed using the ABI Prism 7300 SDS software.

2.5. Immunohistochemistry. NR1, NR2B, and PKCε in rat spinal cord were detected using immunohistochemistry. Antigen retrieval was performed by heating samples in 0.01 M citric acid buffer (pH 6.0) in a microwave oven. After washing with 0.01 M PBS (pH 7.2–7.6) for 3 × 5 min, specimens were treated with 3% H_2O_2 in the dark for 15 min to inactivate endogenous peroxidases. After washing with 0.01 M PBS for 3 × 5 min, specimens were immersed in the diluted anti-NMDAR1 antibody, anti-PKC epsilon antibody, or anti-NMDAR2B antibody (Abcam, UK) and incubated at 4°C overnight. The specimens were warmed up for 30 min, washed with 0.01 M PBS for 3 × 5 min, and incubated with the secondary antibody from the EnVision reagent kit (Gene Tech (Shanghai) Co., Ltd., Shanghai, China) at room temperature for 30 min. After washing with 0.01 M PBS for 3 × 5 min, DAB developing solution (Gene Tech (Shanghai) Co., Ltd., Shanghai, China) was added, the tissues were washed with double-distilled water to terminate the development, and then they were dehydrated, mounted, and observed under a light microscope.

2.6. Western Blot. NR1, NR2B, and PKCε were measured by western blot in spinal cord tissues of rats in all groups. RIPA lysis buffer at the ratio of 100 mg tissue/mL lysis buffer (Beyotime Institute of Biotechnology, China) was used for the extraction of total protein from spinal dorsal horns. The protein concentration was determined using the BCA method with the BCA protein concentration determination reagent kit (Beyotime Institute of Biotechnology, China). Protein standards at 0.5 mg/mL were added to standard wells in a 96-well plate, and the volume was filled up to 40 μL using the standard dilution buffer. The absorbance value at 562 nm of each well was measured. According to the standard curve, the protein concentrations of samples were calculated. The loading mass of samples was 100 μg and the loading volume was 10 μL. Samples were subjected to sodium dodecyl sulfate-polyacrylamide gel electrophoresis (SDS-PAGE) (Bio-Rad, USA) and transferred to a nitrocellulose (NC) membrane (wet transfer). After the transfer was finished, the NC membrane was removed, placed in an incubation box, and blocked in an appropriate amount of 5% BSA on a shaker at room temperature for 1 h. The trimmed NC membrane was placed in a corresponding incubation box and incubated with PKCε rabbit mAb, NMDAR1 rabbit mAb, NMDAR2B rabbit mAb (Cell Signaling Technology, USA), and HRP-labeled β-actin internal control followed by HRP-labeled goat anti-rabbit IgG secondary antibody (Beyotime Institute of Biotechnology, China) (according to the titers of antibodies, they were diluted in 5% BSA at 1 : 1000). The A and B solutions (500 μL each) from the ECL chemiluminescence reagent kit (Pierce) were mixed in a centrifuge tube. The NC membrane incubated with HRP-labeled β-actin was dipped into the A and B solution mix for 1 min. The chemiluminescence solution was removed, and the membrane was automatically exposed in a gel documentation system. The software in the system was used to analyze the target protein bands.

2.7. Statistical Methods. Experimental data were all analyzed using SPSS 19.0. If experimental data conformed to the normal distribution and had homogeneous variances, the statistical description was presented as $\overline{x} \pm s$. The comparison of mean values between two independent samples was statistically analyzed using the two-sample *t*-test. The comparison of mean values between multiple independent samples was examined using the one-way analysis of variance (ANOVA). $P < 0.05$ implied statistical significance.

3. Experimental Results

3.1. AWR Scores of Rats in Each Group after Moxibustion Intervention. After moxibustion, under different pressure levels of CRD stimulation, the AWR scores were significantly different in all intergroup comparisons ($P < 0.001$). Multiple comparisons using the Nemenyi method showed that, with the gradual increase of the stimulation intensity, the AWR scores of rats in each group increased accordingly. Under the same intensity of pressure stimulation, the AWR score in the model group significantly increased compared to the normal group ($P < 0.001$). Compared to the model group, the AWR scores in the moxibustion group and the Ro 25-6981 group both significantly decreased ($P < 0.001$). Figure 2 shows that moxibustion significantly decreased the AWR score of IBS visceral hyperalgesia rats and effectively relieved the IBS visceral hyperalgesia status of rats.

3.2. Pathology of Colon Tissues (HE Stain). The observation of colon tissues under a light microscope showed that the overall structure of colon tissues of rats in the model group was clear (Figure 3). There were no abnormal pathological changes such as hyperplasia, erosions, or ulcers. There was no significant inflammatory cell infiltration and no obvious interstitial edema. The mucosal epithelium was complete, the glands in the lamina propria were arranged orderly, and the distribution of submucosa layer and muscular layer was regular. These results conformed to the clinical characteristics of IBS that there was abdominal pain but there were no obvious histopathological changes.

3.3. Expression of NR1, NR2B, and PKCε mRNA in Spinal Cord. The above experiments showed that the NR1, NR2B, and PKCε receptor proteins played important roles in the pathogenesis of visceral pain and the relief of visceral pain by moxibustion. In particular, intrathecal injection of Ro 25-6981 inhibited the expression of the NR1 and NR2B subtypes; at the same time, the visceral hyperalgesia was also significantly decreased. To observe whether the mRNAs of the NR1, NR2B, and PKCε subtypes also changed during this process, real-time PCR was used.

Real-time PCR showed that NR1 and NR2B were upregulated in spinal cord tissues of rats in the model group compared to the normal group ($P < 0.001$) (Figures 4(a) and 4(b)); the level of upregulation of NR2B mRNA was higher than that of NR1 mRNA. Compared to the model group, moxibustion (Tianshu and Shangjuxu) and intrathecal injection of Ro 25-6981 both inhibited the expression of NR1 and NR2B mRNA in the spinal cord of rats ($P < 0.001$). The comparison between the moxibustion group and the Ro 25-6981 group did not show a significant difference ($P > 0.05$).

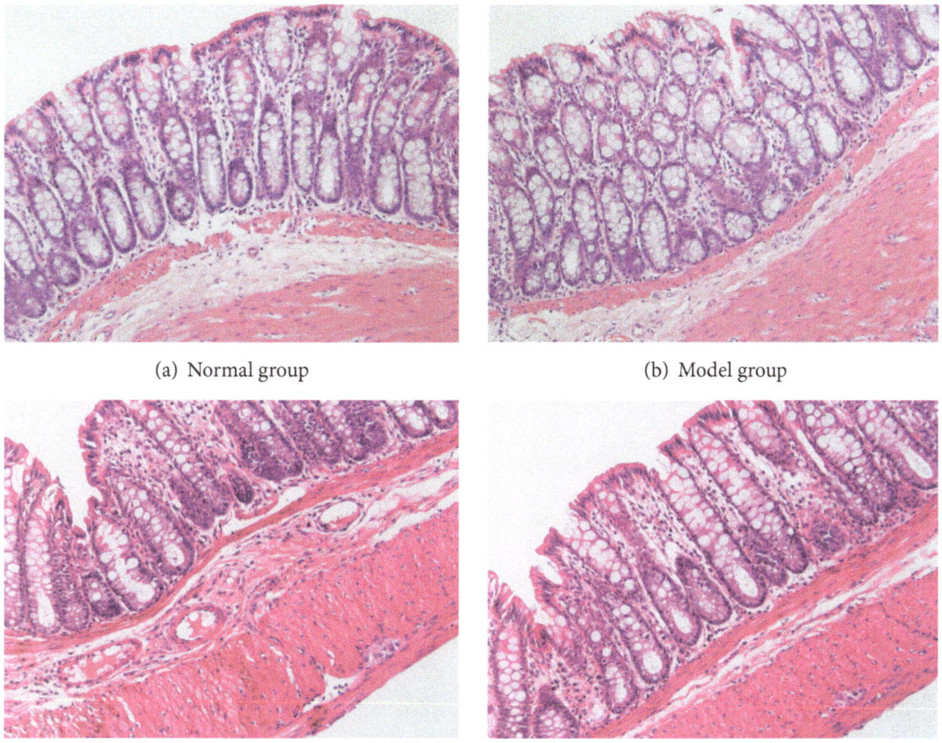

(a) Normal group

(b) Model group

(c) Ro 25-6981 group

(d) Moxibustion group

FIGURE 3: Pathology of colon tissues (HE stain ×200). The observation of colon tissues under a light microscope showed that the overall structure of colon tissues of rats in the model group was clear. There were no abnormal pathological changes such as hyperplasia, erosions, or ulcers. There was no significant inflammatory cell infiltration and no obvious interstitial edema. The mucosal epithelium was complete, the glands in the lamina propria were arranged orderly, and the distribution of submucosa layer and muscular layer was regular.

Based on the inhibitory effects of moxibustion and the NMDA receptor antagonist Ro 25-6981 on NR1 and NR2B mRNA and protein in the spinal dorsal horn, we observed whether moxibustion also had regulatory effects on PKCε mRNA in the central spinal dorsal horns. The effects of moxibustion and Ro 25-6981 on PKCε mRNA in the spinal cord tissues in rats were observed using real-time PCR. Compared to the normal group, PKCε mRNA expression significantly increased in the model group ($P < 0.001$). Compared to the model group, PKCε mRNA expression in the moxibustion group and the Ro 25-6981 group significantly decreased ($P < 0.001$) (Figure 4(c)), suggesting that PKCε mRNA expression significantly increased in the spinal cord of IBS visceral hyperalgesia rats and that moxibustion mitigates this increase.

3.4. Immunohistochemistry for NR1, NR2B, and PKCε in Spinal Dorsal Horn. The immunohistochemistry was performed in spinal tissues with positive expression of NR1, NR2B, and PKCε to detect their localization and for semiquantitative detection. Each pairwise comparison between groups showed significantly different levels of positive immunoactive expression of NR1 subtypes in the cell membrane and cytoplasm of neurons in the spinal dorsal horn ($P < 0.001$) (Figures 5(a)–5(d)). As shown in Figure 5(e), the expression was concentrated in layers I and II of the spinal dorsal horn. The positive expression of the NR1 subtype was yellow to brown, and the cell nucleus was blue. In the normal group, NR1 had weak expression in layers I and II; the color was light and the distribution was sparse (Figure 5(a)). In the model group, the NR1-positive staining was darker than that in the normal group ($P < 0.001$) and the distribution was denser (Figure 5(b)). In the Ro 25-6981 and moxibustion groups, the NR1-positive expression was weaker than that in the model group ($P < 0.001$); the staining was lighter and the distribution was sparser (Figures 5(c) and 5(d)). The comparison between the moxibustion group and the Ro 25-6981 group did not show a significant difference ($P > 0.05$).

Positive immunoactive expression of NR2B in the cytoplasm and cell membrane of spinal dorsal horn neurons was also different in each group ($P < 0.001$) (Figures 5(f) and 5(i)). NR2B stained yellowish brown. Figure 5(j) shows that its location was similar to that of the NR1 subtype: it was concentrated in layers I and II of the dorsal horn. In the normal group, NR2B had weak expression in layers I and II; the color was light and the distribution was sparse (Figure 5(f)). The NR2B-positive staining in the model group was darker than that in the normal group ($P < 0.001$) and the distribution was denser (Figure 5(g)). The NR2B-positive expression in spinal cord of rats in the Ro 25-6981 group and the moxibustion group significantly decreased compared to the model group ($P < 0.001$); the color was lighter and the distribution was sparser (Figures 5(h) and 5(i)).

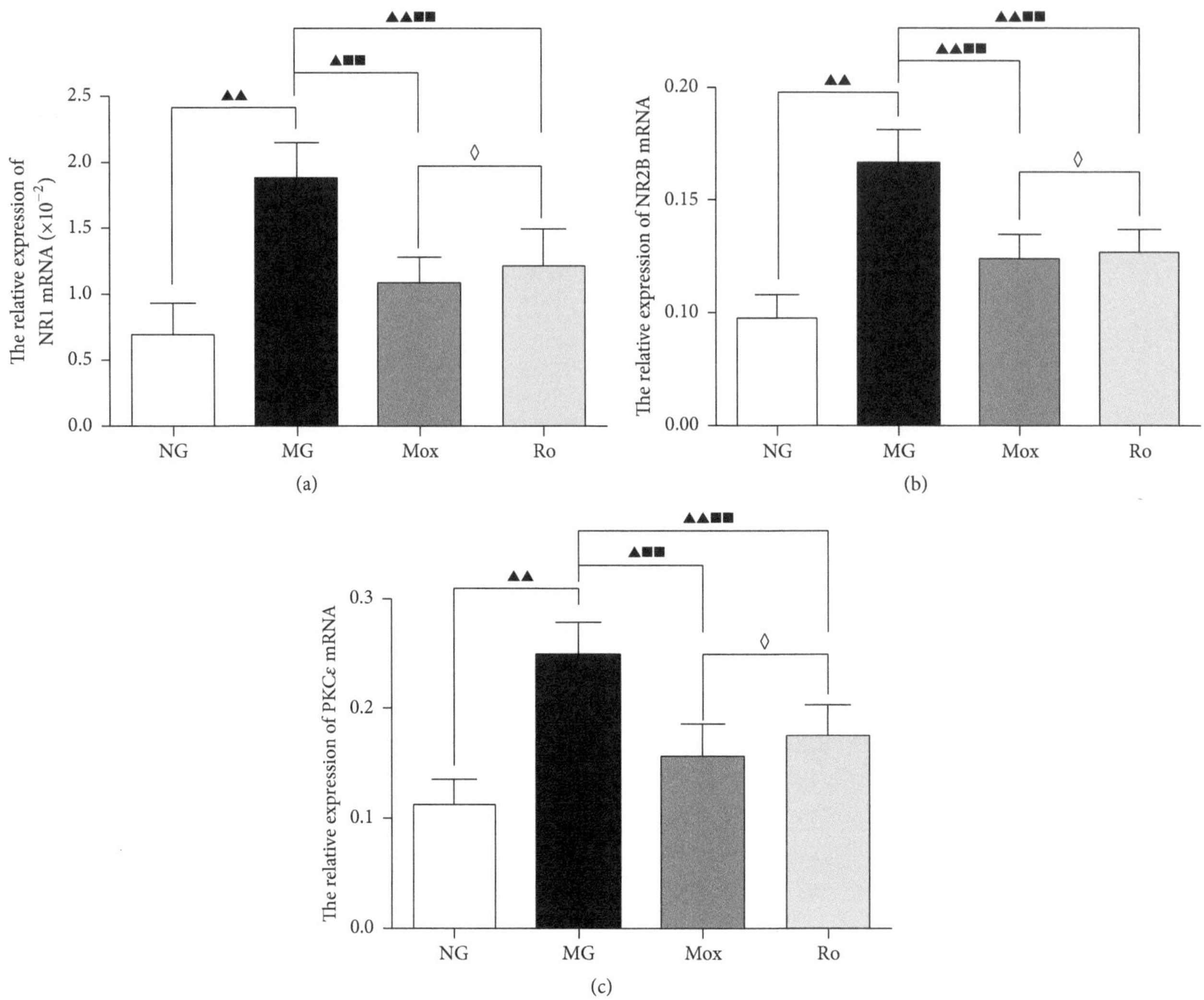

FIGURE 4: NR1 mRNA expression in the spinal cord was significantly different between all groups ($P < 0.001$) except the moxibustion versus the Ro 25-6981 group ($P > 0.05$) (a). NR2B (b) and PKCε (c) followed the same pattern. Pairwise comparisons by LSD t-test. Compared to the normal group, ▲▲$P < 0.001$ and ▲$P < 0.01$; compared to the model group, ■■$P < 0.001$; compared to the Ro 25-6981 group, ◊$P > 0.05$.

These results suggest that NR1 expression in spinal cord in IBS visceral hyperalgesia rats significantly increases and that moxibustion could significantly reduce the expression of NR1 and NR2B in IBS visceral hyperalgesia rats.

Immunohistochemistry for PKCε in the spinal dorsal horn neurons showed different levels of immunoactive expression in the cell membrane and cytoplasm between all four groups ($P < 0.001$) (Figures 5(k) and 5(n)). As shown in Figure 5(o), the expression was again concentrated in layers I and II. The expression of the PKCε subtype was yellow to yellowish brown, and the nucleus was blue. The PKCε-positive staining in the model group was darker than that in the normal group ($P < 0.001$) and the distribution was denser (Figures 5(k) and 5(l)). The PKCε-positive staining in the Ro 25-6981 and moxibustion groups decreased compared to the model group ($P < 0.001$); the color was lighter and the distribution was sparser (Figures 5(m) and 5(n)). The comparison between the moxibustion group and the Ro 25-6981 group did not show a significant difference ($P > 0.05$). The expression change of the PKCε subtype had a similar trend to that of the NR1 and NR2B subtypes, suggesting that PKCε expression in the spinal cord of IBS visceral hyperalgesia rats significantly increases and that moxibustion mitigates this increase.

3.5. Western Blot for NR1, NR2B, and PKCε in Spinal Dorsal Horn. Based on the above localization and semiquantitative detection, western blot was performed to quantify NR1, NR2B, and PKCε in the spinal dorsal horn in all four groups.

Detection of NR1 and NR2B in the spinal cord using western blot showed increased expression in the model group compared to the normal group ($P < 0.001$) (Figures 6(b) and 6(d)). Compared to the model group, moxibustion on the Tianshu and Shangjuxu acupoints and Ro 25-6981 treatment both downregulated NR1 and NR2B proteins in spinal cord ($P < 0.05$). The comparison between the moxibustion group and the Ro 25-6981 group did not show a significant difference ($P > 0.05$). These results suggest that the expression of

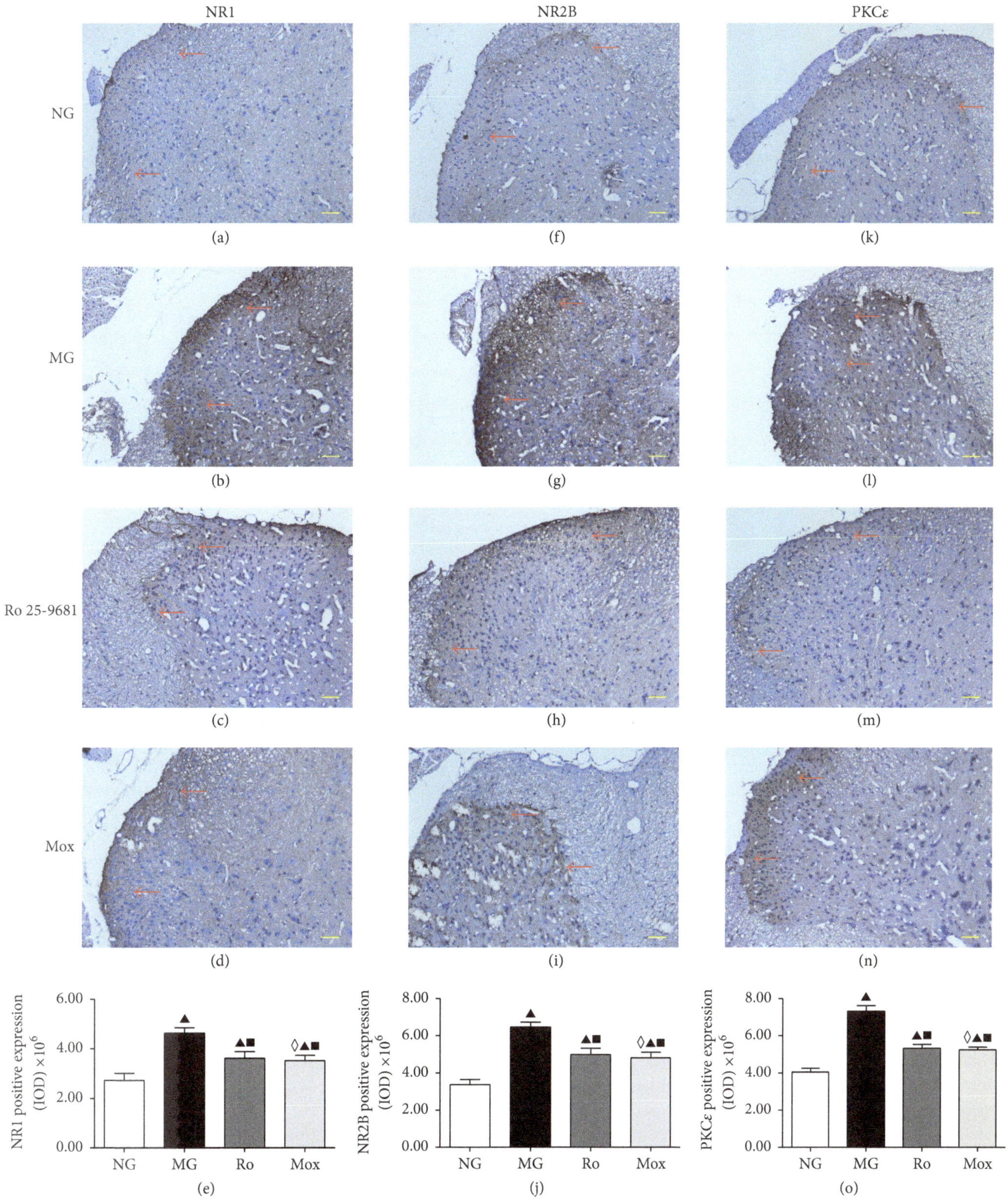

FIGURE 5: The differences in the expression of NR1 ((a) and (d)), NR2B ((f)–(i)), and PKCε ((k)–(n)) in spinal cord were statistically significant between all groups ($P < 0.001$) ((e), (j), and (o)). The least significant difference (LSD) t-test was performed for pairwise comparison, and the results showed that the expression of NR1, NR2B, and PKCε in the model group significantly increased compared to the normal group ($P < 0.001$) ((b), (g), and (l)). Compared to the model group, the expression of NR1, NR2B, and PKCε in the moxibustion group ((d), (i), and (n)) and the Ro 25-6981 group ((c), (h), and (m)) significantly decreased ($P < 0.001$) ((e), (j), and (o)). Compared to the normal group, ▲$P < 0.001$; compared to the model group, ■$P < 0.001$. The comparison between the moxibustion group and the Ro 25-6981 group did not show a significant difference (◊$P > 0.05$) (magnification ×200).

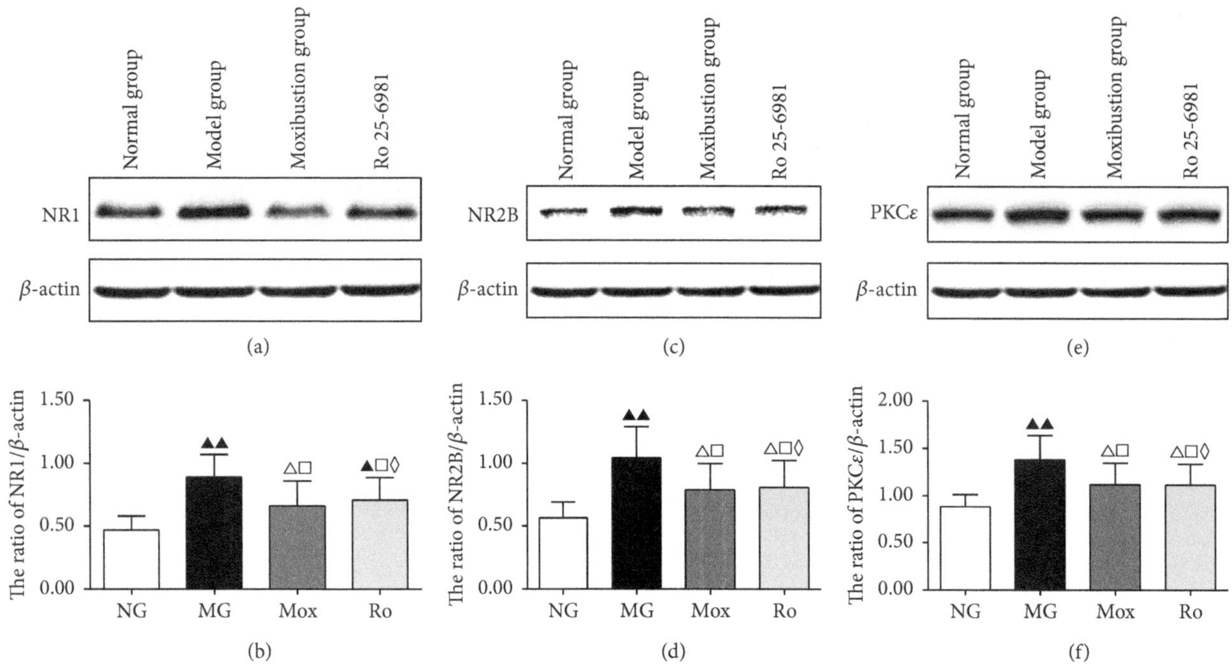

FIGURE 6: The levels of NR1 and NR2B proteins in spinal cord of rats were different between all groups ($P < 0.001$) ((a), (b), (c), and (d)). Further pairwise comparison using the LSD t-test showed that the expression of NR1 and NR2B proteins in the model groups significantly increased compared to the normal group ($P < 0.001$). Compared to the model group, NR1 and NR2B proteins in the moxibustion group and Ro 25-6981 group both significantly decreased ($P < 0.05$). PKCε showed a similar pattern. ((e) and (f)) compared to the normal group, $^{▲▲}P < 0.001$, $^{▲}P < 0.01$, and $^{\triangle}P < 0.05$; compared to the model group, $^{\square}P < 0.05$; compared to the Ro 25-6981 group, $^{\lozenge}P > 0.05$.

NR1 and NR2B protein significantly increases in the spinal cord of IBS visceral hyperalgesia rats and that moxibustion on the Tianshu and Shangjuxu acupoints reverses this increase.

Detection of PKCε in the spinal cord showed a significant increase in the model group compared to the normal group ($P < 0.001$) (Figure 6(f)). Compared to the model group, moxibustion on the Tianshu and Shangjuxu acupoints and Ro 25-6981 both downregulated PKCε in spinal cord ($P < 0.05$). The comparison between the moxibustion group and the Ro 25-6981 group did not show a significant difference ($P > 0.05$). These results suggest that the expression of PKCε protein significantly increases in the spinal cord of IBS visceral hyperalgesia rats and that moxibustion on the Tianshu and Shangjuxu acupoints reversed this increase.

4. Discussion

Central sensitization is considered a key factor in the process of development and progression of visceral hypersensitivity and visceral hyperalgesia. The spinal dorsal horn is the first relay station of the transmission of pain signals into the central nervous system. It can both directly regulate pain messages and receive the downward regulatory signals from the central nervous system above the spinal cord to regulate the transmission of nociceptive signals received by internal organs. Therefore, the spinal dorsal horn has received extensive attention in the studies of central sensitization. Moxibustion on the Tianshu acupoint can significantly reduce the AWR score of IBS rats and improve the abnormally high PK1 and PKR1 in spinal cord and colon tissues [27, 28]. Moxibustion treatment can increase the levels of endogenous opioid peptides (dynorphin, endomorphin, enkephalins, and orphanin), suggesting that these peptides at the spinal cord level might be involved in the analgesic effect of moxibustion [29, 30]. The analgesic mechanism of moxibustion is more complex, involving the nervous-endocrine-immune aspects and being associated with parameters such as acupoint specificity, stimulation time, and temperature.

Boyce et al. [31] showed that the distribution of NR2B is mainly limited to the spinal dorsal horns, especially layers I and II. Nagy et al. [32] used the pepsin digestion technique to expose antigens and observed the distribution of NR2B in layers I and II during visceral pain. NR1 is distributed throughout the central nervous system. The expression level of NR1 significantly increases in lamina layers I and II of the spinal cord dorsal horn in rats with visceral hypersensitivity induced by intracolonic trinitrobenzene sulfonic acid (TNBS) [33]. The NR2B subunit plays an important role in the transmission of nociceptive messages at the spinal cord level and the generation and maintenance of hyperalgesia [34]. In the thoracolumbar segment and lumbosacral segment of rats in the IBS model, the expression of NR2B protein significantly increases [35], indicating that the chronic visceral hyperalgesia in IBS-like rats might be associated with the increased NR2B subunit in these two segments. These results suggest that NR2B might play an important role in the process of transmission of chronic visceral pain signals.

We used the CRD stimulation method to prepare a rat model of IBS visceral hyperalgesia. The behavioral tests showed that, under different pressure levels of CRD stimulation, the AWR scores in the model groups all significantly increased, indicating visceral hypersensitivity. HE staining results also suggested that the colon in the model group did not have obvious pathological changes, which confirmed the clinical characteristics of IBS of abdominal pain but no significant histopathological changes. The expression of NR1 protein and mRNA in layers I and II of the spinal dorsal horn was higher than in normal rats (Figures 4(a), 5(b), and 6(b)). The analysis of NR2B protein and mRNA produced similar results (Figures 4(b), 5(g), and 6(d)). However, the expression levels of NR2B protein and mRNA were significantly higher than those of NR1. Combined with the observation of the behavioral scores of rats (Figure 2), these results indicate that NR1 and NR2B might play a role in the pathogenesis of the increase of visceral sensitivity.

The NMDA receptor in the central nervous system is involved in the formation of visceral hyperalgesia-central sensitization [36, 37]. Intrathecal injection of NMDA enhances the pain reaction of animals induced by internal organ stimulation in a dose-dependent manner. Electrophysiological experiments also suggest that NMDA induces the enhancement of discharge by neurons upon CRD stimulation, which is also combined with a strong afterdischarge [38]. Intrathecal injection of specific NMDA receptor antagonists could relieve visceral hypersensitivity in rats [39]. To further validate this result, we performed intrathecal injection of the NMDA receptor antagonist Ro 25-6981 to block the NMDA receptor function above the spinal cord level. First, the AWR score of the visceral reflex of IBS rats was measured. Intrathecal injection of Ro 25-6981 significantly decreases the visceral hyperalgesia (Figure 2). Detection of NR1 and NR2B in the spinal dorsal horns of rats in the Ro 25-6981 group also showed decreased NR1 and NR2B mRNA (Figures 4(a), 4(b), 5(e), 5(j), 6(b), and 6(c)). After moxibustion treatment, the visceral hyperalgesia of rats in the model group was significantly relieved (Figure 2). We speculated that moxibustion exerted its analgesic effect through the regulation of NR1 and NR2B function. We therefore detected the mRNA expression of NR1 and NR2B in the spinal dorsal horn and found that moxibustion mitigated the increases in NR1 and NR2B mRNA seen in the model rats (Figures 4(a), 4(b), 5(e), 5(j), 6(b), and 6(d)). These results indicate that, by inhibiting NR1 and NR2B expression in layers I and II of the dorsal horn, moxibustion inhibits the binding between excitatory glutamate and NMDA receptor and decreases the number of activated ion channels, thus inhibiting the function of the regulatory region of PKC and eventually relieving visceral pain. In this study, the efficacy of moxibustion on the relief of visceral pain was slightly better than that of the intrathecal injection of Ro 25-6981. One possible reason was that moxibustion also relieved visceral pain through other pathways.

Activated PKC can phosphorylate many receptors and ion channels, including NMDA receptor. As a subtype of PKC, PKCε plays a certain regulatory role in the process of transduction of pain signals at the spinal cord level. Sweitzer et al. [40] showed that PKCε might regulate the phenomenon of hypersensitive response or excessive pain reaction to stimulation presented by patients after morphine withdrawal in clinical setting. Zhang et al. [41] used western blot to study the function of PKCε in visceral pain through a rat model of visceral pain. They found that PKCε is activated during the process of visceral pain, suggesting that PKCε might be involved in the development of visceral pain. In the present study, layers I and II of the spinal dorsal horn of IBS rats induced by mechanical CRD stimulation had upregulated PKCε protein and mRNA (Figures 4(c), 5(o), and 6(f)). Our previous experiments had already shown that moxibustion could regulate the stage of binding between excitatory glutamate and the NR1 and NR2B subtypes of the NMDA receptor; the intrathecal injection of the NMDA receptor antagonist downregulated PKCε in layers I and II of the spinal dorsal horn (Figure 5(o)). These results indicate that the function of PKCε is affected after the NMDA receptor is inhibited. We speculated that moxibustion also regulates PKCε activation to exert its effects on relieving visceral pain. In the group treated by moxibustion on the Tianshu and Shangjuxu acupoints seven times, PKCε protein and mRNA were downregulated in layers I and II of the spinal cord dorsal horn (Figures 4(c), 5(o), and 6(f)), indicating that PKCε is involved in the relief of visceral pain by moxibustion.

In summary, by decreasing the expression of NR1, NR2B, and PKCε in spinal cord of IBS visceral hyperalgesia rats, moxibustion reduced the transduction of visceral hyperalgesia signals and inhibited the process of central sensitization, which might be an important mechanism by which moxibustion relieves the IBS visceral hyperalgesia status.

Competing Interests

The authors declare that they have no competing interests regarding the publication of this paper.

Authors' Contributions

L. Y. Tan, H. R. Liu, and H. G. Wu designed and performed the experiments; L. D. Wang, J. M. Zhao, R. J. Huang, Z. H. Hu, and K. Wang analyzed the data; and L. D. Wang and Z. J. Weng wrote the paper. L. D. Wang, J. M. Zhao, and R. J. Huang contributed equally to this work.

Acknowledgments

This research was funded by the National Natural Science Foundation of China (no. 812027520), the National Basic Research Program of China (973 Program, no. 2015CB554500), and Key Project of Chinese Ministry of Education (no. 20123107110008).

References

[1] Q. Zhou, D. D. Price, C. S. Callam, M. A. Woodruff, and G. N. Verne, "Effects of the N-methyl-D-aspartate receptor on temporal summation of second pain (Wind-up) in irritable bowel syndrome," *The Journal of Pain*, vol. 12, no. 2, pp. 297–303, 2011.

[2] M. Yang, "Progress in the studies of visceral hypersensitivity-central sensitization," *Chongqing Medicine*, vol. 38, no. 15, pp. 1958–1960, 2009.

[3] Y. M. Wang, Y. Y. Xia, and Y. Min, "Voltage-gated calcium channel as a target for new analgesic drugs," *World Clinical Drugs*, vol. 31, no. 7, pp. 433–437, 2010.

[4] J. Shi, M. Liu, L. Lan et al., "Application of moxibustion in the treatment of functional gastrointestinal diseases," *Journal of Traditional Chinese Medicine*, vol. 53, no. 18, article 1605, 2012.

[5] S. Y. Wang, X. Chen, and Q. G. Gao, "Clinical observation of treatment of irritable bowel syndrome (IBS) using moxibustion," *Journal of Clinical Acupuncture and Moxibustion*, vol. 19, no. 10, pp. 43–44, 2003.

[6] Q. Li, N. Li, H. R. Liu et al., "Clinical and experimental studies on moxibustion for treatment of irritable bowel syndrome," *Chinese Archives of Traditional Chinese Medicine*, vol. 25, no. 12, pp. 2224–2227, 2010.

[7] H. B. Zheng, Y. Chen, J. Chen et al., "Application of data mining methods to the studies of selection of points in the treatment of irritable bowel syndrome using acupuncture and moxibustion," *Lishizhen Medicine and Materia Medica Research*, vol. 24, no. 3, pp. 701–702, 2013.

[8] X. M. Qiu and X. Z. Chen, "Analysis of acupoint selection and formula rules of irritable bowel syndrome treated by acupuncture and moxibustion," *Journal of Clinical Acupuncture and Moxibustion*, vol. 29, no. 5, pp. 48–50, 2013.

[9] G. Y. Han and J. H. Sun, "Acupoint selection rules of acupuncture therapies for irritable bowel syndrome preliminary exploration," *Journal of Liaoning University of TCM*, vol. 13, no. 5, pp. 213–216, 2011.

[10] M. Narita, K. Miyoshi, M. Narita, and T. Suzuki, "Changes in the function of NMDA receptor NR2B subunit in spinal cord of rats with neuropathy following chronic ethanol consumption," *Life Sciences*, vol. 80, no. 9, pp. 852–859, 2007.

[11] X.-Q. Luo, Q.-Y. Cai, Y. Chen et al., "Tyrosine phosphorylation of the NR2B subunit of the NMDA receptor in the spinal cord contributes to chronic visceral pain in rats," *Brain Research*, vol. 1542, pp. 167–175, 2014.

[12] Y. Ji, G. Bai, D.-Y. Cao, and R. J. Traub, "Estradiol modulates visceral hyperalgesia by increasing thoracolumbar spinal GluN2B subunit activity in female rats," *Neurogastroenterology and Motility*, vol. 27, no. 6, pp. 775–786, 2015.

[13] Q. P. Ma and C. J. Woolf, *The NMDA Receptor, Pain and Central Sensitization*, Birkhäuser, Basel, Switzerland, 2002.

[14] F. Labombarda, M. F. Coronel, M. J. Villar, A. F. D. Nicola, and S. L. González, "Neuropathic pain and temporal expression of preprodynorphin, protein kinase C and N-methyl-d-aspartate receptor subunits after spinal cord injury," *Neuroscience Letters*, vol. 447, no. 2-3, pp. 115–119, 2008.

[15] J. Li, L. Li, L. Zhao, K. T. Ma, and J. Q. Si, "N-methyl-D-aspartate receptor and pain," *Journal of Baotou Medical College*, vol. 25, no. 5, pp. 106–108, 2009.

[16] Y. Zhang, L. Zhang, F. Wang et al., "Activation of M3 muscarinic receptors inhibits T-type Ca^{2+} channel currents via pertussis toxin-sensitive novel protein kinase C pathway in small dorsal root ganglion neurons," *Cellular Signalling*, vol. 23, no. 6, pp. 1057–1067, 2011.

[17] G. Mo, R. Grant, D. O'Donnell, D. S. Ragsdale, C.-Q. Cao, and P. Séguéla, "Neuropathic Nav1.3-mediated sensitization to P2X activation is regulated by protein kinase C," *Molecular Pain*, vol. 7, no. 1, article 14, 2011.

[18] E. D. Al-Chaer, M. Kawasaki, and P. J. Pasricha, "A new model of chronic visceral hypersensitivity in adult rats induced by colon irritation during postnatal development," *Gastroenterology*, vol. 119, no. 5, pp. 1276–1285, 2000.

[19] W. M. Li, K. M. Cui, and G. C. Wu, "The therapeutic effect of electro-acupuncture on irritable bowel syndrome in rats," *Shanghai Journal of Acupuncture and Moxibustion*, vol. 25, no. 3, pp. 43–47, 2006.

[20] C. Li, *Experimental Acupuncture*, China Press of Traditional Chinese Medicine, Beijing, China, 2007.

[21] C. H. Li, Y. Q. Liu, P. Zhang et al., "Progress on acupuncture acupoint location research domestically during the 11th five-year," *Chinese Archives of Traditional Chinese Medicine*, vol. 31, no. 2, pp. 261–262, 2013.

[22] H. J. Wang and L. X. Ji, "Positioning of "Shenque" acupoint in rats," *Acupuncture Research*, vol. 32, no. 5, p. 312, 2007.

[23] H.-R. Liu, L. Qi, L.-Y. Wu et al., "Effects of moxibustion on dynorphin and endomorphin in rats with chronic visceral hyperalgesia," *World Journal of Gastroenterology*, vol. 16, no. 32, pp. 4079–4083, 2010.

[24] X. X. Qu, M. J. Li, J. Cai et al., "The analgesic effects of intrathecal administration of Ro 25-6981 on neuropathic pain in rats: study on the electrophysiological mechanisms," *Chinese Journal of Pain Medicine*, vol. 14, no. 2, pp. 87–90, 2008.

[25] X.-X. Qu, J. Cai, M.-J. Li et al., "Role of the spinal cord NR2B-containing NMDA receptors in the development of neuropathic pain," *Experimental Neurology*, vol. 215, no. 2, pp. 298–307, 2009.

[26] M. Jiang, X. P. Gu, Z. L. Ma et al., "The analgesic effects of intrathecal administration of Ro 25-6981 on incision pain in rats," *International Journal of Anesthesiology and Resuscitation*, vol. 32, no. 2, pp. 162–164, 2011.

[27] C. Zhao, L. Qi, L. Wu et al., "Suspended moxibustion at Tianshu (ST25) inhibits prokineticin 1 and prokineticin receptor 1 expression in the spinal cord of rats with chronic visceral hypersensitivity," *Neural Regeneration Research*, vol. 7, no. 15, pp. 1145–1150, 2012.

[28] L. Wu, C. Bao, L. Ge et al., "Mild moxibustion at Tianshu (ST 25) decreases expression of prokineticin-1 and prokineticin receptor-1 in colon tissue of rats with chronic visceral hyperalgesia," *Neural Regeneration Research*, vol. 6, no. 33, pp. 2600–2604, 2011.

[29] H.-G. Wu, L. Qi, H.-R. Liu et al., "Warming moxibustion relieves chronic visceral hyperalgesia in rats: relations to spinal dynorphin and orphanin-FQ system," *Evidence-Based Complementary and Alternative Medicine*, vol. 2013, Article ID 920675, 10 pages, 2013.

[30] T. Yi, L. Qi, H. Wu, X. Ma, H. Liu, and X. Wang, "Analgesic action of suspended moxibustion in rats with chronic visceral hyperalgesia correlates with enkephalins in the spinal cord," *Neural Regeneration Research*, vol. 7, no. 3, pp. 219–222, 2012.

[31] S. Boyce, A. Wyatt, J. K. Webb et al., "Selective NMDA NR2B antagonists induce antinociception without motor dysfunction: correlation with restricted localisation of NR2B subunit in dorsal horn," *Neuropharmacology*, vol. 38, no. 5, pp. 611–623, 1999.

[32] G. G. Nagy, M. Watanabe, M. Fukaya, and A. J. Todd, "Synaptic distribution of the NR1, NR2A and NR2B subunits of the N-methyl-D-aspartate receptor in the rat lumbar spinal cord revealed with an antigen-unmasking technique," *European Journal of Neuroscience*, vol. 20, no. 12, pp. 3301–3312, 2004.

[33] Q. Zhou, D. D. Price, R. M. Caudle, and G. N. Verne, "Spinal NMDA NR1 subunit expression following transient TNBS colitis," *Brain Research*, vol. 1279, pp. 109–120, 2009.

[34] P.-H. Tan, L.-C. Yang, H.-C. Shih, K.-C. Lan, and J.-T. Cheng, "Gene knockdown with intrathecal siRNA of NMDA receptor

NR2B subunit reduces formalin-induced nociception in the rat," *Gene Therapy*, vol. 12, no. 1, pp. 59–66, 2005.

[35] C. Lin, G.-W. Lin, W. Zheng, A.-Q. Chen, and C.-X. Yu, "Effect of NMDA receptors NR2B subunit on chronic visceral hypersensitivity," *Chinese Pharmacological Bulletin*, vol. 24, no. 8, pp. 1015–1018, 2008.

[36] D. Grundy, "What activates visceral afferents?" *Gut*, vol. 53, supplement 2, pp. 115–118, 2004.

[37] N. Lü, M. Han, Z.-L. Yang, Y.-Q. Wang, G.-C. Wu, and Y.-Q. Zhang, "Nociceptin/Orphanin FQ in PAG modulates the release of amino acids, serotonin and norepinephrine in the rostral ventromedial medulla and spinal cord in rats," *Pain*, vol. 148, no. 3, pp. 414–425, 2010.

[38] R. Kolhekar, S. T. Meller, and G. F. Gebhart, "Characterization of the role of spinal N-methyl-D-aspartate receptors in thermal nociception in the rat," *Neuroscience*, vol. 57, no. 2, pp. 385–395, 1993.

[39] A. C. Soliman, J. S. C. Yu, and T. J. Coderre, "mGlu and NMDA receptor contributions to capsaicin-induced thermal and mechanical hypersensitivity," *Neuropharmacology*, vol. 48, no. 3, pp. 325–332, 2005.

[40] S. M. Sweitzer, S. M. E. Wong, A. Tjolsen, C. P. Allen, D. Mochly-Rosen, and J. J. Kendig, "Exaggerated nociceptive responses on morphine withdrawal: roles of protein kinase C ε and γ," *Pain*, vol. 110, no. 1-2, pp. 281–289, 2004.

[41] Y. B. Zhang, C. Y. Gao, J. J. Li et al., "Changes to PKC and PKCε in the spinal cord in visceral inflammatory pain induced by formalin in the rat," *The Chinese Journal of Pain*, vol. 11, no. 2, pp. 91–95, 2005.

3

The Study of Misclassification Probability in Discriminant Model of Pattern Identification for Stroke

Mi Mi Ko[1] and Honggie Kim[2]

[1] *KM Fundamental Research Division, Korea Institute of Oriental Medicine, Daejeon 305-811, Republic of Korea*
[2] *Department of Information and Statistics, Chungnam National University, Daejeon 305-764, Republic of Korea*

Correspondence should be addressed to Honggie Kim; honggiekim@cnu.ac.kr

Academic Editor: Chris Zaslawski

Background. Pattern identification (PI) is the basic system for diagnosis of patients in traditional Korean medicine (TKM). The purpose of this study was to identify misclassification objects in discriminant model of PI for improving the classification accuracy of PI for stroke. *Methods.* The study included 3306 patients with stroke who were admitted to 15 TKM hospitals from June 2006 to December 2012. We derive the four kinds of measure (D, R, S, and C score) based on the pattern of the profile graphs according to classification types. The proposed measures are applied to the data to evaluate how well those detect misclassification objects. *Results.* In 10–20% of the filtered data, misclassification rate of C score was highest compared to those rates of other scores (42.60%, 41.15%, resp.). In 30% of the filtered data, misclassification rate of R score was highest compared to those rates of other scores (40.32%). And, in 40–90% of the filtered data, misclassification rate of D score was highest compared to those rates of other scores. Additionally, we can derive the same result of C score from multiple regression model with two independent variables. *Conclusions.* The results of this study should assist the development of diagnostic standards in TKM.

1. Introduction

Due to the development of modern medicine, the average lifespan for human beings is anticipated to rise beyond 85 years of age within the following 20 years [1]. In the meantime, since the rate of aging in South Korea is expected to surge up to 35.1% by 2050, ranking 2nd in the world close to Japan (37.7%), geriatric diseases and the health of the elderly have emerged as one of the most critical social problems of improving the quality of life in the future [2]. In particular, stroke is one of the representative geriatric diseases, along with dementia. Personal and social insecurities caused by the disease have continued to grow. In addition, stroke ranks as the top mortality risk to Koreans among the single diseases and contributes to more than 70% of the in-patients at traditional Korean medical hospitals [3, 4]. In traditional Korean medicine (TKM), specific or nonspecific symptoms of patients are diagnosed by observing, listening, asking, and feeling their pulse under the diagnostic system of pattern identification (PI) in order to determine the cause, nature, treatment method, and treatment drugs of a disease [5–7]. This PI diagnosis collects specific or nonspecific symptoms of patients and classifies them into one of the hundreds of symptom classes. It is the essential core technology forming the backbone of diagnosis and treatment in oriental medicine. However, the PI diagnosis holds limited objectivity and reproducibility due to the lack of standardized measurement indices, and objectification problems have always arisen with respect to personal deviations among TKM physicians based on their knowledge and experience [6–8].

As the necessity for the standardization of diagnostic systems has recently come to the fore, studies have been underway to objectify diagnosis.

In the study titled "Fundamental Study for the Standardization and Objectification of Pattern Identification in Traditional Korean Medicine for Stroke (SOPI-Stroke)," which was conducted over 9 years from 2005 to 2013, the Korea Institute of Oriental Medicine (KIOM) proposed a standardization plan for PI/syndrome differentiation of stroke, established stroke PI diagnostic indices, built a database system relating

TABLE 1: Results using the classification of discriminant model.

		Classification result N (%)				
		QD	DP	YD	FH	Total
Physician's diagnosis	QD	498 (66.94)	115 (15.46)	95 (12.77)	36 (4.84)	744 (22.50)
	DP	118 (10.61)	783 (70.41)	69 (6.21)	142 (12.77)	1112 (33.64)
	YD	70 (14.64)	55 (11.51)	276 (57.74)	77 (16.11)	478 (14.46)
	FH	46 (4.73)	147 (15.12)	127 (13.07)	652 (67.08)	972 (29.40)
	Total	732 (22.14)	1100 (33.27)	567 (17.15)	907 (27.44)	3306 (100.00)

QD: Qi deficiency pattern; DP: Dampness-phlegm pattern; YD: Yin deficiency pattern; FH: Fire-heat pattern.

to TKM clinical technologies by setting up a clinical index database, and founded a scientific basis for stroke and PI by discovering stroke and PI biological indices, to which the latest research methods, such as OMICS, were applied. Studies were carried out to discover biological indices that could be helpful to stroke prevention by finding out what the stroke risk factors were [9–16].

Consequently, the purpose of this study was to identify misclassification objects in discriminant model of PI for improving the classification accuracy of PI for stroke patients. Although current TKM PI diagnostic tools for stroke were developed after several years of research and prepared for public release, the tools still need corrections and modifications in many aspects [17–19]. In this study, the key topics for discussion involve appropriate statistical methods to reduce the probability of diagnostic misclassification.

2. Methods

2.1. Subjects. The study included 3306 patients with stroke who were admitted to 15 oriental medical university hospitals from June 2006 to December 2012. Each patient provided informed consent to undergo procedures that were approved by the respective institutions' Institutional Review Boards (IRB). Informed consent of all the study patients was obtained after a thorough explanation of the details. We enrolled stroke patients for enrollment within 30 days of the onset of their symptoms, provided that their diagnosis was confirmed by an imaging diagnosis such as computerized tomography (CT) or magnetic resonance imaging (MRI). Patients with traumatic stroke such as subarachnoid, subdural, and epidural hemorrhage were excluded from the study.

2.2. Measured Variables. Each patient was seen by two experts at the same department within each site. All experts who were well trained in standard operation procedures (SOPs) were participating in this study. The experts had at least three years of clinical experiences with stroke after finishing regular college education about TKM for six years. The examination parameters were extracted from parts of a case report form (CRF) for the standardization of stroke diagnosis that had been developed by an expert committee organized by the KIOM [7, 11, 12].

2.2.1. The Korean Standard PI for Stroke-3. PI process for differentiating stroke with four TKM types: the Fire-heat (FH) pattern, Dampness-phlegm (DP) pattern, Yin deficiency (YD) pattern, and Qi deficiency (QD) p attern [11, 12]. The F H p attern i s c haracterized b y a ny s ymptom of heat or fire t hat i s c ontracted e xternally o r engendered internally. The D P p attern i s c haracterized b y impeding Qi movement and its turbidity, heaviness, stickiness, and downward-flowing p roperties. Th e QD pa ttern is characterized by qi deficiency w ith d iminished i nternal organ function, which is marked by shortness of breath, lassitude, listlessness, spontaneous sweating, a pale tongue, and a weak pulse. The Y D p attern i s c haracterized b y y in deficiency with diminished moistening and the inability to restrain yang, which is usually manifested as fever [7, 9–13, 20]. The Korean Standard PI for Stroke-3 consists of 44 clinical indices and each clinical index belongs to its respective PI.

2.3. Statistical Methods. After determining 12 different types of misclassification through discriminant analysis, we plotted it on the profile graphs according to types. And then we derive the four kinds of measure (*D*, *R*, *S*, and *C* score) based on the pattern analysis of the profile graphs. The proposed measures are applied to the stroke data to evaluate how well those detect misclassification objects.

2.3.1. Types of Misclassification. According to the results from the discriminant model classification, 2,209 patients posted correct classifications out of the total of 3,306 patients (66.82%) (Table 1). Out of the 3,306 patients, 1,097 were misclassified (33.2%) and the misclassification types are summarized in Table 2. To analyze the misclassification types, 44 clinical indices of the Korean Standard PI for Stroke-3 were grouped into four upper-class variables (QD, DP, YD, and FH pattern indices). In addition, the average and standard deviation of each upper-class variable was used to attain standardized scores, after which the misclassification types were analyzed (Figure 1).

2.3.2. The Profile Graphs. With 12 misclassification types and 4 correct classification types categorized by the discriminant analysis, the profile graphs were drawn. Specifically, two of the 4 patterns were selected and the correct classification types and misclassification types for each pattern were collected from the TKM physicians and divided. For instance, as described in Figure 2, patients applicable to two misclassification types (FHQD and QDFH) were grouped together.

Table 2: The mean values of the standardized scores for upper-class variables according to misclassification type.

	Types of misclassification	N (%)	Z_{QD}	Z_{DP}	Z_{YD}	Z_{FH}
1	DPFH[#]	142 (12.94)	−0.565	−0.113	−0.251	0.648
2	DPQD	118 (10.76)	1.004	−0.001	−0.312	−0.492
3	DPYD	69 (6.29)	0.118	−0.060	0.902	0.085
4	FHDP	147 (13.40)	−0.426	0.610	−0.114	0.069
5	FHQD	46 (4.19)	0.907	−0.494	−0.233	0.096
6	FHYD	127 (11.58)	−0.291	−0.596	0.956	0.184
7	QDDP	115 (10.48)	0.111	0.605	−0.394	−0.456
8	QDFH	36 (3.28)	0.075	−0.500	−0.373	0.560
9	QDYD	95 (8.66)	0.512	−0.487	0.808	−0.299
10	YDDP	55 (5.01)	−0.229	0.529	−0.153	−0.336
11	YDFH	77 (7.02)	−0.393	−0.525	0.133	0.568
12	YDQD	70 (6.38)	0.914	−0.492	0.240	−0.337
Total		1097 (100.00)	0.067	−0.063	0.110	0.017

QD: Qi deficiency pattern; DP: Dampness-phlegm pattern; YD: Yin deficiency pattern; FH: Fire-heat pattern; DPFH[#]: physician's diagnosis- Dampness-phlegm pattern, classification result, Fire-heat pattern; Z_{QD}: the standardized scores for upper-class variables according to Qi deficiency pattern; Z_{DP}: the standardized scores for upper-class variables according to Dampness-phlegm pattern; Z_{YD}: the standardized scores for upper-class variables according to Yin deficiency pattern; Z_{FH}: the standardized scores for upper-class variables according to Fire-heat pattern.

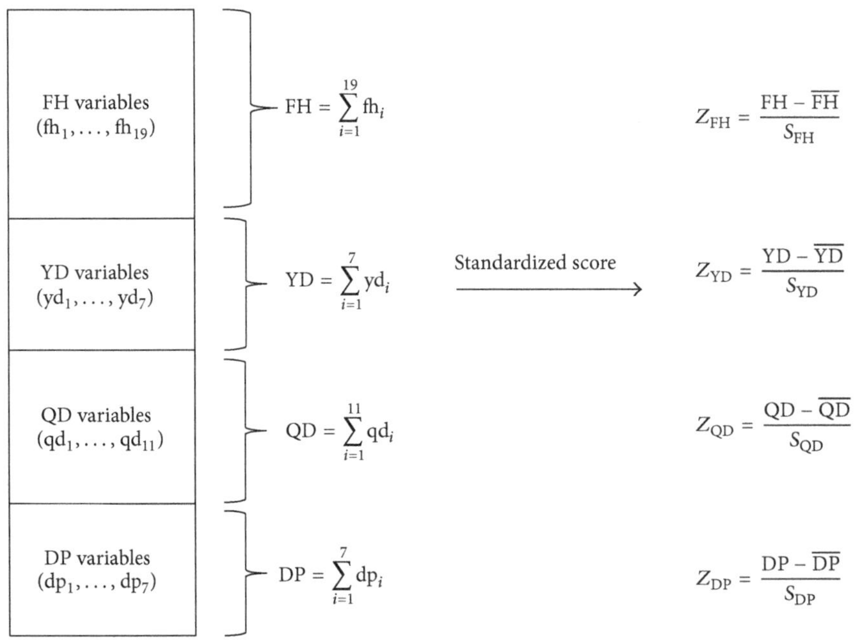

Figure 1: Process of grouping of explanatory variables and standardized scores generation. The mean and standard deviation of each upper-class variable were used to attain standardized scores, after which the misclassification types were analyzed. QD: Qi deficiency pattern; DP: Dampness-phlegm pattern; YD: Yin deficiency pattern; FH: Fire-heat pattern.

Next, the upper-class variable scores of each patient were used to draw a profile plot. At this point, it was critical to arrange the pattern scores of correct classification on the edges and those of the other two pattern scores inside. The profile graphs of the misclassification types (FHQD, QDFH, etc.) and the correct classification types (e.g., FH, QD, YD, and DP) are depicted in Figures 2–7 and the relevant statistics are in Table 3. As illustrated in Figures 2–7, two misclassification types demonstrate a U-shaped pattern and correct classification types an L-shaped or flipped-L-shaped pattern.

2.3.3. Derived Four Measures (D, R, S, and C Scores). In the profile graphs, misclassification observations in most of the 6 cases displayed a bathtub or U-shaped pattern since pattern scores corresponding to actual patterns would be relatively high and the misclassification of a pattern is highly probable if relatively higher scores were observed in the other pattern.

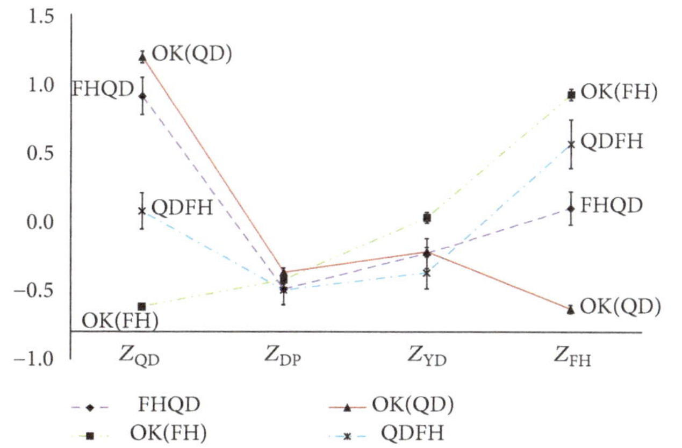

FIGURE 2: The profiles graphs of the FH and QD. Z_{FH}: the standardized scores for upper-class variables according to Fire-heat pattern; Z_{QD}: the standardized scores for upper-class variables according to Qi deficiency pattern; Z_{DP}: the standardized scores for upper-class variables according to Dampness-phlegm pattern; Z_{YD}: the standardized scores for upper-class variables according to Yin deficiency pattern; OK: the correct classification types.

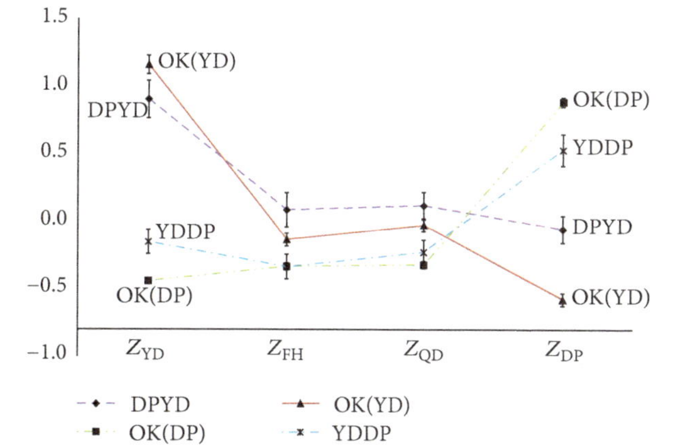

FIGURE 4: The profiles graphs of the DP and YD. Z_{FH}: the standardized scores for upper-class variables according to Fire-heat pattern; Z_{QD}: the standardized scores for upper-class variables according to Qi deficiency pattern; Z_{DP}: the standardized scores for upper-class variables according to Dampness-phlegm pattern; Z_{YD}: the standardized scores for upper-class variables according to Yin deficiency pattern; OK: the correct classification types.

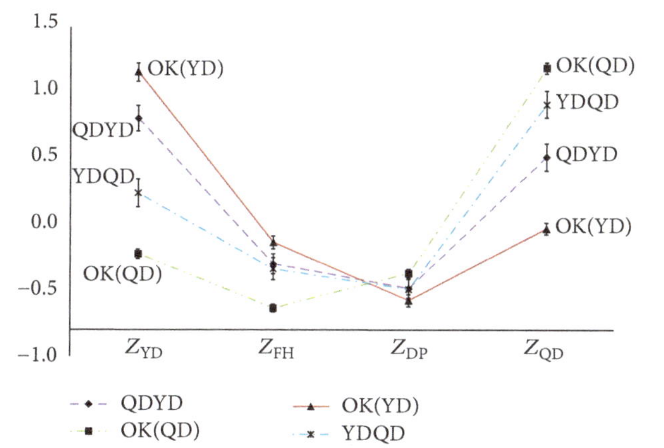

FIGURE 3: The profiles graphs of the QD and YD. Z_{FH}: the standardized scores for upper-class variables according to Fire-heat pattern; Z_{QD}: the standardized scores for upper-class variables according to Qi deficiency pattern; Z_{DP}: the standardized scores for upper-class variables according to Dampness-phlegm pattern; Z_{YD}: the standardized scores for upper-class variables according to Yin deficiency pattern; OK: the correct classification types.

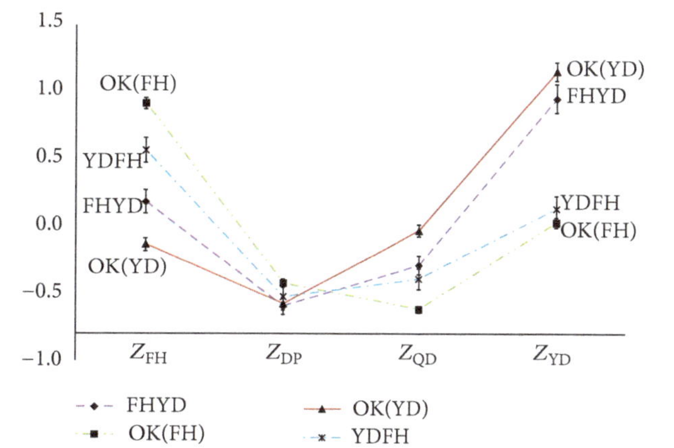

FIGURE 5: The profiles graphs of the FH and YD. Z_{FH}: the standardized scores for upper-class variables according to Fire-heat pattern; Z_{QD}: the standardized scores for upper-class variables according to Qi deficiency pattern; Z_{DP}: the standardized scores for upper-class variables according to Dampness-phlegm pattern; Z_{YD}: the standardized scores for upper-class variables according to Yin deficiency pattern; OK: the correct classification types.

In the meantime, correct classification observations showed an L-shaped (or flipped-L-shaped) pattern. Although actual patterns are unknown due to the lack of direct diagnoses from TKM physicians, if a new patient establishes a bathtub-shaped profile simply with 4 upper-class pattern scores (obligatory two high scores and two low scores), this patient is likely to be misclassified through the future discriminant model. Criteria were designed to assess how close a pattern score profile would be to a bathtub shape through various arrangements and simple calculations of the four pattern scores and applied to already discriminated data. By doing so, comparison was conducted to investigate how much misclassification was estimated and how much discrimination rates improved when the estimated misclassification observations were eliminated beforehand.

(1) D Score. Analyzing correct classification and misclassification types with profile graphs, the D value was derived considering that a difference between the maximum value $Z_{(1)}$ and the second-largest value $Z_{(2)}$ of misclassification was smaller than that of correct classification, and classification by the value was attempted (Figure 8). Namely, under the hypothesis that the smaller the D value was, the closer the profile graph was to a bathtub shape and the higher the probability of the respective observations corresponding to misclassification was, the D values were applied to the clinical stroke data.

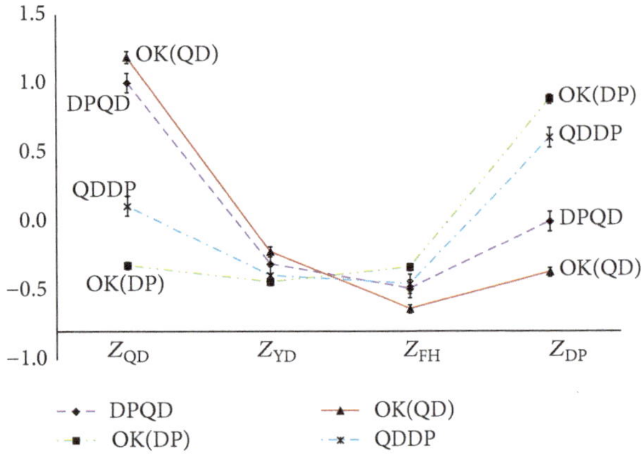

FIGURE 6: The profiles graphs of the DP and QD. Z_{FH}: the standardized scores for upper-class variables according to Fire-heat pattern; Z_{QD}: the standardized scores for upper-class variables according to Qi deficiency pattern; Z_{DP}: the standardized scores for upper-class variables according to Dampness-phlegm pattern; Z_{YD}: the standardized scores for upper-class variables according to Yin deficiency pattern; OK: the correct classification types.

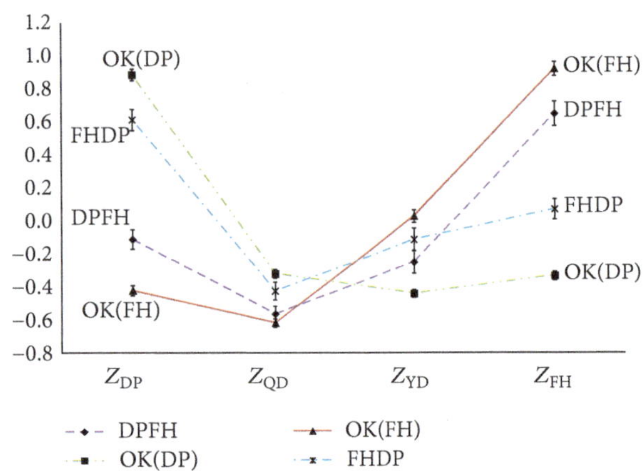

FIGURE 7: The profiles graphs of the DP and FH. Z_{FH}: the standardized scores for upper-class variables according to Fire-heat pattern; Z_{QD}: the standardized scores for upper-class variables according to Qi deficiency pattern; Z_{DP}: the standardized scores for upper-class variables according to Dampness-phlegm pattern; Z_{YD}: the standardized scores for upper-class variables according to Yin deficiency pattern; OK: the correct classification types.

After sorting the data by the D value in descending order and investigating the frequency and rates of misclassification over 10% intervals (Figure 9), the misclassification probability of the 10% ($N = 331$) filtered data reached 40.79% ($N_m = 135$, $\text{Mean}_m = 0.058$), which was 7.61% p higher than the previously calculated misclassification probability (33.18%) of the total data. The misclassification probabilities of the data filtered from 20% to 90% were lower than that of the 10% filtered data but higher than that of the total data (33.18%). In the data filtered at 10%, 20%, 40%, and 50%, average D values of the misclassifications and correct classifications were barely different from each other, even though the average D values of the misclassifications tended to be higher than those of the correct classifications. In the other data groups, the average D values of the correct classifications were higher than those of the misclassifications (Table 4). Meanwhile, examining the frequencies and rates of the correct classifications in the data selected for D values, the misclassification probability of the correct classifications in the 90% ($N = 2975$) selected data recorded 67.66% ($N_c = 2013$, % of $N_m = 32.34\%$), which was 0.86% p higher than those of the previously calculated correct classifications (66.8%) of the total data. In the 80% ($N = 2645$) selected data, the misclassification probabilities of correct classifications reached 68.28% ($N_c = 1806$, % of $N_m = 31.72\%$), which was 0.62% p higher than those in the 90% selected data. In the data selected from 70% to 10%, the correct classifications gradually increased (Table 4).

(2) R Score. Analyzing correct classification and misclassification types with profile graphs, the R value was derived considering that a difference between the maximum value $Z_{(1)}$ and the minimum value $Z_{(4)}$ of misclassification was smaller than that of correct classification, and classification by the value was attempted (Figure 10). Namely, under the hypothesis that the larger the R value was, the closer the profile graph was to an L-shaped or flipped-L-shaped pattern, and the higher the probability of the respective observations corresponding to correct classification was the R values were applied to the clinical stroke data in the same way as previously (Table 5).

(3) S Score. Analyzing correct classification and misclassification types with profile graphs, the S value was derived considering that the second-largest value $Z_{(2)}$ of misclassification was higher than that of correct classification, and classification by the value was attempted (Figure 11). Namely, under the hypothesis that the larger the S value was, the closer the profile graph was to a bathtub (or U) shape and the higher the probability of the respective observations corresponding to misclassification was, the S values were applied to the clinical stroke data. In this case, the frequency and rates of misclassification over 10% intervals were investigated after sorting the data by the S value in ascending order (Table 6).

(4) C Score. Analyzing correct classification and misclassification types with profile graphs, the C value was derived considering that a difference between the sum of $Z_{(1)}$ and $Z_{(2)}$ and the sum of $Z_{(3)}$ and $Z_{(4)}$ of misclassification was larger than that of correct classification, and classification by the value was attempted (Figure 12). Namely, under the hypothesis that the larger the C value was, the closer the profile graph was to a bathtub (or U) shape, the higher the probability of the respective observations corresponding to misclassification was, the C values were applied to the clinical stroke data in the same way as previously (Table 7).

3. Results

3.1. Estimated Misclassification Probability and Discrimination Rate according to Proposed Four Scores. Table 8 summarizes the misclassification probabilities after the data was sorted

TABLE 3: Summary of Z scores according to the profile graphs for PI classification types.

	Classification types	N	Z scores (mean ± SE)			
			Z_{QD}	Z_{DP}	Z_{YD}	Z_{FH}
FH, QD classification types	FHQD	46	0.907 ± 0.137	−0.494 ± 0.110	−0.233 ± 0.109	0.097 ± 0.120
	OK(FH)	652	−0.620 ± 0.025	−0.425 ± 0.031	0.028 ± 0.038	0.919 ± 0.042
	OK(QD)	498	1.189 ± 0.043	−0.372 ± 0.033	−0.223 ± 0.035	−0.637 ± 0.030
	QDFH	36	0.075 ± 0.130	−0.500 ± 0.107	−0.373 ± 0.118	0.560 ± 0.175
	Total	1232	0.189 ± 0.034	−0.408 ± 0.022	−0.095 ± 0.025	0.249 ± 0.034
QD, YD classification types	QDYD	95	0.513 ± 0.103	−0.487 ± 0.072	0.808 ± 0.099	−0.300 ± 0.078
	OK(QD)	498	1.189 ± 0.043	−0.372 ± 0.033	−0.223 ± 0.035	−0.637 ± 0.030
	OK(YD)	276	−0.031 ± 0.045	−0.579 ± 0.046	1.159 ± 0.068	−0.135 ± 0.048
	YDQD	70	0.914 ± 0.102	−0.493 ± 0.090	0.240 ± 0.105	−0.337 ± 0.085
	Total	939	0.742 ± 0.034	−0.454 ± 0.024	0.322 ± 0.036	−0.433 ± 0.025
DP, YD classification types	DPYD	69	0.118 ± 0.097	−0.060 ± 0.101	0.903 ± 0.139	0.085 ± 0.127
	OK(DP)	783	−0.323 ± 0.027	0.883 ± 0.034	−0.443 ± 0.024	−0.336 ± 0.026
	OK(YD)	276	−0.031 ± 0.045	−0.579 ± 0.046	1.159 ± 0.068	−0.135 ± 0.048
	YDDP	55	−0.229 ± 0.090	0.529 ± 0.116	−0.153 ± 0.090	−0.336 ± 0.092
	Total	1183	−0.225 ± 0.022	0.471 ± 0.032	0.022 ± 0.032	−0.264 ± 0.023
FH, YD classification types	FHYD	127	−0.291 ± 0.069	−0.597 ± 0.063	0.956 ± 0.108	0.184 ± 0.087
	OK(FH)	652	−0.620 ± 0.025	−0.425 ± 0.031	0.028 ± 0.038	0.919 ± 0.042
	OK(YD)	276	−0.031 ± 0.045	−0.579 ± 0.046	1.159 ± 0.068	−0.135 ± 0.048
	YDFH	77	−0.393 ± 0.077	−0.525 ± 0.086	0.133 ± 0.095	0.568 ± 0.093
	Total	1132	−0.424 ± 0.022	−0.489 ± 0.023	0.415 ± 0.034	0.555 ± 0.032
DP, QD classification types	DPQD	118	1.004 ± 0.071	−0.001 ± 0.071	−0.312 ± 0.070	−0.492 ± 0.064
	OK(DP)	783	−0.323 ± 0.027	0.883 ± 0.034	−0.443 ± 0.024	−0.336 ± 0.026
	OK(QD)	498	1.189 ± 0.043	−0.372 ± 0.033	−0.223 ± 0.035	−0.637 ± 0.030
	QDDP	115	0.111 ± 0.070	0.605 ± 0.071	−0.395 ± 0.067	−0.456 ± 0.069
	Total	1514	0.311 ± 0.028	0.380 ± 0.027	−0.357 ± 0.019	−0.456 ± 0.018
DP, FH classification types	DPFH	142	−0.565 ± 0.047	−0.113 ± 0.059	−0.251 ± 0.069	0.648 ± 0.076
	OK(DP)	783	−0.323 ± 0.027	0.883 ± 0.034	−0.443 ± 0.024	−0.336 ± 0.026
	OK(FH)	652	−0.620 ± 0.025	−0.425 ± 0.031	0.028 ± 0.038	0.919 ± 0.042
	FHDP	147	−0.426 ± 0.054	0.610 ± 0.064	−0.114 ± 0.068	0.069 ± 0.061
	Total	1724	−0.464 ± 0.017	0.283 ± 0.026	−0.221 ± 0.020	0.254 ± 0.026

PI: pattern identification; QD: Qi deficiency pattern; DP: Dampness-phlegm pattern; YD: Yin deficiency pattern; FH: Fire-heat pattern; OK: the correct classification types; Z_{QD}: the standardized scores for upper-class variables according to Qi deficiency pattern; Z_{DP}: the standardized scores for upper-class variables according to Dampness-phlegm pattern; Z_{YD}: the standardized scores for upper-class variables according to Yin deficiency pattern; Z_{FH}: the standardized scores for upper-class variables according to Fire-heat pattern.

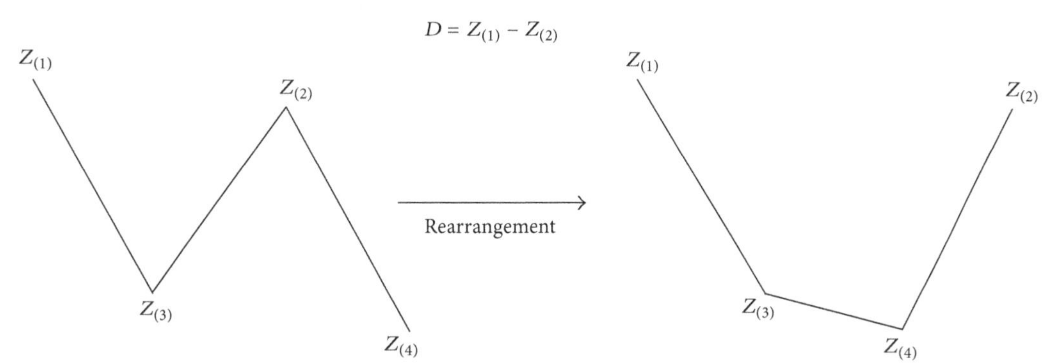

FIGURE 8: Derived D values based on the pattern analysis of the profile graphs. Under the hypothesis that the smaller the D value was, the closer the profile graph was to a bathtub (or U) shape, and the higher the probability of the respective observations corresponding to misclassification was.

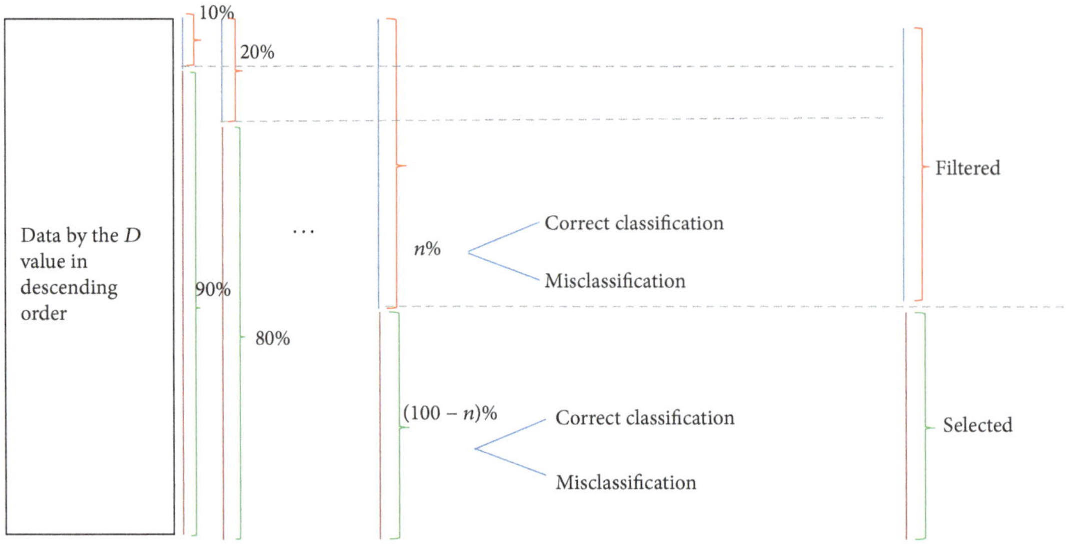

FIGURE 9: Data filtering and selection method. Data were ranged according to each four measures (D, R, S, and C values) in descending or ascending order by increasing data by 10% intervals.

according to the 4 criteria and investigating the misclassification probability over 10% intervals. If the data were filtered 10–20%, the C score marked 42.60% and 41.15%, respectively, indicating the highest misclassification probability among the criteria. If the data were filtered 30%, the R score stands at 40.32% and the C score at 39.92%. If the data were filtered 40~90%, the misclassification probability of the D score was the highest.

For the data previously selected by 4 scores (D, R, S, and C), discrimination rates were compared. Having the 4 QD, DP, YD, and FH patterns set as reaction variables for the entire clinical stroke data and 44 clinical indices of the *Korean Standard PI for Stroke-3* as independent variables, the discriminant analysis was conducted to calculate the discrimination accuracy (Table 9). If the data were selected at 90%, the discrimination rate of the D score increased to 68.2%, which was the largest increase among the four scores. If the data were selected at 80%, the C score reached 69.0%, making the largest increase. If the data were selected at 70%, the R score posted 70.0%, demonstrating the largest increase in the discrimination rate among the four scores. If the data were selected at 60–10%, the D score recorded the largest increase in the discrimination rate among the four scores.

3.2. Similarities between Secondary Curvature Function and C Score

3.2.1. Curvature Created by $Z_{(1)}$, $Z_{(2)}$, $Z_{(3)}$, and $Z_{(4)}$ Scores. First of all, assume four scores, $Z_{(1)}$, $Z_{(2)}$, $Z_{(3)}$, and $Z_{(4)}$, as dependent variables observed in the x values (e.g., 1, 2, 3, and 4) having equal intervals, as shown in the profile graphs. In addition, assume that $Z_{(1)}$ is a dependent variable when $x = 1$, $Z_{(2)}$ when $x = 4$, $Z_{(3)}$ when $x = 2$, and $Z_{(4)}$ when $x = 3$. This assumption is illustrated in Figure 13.

3.2.2. Estimation of Secondary Curvature. Considering the quadratic curve regression model passing through the four points $(1, Z_{(1)})$, $(2, Z_{(3)})$, $(3, Z_{(4)})$, and $(4, Z_{(2)})$, $Y = \beta_0 + \beta_1 X + \beta_2 X^2 + \epsilon$, the coefficient of β_2 is the secondary curvature value that we wanted. Namely, the larger the β_2 is, the stronger the bathtub shape becomes, boosting the misclassification probability. Assuming that the estimates of β_0, β_1, and β_2 are b_0, b_1, and b_2, these estimates satisfy the following normal equation [21]:

$$\left(X'X\right) b = X'Y. \tag{1}$$

Here

$$X = \begin{bmatrix} 1 & 1 & 1^2 \\ 1 & 2 & 2^2 \\ 1 & 3 & 3^2 \\ 1 & 4 & 4^2 \end{bmatrix},$$

$$b = \begin{bmatrix} b_0 \\ b_1 \\ b_2 \end{bmatrix}, \tag{2}$$

$$Y = \begin{bmatrix} Z_{(1)} \\ Z_{(2)} \\ Z_{(3)} \\ Z_{(4)} \end{bmatrix}.$$

According to Neter et al. [21], a general two-variable regression model,

$$Y_i = \beta_0 + \beta_1 X_{i1} + \beta_2 X_{i2} + \epsilon_i, \tag{3}$$

TABLE 4: Types of classifications distribution of filtered/selected data by D value.

Filtered%	Type of classifications distribution of filtered data by D value						Selected%	Type of classifications distribution of selected data by D value					
	N_m (%)	N_c (%)	N_t (%)	$Mean_m$	$Mean_c$	$Mean_t$		N_m (%)	N_c (%)	N_t (%)	$Mean_m$	$Mean_c$	$Mean_t$
10%	135 (40.79)	196 (59.21)	331 (100)	0.058	0.053	0.055	10%	42 (12.69)	289 (87.31)	331 (100)	2.399	2.531	2.515
20%	258 (39.03)	403 (60.97)	661 (100)	0.124	0.125	0.125	20%	119 (18.00)	542 (82.00)	661 (100)	1.913	2.112	2.076
30%	382 (38.51)	610 (61.49)	992 (100)	0.184	0.184	0.184	30%	232 (23.39)	760 (76.61)	992 (100)	1.585	1.870	1.804
40%	525 (39.71)	797 (60.29)	1322 (100)	0.252	0.242	0.246	40%	338 (25.57)	984 (74.43)	1322 (100)	1.397	1.668	1.599
50%	647 (39.14)	1006 (60.86)	1653 (100)	0.319	0.319	0.319	50%	450 (27.22)	1203 (72.78)	1653 (100)	1.244	1.508	1.436
60%	759 (38.26)	1225 (61.74)	1984 (100)	0.387	0.402	0.396	60%	572 (28.83)	1412 (71.17)	1984 (100)	1.107	1.375	1.298
70%	865 (37.38)	1449 (62.62)	2314 (100)	0.460	0.492	0.480	70%	715 (30.90)	1599 (69.10)	2314 (100)	0.973	1.265	1.175
80%	978 (36.98)	1667 (63.02)	2645 (100)	0.550	0.593	0.578	80%	839 (31.72)	1806 (68.28)	2645 (100)	0.875	1.154	1.065
90%	1055 (35.46)	1920 (64.54)	2975 (100)	0.630	0.731	0.695	90%	962 (32.34)	2013 (67.66)	2975 (100)	0.788	1.055	0.969

N_m: number of misclassification types; N_c: number of correct classification types; N_t: number of total classification types; $Mean_m$: mean of misclassification type; $Mean_c$: mean of correct classification type; $Mean_t$: mean of total classification type.

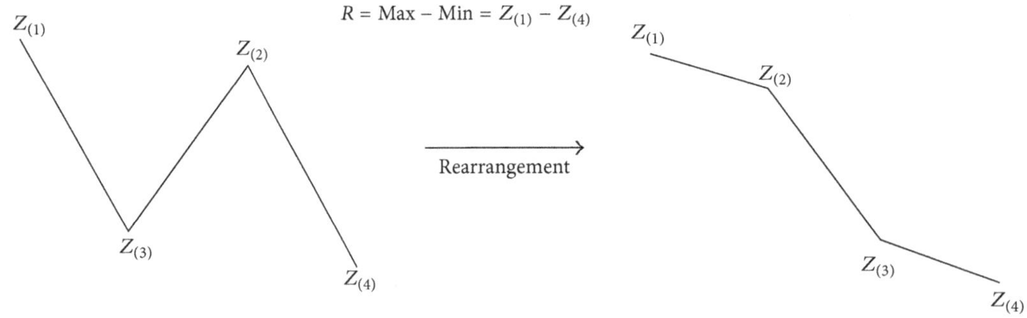

FIGURE 10: Derived R values based on the pattern analysis of the profile graphs. Under the hypothesis that the larger the R value was, the closer the profile graph was to an L-shaped or flipped-L-shaped pattern, the higher the probability of the respective observations corresponding to correct classification was.

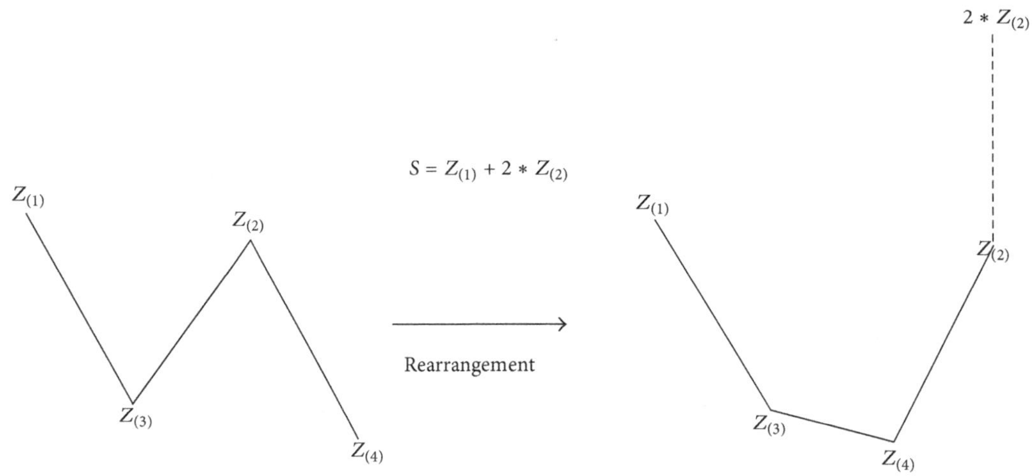

FIGURE 11: Derived S values based on the pattern analysis of the profile graphs. Under the hypothesis that the larger the S value was, the closer the profile graph was to a bathtub (or U) shape, the higher the probability of the respective observations corresponding to misclassification was.

has a normal equation

$$\left(X'X\right) b = X'Y, \tag{4}$$

which is equal to

$$\begin{bmatrix} n & \sum X_{i1} & \sum X_{i2} \\ \sum X_{i1} & \sum X_{i1}^2 & \sum X_{i1}X_{i2} \\ \sum X_{i2} & \sum X_{i2}X_{i1} & \sum X^2_{i2} \end{bmatrix} \begin{bmatrix} b_0 \\ b_1 \\ b_2 \end{bmatrix} = \begin{bmatrix} \sum Y_i \\ \sum X_{i1}Y_i \\ \sum X_{i2}Y_i \end{bmatrix}, \tag{5}$$

and the following normal equations,

$$\begin{gathered} \sum Y_i = nb_0 + b_1 \sum X_{i1} + b_2 \sum X_{i2}, \\ \sum X_{i1}Y_i = b_0 \sum X_{i1} + b_1 \sum X_{i1}^2 + b_2 \sum X_{i1}X_{i2} \\ \sum X_{i2}Y_i = b_0 \sum X_{i2} + b_1 \sum X_{i1}X_{i2} + b_2 \sum X_{i2}^2, \end{gathered} \tag{6}$$

are obtained. In this case, the equations are

$$\begin{gathered} X_{i1} = i, \quad i = 1, 2, 3, 4, \\ X_{i2} = i^2, \quad i = 1, 2, 3, 4, \\ Y_1 = Z_{(1)}, \\ Y_2 = Z_{(3)}, \\ Y_3 = Z_{(4)}, \\ Y_4 = Z_{(2)}. \end{gathered} \tag{7}$$

Now, if

$$\begin{gathered} S_1 = Z_{(1)} + Z_{(2)} + Z_{(3)} + Z_{(4)}, \\ S_2 = Z_{(1)} + 2Z_{(3)} + 3Z_{(4)} + 4Z_{(2)}, \\ S_3 = Z_{(1)} + 4Z_{(3)} + 9Z_{(4)} + 16Z_{(2)}, \end{gathered} \tag{8}$$

TABLE 5: Types of classifications distribution of filtered/selected data by R value.

Filtered%	Type of classifications distribution of filtered data by R value						Selected%	Type of classifications distribution of selected data by R value					
	N_m (%)	N_c (%)	N_t (%)	$Mean_m$	$Mean_c$	$Mean_t$		N_m (%)	N_c (%)	N_t (%)	$Mean_m$	$Mean_c$	$Mean_t$
10%	135 (40.79)	196 (59.21)	331 (100)	0.674	0.677	0.676	10%	65 (19.64)	266 (80.36)	331 (100)	3.790	3.882	3.864
20%	261 (39.49)	400 (60.51)	661 (100)	0.847	0.864	0.858	20%	160 (24.21)	501 (75.79)	661 (100)	3.247	3.418	3.376
30%	400 (40.32)	592 (59.68)	992 (100)	0.991	0.990	0.990	30%	254 (25.60)	738 (74.40)	992 (100)	2.967	3.116	3.078
40%	507 (38.35)	815 (61.65)	1322 (100)	1.099	1.130	1.118	40%	371 (28.06)	951 (71.94)	1322 (100)	2.719	2.905	2.853
50%	623 (37.69)	1030 (62.31)	1653 (100)	1.212	1.252	1.234	50%	474 (28.68)	1179 (71.32)	1653 (100)	2.542	2.710	2.662
60%	726 (36.59)	1258 (63.41)	1984 (100)	1.310	1.369	1.347	60%	590 (29.74)	1394 (70.26)	1984 (100)	2.377	2.556	2.503
70%	843 (36.43)	1471 (63.57)	2314 (100)	1.431	1.486	1.466	70%	697 (30.12)	1617 (69.88)	2314 (100)	2.243	2.411	2.360
80%	937 (35.43)	1708 (64.57)	2645 (100)	1.537	1.623	1.593	80%	836 (31.61)	1809 (68.39)	2645 (100)	2.080	2.288	2.222
90%	1032 (34.69)	1943 (65.31)	2975 (100)	1.660	1.777	1.736	90%	962 (32.34)	2013 (67.66)	2975 (100)	1.942	2.162	2.091

N_m: number of misclassification types; N_c: number of correct classification types; N_t: number of total classification types; $Mean_m$: mean of misclassification types; $Mean_c$: mean of correct classification types; $Mean_t$: mean of total classification types.

Table 6: Types of classifications distribution of filtered/selected data by S value.

Filtered%	Type of classifications distribution of filtered data by S value						Selected%	Type of classifications distribution of selected data by S value					
	N_m (%)	N_c (%)	N_t (%)	$Mean_m$	$Mean_c$	$Mean_t$		N_m (%)	N_c (%)	N_t (%)	$Mean_m$	$Mean_c$	$Mean_t$
10%	120 (36.25)	211 (63.75)	331 (100)	5.587	5.763	5.699	10%	100 (30.21)	231 (69.79)	331 (100)	−1.678	−1.625	−1.641
20%	234 (35.40)	427 (64.60)	661 (100)	4.620	4.673	4.654	20%	205 (31.01)	456 (68.99)	661 (100)	−1.159	−1.162	−1.161
30%	333 (33.57)	659 (66.43)	992 (100)	4.051	3.975	4.000	30%	312 (31.45)	680 (68.55)	992 (100)	−0.792	−0.804	−0.800
40%	435 (32.90)	887 (67.10)	1322 (100)	3.580	3.475	3.509	40%	431 (32.60)	891 (67.40)	1322 (100)	−0.469	−0.516	−0.501
50%	554 (33.51)	1099 (66.49)	1653 (100)	3.126	3.085	3.099	50%	543 (32.85)	1110 (67.15)	1653 (100)	−0.167	−0.226	−0.207
60%	666 (33.57)	1318 (66.43)	1984 (100)	2.768	2.731	2.743	60%	662 (33.37)	1322 (66.63)	1984 (100)	0.127	0.043	0.071
70%	785 (33.92)	1529 (66.08)	2314 (100)	2.405	2.411	2.409	70%	764 (33.02)	1550 (66.98)	2314 (100)	0.382	0.335	0.351
80%	892 (33.72)	1753 (66.28)	2645 (100)	2.106	2.093	2.097	80%	863 (32.63)	1782 (67.37)	2645 (100)	0.649	0.642	0.644
90%	997 (33.51)	1978 (66.49)	2975 (100)	1.814	1.777	1.789	90%	977 (32.84)	1998 (67.16)	2975 (100)	0.993	0.963	0.973

N_m: number of misclassification types; N_c: number of correct classification types; N_t: number of total classification types; $Mean_m$: mean of misclassification type; $Mean_c$: mean of correct classification type; $Mean_t$: mean of total classification type.

TABLE 7: Types of classifications distribution of filtered/selected data by C value.

Filtered%	Type of classifications distribution of filtered data by C value						Selected%	Type of classifications distribution of selected data by C value					
	N_m (%)	N_c (%)	N_t (%)	Mean_m	Mean_c	Mean_t		N_m (%)	N_c (%)	N_t (%)	Mean_m	Mean_c	Mean_t
10%	141 (42.60)	190 (57.40)	331 (100)	0.846	0.845	0.845	10%	84 (25.38)	247 (74.62)	331 (100)	5.037	5.134	5.110
20%	272 (41.15)	389 (58.85)	661 (100)	1.066	1.085	1.078	20%	177 (26.78)	484 (73.22)	661 (100)	4.345	4.463	4.431
30%	396 (39.92)	596 (60.08)	992 (100)	1.240	1.267	1.256	30%	273 (27.52)	719 (72.48)	992 (100)	3.928	4.040	4.009
40%	516 (39.03)	806 (60.97)	1322 (100)	1.392	1.426	1.413	40%	370 (27.99)	952 (72.01)	1322 (100)	3.636	3.737	3.708
50%	619 (37.45)	1034 (62.55)	1653 (100)	1.520	1.588	1.562	50%	478 (28.92)	1175 (71.08)	1653 (100)	3.378	3.498	3.463
60%	727 (36.64)	1257 (63.36)	1984 (100)	1.664	1.746	1.716	60%	581 (29.28)	1403 (70.72)	1984 (100)	3.161	3.281	3.246
70%	824 (35.61)	1490 (64.39)	2314 (100)	1.799	1.911	1.871	70%	701 (30.29)	1613 (69.71)	2314 (100)	2.945	3.098	3.051
80%	920 (34.78)	1725 (65.22)	2645 (100)	1.941	2.082	2.033	80%	825 (31.19)	1820 (68.81)	2645 (100)	2.746	2.928	2.871
90%	1013 (34.05)	1962 (65.95)	2975 (100)	2.105	2.285	2.224	90%	956 (32.13)	2019 (67.87)	2975 (100)	2.548	2.769	2.698

N_m: number of misclassification types; N_c: number of correct classification types; N_t: number of total classification types; Mean_m: mean of misclassification type; Mean_c: mean of correct classification type; Mean_t: mean of total classification type.

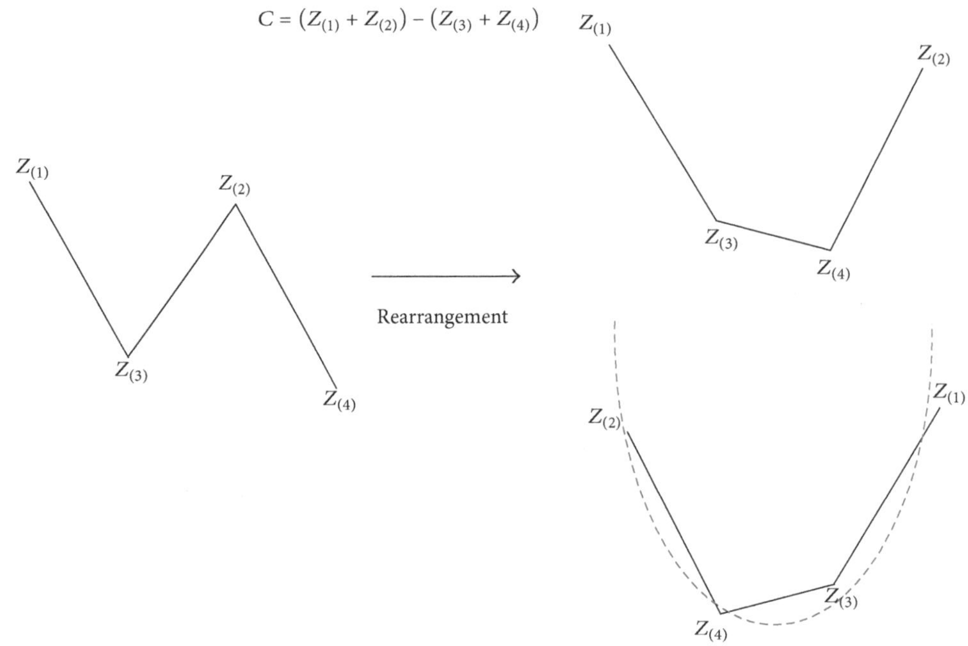

FIGURE 12: Derived C values based on the pattern analysis of the profile graphs. Under the hypothesis that the larger the C value was, the closer the profile graph was to a bathtub (or U) shape, the higher the probability of the respective observations corresponding to misclassification was.

TABLE 8: Misclassification rate distribution of the filtered data according to four measures.

Filtered%	N	D	R	S	C
10%	331	40.79	40.79	36.25	42.60
20%	661	39.03	39.49	35.40	41.15
30%	992	38.51	40.32	33.57	39.92
40%	1322	39.71	38.35	32.90	39.03
50%	1653	39.14	37.69	33.51	37.45
60%	1984	38.26	36.59	33.57	36.64
70%	2314	37.38	36.43	33.92	35.61
80%	2645	36.98	35.43	33.72	34.78
90%	2975	35.46	34.69	33.51	34.05

the normal equations should be equal to

$$\begin{aligned} S_1 &= 4b_0 + 10b_1 + 30b_2, \\ S_2 &= 10b_0 + 30b_1 + 100b_2, \\ S_3 &= 30b_0 + 100b_1 + 354b_2 \end{aligned} \tag{9}$$

and, ultimately, we obtain

$$\begin{aligned} \therefore b_2 &= \frac{5}{4}\left(S_1 - S_2 + \frac{S_3}{5}\right) \\ &= \frac{1}{4}\left\{(Z_{(1)} + Z_{(2)}) - (Z_{(3)} + Z_{(4)})\right\}. \end{aligned} \tag{10}$$

Certainly, the values of b_0 and b_1 may be obtained but omitted herein because they are meaningless. In (10), $Z_{(1)}$ and $Z_{(2)}$ are symmetric, and so are $Z_{(3)}$ and $Z_{(4)}$. Namely, when the curvature creates the largest profile with the 4 points, the curvature will not have any changes even if the largest and the second largest scores were switched. This also holds true for the smallest and the second smallest scores.

In the meantime, the b_2 value equals 1/4 of the C score among the 4 criteria obtained. Namely, the previously used C score was equal to $Z_{(3)}$ and $Z_{(4)}$ was simply subtracted from the total of $Z_{(1)}$ and $Z_{(2)}$, which was the same as the secondary curvature created by the 4 scores.

4. Discussion

In TKM, a PI diagnostic system—one of the core technologies in the diagnosis and treatment of oriental medicine—is used to determine the cause and nature of a disease, treatment methods, and treatment drugs for the patients [5–7]. However, the PI diagnosis holds limited objectivity and reproducibility due to the lack of standardized measurement indices. Objectification problems have always arisen with respect to personal deviations among TKM physicians. As the demand for the reestablishment and development of TKM has increased, studies on the establishment of a scientific basis for and the standardization of PI have been actively conducted [7, 12].

In this study, the clinical data of PI diagnosis for stroke were used to analyze and quantify the profile patterns of the misclassification types by applying the proposed scores to the comparative analysis. This was intended to boost the correct classification of objects by detecting those objects with a high probability of actual misclassification and deferring discrimination. Misclassification types were discerned by a discriminant analysis on the actual clinical data of PI diagnosis for stroke and quantified by a profile pattern analysis. The

TABLE 9: Discriminant rate distribution of the selected data according to four measures.

		Discriminant rate			
	N	D	R	S	C
100%	3306	66.82	66.82	66.82	66.82
90%	2975	**68.24 (+1.42)**	67.63 (+0.81)	66.92 (+0.10)	67.53 (+0.71)
80%	2645	68.62 (+0.38)	68.47 (+0.84)	67.15 (+0.23)	**69.04 (+1.51)**
70%	2314	69.53 (+0.91)	**69.97 (+1.50)**	66.98 (−0.17)	69.49 (+0.45)
60%	1984	**71.98 (+2.45)**	70.82 (+0.85)	66.94 (−0.04)	71.22 (+1.73)
50%	1653	**73.32 (+1.34)**	73.08 (+2.26)	69.03 (+2.09)	71.81 (+0.59)
40%	1322	**75.34 (+2.02)**	74.28 (+1.20)	68.68 (−0.35)	73.75 (+1.94)
30%	992	**77.32 (+1.98)**	76.81 (+2.53)	70.26 (+1.58)	75.81 (+2.06)
20%	661	**83.36 (+6.04)**	80.94 (+4.13)	73.83 (+3.57)	77.61 (+1.80)
10%	331	**89.12 (+5.76)**	87.01 (+6.07)	75.83 (+2.00)	82.78 (+5.17)

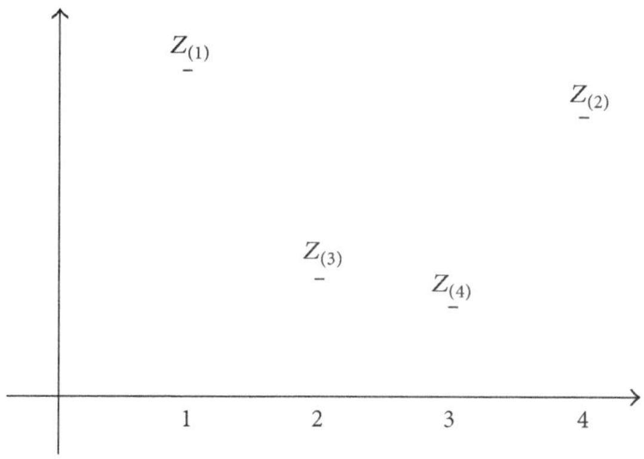

FIGURE 13: Curvature created by Z scores ($Z_{(1)}$, $Z_{(2)}$, $Z_{(3)}$, and $Z_{(4)}$). $Z_{(1)}$, $Z_{(2)}$, $Z_{(3)}$, and $Z_{(4)}$, as dependent variables observed in the x values having equal intervals. $Z_{(1)}$ is a dependent variable when $x = 1$, $Z_{(2)}$ when $x = 4$, $Z_{(3)}$ when $x = 2$, and $Z_{(4)}$ when $x = 3$.

proposed criteria of each standard were applied to the data already discriminated by the previous discriminant analysis in order to compare how well the misclassification had been estimated and how much the discrimination rate had improved when the estimated misclassification observations were removed in advanced. Particularly, the C score delivered the same results as those from the discrimination of misclassification observations through a secondary curvature. Going forward, the following studies must be performed. First of all, 4 criteria to estimate misclassification were proposed in this study and applied to the actual clinical data, producing the possibility of better estimation of partial misclassification. Nonetheless, it was difficult to notably enhance discrimination rates and additional research appears to be necessary. In addition, 4 pattern groups with a different sample size were used in this study. Hence, the effects of different sample sizes need to be investigated.

Conflict of Interests

The authors declare that there is no conflict of interests regarding the publication of this paper.

Acknowledgment

This research was supported by a grant from the Korea Institute of Oriental Medicine (K13130, K16111).

References

[1] Social Statistics Office, *2012 Statistics on the Aged*, Korean Statistical Information Service, Seoul, Republic of Korea, 2012.

[2] H. S. Jeong, *Progress of Aging Population and Policy Responses in Japan*, Research Department, The Bank of Korea, Seoul, South Korea, 2007 (Korean), http://public.bokeducation.or.kr/ecostudy/publishList.do?&bbsId=22&mode=view&contentId=2655&cPage=19.

[3] Social Statistics Office, *Statistics on the Cause of Death*, Korean Statistical Information Service, Seoul, Republic of Korea, 2010.

[4] Division of Statistical Analysis in the Institute of Health Insurance Policy, *The Status of Health Insurance Benefits of the Inpatients Frequent Diseases on Classified Subdivision of Diseases in Traditional Korean Medicine 2009*, The National Health Insurance Corporation, Seoul, Republic of Korea, 2010.

[5] WHO Western Pacific Region, *WHO International Standard Terminologies on Traditional Medicine in the Western Pacific Region*, World Health Organization (WHO), Geneva, Switzerland, 2007.

[6] S. S. Shin, S. M. Choi, M. K. Shin, and K. S. Yang, *A Study of Standardization of Diagnoses and Diagnostic Requirements in Traditional Korean Medicine III*, Korea Institute of Oriental Medicine, Seoul, Republic of Korea, 1997.

[7] T.-Y. Park, J. A. Lee, M. H. Cha et al., "The fundamental study for the Standardization and Objectification of Pattern Identification in traditional Korean medicine for stroke (SOPI-Stroke): an overview of phase I," *European Journal of Integrative Medicine*, vol. 4, no. 2, pp. e125–e131, 2012.

[8] M. M. Ko, J. A. Lee, K. J. Yun, S. S. You, and M. S. Lee, "Perception of pattern identification in traditional medicine: a survey of Korean medical practitioners," *Journal of Traditional Chinese Medicine*, vol. 34, no. 3, pp. 369–372, 2014.

[9] J. K. Kim, I. C. Seol, I. Lee, K. Oh, B. C. Yu, and S. M. Choi, "Report on the Korean standard differentiation of the symptoms and signs for the stoke-1," *Korean Journal of Oriental Physiology & Pathology*, vol. 20, pp. 229–234, 2006.

[10] H. Y. Go, Y. K. Kim, B. K. Kang et al., "Report on the Korean standard differentiation of the symptoms and signs for the

stoke-2," *Korean Journal of Oriental Physiology & Pathology*, vol. 20, pp. 1789–1791, 2006.

[11] J. A. Lee, J. S. Lee, M. M. Ko et al., "Report on the Korean standard pattern identifications for stroke-III," *The Journal of Korean Oriental Internal Medicine*, vol. 32, pp. 232–242, 2011.

[12] J. A. Lee, M. H. Cha, B.-K. Kang et al., "Fundamental study for the standardization and objectification of pattern identification in traditional Korean medicine for stroke (SOPI-Stroke): an overview of the second and third stages," *European Journal of Integrative Medicine*, vol. 7, no. 4, pp. 378–383, 2015.

[13] B.-K. Kang, T.-W. Moon, J. A. Lee, T.-Y. Park, M. M. Ko, and M. S. Lee, "The fundamental study for the standardisation and objectification of pattern identification in traditional Korean medicine for stroke (SOPI-Stroke): development and interobserver agreement of the Korean standard pattern identification for stroke (K-SPI-Stroke) tool," *European Journal of Integrative Medicine*, vol. 4, no. 2, pp. e133–e139, 2012.

[14] I. C. Kim, M. H. Cha, D. M. Kim et al., "A functional promoter polymorphism −607G>C of WNT10B is associated with abdominal fat in Korean female subjects," *Journal of Nutritional Biochemistry*, vol. 22, no. 3, pp. 252–258, 2011.

[15] M. M. Ko, T.-Y. Park, J. H. Lim, M. H. Cha, and M. S. Lee, "WNT10B polymorphism in Korean stroke patients with Yin deficiency pattern," *Evidence-Based Complementary and Alternative Medicine*, vol. 2012, Article ID 798131, 6 pages, 2012.

[16] J. H. Lim, M. M. Ko, J. S. Lee et al., "Genetic association of SNPs located at PON1 gene with dampness and phlegm pattern identification among Korea stroke patients," *The Journal of Korean Oriental Internal Medicine*, vol. 31, pp. 752–762, 2010.

[17] B. K. Kang, K. W. Kang, S. W. Park et al., "The discrimination model for the pattern identification diagnosis of the stroke," *Korean Journal of Oriental Internal Medicine*, vol. 13, no. 2, pp. 59–63, 2007.

[18] B. K. Kang, J. S. Lee, S. Y. Kim et al., "The discrimination model IV for syndrome differentiation diagnosis in stroke patients," *Journal of the Korean Data Analysis Society*, vol. 11, no. 6, pp. 2995–3007, 2009.

[19] B. K. Kang, M. M. Ko, J. A. Lee, T. Y. Park, and Y. G. Park, "Discriminant modeling for pattern identification using the Korean standard PI for stroke-III," *Korean Journal of Oriental Physiology & Pathology*, vol. 25, no. 6, pp. 1–6, 2011.

[20] J. A. Lee, T.-Y. Park, J. S. Lee et al., "Developing indicators of pattern identification in patients with stroke using traditional Korean medicine," *BMC Research Notes*, vol. 5, article 136, 2012.

[21] J. Neter, W. Wasserman, and M. H. Kutner, *Applied Linear Statistical Models*, CRC Press, Philadelphia, Pa, USA, 3rd edition, 1990.

4

Effect of Yi Gong San Decoction on Iron Homeostasis in a Mouse Model of Acute Inflammation

Qin Zheng,[1] Yu Guan,[2] Lemin Xia,[1] Zhicheng Wang,[3] Yiling Jiang,[1] Xiaofeng Zhang,[2] Jianying Wang,[4] Guohua Wang,[2] Yiqiong Pu,[4] Jing Xia,[2] and Meihong Luo[1]

[1] *Department of Hematology, Shanghai Baoshan Hospital of Integrated Traditional Chinese and Western Medicine (Baoshan Branch of Shuguang Hospital Affiliated to Shanghai University of Traditional Chinese Medicine), Shanghai 201999, China*
[2] *Department of Central Laboratory Medicine, Shanghai Municipal Hospital of Traditional Chinese Medicine, Shanghai University of Traditional Chinese Medicine, Shanghai 200071, China*
[3] *Department of Laboratory Medicine, Huashan Hospital, Shanghai Medical College, Fudan University, Shanghai 200040, China*
[4] *College of Pharmacy, Shanghai University of Traditional Chinese Medicine, Shanghai 201203, China*

Correspondence should be addressed to Meihong Luo; lmh021009@163.com

Academic Editor: Luciana Dini

We investigated the effect of Yi Gong San (YGS) decoction on iron homeostasis and the possible underlying mechanisms in a mouse model of acute inflammation in this study. Our findings suggest that YGS regulates iron homeostasis by downregulating the level of HAMP mRNA, which may depend on regulation of the IL-6/STAT3 or BMP/HJV/SMAD pathway during acute inflammation.

1. Introduction

Iron plays a pivotal role in cell survival and proliferation. It is thus an important source of nutrition in the competition between microbial pathogens and their hosts [1]. In humans, host defense responses to infectious agents modulate local and systemic iron availability, which disrupts infections such as malaria and tuberculosis [2]. Increased production of inflammatory cytokines can directly induce changes in iron homeostasis, which are characterized by reduction of both iron absorption and macrophage iron release. Hepatic bactericidal protein (hepcidin) provides a first line of defense at mucosal barriers, although it is less potent than many other antimicrobial peptides. Hepcidin impairs iron absorption and macrophage iron release and acts as a major hormonal regulator of iron homeostasis [1, 3]. The bone morphogenic protein (BMP)/hemojuvelin (HJV)/SMAD pathway is the major regulator of hepcidin expression that responds to iron status. Additionally, inflammation stimulates hepcidin via the interleukin- (IL-) 6/STAT3 pathway with support by activation of the BMP/HJV/SMAD pathway [4]. The expression of hepcidin in isolated primary hepatocytes increases in response to infection/inflammation stimulated by IL-6, IL-1, and LPS [5]. LPS is a component of the outer membrane of Gram-negative bacteria and elicits a potent inflammatory response when administered intravenously or intraperitoneally [6]. LPS induces hepcidin and causes hypoferraemia within hours of administration in both humans [7] and mice [3, 8]. Therefore, we investigated iron homeostasis in a mouse model of LPS-induced acute inflammation.

YGS originated from *Pediatric Medicine Card Straight Strategics*, a classic book of traditional Chinese medicine (TCM) that was written approximately 900 years ago. It has the functions of tonifying splenic Qi and gasification stagnation. YGS is based on Si Jun Zi decoction (SJZD) combined with Citri Unshius Pericarpium. SJZD can decrease serum levels of IL-6, CRP, and TNF. Early application of SJZD during enteral nutritional therapy can enhance the immune function of patients with gastrointestinal tumours [9]. In addition, YGS has been traditionally used in Korea to treat a variety of inflammatory diseases; pretreatment with YGS inhibited TNF-α and IL-6 production by LPS-stimulated mouse peritoneal macrophages [10]. Thus, YGS may maintain iron homeostasis by regulating the production of inflammatory cytokines. This study aimed to determine the effect of YGS on iron homeostasis and elucidate the underlying mechanisms to facilitate its clinical application.

2. Materials and Methods

2.1. Animals. Six-week-old C57BL/6 female mice were purchased from SLRC Laboratory Animals (Shanghai, China). The mice were housed in an environmentally controlled animal care facility and were used for experiments after 4 days of acclimation. Experiments were carried out according to the China Council on Animal Care guidelines after approval by the Institutional Animal Care Committee of Shanghai University of Traditional Chinese Medicine, Shanghai, China.

2.2. Preparation of YGS. YGS is composed of five different herbs: Ginseng Radix et Rhizoma (Ren-Shen), Glycyrrhizae Radix et Rhizoma (Gan-Cao), Citri Reticulatae Pericarpium (Chen-Pi), Atractylodis Macrocephalae Rhizoma (Bai-Zhu), and Poria (Fu-Ling). All of the five herbs were provided by our hospital pharmacy. After being soaked together for 1 h, the five herbs in equal dose were water decocted for 20 min, concentrated by distillation, dried through 60°C vacuum decompression, and homogenised into 100-mesh powders. 1 g dry powder was equal to 4.1 g herb (performed at the College of Pharmacy, Shanghai University of Traditional Chinese Medicine, Shanghai, China). The dosage given to mice was 10.57 g/kg which was equally effective to clinical routine dosage (each herb 15 g, total 75 g), calculated according to the surface area formula. The powder was dissolved in double-distilled water to a final concentration of 1.057 g/mL.

2.3. Multicomponent Analysis of YGS Powder

2.3.1. Sample Preparation. 0.3 g of accurately weighed fine powder was placed in a 50 mL centrifuge tube and ultrasonically extracted with 25 mL of 50% methanol (v/v) for 20 min. After centrifugation at 14000 rpm for 10 min, the supernatant was obtained and used as the test solution.

2.3.2. UPLC/QTOF MS Conditions. Chromatographic separation was performed on Waters ACQUITY I-Class UPLC (Waters, Milford, MA, USA) equipped with a binary solvent manager, a sample manager, and a column manager. A Waters HSS T3 column (2.1 × 100 mm, 1.7 μm) together with a Waters on-line filtrate 35°C was used. The mobile phase consisted of acetonitrile (B) and water containing 0.1% formic acid (v/v) (A) following a gradient elution program: 0–2 min: 15%–25% (B); 2–18 min: 25%–47% (B); 18–18.5 min: 47%–75% (B); 18.5–20 min: 75%–90% (B); 20–22 min: 90% (B); 22–22.1 min: 90%–15% (B); 22.1–26 min : 15% (B). The flow rate was set at 0.4 mL/min. 2 μL of the test solution was injected for UPLC analysis.

High-accuracy mass spectrometric data were recorded on a Waters Xevo G2-S QTOF mass spectrometer (Waters, Manchester, UK). Tune parameters were set for MS^E experiments: capillary voltage, 2.5 kV (negative mode) and 2.0 KV (positive mode); sampling cone, 60 V; source offset voltage, 60 V; source temperature, 120°C; desolvation temperature, 450°C (negative mode) and 350°C (positive mode); cone gas flow, 30 L/h (negative mode) and 20 L/h (positive mode); desolvation gas, 900 L/h (negative mode) and 800 L/h (positive mode). The mass analyzer scanned over a mass range of 100–1500 Da within 0.1 s under a low collision energy at 6 V. High collision energy ramp of 20–90 V for negative mode and 40–90 V for positive mode was employed. Data calibration was performed using an external reference (LockSpray™) constant infused at 1 ng/μL of leucine enkephalin (LE; Sigma-Aldrich, St. Louis, MO, USA) at a flow rate of 5 μL/min, and with reference to the ion *m/z* 554.2615. Data acquisition was controlled by MassLynx V4.1 software (Waters Corporation, Milford, USA). Automatic metabolites characterization was performed using UNIFI 1.8 (Waters, Milford, USA) by the search of the TCM library.

2.4. Detection of Total Iron Concentration in YGS Powder. Total iron concentration in YGS Powder was determined by using an Agilent Technologies 7700 Series ICP-MS system equipped with ASX-500 Series ICP-MS Autosampler. The procedure was performed as previously described [11].

2.5. Animal Model. To induce acute inflammation, mice were injected with LPS (*Escherichia coli* serotype O127:B8, 1.5 mg/kg intraperitoneally; Sigma-Aldrich, Inc., USA) and sacrificed at 3, 6, 9, and 12 h thereafter. A CTL group was also established. All animals were given an equivalent volume of double-distilled water via intragastric administration for 7 successive days before being injected with LPS. To evaluate the effect of YGS on iron homeostasis *in vivo* and the underlying mechanisms, YGS (10.57 g/kg) was given to mice via intragastric administration for 7 successive days. Mice were injected with LPS on the following day and sacrificed at 3, 6, 9, and 12 h. A YGS control group was also established.

2.6. Specimen Collection. Mice were immediately killed with isoflurane, and blood was collected into serum separator tubes through cardiac puncture. The abdomen was then opened and liver samples were taken for tissue iron determination and ribonucleic acid (RNA) and protein isolation. Samples were stored at −80°C for later analysis.

2.7. Determination of Liver Iron. Liver tissue was processed as follows. About 100 to 200 mg of liver tissue was accurately weighed in a 1.5 mL centrifuge tube. Following the addition of 1 mL nitric acid solution, each centrifuge tube was vortex mixed after blending into the microwave digestion instrument resolution organisation and made up to 1.5 mL using nitric acid solution. Samples were then centrifuged at room temperature at 12,000 rpm for 3 min and then transferred to 96-well plates. After incubation for 10 min at room temperature, an ultraviolet spectrophotometer was used to determine the OD at 535 nm of the samples. Iron content was calculated using the following formula: iron concentration (μg/g wet weight) = $[(A_t - A_b) * (n + 0.75W) * \text{Fes}\,(1 + V_e)]/[(A_s - A_b) * W * V_e \times 1.1]$ (A_T = sample absorbance; A_b = absorbance blank hole; A_s = standard absorbance; Fes = standard iron content

TABLE 1: PCR primers, product sizes, and annealing temperatures.

Gene	PCR primer sequence	Temperature (°C)
β-actin	5′-AGCTGAGAGGAAATCGTGCG-3′ 5′-GTGCCACCAGACAGCACTGTG-3′	59.8
HAMP	5′-AGCACCACCTATCTCCATCAAC-3′ 5′-TGTCTCTCTTCCTTCTCTTCTGC-3′	57.0
IL-6	5′-GGAGAGGAGACTTCACAGAGGA-3′ 5′-ATTTCCACGATTTCCCAGAGA-3′	57.0
BMP6	5′-CAGGAGCATCAGCACAGAGA-3′ 5′-GTCACCACCCACAGATTGC-3′	59.8
HJV	5′-TGCTAACCTTGGGAGTCACG-3′ 5′-TCCTCTGCTACCCTGATGGA-3′	59.8

(μg); W = wet weight; n = join tissue samples of acid volume (mL); V_e = acid extraction volume (mL)).

2.8. Determination of Serum Iron Levels. About 200 μL of whole blood from the posterior orbital venous plexus was placed in serum separation tubes and centrifuged at 3000 rpm for 25 min at 4°C to separate the serum; approximately 40 μL of serum was produced from each sample. In accordance with the manufacturer's instructions, 50 μL of liquid iron buffer was added to the wells of a 96-well plate, as were 10 μL aliquots of the standard and the test samples. A trace ultraviolet spectrophotometer A1 value wavelength (560 nm) was used. We added 1 μL of iron chromogenic agent in each hole, 37°C, 10 min, using trace ultraviolet spectrophotometer A2 value wavelength (560 nm). Serum iron (μg/dL) was calculated using the following formula: 500 × (A2a − A1a)/(A2b − A1b) (A2a, A2 specimens; A1a, A1 specimens; A2b, A2 standard samples; A1b, A1 standard samples). Serum and liver iron levels were measured by colourimetric assay (MI 48188, Pointe Scientific Inc., USA) using a NanoDrop2000 Spectrophotometer (Thermo Scientific Inc., USA).

2.9. IL-6 Assay. Serum IL-6 levels were determined using an ELISA kit according to the manufacturer's instructions (mouse IL-6 ELISA kit, M6000B; R&D Systems, Inc., USA). A standard dilution series of 3.12, 6.25, 12.5, 25, 50, and 100 pg/L was created. To each well of a 96-well plate was added 100 μL of standard diluent RDIW together with 100 μL of standard or sample. Following incubation at room temperature for 2 h, liquid was aspirated and wells were washed four times. Next, 200 μL of IL-6 polymer was added, followed by incubation at room temperature for 2 h. Liquid was aspirated and wells were washed four times. Next, 200 μL of substrate solution was added to each well, followed by incubation in the dark at a room temperature for 20 min. Next, 50 μL of liquid was added to each well, and the plates were incubated at room temperature for 30 min. IL-6 levels were then determined using an ultraviolet spectrophotometer to read OD values (450 nm wavelength, calibration wavelengths of 540 and 570 nm). The standard curve was used to calculate IL-6 levels.

2.10. Determination of mRNA Levels. Total RNA was isolated using RNAiso Plus (D9108A, TaKaRa Bio Inc., Japan) and reverse-transcribed by PrimeScript reverse transcriptase using a real-time polymerase chain reaction (RT-PCR) system (TaKaRa Bio Inc., Japan). β-actin, HAMP, IL-6, BMP6, and HJV mRNA levels were measured using CFX96 RT-PCR Detection System (Bio-Rad, Inc., USA) with SYBR Premix Ex Taq Kit (DRR420A, Bio-Rad, Inc., USA). Expression levels were normalised to that of the housekeeping gene β-actin. The primers used are shown in Table 1.

2.11. Sodium Dodecyl Sulfate- (SDS-) Polyacrylamide Gel Electrophoresis and Western Blot Analysis. Livers were removed, rinsed in ice-cold phosphate-buffered saline, and used to prepare total protein extracts with RIPA Lysis Buffer (Beyotime Institute of Biotechnology, China) plus 1 mM phenylmethanesulfonyl fluoride and 0.1 to 2.0 mM sodium orthovanadate (Beyotime Institute of Biotechnology, China). Total protein extracts were separated in a 10% SDS-polyacrylamide gel and blotted onto nitrocellulose membranes (Bio-Rad, Inc., USA). The membranes were immunoblotted with antibodies to the following: phospho-STAT3, STAT3, β-actin, phospho-SMAD1/5/8, SMAD5 (Cell Signaling Technology, Inc., USA), and HJV (R&D Systems, Inc., USA). Anti-rabbit IgG, anti-mouse IgG, and anti-goat IgG (Cell Signaling Technology, Inc., USA) were used as secondary antibodies. Antigen-antibody complexes were visualised using an Immune-Star™ Western C™ Kit (Bio-Rad, Inc., USA) and analyzed using Image Lab™ software (Bio-Rad, Inc., USA).

2.12. Statistical Analysis. All statistical analyses were performed using SPSS 22.0 software (IBM Inc., USA). Multiple comparisons were performed by one-way analysis of variance (ANOVA) followed by the Bonferroni correction. If data could not be compared using an equal variance t-test, a Kruskal-Wallis test and one-way ANOVA were used, followed by Student-Newman-Keuls or the Dunn *post hoc* test. Correlation coefficients were determined using Spearman's rank-order correlation method.

3. Results

3.1. Multicomponent of YGS Powder. By optimizing the gradient elution program, satisfactory separation of major peaks was achieved in both negative and position ion modes, as

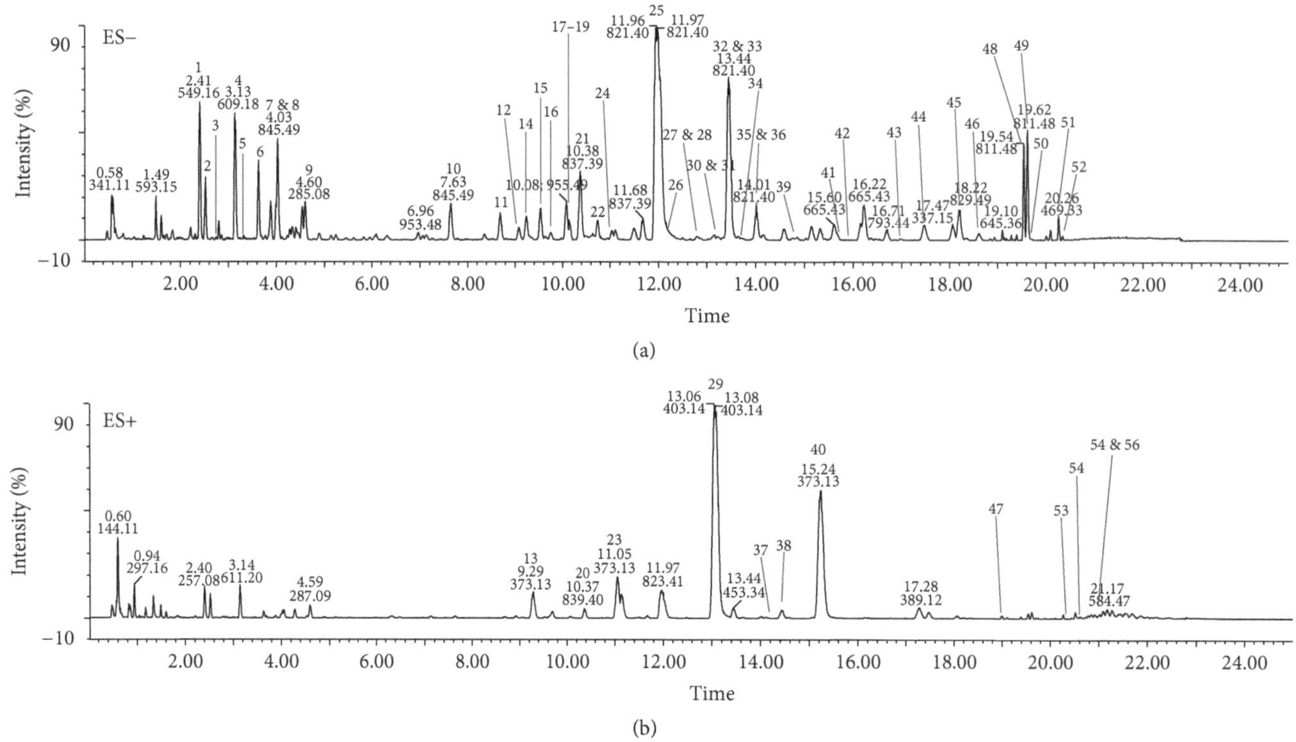

FIGURE 1: Base peak chromatograms of YGSP in negative mode (a) and positive mode (b).

shown in Figure 1. The obtained MS^E data were further imported into UNIFI software for automatic components characterization. By comparison with the TCM library, 56 peaks were identified or tentatively characterized by element composition and fragment matching analyses (Table 2). Among them, 24 saponins should be from Glycyrrhizae Radix et Rhizoma, 19 saponins from Ginseng Radix et Rhizoma, 5 compounds from Citri Reticulatae Pericarpium, 5 from Poria, and 3 from Atractylodis Macrocephalae Rhizoma.

In contrast, compounds **7**, **8**, **15**, **25**, **32**, and **35**, from Glycyrrhizae Radix et Rhizoma or Ginseng Radix et Rhizoma, gave strong ion response in the negative ion mode, whilst the protonated precursors of compounds **23**, **29**, and **40**, from Citri Reticulatae Pericarpium, were strong in positive ion mode. These compounds with strong responses as well as abundant secondary product ions lead to credible identification results. However, the compounds characteristic of Poria and Atractylodis Macrocephalae Rhizoma generated rather weak signals of precursor ions, without MS/MS fragments.

3.2. The Iron Element Level in YGS Decoction Could Not Directly Affect the Results. The iron concentration in YGS Powder was 2.56 mg per 100 g lyophilized powder weight. The dosage of YGS decoction given to the mice was 10.57 g/kg. The weight of the mice was from 18 g to 20 g. So, the iron taken by the mice from YGS decoction was not over 0.0015 mg. Mice were fed a standard iron rodent laboratory diet (232 mg iron/kg). Thus, precious little iron in YGS decoction could not directly affect the results.

3.3. YGS Increased Serum Iron by Decreasing Liver Iron Retention. In light of the influence of YGS on imbalanced iron homeostasis mediated by LPS, serum and liver iron concentrations were determined following preventive intervention with YGS. YGS alone had no significant effect on serum or liver iron levels. However, when compared with the LPS-treated control, YGS pretreatment significantly reduced the ability of LPS to decrease the serum iron level (Figure 2(a)) and iron retention in the liver (Figure 2(b)) at both 3 and 6 h after LPS injection ($P < 0.05$). Therefore, 3 and 6 h were used in subsequent analyses.

3.4. YGS Blockade of LPS-Mediated Hepcidin Induction via the IL-6/STAT3 Signaling Pathway. LPS injection leads to the production of the inflammatory cytokine IL-6 [12], which has been identified as a major inducer of hepcidin through the IL-6/STAT pathway [3]. Inhibiting LPS-induced secretion of IL-6 decreases hepcidin levels. Hence, in this study, a mouse model was used to evaluate the effect of YGS on LPS-induced IL-6 release. Compared with the LPS-treated control, YGS pretreatment significantly reduced the ability of LPS to increase serum IL-6 levels (Figure 3(a)) at 3 h, as well as IL-6 mRNA expression (Figure 3(b)) at both 3 and 6 h ($P < 0.05$). Hence, YGS blocked IL-6 increase after LPS injection *in vivo*. LPS-mediated HAMP mRNA expression (Figure 3(c)) was

TABLE 2: Information of 56 compounds identified from YGNP by UPLC/QTOF MS.

Number	Retention time (min)	Identification	TCM
1	2.42	Licurazide or its isomer	GC
2	2.52	Isoliquiritin or its isomer	GC
3	2.75	Ferulic acid	GC
4	3.14	Hesperidin or neohesperidin	CP
5	3.32	20-*O*-Glucopyranosyl ginsenoside Rf	RS
6	3.63	Licurazide or its isomer	GC
7	4.01	Ginsenoside Re	RS
8	4.03	Ginsenoside Rg1	RS
9	4.60	Licochalcone B	GC
10	7.64	Ginsenoside Rf	RS
11	8.74	Uralsaponin U/N or licorice saponin G2	GC
12	9.08	Ginsenoside 20(*S*)-Rg2	RS
13	9.28	Sinensetin or its isomer	CP
14	9.31	Ginsenoside Ra1 or Ra2	RS
15	9.53	Ginsenoside Rb1	RS
16	9.81	Ginsenoside F1	RS
17	10.13	Ginsenoside Ro	RS
18	10.14	Ginsenoside Ra2	RS
19	10.15	Ginsenoside Rb2, Rb3, or Rc	RS
20	10.37	Glabrolide or isoglabrolide	GC
21	10.42	Uralsaponin U/N or licorice saponin G2	GC
22	10.74	Ginsenoside Rb2, Rb3, or Rc	RS
23	11.05	Sinensetin or its isomer	CP
24	11.08	Uralsaponin U/N or licorice saponin G2	GC
25	11.95	Glycyrrhizic acid or its isomer	GC
26	12.08	Ginsenoside Rd	RS
27	12.80	Glycyrrhizic acid or its isomer	GC
28	12.82	Licorice saponin K2 or its isomer	GC
29	13.07	Nobiletin	CP
30	13.17	Ginsenoside Ro	RS
31	13.22	Licoflavone A or its isomer	GC
32	13.44	Glycyrrhizic acid or its isomer	GC
33	13.48	Licorice saponin K2 or its isomer	GC
34	13.64	Licobenzofuran	GC
35	14.01	Glycyrrhizic acid or its isomer	GC
36	14.04	Licorice saponin K2 or its isomer	GC
37	14.11	Atractylenolide I or its isomer	BZ
38	14.61	Uralsaponin C/P or licorice saponin J2	GC
39	14.75	Ginsenoside Rg3 or its isomer	RS
40	15.23	Sinensetin or its isomer	CP
41	15.68	Uralsaponin V/W or licorice saponin C2	GC
42	15.89	Poricoic B or its isomer	FL
43	16.99	Licoflavone A or its isomer	GC
44	17.47	Licoflavone A or its isomer	GC
45	18.20	Ginsenoside 20(S)-Rg3	RS
46	18.61	Ginsenoside 20(R)-Rg3	RS
47	18.99	3β-Hydroxyatractylon or atractylenolide II	BZ
48	19.54	Ginsenoside Rg4 or Rg6	RS
49	19.62	Ginsenoside Rg4 or Rg6	RS
50	19.71	Stractylenolide I or its isomer	BZ

Table 2: Continued.

Number	Retention time (min)	Identification	TCM
51	20.27	Glycyrrhetinic acid or its isomer	GC
52	20.36	Glycyrrhetinic acid or its isomer	GC
53	20.44	Poricoic B or its isomer	FL
54	20.63	Dehydropachymic acid	FL
55	21.03	Pachymic acid	FL
56	21.09	Trametenolic acid or its isomer	FL

Note: GC (Gan-Cao): Glycyrrhizae Radix et Rhizoma; RS (Ren-Shen): Ginseng Radix et Rhizoma; CP (Chen-Pi): Citri Reticulatae Pericarpium; FL (Fu-Ling): Poria; BZ (Bai-Zhi): Atractylodis Macrocephalae Rhizoma.

also significantly decreased by YGS at both 3 and 6 h ($P < 0.05$), although YGS alone did not significantly reduce HAMP mRNA levels. YGS inhibited STAT3 phosphorylation only at 3 h ($P < 0.05$) (Figures 3(d) and 3(e)).

3.5. BMP/HJV/SMAD Signaling Pathway May Contribute to Maintenance of Iron Homeostasis by YGS. There is a crosslink between the iron and cytokine-dependent pathways of hepcidin upregulation. The integrity of the BMP/HJV/SMAD pathway is required to activate hepcidin [13]. Hence, we determined whether YGS downregulates hepcidin through BMP/HJV/SMAD pathway. Compared with the CTL group, LPS resulted in a significant increase in the liver HJV mRNA level (Figure 4(b)) and P-SMAD1/5/8 (Figures 4(c) and 4(d)) and HJV (Figures 4(c) and 4(e)) protein levels at both 3 and 6 h, and BMP6 mRNA expression (Figure 4(a)) only at 6 h ($P < 0.05$). Moreover, YGS pretreatment significantly inhibited the increase in the BMP mRNA level (Figure 4(a)) and P-SMAD1/5/8 (Figures 4(c) and 4(d)) and HJV (Figures 4(c) and 4(e)) protein levels only at 6 h ($P < 0.05$).

4. Discussion

Metabolic iron homeostasis is regulated by several factors but is most closely related to hepcidin, the central mediator of iron homeostasis. As it binds to its target iron-export protein, ferroportin (Fpn), hepcidin stimulates internalisation and degradation of Fpn and reduces the quantity of Fpn on the small intestinal mucosa and in macrophages [14]. This process serves to control dietary iron absorption, iron release from storage sites, and iron bioavailability in the body, therefore regulating the balance among iron absorption, iron utilisation, and iron storage [15].

In inflammatory conditions, hepcidin is augmented by increased levels of the inflammatory factor IL-6. Upon binding to its membrane-bound receptor glycoprotein (gp)80 on hepatocytes, IL-6 further interacts with the gp130 membrane glycoprotein to induce STAT3 (signal transducer and activator of transcription) phosphorylation [12]. Phosphorylated STAT3 enters the nucleus and upregulates transcription of the gene encoding hepcidin. This increases the circulating hepcidin level, followed by enhanced Fpn internalisation and degradation [1]. As a result, dietary iron absorption and iron release from storage sites are restricted.

The spleen is a larger concept in TCM than in Western medicine. According to TCM theory, the spleen has the central function of transporting and transforming nutrient substances, and this function plays a major role in erythropoiesis. Hence, it is plausible that iron absorption, transport, and transformation are controlled by the spleen. Furthermore, we hypothesised that an imbalance of iron homeostasis might be improved by promoting movement of splenic Qi [16]. YGS, a representative TCM prescription for promoting the movement of splenic Qi, was investigated because it has been reported to regulate the expression of inflammatory factors.

We first investigated the effect of YGS on LPS-induced imbalanced iron homeostasis in mice. Injection of 1.5 mg/kg of LPS into mice resulted in serum iron deficiency and liver iron retention within 3, 6, 9, or 12 h. Both the minimum serum iron level and maximum liver iron level occurred at 6 h. Serum and liver iron levels differed significantly between groups with and without YGS pretreatment before LPS injection, particularly at 3 and 6 h. Thus, YGS pretreatment blocked the ability of LPS to decrease serum iron levels and increase liver iron levels. This finding suggests that YGS can adjust the abnormal iron distribution under inflammatory conditions.

We next investigated the mechanisms underlying the maintenance of iron homeostasis by YGS. LPS injection leads to the production of the inflammatory cytokine IL-6, which is a major hepcidin inducer [12]. Inhibition of LPS-induced secretion of IL-6 decreases hepcidin levels. IL-6 directly regulates hepcidin through induction and subsequent promoter binding of STAT3, which is necessary for IL-6-mediated hepcidin induction [17]. Hence, we first investigated the STAT3 pathway. We observed the downregulation of IL-6 mRNA in mice pretreated with YGS prior to LPS administration at both 3 and 6 h. However, serum IL-6 was downregulated only at 3 h. The kinetics of mRNA and protein levels differed, likely because serum IL-6 protein has a longer half-life than IL-6 mRNA [18]. In addition, the use of incremental doses or prolonged delivery of YGS may result in more persistent downregulation of serum IL-6 levels; this warrants further research.

As expected, HAMP mRNA levels at 3 h were downregulated due to the decreased IL-6 mRNA and protein levels. p-STAT3 levels also decreased at 3 h, which indicates that YGS may maintain iron homeostasis by regulating IL-6/STAT3/hepcidin pathway. However, HAMP mRNA levels at 6 h were also downregulated by YGS pretreatment, although serum IL-6 and p-STAT3 levels were unaffected.

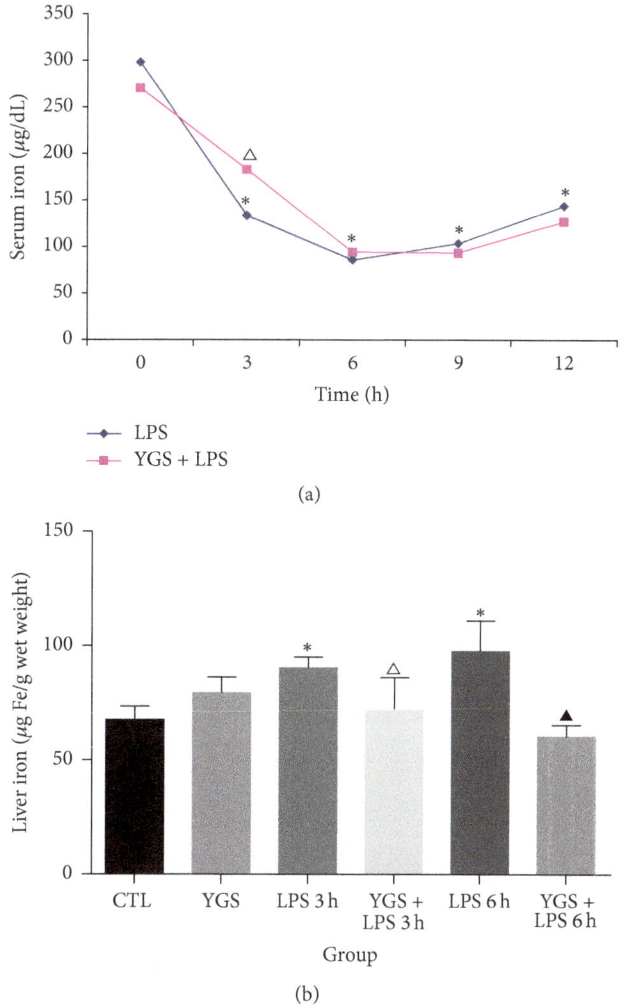

Figure 2: Effects of YGS on LPS-induced imbalanced iron homeostasis. (a) Colourimetric analysis of serum iron levels at 3, 6, 9, and 12 h after LPS administration. (b) Colourimetric analysis of liver iron levels at 3 and 6 h after LPS administration. This experiment was repeated twice, and the results are shown as mean plus or minus SD; $n = 6$. $^{*}P < 0.05$ versus the control group; $^{\triangle}P < 0.05$ versus the LPS 3 h group; $^{\blacktriangle}P < 0.05$ versus the LPS 6 h group.

Therefore, YGS may have inhibited inflammation caused by hepcidin production via another signaling pathway.

The BMP signaling pathway is involved in regulating hepcidin expression in the liver. BMPs are potent inducers of hepcidin production. The interactions of BMPs with BMP receptors result in the phosphorylation of a subset of SMAD proteins (SMAD1/5/8) and subsequent formation of a heteromeric complex with SMAD4, which translocates to the nucleus and induces the transcription of target genes [19]. HJV, a member of the repulsive guidance molecule (RGM) family, acts as a BMP coreceptor and triggers the binding of BMP ligands to BMP receptors to enhance hepcidin expression. Regulation of BMP/HJV/SMAD signaling occurs also after the phosphorylation of SMAD1/5/8, which ensures fine-tuning at the cytosolic level. STAT3-inducible hepcidin expression is also influenced by BMP-dependent SMAD activation. The BMP/HJV/SMAD signaling pathway modulates IL-6-inducible STAT3 pathway [12]. Thus, it may cooperate and enhance IL-6-dependent stimulation and may represent a connecting component between iron status and inflammation.

As mentioned earlier, we further explored BMP/HJV/SMAD pathway. BMP6 mRNA and P-SMAD1/5/8 and HJV protein levels were downregulated at 6 h by YGS pretreatment, which was correlated with the HAMP mRNA levels. Thus, we speculated that regulation of the BMP/HJV/SMAD pathway by YGS may contribute to the downregulation of hepcidin, resulting in the restoration of iron homeostasis. Our findings show that YGS regulates iron homeostasis by downregulating HAMP mRNA, which may depend on the regulation of the IL-6/STAT3 or BMP/HJV/SMAD pathway during acute inflammation.

Anaemia of chronic disease (ACD) is the most common anaemia secondary to various chronic infections, chronic inflammation, and malignancies. Increased production of inflammatory cytokines can directly induce changes in iron homeostasis, which are characterized by the reduction of both iron absorption and macrophage iron release, resulting in ACD [20, 21]. In contrast to iron deficiency anaemia, hypoferraemia in ACD is not due to iron deficiency; instead, the impaired iron absorption and utilisation regulatory mechanisms result in imbalanced iron homeostasis [22]. The changes of iron metabolism in the mice caused by LPS injection through hepcidin-induced inflammation pathway, which is one of the important ACD pathogenesis, imitate ACD pathological state although the mice can not be anaemic [6, 23]. So, if YGS decoction could improve this mimic ACD pathological state, it is possible to be used to prevent or treat ACD. Further studies on the YGS decoction are maybe important in science and application.

Competing Interests

The authors declare that they have no competing interests.

Authors' Contributions

Qin Zheng and Yu Guan contributed equally to this work. Meihong Luo designed and performed the research, analyzed data, and wrote this paper; Qin Zheng and Yu Guan performed research, analyzed data, and wrote the paper; Lemin Xia, Zhicheng Wang, Yiling Jiang, Xiaofeng Zhang, Jianying Wang, Guohua Wang, Yiqiong Pu, and Jing Xia performed the research.

Acknowledgments

The authors acknowledge the technical help of Huan Zhao, Renye Que, and Yanting Shen. This work was supported by grants from National Natural Sciences Foundation of China (Grant nos. 81102569 and 81500676), Science & Technol-

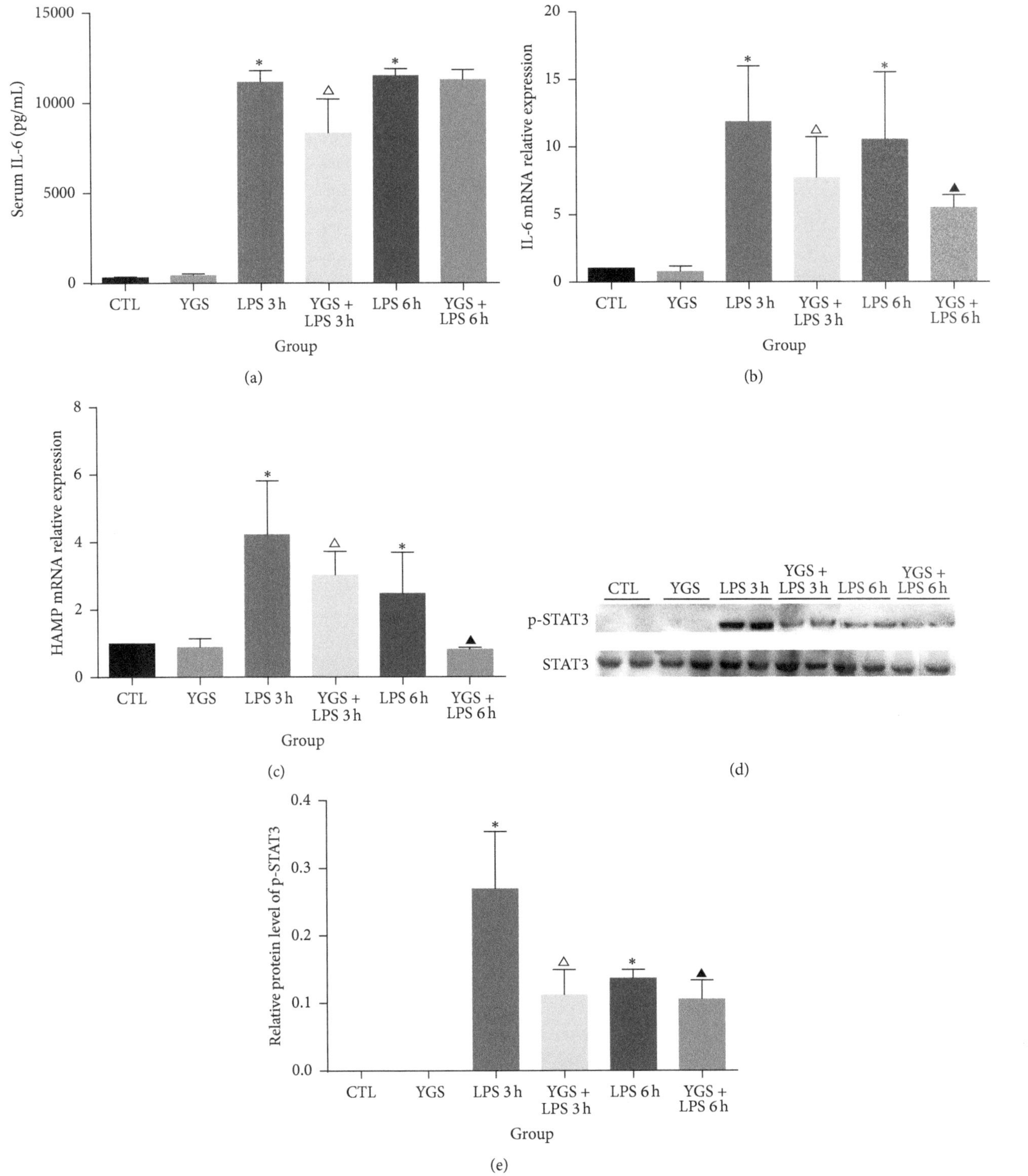

FIGURE 3: Levels of serum and liver IL-6 protein and liver HAMP mRNA and p-STAT3 protein. (a) ELISA of serum IL-6 levels. (b) Real-time PCR analysis of liver IL-6 and HAMP mRNA levels. (c) Western blotting analysis of p-STAT3 and STAT3 protein levels. (d, e) Western blotting analysis of p-STAT3/STAT3 protein levels expressed as densitometry values. This experiment was repeated twice, and the results are shown as mean plus or minus SD; $n = 6$. $^{*}P < 0.05$ versus the control group; $^{\triangle}P < 0.05$ versus the LPS 3 h group; $^{\blacktriangle}P < 0.05$ versus the LPS 6 h group.

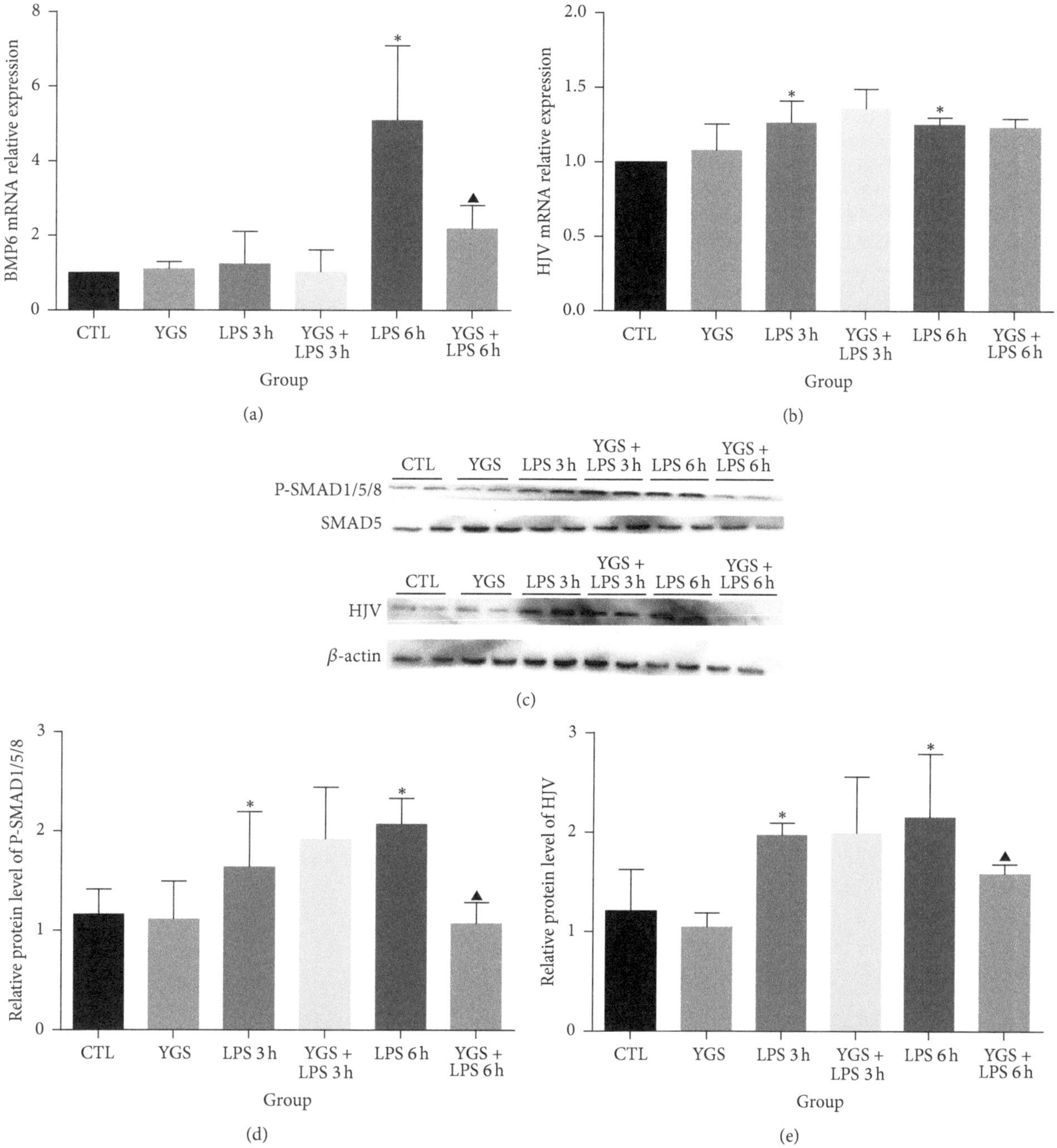

FIGURE 4: Hepatic levels of BMP6 and HJV mRNA and p-SMAD1/5/8 and HJV protein. Real-time PCR analysis of liver BMP6 (a) and HJV (b) mRNA levels at 3 and 6 h after LPS administration. Western blotting analysis of p-SMAD1/5/8 (c, d) and HJV (c, e) protein levels expressed as densitometry values. This experiment was repeated twice, and the results are shown as means plus or minus SD; $n = 6$. $^{*}P < 0.05$ versus the control group; and $^{▲}P < 0.05$ versus the LPS 6 h group.

ogy Commission of Shanghai Municipality grants (Grant no. 13ZR1440000), and Shanghai Municipal Commission of Health and Family Planning (Grant no. 201440587).

References

[1] B. Silva and P. Faustino, "An overview of molecular basis of iron metabolism regulation and the associated pathologies," *Biochimica et Biophysica Acta—Molecular Basis of Disease*, vol. 1852, no. 7, pp. 1347–1359, 2015.

[2] S. Yun and N. D. Vincelette, "Update on iron metabolism and molecular perspective of common genetic and acquired disorder, hemochromatosis," *Critical Reviews in Oncology/Hematology*, vol. 95, no. 1, pp. 12–25, 2015.

[3] A. Pagani, A. Nai, G. Corna et al., "Low hepcidin accounts for the proinflammatory status associated with iron deficiency," *Blood*, vol. 118, no. 3, pp. 736–746, 2011.

[4] M. Poli, M. Asperti, P. Ruzzenenti, M. Regoni, and P. Arosio, "Hepcidin antagonists for potential treatments of disorders with hepcidin excess," *Frontiers in Pharmacology*, vol. 5, article 86, 2014.

[5] X. Wu, L.-M. Yung, W.-H. Cheng et al., "Hepcidin regulation by BMP signaling in macrophages is lipopolysaccharide dependent," *PLoS ONE*, vol. 7, no. 9, Article ID e44622, 2012.

[6] S. Rivera and T. Ganz, "Animal models of anemia of inflammation," *Seminars in Hematology*, vol. 46, no. 4, pp. 351–357, 2009.

[7] E. H. J. M. Kemna, A. E. R. Kartikasari, L. J. H. van Tits, P. Pickkers, H. Tjalsma, and D. W. Swinkels, "Regulation of hepcidin: insights from biochemical analyses on human serum samples," *Blood Cells, Molecules, and Diseases*, vol. 40, no. 3, pp. 339–346, 2008.

[8] S. Lasocki, S. Millot, V. Andrieu et al., "Phlebotomies or erythropoietin injections allow mobilization of iron stores in a mouse model mimicking intensive care anemia," *Critical Care Medicine*, vol. 36, no. 8, pp. 2388–2394, 2008.

[9] C. Liang, S.-H. Zhang, and Z.-D. Cai, "Effects of early intestinal application of sijunzi decoction on immune function in post-operational patients of gastrointestinal tumor," *Zhongguo Zhong Xi Yi Jie He Za Zhi*, vol. 25, no. 12, pp. 1070–1073, 2005.

[10] S.-J. Kim, H.-J. Shin, B.-J. Lee et al., "The antiinflammatory mechanism of igongsan in mouse peritoneal macrophages via suppression of NF-κB/caspase-1 activation," *Phytotherapy Research*, vol. 28, no. 5, pp. 736–744, 2014.

[11] L. Sun, Y. Yu, T. Huang et al., "Associations between ionomic profile and metabolic abnormalities in human population," *PLoS ONE*, vol. 7, no. 6, Article ID e38845, 2012.

[12] E. Nemeth, S. Rivera, V. Gabayan et al., "IL-6 mediates hypoferremia of inflammation by inducing the synthesis of the iron regulatory hormone hepcidin," *Journal of Clinical Investigation*, vol. 113, no. 9, pp. 1271–1276, 2004.

[13] L. Kautz, D. Meynard, A. Monnier et al., "Iron regulates phosphorylation of Smad1/5/8 and gene expression of Bmp6, Smad7, Id1, and Atoh8 in the mouse liver," *Blood*, vol. 112, no. 4, pp. 1503–1509, 2008.

[14] M. Cankurtaran, B. B. Yavuz, M. Halil, Z. Ulger, I. C. Haznedaroğlu, and S. Arıoğul, "Increased ferritin levels could reflect ongoing aging-associated inflammation and may obscure underlying iron deficiency in the geriatric population," *European Geriatric Medicine*, vol. 3, no. 5, pp. 277–280, 2012.

[15] L. Viatte and S. Vaulont, "Hepcidin, the iron watcher," *Biochimie*, vol. 91, no. 10, pp. 1223–1228, 2009.

[16] M. H. Luo, "From theory of the spleen transporting and transforming blood to discuss TCM pathogensis and treatment of chronic anemia," *Journal of Traditional Chinese Medicine*, vol. 54, no. 18, pp. 1556–1557, 2015.

[17] D. M. Wrighting and N. C. Andrews, "Interleukin-6 induces hepcidin expression through STAT3," *Blood*, vol. 108, no. 9, pp. 3204–3209, 2006.

[18] L. E. DeForge and D. G. Remick, "Kinetics of TNF, IL-6, and IL-8 gene expression in LPS-stimulated human whole blood," *Biochemical and Biophysical Research Communications*, vol. 174, no. 1, pp. 18–24, 1991.

[19] M. W. Hentze, M. U. Muckenthaler, B. Galy, and C. Camaschella, "Two to tango: regulation of mammalian iron metabolism," *Cell*, vol. 142, no. 1, pp. 24–38, 2010.

[20] I. Theurl, A. Schroll, M. Nairz et al., "Pathways for the regulation of hepcidin expression in anemia of chronic disease and iron deficiency anemia in vivo," *Haematologica*, vol. 96, no. 12, pp. 1761–1769, 2011.

[21] R. Sakamori, T. Takehara, T. Tatsumi et al., "STAT3 signaling within hepatocytes is required for anemia of inflammation in vivo," *Journal of Gastroenterology*, vol. 45, no. 2, pp. 244–248, 2010.

[22] I. Theurl, E. Aigner, M. Theurl et al., "Regulation of iron homeostasis in anemia of chronic disease and iron deficiency anemia: diagnostic and therapeutic implications," *Blood*, vol. 113, no. 21, pp. 5277–5286, 2009.

[23] L. Yuan, L. Geng, L. Ge et al., "Effect of iron liposomes on anemia of inflammation," *International Journal of Pharmaceutics*, vol. 454, no. 1, pp. 82–89, 2013.

5

Evaluation of Medicinal Categorization of *Atractylodes japonica* Koidz. by Using Internal Transcribed Spacer Sequencing Analysis and HPLC Fingerprinting Combined with Statistical Tools

Jung-Hoon Kim,[1] Eui-Jeong Doh,[2,3] and Guemsan Lee[2]

[1] *Division of Pharmacology, School of Korean Medicine, Pusan National University, Yangsan 626-870, Republic of Korea*
[2] *Department of Herbology, College of Korean Medicine, Wonkwang University, Iksan 570-749, Republic of Korea*
[3] *Center for Metabolic Function Regulation, Wonkwang University, Iksan 570-749, Republic of Korea*

Correspondence should be addressed to Guemsan Lee; rasfin@wku.ac.kr

Academic Editor: Salih Mollahaliloglu

Atractylodes rhizomes have been used as the herbal medicine "Changchul" or "Baekchul," according to their clinical purpose, in Korea, China, and Japan. Among the *Atractylodes* species, the medicinal use of *Atractylodes japonica* has been controversial, as it is categorized as both Changchul and Baekchul in those countries, and, moreover, parts of the rhizome have been differently used, depending on age of the plant, in Korea. Chromatographic fingerprinting by using HPLC combined with chemometric analyses and internal transcribed spacer (ITS) sequencing analysis were conducted to classify and identify 34 crude drugs derived from *Atractylodes* rhizomes. The identification of the samples, authenticated by their morphological features as *A. japonica* Koidz. (Changchul and Baekchul), *A. chinensis* Koidz., and *A. macrocephala* Koidz., was confirmed as *A. japonica*, *A. chinensis*, and *A. macrocephala* by ITS sequencing. The results from chemometric analyses showed that the chemical components of the crude drugs from *A. japonica* were significantly different from those from *A. macrocephala* but were similar to those from *A. chinensis*. The analyses also suggested that the categorization by age of *A. japonica* as Changchul or Baekchul is not recommended. The results indicate that *A. japonica* should be categorized as "Changchul" and should not be further categorized by age.

1. Introduction

The genus *Atractylodes* (Asteraceae) are perennial herbs distributed in Korea, China, and Japan. Their dried rhizomes have been classified into two kinds of herbal medicines according to their clinical purpose, "Baekchul" (Baizhu in Chinese, Byakujutsu in Japanese) and "Changchul" (Cangzhu in Chinese, Soujutsu in Japanese) [1]. In medicinal applications in Korea, Japan, and China, the rhizomes of *A. lancea* DC. and *A. chinensis* Koidz. have been classified as Changchul, while that of *A. macrocephala* Koidz. has been classified as Baekchul in the pharmacopeias of Korea, China, and Japan [2–4].

However, there has been disagreement between countries in classifying the rhizome of *A. japonica* Koidz.: Korean and Japanese pharmacopeias, as well as some studies from Korea and Japan, have classified the rhizome of *A. japonica* as Baekchul, whereas Chinese studies have classified it as "Gwan-Changchul" (Guan-Cangzhu in Chinese), a type of Changchul, which is not even listed in the Chinese pharmacopeia [5, 6]. Moreover, *A. japonica* is recorded as a synonym of *A. lancea* in the *Flora of China* [7]. Confusion also occurs in local herbal markets in Korea, where the rhizomes of *A. japonica* have been used as Changchul when the fibrous substance has formed after it has grown over two years [8]. The dried rhizomes of *Atractylodes* species can be identified by their morphological features; however, it is difficult to discriminate them by macroscopic observation, a subjective method, due to their morphological similarity. Consequently, the misuse of *Atractylodes* rhizomes may occur when identification is based only on their morphological features. Therefore, strict classification is required for the exact use of *Atractylodes* rhizomes for medicinal purposes.

Genetic identification achieved by hybridization, polymerase chain reaction (PCR), and sequencing techniques is considered more objective, precise, and reliable method for identifying and authenticating herbal species [9, 10]. Internal transcribed spacer (ITS) regions, which are rapidly evolving regions of nuclear ribosomal DNA, have been widely used for the identification of plant materials, and phylogenetic analysis using ITS regions has been conducted to investigate the genetic variability of complicated herbal species [11–13]. It has been reported that the four species of *Atractylodes* (*A. japonica*, *A. macrocephala*, *A. lancea*, and *A. chinensis*) can be distinguished by their different genotypes on ITS sequences [14]. In contrast, one study conducted by PCR-restriction fragment length polymorphism (PCR-RFLP) analysis of the ITS region on nucleotide ribosome DNA (nrDNA) reported that *A. japonica* is not different from *A. macrocephala* [15]. Other studies have demonstrated that the geographical distributions, morphological features, and genetic differentiation between *A. lancea* and *A. chinensis* were not consistent, and *A. japonica* was most closely related to *A. lancea*, according to the results from ITS and *trnL-F* sequences [16, 17]. The results of these studies demonstrate that the classification of *Atractylodes* rhizomes, particularly that of *A. japonica*, remains controversial.

Chemical fingerprinting by using HPLC is an effective and reliable method for the investigation of chemical components in herbal medicines, owing to its high separation efficiency and high detection sensitivity [18]. HPLC fingerprinting also enables a systematic and comprehensive approach to the identification and quantification of the components in herbal medicines [19]. HPLC fingerprinting, combined with chemometric statistical analysis, has been widely used for the quality control of herbal medicines and related herbal products [20, 21]. Moreover, such techniques have also been used to discriminate interspecies differences in herbal medicines, by incorporating principal components analysis (PCA) [22–24]. In previous studies, *A. lancea* was chemically differentiated from *A. chinensis* by HPLC fingerprinting combined with PCA or orthogonal partial least squares-discriminant analysis [25, 26]. However, the chemical discrimination of *Atractylodes* species, using HPLC fingerprinting and chemometric analysis, has not been conducted.

In the present study, chromatographic fingerprinting and chemometric statistical analyses, including PCA, hierarchical clustering analysis (HCA) analysis, and Pearson's correlation coefficient analysis were conducted to classify the crude drugs derived from *Atractylodes* rhizomes. The ITS sequences from nrDNA were also examined to identify the *Atractylodes* species.

2. Materials and Methods

2.1. Plant Materials and Reagents. Thirty-four samples of crude drugs from *Atractylodes* rhizomes were collected or purchased from the wild, agricultural fields, or local markets in Korea and China. The samples were authenticated by their morphological features through identification criteria by authors. Fifteen rhizomes were identified as *A. chinensis* (coded as "AC"); seven samples of Baekchul and five samples of Changchul were "young" and "aged" dried rhizomes of *A. japonica* (coded as "AJB" and "AJC," resp.); and seven rhizomes were identified as *A. macrocephala* (coded as "AM") (Table 1). The voucher specimens have been deposited in the herbarium of the College of Korean Medicine, Woosuk University (Jeonju, Jeonbuk, Korea).

Nine specimens (coded as Arabic number) of *Atractylodes* plants were collected as species reference samples for identification of *Atractylodes* rhizomes in Table 1 and those samples were deposited in the Korea Institute of Oriental Medicine as voucher specimens. The classification result of nine dried-voucher specimens is shown in Table 2.

2.2. Preparation of Genomic DNA. The genomic DNA was extracted from the crude drugs of *Atractylodes* rhizomes according to the manuals of NucleoSpin® Plant II kit (Macherey-Nagel, Dueren, Germany). For some samples, 10% cetyl trimethyl ammonium bromide (CTAB) and 0.7 M NaCl were used to remove the phenolic compounds and polysaccharides.

2.3. PCR Amplification. For ITS amplification, PCR was performed using T-personal cycler (Biometra, Germany). In brief, 600 nM of primer set of ITS1 (5′-TCCGTAGGTGAACCTGCGG-3′) and ITS4 (5′-TCCTCCGCTTATTGATATGC-3′) [27], 1x BluePreMIX-HF (Macrogen, Korea), and 50 ng of genomic DNA were used for PCR amplification. PCR cycling conditions which were followed by predenaturation process (95°C, 5 min) were as follows: denaturation process (95°C, 30 s); annealing process (52°C, 30 s); extension process (72°C, 40 s) × 36 cycles; and final extension process (72°C, 5 min). The amplified PCR product was separated from other gradients using 1.5% agarose gel electrophoresis after the staining by the addition of Safe-white™ (abm, Canada). Amplified products were analyzed using MyImage (Seoulin Biotechnology, Korea).

2.4. Determination of DNA Sequence of PCR Product. PCR product separated from agarose gel was cloned using MG™ TOPcloner TA kit (Macrogen, Korea) and DNA sequence of cloned PCR product was determined through the interpretation performed by Macrogen (Korea).

2.5. Analysis of DNA Sequence and Preparation of Dendrogram. DNA sequence was analyzed using ClustalW multiple sequence alignment (Bioedit, v7.0.9; available at http://www.mbio.ncsu.edu/BioEdit/page2.html) and the phylogenetic tree was created by using DNADist (Bioedit). To study the relationship of *Atractylodes*, the nucleotide sequences of the genera *Atractylis* and *Carlina* deposited in NCBI GenBank were used. The genera *Brachylaena*, *Cardopatium*, *Cirsium*, *Echinops*, *Phonus*, and *Tarchonanthus* were also used as reference for phylogenetic relationship. *Magnolia heptapeta*,

TABLE 1: Morphological identification of the crude drugs of *Atractylodes* rhizomes.

Code	Species	Origin	Code	Species	Origin
AC-1	*A. chinensis* Koidz.	China	AJB-3	*A. japonica* Koidz.	China
AC-2	*A. chinensis* Koidz.	China	AJB-4	*A. japonica* Koidz.	Unclear
AC-3	*A. chinensis* Koidz.	China	AJB-5	*A. japonica* Koidz.	Unclear
AC-4	*A. chinensis* Koidz.	China	AJB-6	*A. japonica* Koidz.	Unclear
AC-5	*A. chinensis* Koidz.	China	AJB-7	*A. japonica* Koidz.	Korea
AC-6	*A. chinensis* Koidz.	Korea	AJC-1	*A. japonica* Koidz.	Korea
AC-7	*A. chinensis* Koidz.	Korea	AJC-2	*A. japonica* Koidz.	Unclear
AC-8	*A. chinensis* Koidz.	China	AJC-3	*A. japonica* Koidz.	Unclear
AC-9	*A. chinensis* Koidz.	China	AJC-4	*A. japonica* Koidz.	Korea
AC-10	*A. chinensis* Koidz.	China	AJC-5	*A. japonica* Koidz.	Unclear
AC-11	*A. chinensis* Koidz.	China	AM-1	*A. macrocephala* Koidz.	China
AC-12	*A. chinensis* Koidz.	China	AM-2	*A. macrocephala* Koidz.	China
AC-13	*A. chinensis* Koidz.	China	AM-3	*A. macrocephala* Koidz.	China
AC-14	*A. chinensis* Koidz.	China	AM-4	*A. macrocephala* Koidz.	China
AC-15	*A. chinensis* Koidz.	China	AM-5	*A. macrocephala* Koidz.	China
AJB-1	*A. japonica* Koidz.	Korea	AM-6	*A. macrocephala* Koidz.	China
AJB-2	*A. japonica* Koidz.	Korea	AM-7	*A. macrocephala* Koidz.	China

TABLE 2: Identification of dried-voucher specimens coded as Arabic numbers.

Number	Identification
1	*A. japonica* Koidzumi
2	*A. lancea* de Candolle
3	*A. lancea* de Candolle
4	*A. macrocephala* Koidzumi
5	*A. japonica* Koidzumi
6	*A. japonica* Koidzumi
8	*A. lancea* de Candolle
9	*A. japonica* Koidzumi
17	*A. japonica* Koidzumi

TABLE 3: The GenBank accession number of species that are used in phylogenetic tree analysis.

Species	GenBank accession number
Atractylis cancellata	AY826231.1
Atractylis arabica	KF850563.1
Atractylis carduus	AY826232.1
Atractylis arbuscula	KF301215.1
Carlina falcata	AY826243.1
Carlina vulgaris	KF301217.1
Carlina acanthifolia	KF301216.1
Echinops viscosus	AY826283.1
Phonus riphaeus	AY826310.1
Cirsium palustre	EU143268.1
Cardopatium corymbosum	AY826238.1
Tarchonanthus camphoratus	AY826340.1
Brachylaena discolor	AY826236.1
Magnolia heptapeta	AY858638.1
Zanthoxylum rhoifolium	KC502933.1
Lilium cernuum	HQ686064.1

Zanthoxylum rhoifolium, and *Lilium cernuum* were used as out-groups in the phylogenetic analyses, based on previous studies [28, 29]. ITS sequences of these taxa were collected from GeneBank in NCBI (the accession numbers were shown in Table 3).

2.6. Preparation of Samples for HPLC Analysis. The dried powder of the rhizomes (100 mg) was weighed and then extracted by sonication with 2 mL of ethanol (HPLC grade; Phillipsburg, NJ, USA) for 40 min. The extract was filtered through a 0.45 μm membrane filter (Adventec, Tokyo, Japan) and concentrated in vacuum oven at 45°C. Concentrated extract was dissolved with methanol at the concentration of 5000 μg/mL and filtered through a 0.45 μm membrane filter, prior to HPLC injection.

2.7. HPLC Conditions for Chromatographic Fingerprinting. An Agilent 1260 liquid chromatography system (Agilent Technologies, Palo Alto, CA, USA) equipped with an autosampler, degasser, quaternary solvent pump, and diode array detector (DAD) was used for chromatographic fingerprinting. The data were processed by using Chemstation software (Agilent Technologies Inc., USA). The separation of compounds was carried out on a Capcell Pak Mg II C_{18} column (4.6 mm × 250 mm, 5 μm; Shiseido, Tokyo, Japan) with Mg II C_{18} guard cartridge (4.0 mm × 10 mm, S-5; Shiseido, Tokyo, Japan) at 35°C. The flow rate was 1 mL/min and the injection volume was 10 μL. The mobile phase consisted of solvent A (HPLC-grade water; Phillipsburg, NJ, USA) and solvent B (HPLC-grade acetonitrile; Phillipsburg, NJ, USA), with the following gradient elution, 20% (B) over 0–2 min, 20–55% (B) over 2–10 min, 55% (B) over 10–13 min, 55–60%

(B) over 13–35 min, 60% (B) over 35–38 min, and 60–75% (B) over 38–50 min, held for 2 min, and then reequilibrated to 20% until the end of the analysis. Detection was performed using a UV detector at the wavelengths of 255, 275, 295, 315, and 340 nm.

2.8. Chemometric Statistical Analysis. The 34 samples that were genetically identified and recoded were used for PCA, HCA, and Pearson's correlation analysis. Total 27 peaks were selected as "reference peaks," and their absolute area was calculated by peak area integration. The 27 reference peaks for the chromatographic fingerprinting, which were representative and >1.0% of total peak area, were chosen at their optimal UV absorption. The absolute area of chosen peak was calculated for chromatographic fingerprinting. A matrix composed of the rows (*Atractylodes* sample) and columns (absolute area of each reference peak) was used for construction of PCA plot, HCA dendrogram, and Pearson's correlation analysis, which were conducted using open-source software R (v.3.1.1).

3. Results

3.1. ITS Genotype and Genetic Identification of Atractylodes Rhizomes. The amplification of internal transcribed spacer (ITS) region produced overall 733 bp of nucleotide sequences from 34 samples listed in Table 1 and nine dried-voucher specimens (Figure 1). The determined ITS nucleotide sequence of samples were confirmed by using DNA sequence registered in NCBI GenBank as well as previous paper [14] with comparison of the accession numbers: *A. japonica* (AB219405), *A. macrocephala* (AB219406), *A. lancea* (AB219407), *A. chinensis* (AB219408), and *A. koreana* (AB219409). As presented in Table 4, there was nucleotide substitutions observed on 37 sites on the ITS regions of *Atractylodes* samples. Type 1, ITS sequence of *A. japonica*, showed multiple sequences comparing to other species, while types 2 and 3 were the genotypes of *A. macrocephala* and *A. lancea*, respectively. Type 4, the genotype of *A. chinensis*, was identical to type 5, the genotype of *A. koreana*.

All 7 samples labelled as "AM" were determined as *A. macrocephala* and the difference of DNA sequence between samples was not observed. Among 15 samples labelled as "AC," AC-1, AC-2, AC-4, AC-5, AC-6, and AC-11 were determined as *A. chinensis*, whereas the rest were *A. japonica*. The sequence of AC-1 was different from that of type 4 by 1 bp (A → G) at nucleotide position, 128 bp, which indicates intraspecific variation. All 7 samples labelled as "AJB" as well as 5 samples labelled as "AJC" were determined as *A. japonica*. AC-13 and AJB-5 were different form that of type 1 by 1 bp (G → A), at nucleotide position, 80 bp. AJC-2, AJC-3, and AJC-5 have 2 different nucleotide positions at 80 bp (G → A) and 481 bp (C → T), showing intraspecific variation.

3.2. Genetic Relationship of the Atractylodes. Nine dried-voucher specimens were confirmed as *A. japonica*, *A. lancea*, and *A. macrocephala*. Thirty-four samples of *Atractylodes* rhizomes were identified as *A. chinensis*, *A. japonica*, and *A. macrocephala*. Phylogenetic classification based on ITS region was constructed and the inferred evolutionary relationships among *Atractylodes* rhizomes were represented on phylogenetic tree. The genus *Atractylodes* is well separated from other close genera and out-groups. The samples of *A. japonica*, *A. lancea*, and *A. chinensis* formed *A. lancea* complex, whereas those of *A. macrocephala* formed their own complex, namely, *A. macrocephala* complex. Five AC samples, AC-2, AC-4, AC-5, AC-6, and AC-11, were involved in *A. chinensis* group. AJB, AJC samples, and the rest AC samples were contained in *A. japonica* group (Figure 2).

Comparing the genotypes listed in Figures 1 and 2 and Table 4, the species of 34 samples in Table 1 of *Atractylodes* rhizomes were recoded as shown in Table 5.

3.3. HPLC Fingerprinting of Atractylodes Samples. Through macroscopic observation of the results of HPLC fingerprinting, the chromatograms of *A. japonica* samples (AJBs + AJCs + AJs) and *A. chinensis* samples (ACs) showed peak patterns similar to each other, whereas the chromatograms of *A. macrocephala* samples (AMs) represented different peak patterns compared with those of *A. japonica* and *A. chinensis* samples. Moreover, chromatographic difference between Baekchul samples (AJBs) and Changchul samples (AJCs) was not apparently distinguished (Figures 3 and 4).

3.4. Chemometric Statistical Analysis of Atractylodes Samples. The results of the chromatographic fingerprinting were further analyzed using principle component analysis (PCA), hierarchical clustering analysis (HCA), and Pearson's correlation analysis to evaluate the correlations between the samples whose code names were redetermined by genetic identification as listed in Table 5.

Principle component 1 (PC1) score divided the samples of "*A. japonica* + *A. chinensis*" group in the positive plot with exception of AC-6, AJ-9, and AJC-5, while "*A. macrocephala*" group was in the negative plot. PC2 score further differentiated the samples having positive PC1 scores into positive PC2 plot (AC-1, AC-3, AC-5, AJ-1, AJ-2, AJ-6, AJ-7, AJ-8, AJB-2, AJB-3, AJB-7, AJC-1, and AJC-2) and negative PC2 plot (AC-2, AC-4, AJ-3, AJ-4, AJ-5, AJB-1, AJB-4, AJB-5, AJB-6, AJC-3, and AJC-4) and samples having negative PC1 scores into positive PC2 (AM-1, AM-5, AM-6, and AM-7) and negative PC2 (AM-2, AM-3, and AM-4) (Figure 5).

HCA results also showed similar result obtained from PCA. Below the height of 30000, while the samples of *A. macrocephala* formed their own clustering, those of *A. japonica* and *A. chinensis* were gathered together, where *A. japonica* samples and *A. chinensis* samples were mixed. Therefore, apparent discrimination between *A. japonica* samples and *A. chinensis* samples was not observed. Moreover, as seen in PCA score plot, AJB and AJC samples were not clearly distinguished in HCA dendrogram, as they were grouped undistinguishably within the same levels (Figure 6).

Box plot of average Pearson's correlation coefficient (r) showed two distinct sample groups, the group of *A. macrocephala* samples and the group of *A. japonica* and *A. chinensis* samples. The average coefficients of *A. macrocephala* samples

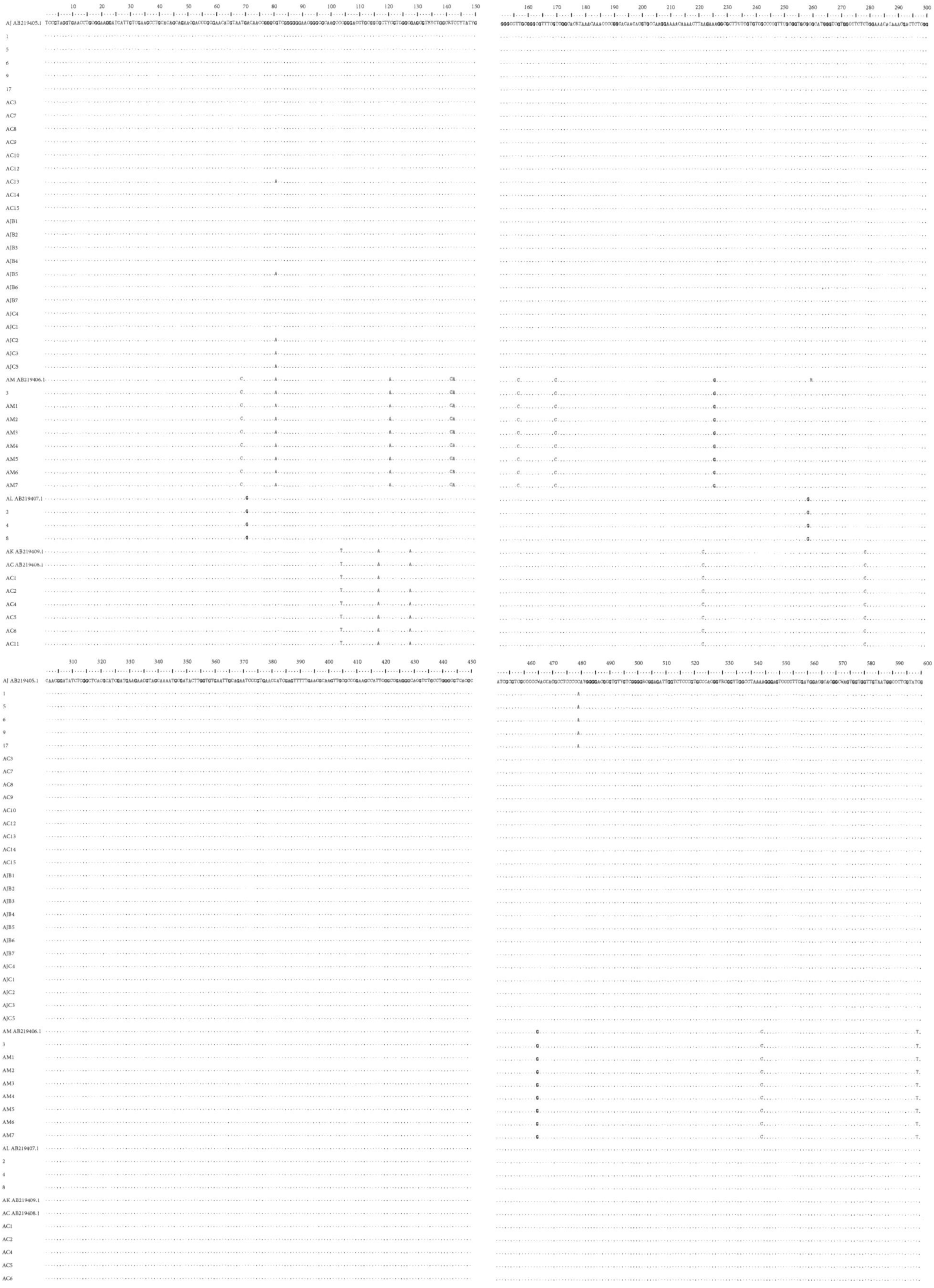

Figure 1: Continued.

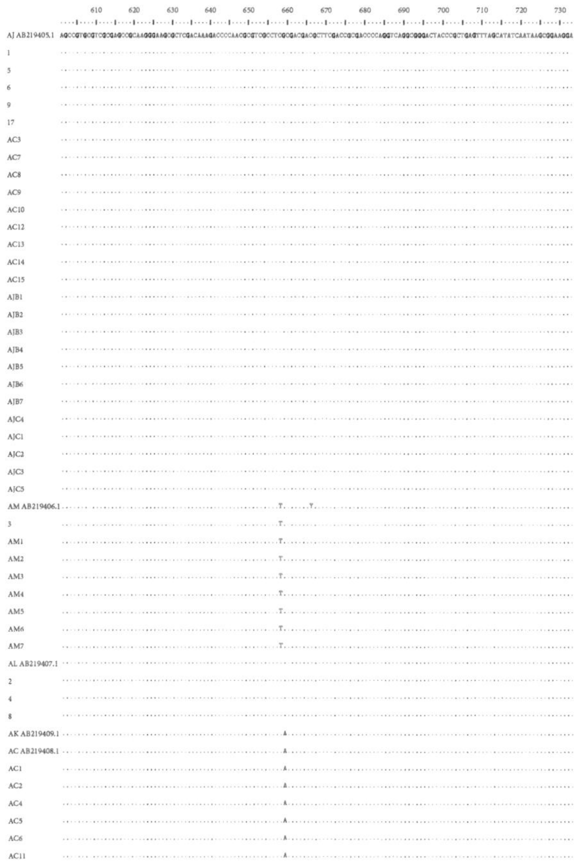

FIGURE 1: Multiple alignments of ITS nucleotide sequence among the sample listed in Table 1. The dots indicate the consensus nucleotide, and the dashes represent the gaps. AB219405.1 accession numbers of NCBI GenBank for the nucleotide sequences of the ITS for *Atractylodes japonica*; AB219409.1 and AB210407.1 accession numbers of NCBI GenBank for the nucleotide sequences of the ITS for *A. koreana* and *A. lancea*, respectively; AB219406.1 accession number of NCBI GenBank for the nucleotide sequence of ITS for *A. macrocephala*; and AB219408.1 accession number of NCBI GenBank for the nucleotide sequence of ITS for *A. chinensis*. The samples with Arabic number were dried-voucher specimens deposited in the Korea Institute of Oriental Medicine.

ranged from −0.2 to 0.0, whereas those of *A. japonica* and *A. chinensis* samples ranged from 0.5 to 1.0, except for AJ-9 showing the average coefficient between 0.0 and 0.2. Furthermore, AJB and AJC samples showed similar values of average Pearson's coefficients (Figure 7).

4. Discussion

Discrimination of herbal medicines according to their therapeutic effect is most important in using herbal medicines as therapeutic agents. To achieve such purpose, correct classification of herbal medicines should be preceded at their species levels. The rhizome of *A. japonica* has been at the center of controversy as it is differently classified in many countries; Korea and Japan have used that as "Baekchul," whereas China has used that as "Changchul." Furthermore, the rhizome of *A. japonica* is further divided into "Baekchul" and "Changchul" by the age; tuberous part grown for less than a year is used as Baekchul, while fibrous part grown for more than two years is used as Changchul. Hence, we classified *Atractylodes* samples which were genetically identified by ITS genotypes using analytical tools combined with chemometric statistics, in order to propose correct categorization of *Atractylodes* rhizomes, especially *A. japonica* rhizomes.

4.1. Genetic Identification of Atractylodes Samples. *Atractylodes*, *Atractylis*, and *Carlina* belong to subtribe Carlininae [28]. ITS sequence of *A. japonica* showing multiple sequences indicates that there are diverse intraspecific variations in *A. japonica* samples. The genotype of *A. chinensis* was identical to that of *A. koreana*. As the distribution of *A. koreana* is limited in Shandong and Liaoning area, *A. koreana* has been possibly derived from *A. chinensis* [14, 17]. The samples of *A. japonica*, *A. lancea*, and *A. chinensis* formed *A. lancea* complex, in accordance with the previous research [17]. *A. japonica* is most closely related to *A. lancea* and next related to *A. chinensis*, as suggested in previous researches [17, 30, 31]. The samples identified as *A. japonica* were obviously separated from those identified as *A. macrocephala* by DNA sequencing analysis [14, 16, 32]. According to the results,

Table 4: Genotypes of ITS nucleotide sequences deposited in the NCBI GenBank for recognition in the *Atractylodes* species.

Nucleotide position	69	71	81	104	117	120	121	128	134	135	141	142	143	145	149	157	170	177	222	226	259	260	279	465	481	494	502	529	530	534	544	560	572	599	658	659	666
Genotype																																					
Type 1	T	A	G	C	G	**Y**	C	G	**M**	**Y**	**R**	T	C	Y	Y	T	T	R	A	A	C	G	T	**W**	**Y**	**Y**	**R**	**Y**	**R**	**Y**	A	**Y**	**W**	C	C	G	C
Type 2	C	A	A	C	G	C	A	G	C	C	G	C	A	C	C	C	C	G	A	G	C	**R**	T	G	C	C	G	C	G	C	C	C	T	T	T	G	**Y**
Type 3	T	G	G	C	G	C	C	G	C	C	G	T	C	C	C	T	T	A	A	A	G	G	T	A	C	C	G	T	G	C	A	C	A	C	C	G	C
Type 4	T	A	G	T	A	C	C	A	C	C	G	T	C	C	T	T	T	G	C	A	C	G	C	T	C	C	G	C	G	C	A	C	T	C	C	A	C
Type 5	T	A	G	T	A	C	C	A	C	C	G	T	C	C	T	T	T	G	C	A	C	G	C	T	C	C	G	C	G	C	A	C	T	C	C	A	C

*Bold characters indicate nucleotide additives, M = A and C; R = A and G; W = A and T; Y = C and T. Type 1 genotype resulted from deposited ITS nucleotide sequences in NCBI Genbank of *Atractylodes japonica*. Type 2 and type 3 represent *A. macrocephala* and *A. lancea*. Type 4 and type 5 represent *A. chinensis* and *A. koreana*.

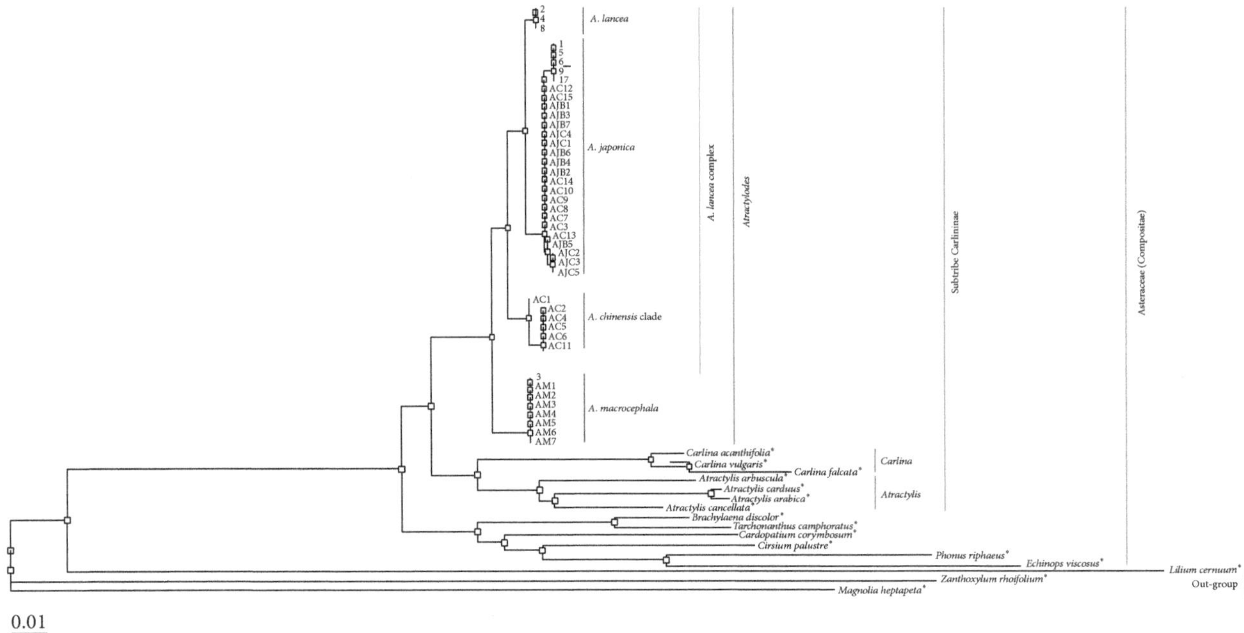

FIGURE 2: Phylogenic tree from DNADist (Neighbor phylogenetic tree) analysis of the ITS nucleotide sequences. The ITS sequences of taxa with "*" such as *Atactylis*, *Carlina*, and out-group were downloaded from Genbank in NCBI. The samples with Arabic number were dried-voucher specimens deposited in the Korea Institute of Oriental Medicine.

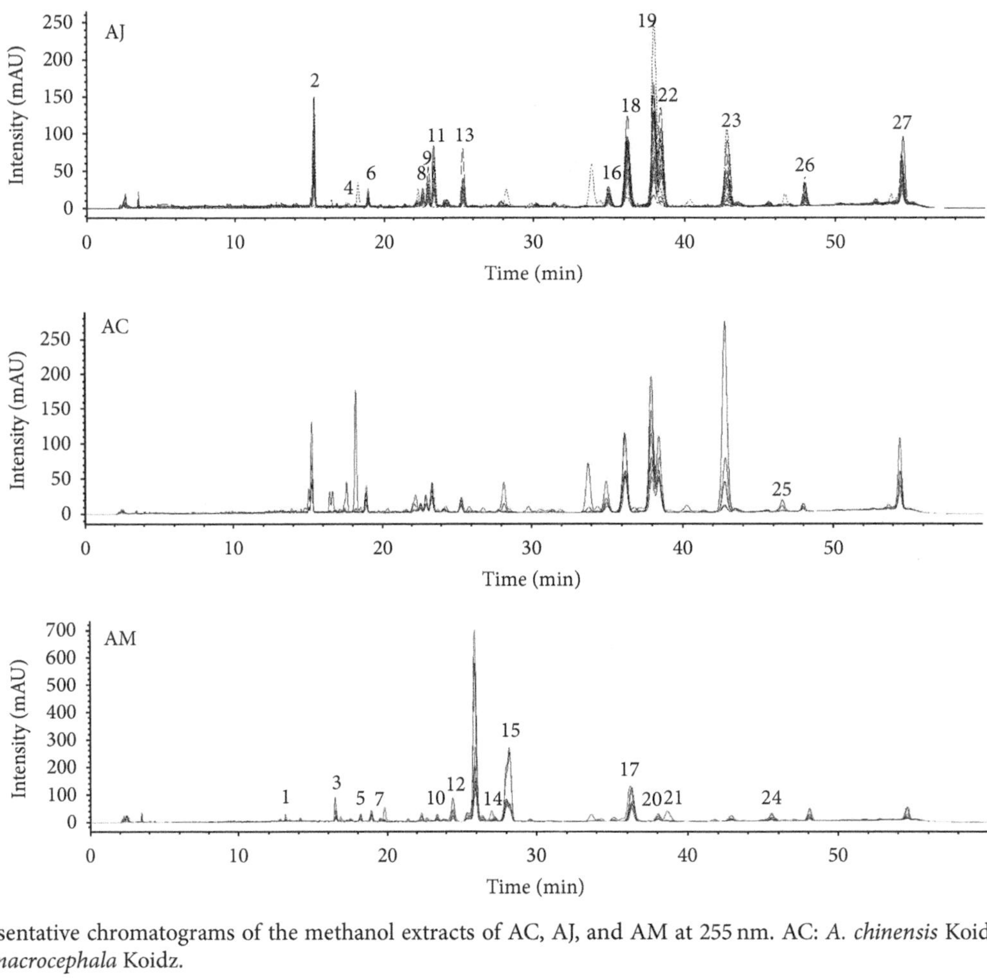

FIGURE 3: Representative chromatograms of the methanol extracts of AC, AJ, and AM at 255 nm. AC: *A. chinensis* Koidz.; AJ: *A. japonica* Koidz.; AM: *A. macrocephala* Koidz.

TABLE 5: Genetic identification of original species of *Atractylodes* rhizomes listed in Table 1.

Code	Genetically identified species	Recode	Code	Genetically identified species	Recode
AC-1	*A. chinensis*	AC-1	AJB-3	*A. japonica*	AJB-3
AC-2	*A. chinensis*	AC-2	AJB-4	*A. japonica*	AJB-4
AC-3	*A. japonica*	AJ-1	AJB-5	*A. japonica*	AJB-5
AC-4	*A. chinensis*	AC-3	AJB-6	*A. japonica*	AJB-6
AC-5	*A. chinensis*	AC-4	AJB-7	*A. japonica*	AJB-7
AC-6	*A. chinensis*	AC-5	AJC-1	*A. japonica*	AJC-1
AC-7	*A. japonica*	AJ-2	AJC-2	*A. japonica*	AJC-2
AC-8	*A. japonica*	AJ-3	AJC-3	*A. japonica*	AJC-3
AC-9	*A. japonica*	AJ-4	AJC-4	*A. japonica*	AJC-4
AC-10	*A. japonica*	AJ-5	AJC-5	*A. japonica*	AJC-5
AC-11	*A. chinensis*	AC-6	AM-1	*A. macrocephala*	AM-1
AC-12	*A. japonica*	AJ-6	AM-2	*A. macrocephala*	AM-2
AC-13	*A. japonica*	AJ-7	AM-3	*A. macrocephala*	AM-3
AC-14	*A. japonica*	AJ-8	AM-4	*A. macrocephala*	AM-4
AC-15	*A. japonica*	AJ-9	AM-5	*A. macrocephala*	AM-5
AJB-1	*A. japonica*	AJB-1	AM-6	*A. macrocephala*	AM-6
AJB-2	*A. japonica*	AJB-2	AM-7	*A. macrocephala*	AM-7

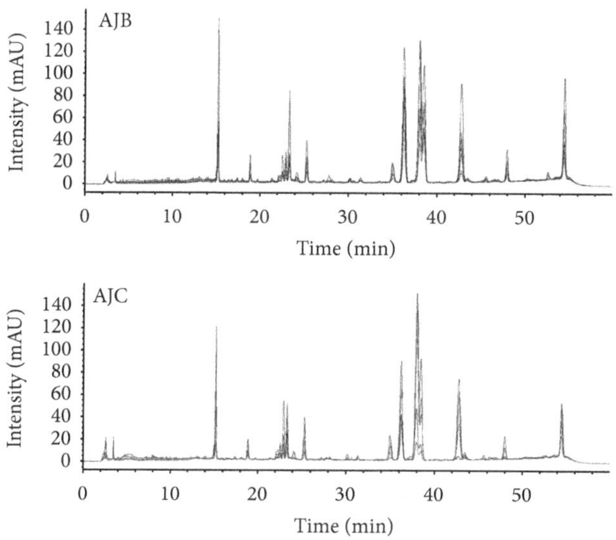

FIGURE 4: Representative chromatograms of the methanol extracts of AJB and AJC at 255 nm. AJB and AJC: *A. japonica* Koidz.

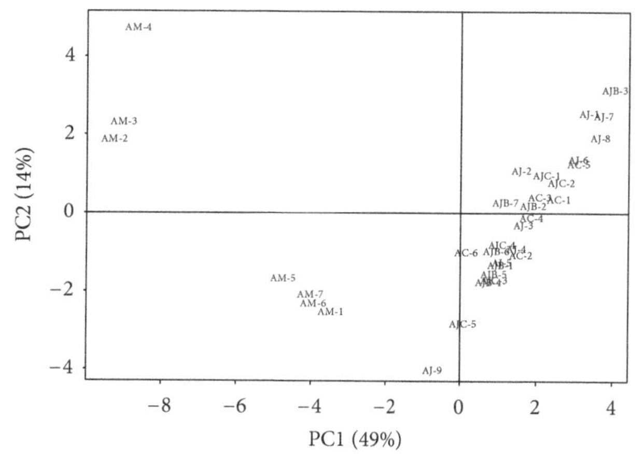

FIGURE 5: Score plot of principal components (PC1 versus PC2) on the variables (absolute area of reference peaks) with *Atractylodes* samples. PC1 and PC2 represent 49% and 14% of the total variance, respectively. AC: *A. chinensis* Koidz.; AJ, AJB, and AJC: *A. japonica* Koidz.; AM: *A. macrocephala* Koidz.

there was difference in classification between morphological identification and genetic identification which might be caused by morphological similarity.

4.2. Classification of Atractylodes Samples Using Chemometric Analysis. Principal components analysis (PCA) was performed for the clustering of the samples and for investigating the relationships among the samples using principal components on the PCA plot. Principal component 1 (PC1) explains most of the variance, and PC2, which is orthogonal to PC1, represents most of the variance not explained by PC1 [33]. HCA is another clustering method which classifies similar objects mathematically into the same group and the classifications were represented as tree diagram called dendrogram [34]. Pearson's correlation coefficient of each sample was calculated to evaluate the correlations between samples ($-1 \leq r \leq +1$; the closer the r is to 1, the more correlated the two fingerprints are) [35].

From the results of PCA, HCA, and Pearson's correlation analysis, the *A. japonica* samples were obviously distinct from *A. macrocephala* samples but distributed close to the *A. chinensis* samples without apparent separation of AJBs and AJCs samples. These results indicate that *A. japonica* is chemically different from *A. macrocephala*; however, the crude drugs derived from *A. japonica* and *A. chinensis* were not clearly distinguishable by their chemical components. These results indicate that the therapeutic effects of *A. japonica* and

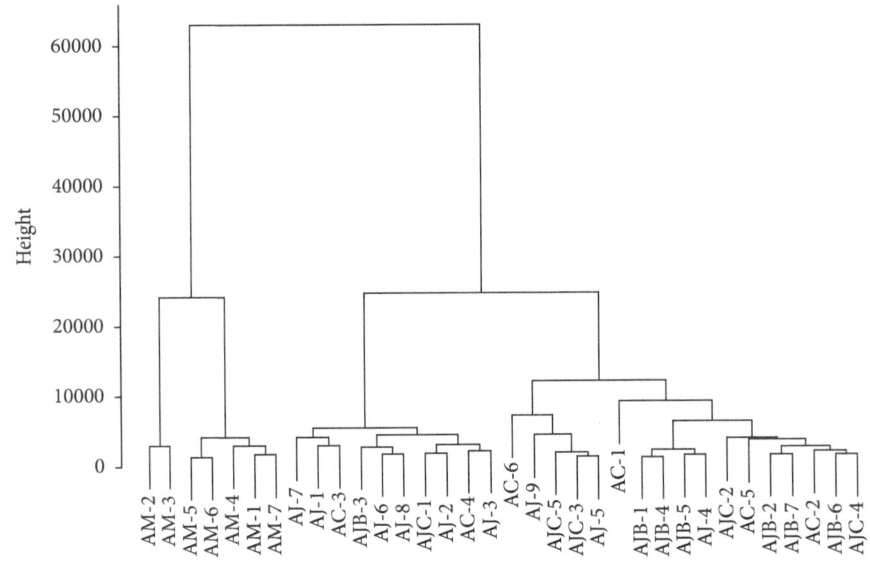

Figure 6: Hierarchical clustering analysis of *Atractylodes* samples. AC: *A. chinensis* Koidz.; AJ, AJB, and AJC: *A. japonica* Koidz.; AM: *A. macrocephala* Koidz.

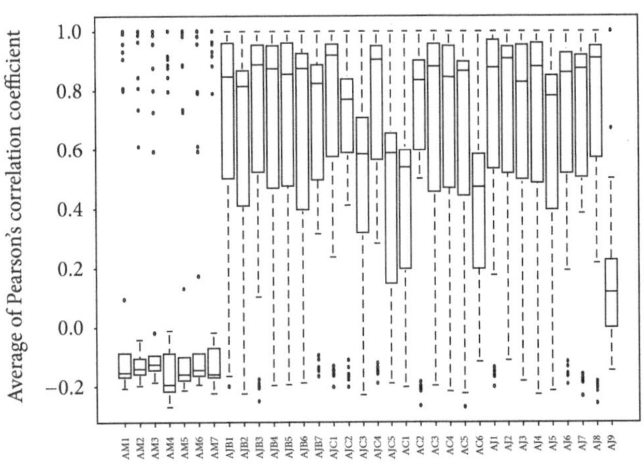

Figure 7: Average coefficients of Pearson's correlation of 34 *Atractylodes* samples. AC: *A. chinensis* Koidz.; AJ, AJB, and AJC: *A. japonica* Koidz.; AM: *A. macrocephala* Koidz.

A. chinensis whose effects can be exerted by the chemical components are thought to be presumably analogous [36], although they are genetically different. Moreover, the separation of *A. japonica* rhizomes as "Baekchul" and "Changchul" is not recommended because they had the closest PC scores, equal levels of hierarchies, and similar Pearson's coefficients [37]; therefore, AJBs and AJCs can be assumed to be the same medicinal parts.

4.3. Assured Medicinal Categorization of Atractylodes japonica Rhizomes. The categorization of *A. japonica* as Baekchul in Korea and Japan, therefore, should be removed, because its relationship to *A. macrocephala*, the only species regarded as Baekchul in China, is not close, which supports the results from previous studies [14, 17, 32, 38]. Moreover, we do not recommend the segregation of *A. japonica* into Baekchul and Changchul, because the segregated crude drugs of *A. japonica* are not distinguishable by their chemical and genetic characteristics. This suggests that there is the lack of chemical or genetic reason to categorize the rhizome of *A. japonica* as Changchul and Baekchul based on plant age.

Therefore, we propose that *A. japonica* should be separated from *A. macrocephala* and should be used as "Changchul" as the Chinese literatures define it, regardless of its age. Further biological and clinical experiments are necessary to confirm the results of the present study.

In conclusion, the 34 crude drugs derived from *Atractylodes* rhizomes were identified using ITS sequencing analysis and classified using HPLC fingerprinting and statistical tools such as PCA, HCA, and Pearson's correlation analysis. The macroscopically authenticated *Atractylodes* samples were genetically identified as *A. japonica*, *A. chinensis*, and *A. macrocephala* by ITS DNA sequencing. The hyphenated HPLC fingerprinting and statistical analyses showed that the chemical components of *A. japonica* were not related to those of *A. macrocephala* but related to those of *A. chinensis*. Moreover, the rhizome of *A. japonica* could not be segregated as Baekchul and Changchul by its age. The results from these chemical and genetic analyses demonstrate that *A. japonica* should be classified as "Changchul" and should not be classified by plant age.

Disclosure

The funders had no role in study design, data collection and analysis, decision to publish, or preparation of the paper.

Competing Interests

The authors declare that they have no competing interests.

Authors' Contributions

J.-H. Kim and E.-J. Doh contributed equally to this work.

Acknowledgments

This study was supported by the Convergence of Conventional Medicine and Traditional Korean Medicine R&D program funded by the Ministry of Health & Welfare through the Korea Health Industry Development Institute (KHIDI) (HI14C0750).

References

[1] D. Bensky, S. Clavey, and E. Stöger, *Chinese Herbal Medicine: Materia Medica*, Eastland Press, Seattle, Wash, USA, 3rd edition, 2004.

[2] The Korea Food and Drug Administration, *The Korean Pharmacopeia*, The Korea Food and Drug Administration, 10th edition, 2013.

[3] The Pharmacopoeia Commission of the Ministry of Health of the People's Republic of China, *The Pharmacopoeia of the People's Republic of China*, China Science and Technology Press, Beijing, China, 10th edition, 2010.

[4] Society of Japanese Pharmacopoeia, *Japanese Pharmacopeia*, vol. 65 of *Labor and Welfare Ministerial Notification*, The Ministry of Health, 2011.

[5] J. Li and W. You, "Analysis of nuclear types in chromosome of Japanese Atractylodes," *Journal of Shenyang Agricultural University*, vol. 18, pp. 75–77, 1987.

[6] E. M. Kang, C. H. Jeong, and K. H. Shim, "Functional properties of Korean *Atractylodes japonica* Koidz," *Korean Journal of Post-Harvest Science and Technology of Agricultural Products*, vol. 8, pp. 86–91, 2001.

[7] Z. Y. Wu, *Flora of China*, vol. 20, Science Press, Beijing, China, 2011.

[8] J. M. Park, K. H. Jang, S. T. Lee et al., "Growth characteristics of *Atractylodes japonica* Koidz. In its native habitat," *Korean Journal of Medicinal Crop Science*, vol. 8, pp. 327–333, 2000.

[9] X. Q. Ma, J. A. Duan, D. Y. Zhu, T. T. X. Dong, and K. W. K. Tsim, "Species identification of *Radix astragali* (Huangqi) by DNA sequence of its 5S-rRNA spacer domain," *Phytochemistry*, vol. 54, no. 4, pp. 363–368, 2000.

[10] B. K. Choo, B. C. Moon, Y. Ji et al., "Development of SCAR markers for the discrimination of three species of medicinal plants, *Angelica decursiva* (*Peucedanum decursivum*), *Peucedanum praeruptorum* and *Anthricus sylvestris*, based on the internal transcribed spacer (ITS) sequence and random amplified polymorphic DNA (RAPD)," *Biological and Pharmaceutical Bulletin*, vol. 32, no. 1, pp. 24–30, 2009.

[11] Y.-Q. Chen, N. Wang, L.-H. Qu, T.-H. Li, and W.-M. Zhang, "Determination of the anamorph of *Cordyceps sinensis* inferred from the analysis of the ribosomal DNA internal transcribed spacers and 5.8S rDNA," *Biochemical Systematics and Ecology*, vol. 29, no. 6, pp. 597–607, 2001.

[12] T. Takamiya, P. Wongsawad, N. Tajima et al., "Identification of *Dendrobium* species used for herbal medicines based on ribosomal DNA Internal transcribed spacer sequence," *Biological and Pharmaceutical Bulletin*, vol. 34, no. 5, pp. 779–782, 2011.

[13] C.-T. Wu, C.-C. Hsieh, W.-C. Lin et al., "Internal transcribed spacer sequence-based identification and phylogenic relationship of I-Tiao-Gung originating from *Flemingia* and *Glycine* (Leguminosae) in Taiwan," *Journal of Food and Drug Analysis*, vol. 21, no. 4, pp. 356–362, 2013.

[14] M. Shiba, K. Kondo, E. Miki et al., "Identification of medicinal Atractylodes based on ITS sequences of nrDNA," *Biological and Pharmaceutical Bulletin*, vol. 29, no. 2, pp. 315–320, 2006.

[15] K. Kondo, M. Shiba, Y. Yotsuyanagi, N. Nishimura, T. Maruyama, and Y. Goda, "Discrimination between *Atractylodes* rhizome (Byaku-jutsu) and *Atractylodes lancea* rhizome (So-jutsu) by the PCR-RFLP analysis of ITS region on nrDNA nrDNA," *Journal of Japanese Botany*, vol. 84, no. 6, pp. 356–359, 2009.

[16] Y.-F. Ge, Y.-Y. Hang, B. Xia, and Y.-L. Wei, "Sequencing of *trn*L-F and analysis of interspecific genetic relationship of five medicinal species in *Atractylodes* DC," *Journal of Plant Resources and Environment*, vol. 16, no. 2, pp. 12–16, 2007.

[17] H.-S. Peng, Q.-J. Yuan, Q.-Q. Li, and L.-Q. Huang, "Molecular systematics of genus atractylodes (Compositae, Cardueae): evidence from internal transcribed spacer (ITS) and trnL-F sequences," *International Journal of Molecular Sciences*, vol. 13, no. 11, pp. 14623–14633, 2012.

[18] D.-Z. Yang, Y.-Q. An, X.-L. Jiang et al., "Development of a novel method combining HPLC fingerprint and multi-ingredients quantitative analysis for quality evaluation of traditional Chinese medicine preparation," *Talanta*, vol. 85, no. 2, pp. 885–890, 2011.

[19] J. Kang, L. Zhou, J. Sun, J. Han, and D.-A. Guo, "Chromatographic fingerprint analysis and characterization of furocoumarins in the roots of *Angelica dahurica* by HPLC/DAD/ESI-MS^n technique," *Journal of Pharmaceutical and Biomedical Analysis*, vol. 47, no. 4-5, pp. 778–785, 2008.

[20] B. Xie, T. Gong, M. Tang et al., "An approach based on HPLC-fingerprint and chemometrics to quality consistency evaluation of Liuwei Dihuang Pills produced by different manufacturers," *Journal of Pharmaceutical and Biomedical Analysis*, vol. 48, no. 4, pp. 1261–1266, 2008.

[21] X. Xu, J. Jiang, Y. Liang, L. Yi, and J. Cheng, "Chemical fingerprint analysis for quality control of *Fructus aurantii immaturus* based on HPLC-DAD combined with chemometric methods," *Analytical Methods*, vol. 2, no. 12, pp. 2002–2010, 2010.

[22] M. Sajewicz, D. Staszek, M. S. Wróbel et al., "The HPLC/DAD fingerprints and chemometric analysis of flavonoid extracts from the selected Sage (*Salvia*) species," *Chromatography Research International*, vol. 2012, Article ID 230903, 8 pages, 2012.

[23] Q.-F. Zhang, H.-Y. Cheung, and L.-B. Zeng, "Development of HPLC fingerprint for species differentiation and quality assessment of *Rhizoma Smilacis Glabrae*," *Journal of Natural Medicines*, vol. 67, no. 1, pp. 207–211, 2013.

[24] W. Tao, J. Duan, R. Zhao et al., "Comparison of three officinal Chinese pharmacopoeia species of *Glycyrrhiza* based on separation and quantification of triterpene saponins and chemometrics analysis," *Food Chemistry*, vol. 141, no. 3, pp. 1681–1689, 2013.

[25] Y. Nakai, K. Yano, M. Shiba et al., "Chemical characterization of rhizomes of *Atractylodes lancea* and *A. chinensis* identified by ITS sequences of nrDNA," *Journal of Japanese Botany*, vol. 81, no. 2, pp. 63–74, 2006.

[26] Y.-G. Xia, B.-Y. Yang, Q.-H. Wang, J. Liang, D. Wang, and H.-X. Kuang, "Species classification and quality assessment of Cangzhu (Atractylodis rhizoma) by high-performance liquid chromatography and chemometric methods," *Journal of Analytical Methods in Chemistry*, vol. 2013, Article ID 497532, 7 pages, 2013.

[27] T. J. White, T. Bruns, S. Lee, and J. Taylor, "Amplification and direct sequencing of fungal ribosomal RNA genes for phylogenetics," in *PCR Protocols: A Guide to Methods and Applications*, M. A. Innis, D. H. Gelfand, J. J. Sninsky, and T. J. White, Eds., pp. 315–322, Academic Press, New York, NY, USA, 1990.

[28] N. Garcia-Jacas, T. Garnatje, A. Susanna, and R. Vilatersana, "Tribal and subtribal delimitation and phylogeny of the cardueae (Asteraceae): a combined nuclear and chloroplast DNA analysis," *Molecular Phylogenetics and Evolution*, vol. 22, no. 1, pp. 51–64, 2002.

[29] A. Susanna, N. Garcia-Jacas, O. Hidalgo, R. Vilatersana, and T. Garnatje, "The Cardueae (Compositae) revisited: insights from ITS, trnL-trnF, and matK nuclear and chloroplast DNA analysis," *Annals of the Missouri Botanical Garden*, vol. 93, no. 1, pp. 150–171, 2006.

[30] H. Mizukami, R. Shimizu, M. Kohjyouma, H. Kohda, F. Kawanishi, and N. Hiraoka, "Phylogenetic analysis of Atractylodes plants based on chloroplast trnK sequence," *Biological and Pharmaceutical Bulletin*, vol. 21, no. 5, pp. 474–478, 1998.

[31] L. P. Guo, L. Q. Huang, M. Wang, X. F. Feng, G. F. Fu, and Y. N. Yan, "A preliminary study on relationship between *Atractylodes lancea* and *A. chinensis* as analyzed by RAPD," *Zhongguo Zhong Yao Za Zhi*, vol. 26, no. 3, pp. 156–158, 2001.

[32] M. K. Huh and K. H. Bang, "Identification of *Atractylodes japonica* and *A. macrocephala* by RAPD analysis and SCAR markers," *Silvae Genetica*, vol. 55, no. 3, pp. 101–105, 2006.

[33] D.-Y. Lee, J.-G. Cho, M.-K. Lee et al., "Discrimination of *Panax ginseng* roots cultivated in different areas in Korea using HPLC-ELSD and principal component analysis," *Journal of Ginseng Research*, vol. 35, no. 1, pp. 31–38, 2011.

[34] Y. Kumooka, "Hierarchical cluster analysis as a tool for preliminary discrimination of ATR-FT-IR spectra of OPP acrylic and rubber-based adhesives," *Forensic Science International*, vol. 189, no. 1–3, pp. 104–110, 2009.

[35] M. Goodarzi, P. J. Russell, and Y. V. Heyden, "Similarity analyses of chromatographic herbal fingerprints: a review," *Analytica Chimica Acta*, vol. 804, pp. 16–28, 2013.

[36] Z.-J. Zhang, "Therapeutic effects of herbal extracts and constituents in animal models of psychiatric disorders," *Life Sciences*, vol. 75, no. 14, pp. 1659–1699, 2004.

[37] J. Lu, J.-S. Wang, and L.-Y. Kong, "Anti-inflammatory effects of Huang-Lian-Jie-Du decoction, its two fractions and four typical compounds," *Journal of Ethnopharmacology*, vol. 134, no. 3, pp. 911–918, 2011.

[38] L. Tian, K.-S. Bi, W.-J. Sun, S.-C. Zhao, G.-F. Wu, and Y. Lu, "Chemical pattern recognition in the Rhizoma of *Atractylodes macrocephala*," *China Journal of Chinese Materia Medica*, vol. 28, no. 2, pp. 143–146, 2003.

6

Methanolic Extract of *Clinacanthus nutans* Exerts Antinociceptive Activity via the Opioid/Nitric Oxide-Mediated, but cGMP-Independent, Pathways

Mohammad Hafiz Abdul Rahim,[1] Zainul Amiruddin Zakaria,[1,2] Mohd Hijaz Mohd Sani,[1] Maizatul Hasyima Omar,[3] Yusnita Yakob,[4] Manraj Singh Cheema,[1,2] Siew Mooi Ching,[5] Zuraini Ahmad,[1] and Arifah Abdul Kadir[6]

[1] *Department of Biomedical Science, Faculty of Medicine and Health Science, Universiti Putra Malaysia, 43400 Serdang, Selangor, Malaysia*
[2] *Integrative Pharmacogenomics Institute (iPROMISE), Faculty of Pharmacy, Universiti Teknologi MARA (UiTM), Puncak Alam Campus, Level 7, FF3, 42300 Bandar Puncak Alam, Selangor, Malaysia*
[3] *Phytochemistry Unit, Herbal Medicine Research Centre, Institute for Medical Research, Jalan Pahang, 50588 Kuala Lumpur, Malaysia*
[4] *Molecular Diagnostics and Protein Unit, Specialised Diagnostics Centre, Institute for Medical Research, Jalan Pahang, 50588 Kuala Lumpur, Malaysia*
[5] *Department of Family Medicine, Faculty of Medicine and Health Science, Universiti Putra Malaysia, 43400 Serdang, Selangor, Malaysia*
[6] *Department of Veterinary Pre-Clinical Sciences, Faculty of Veterinary Sciences, Universiti Putra Malaysia, 43400 Serdang, Selangor, Malaysia*

Correspondence should be addressed to Zainul Amiruddin Zakaria; dr_zaz@yahoo.com

Academic Editor: Haroon Khan

The objectives of the present study were to determine the mechanisms of antinociceptive effect of methanol extract of *Clinacanthus nutans* (Acanthaceae) leaves (MECN) using various animal nociceptive models. The antinociceptive activity of orally administered 10% DMSO, 100 mg/kg acetylsalicylic acid (ASA), 5 mg/kg morphine, or MECN (100, 250, and 500 mg/kg) was determined using the acetic acid-induced abdominal constriction (ACT), formalin-induced paw licking (FT), and hot plate tests (HPT). The role of opioid and nitric oxide/cyclic guanosine monophosphate (NO/cGMP) systems was also investigated. The results showed that MECN produced a significant ($p < 0.05$) antinociceptive response in all nociceptive models with the recorded ED_{50} value of 279.3 mg/kg for the ACT, while, for the early and late phases of the FT, the value was >500 mg/kg or 227.7 mg/kg, respectively. This antinociceptive activity was fully antagonized by naloxone (a nonselective opioid antagonist) but was partially reversed by L-arginine (L-arg; a nitric oxide [NO] precursor), Nω-nitro-L-arginine methyl ester hydrochloride (L-NAME; an NO synthase inhibitor), or their combinations thereof. In contrast, 1H-[1,2,4]oxadiazole[4,3-a]quinoxalin-1-one (ODQ; a soluble guanylyl cyclase inhibitor) enhanced the extract's antinociception. UHPLC analysis revealed the presence of several flavonoid-based compounds with antinociceptive action. In conclusion, MECN exerted the peripherally and centrally mediated antinociceptive activity via the modulation of the opioid/NO-mediated, but cGMP-independent, systems.

1. Introduction

Opioids, such as morphine, and nonsteroidal anti-inflammatory drugs (NSAIDs), such as acetylsalicylic acid, are universally used for the treatment of pain. Although treatments for pain have seen rapid progression, particularly in the field of analgesic drug development, their clinical efficacy and tolerability are often surpassed by the accompanied unwanted adverse effects [1]. Therefore, there is a need to look for an alternative approach to treat pain that has fewer or, possibly, no side effects. Drugs derived from natural sources, especially plants, are vital for the treatment of numerous diseases [2]. The exploration and investigation of plants utilized as pain-relieving agents in traditional ethnomedicine is one of the useful and reasonable strategies in the search for new drugs [3, 4].

Treatment of pain involved the usage of opioids and nonsteroidal anti-inflammatory drugs, and, despite their effectiveness in curing pain, prolonged usage of these classes of drugs has been associated with various unwanted side effects [5]. The risk from NSAID use involves increased GI bleeding and ulceration, increased potential for myocardial infarction, stroke, and Stevens-Johnson syndrome. Opioids, used for moderate-to-severe pain, provide excellent pain relief and are easier to metabolize but have the unwanted effects of sedation, nausea, confusion, and delirium [6]. Other than that, certain types of pain like cancer-related pain are not effectively treated with conventional drugs; thus, patients suffering from this type of pain will seek for alternative treatment [5]. Nowadays the number of patients that are using herbal remedies and complementary and alternative medicine for treatment of pain is growing rapidly [7]. Over the last 20 years, Americans have sought a more "natural" or "holistic" approach to treatment of medical problems in general and pain in particular. Americans spend billions of dollars annually to find a holistic treatment with effective pain relief and few side effects, on complementary and alternative medicine, including herbal therapies [8]. Such increase in popularity and use of CAM by the general public strongly demands that health care professionals have the knowledge to assess, intervene, and advise patients on effective and safe CAM practices [9, 10].

One of the medicinal plants that have gained attention among the scientists is *Clinacanthus nutans* (Burm. f.) Lindau, a plant belonging to the family Acanthaceae. Locally known as "*Belalai Gajah,*" it is a shrub native to the tropical Southeast Asian countries. The fresh leaves are consumed raw as vegetables and mixed with juices and can be used to brew drinks; the dried leaves can be steeped in hot water and served as herbal tea [11]. In Indonesia, Malaysia, and Thailand in particular, the plant is traditionally used in the treatment of skins rashes, insect and snake bites, mental stress, diabetes, rheumatoid arthritis, fever, dysentery, burns, scalds, diarrhea, and herpes skins infections [11]. Scientifically, extracts of *C. nutans* have been shown to exert antibacterial [12], anti-inflammatory [13], antiherpes [14, 15], antioxidant [16], antiproliferative [17], cytotoxic, and antimutagenic [18] activities and demonstrated to affect the immune response when studied *in vivo* (mice) [19] or *in vitro* (human cells) [20]. Moreover, the plant has also been developed into oral-based agent for the treatment of recurrent aphthous stomatitis [21] while the oral toxicity study revealed that *C. nutans* is safe for consumption [22].

Various chemical constituents (i.e., stigmasterol, lupeol, β-sitosterol, betulin, vitexin, isovitexin, schaftoside, isomollupentin-7-O-β-glucopyranoside, orientin, isoorientin, sulfur-containing glucosides, glycoglycerolipids, and monoacylmonogalactosylglycerol) have been isolated and identified from *C. nutans* [11]. However, the bioactivity of some of these compounds still remains to be elucidated. Additionally the presence of *n*-pentadecanol, eicosane, 1-nonadecene, heptadecane, dibutyl phthalate, *n*-tetracosanol-1, heneicosane, behenic alcohol, 1-heptacosanol, 1,2-benzenedicarboxylic acid, mono(2-ethylhexyl) ester, nonadecyl heptafluorobutyrate, eicosanoyl trifluoroacetate, 1,2-benzenedicarboxylic acid, dinonyl ester, phthalic acid, and dodecyl nonyl ester was reported in the chloroform extract of *C. nutans* leaves [19]. Several other compounds have also been identified and further demonstrated to have some degrees of bioactivity. For example, three types of phaeophytins, namely, 13^2-hydroxy-(13^2-*R*)-phaeophytin b, 13^2-hydroxy-(13^2-*S*)-phaeophytin a, and 13^2-hydroxy-(13^2-*R*)-phaeophytin, have been identified from the chloroform extract of *C. nutans* leaves and were reported to exhibit anti-herpes simplex activity [23]. Despite the various reports on pharmacological activity of *C. nutans*, there has been no study on MECN's antinociceptive activity to date. The proposed antinociceptive study is attributed to finding that *C. nutans* exerts anti-inflammatory activity [14] and contains several classes of phytoconstituents (i.e., flavonoids, saponins, and triterpenes) that are strongly associated with antinociceptive activity [13]. Thus, the present study aimed at determining the antinociceptive activity of methanol extract of *C. nutans* (MECN) and to elucidate the possible mechanisms of antinociception involved.

2. Materials and Methods

2.1. Plant Material and Extraction. Fresh *C. nutans* leaves were obtained from Clinnthus Enterprise (Kuala Lumpur, Malaysia) in January 2013. Authentication of the plant was made by Dr. Shamsul Khamis, a botanist from the Institute of Bioscience, Universiti Putra Malaysia, Serdang, Selangor, Malaysia, and a voucher specimen (SK 2679/15) has been deposited at the herbarium of the institute. Extraction was carried out according to the method previously described [24]. To obtain the MECN, 250 g of *C. nutans* leaves, which were dried in an oven at 40°C for 1-2 days and ground into powder form using an electric grinder (RT-08; Rong Tsong Precision Technology, Taichung, Taiwan), was soaked in methanol (Fisher Scientific, Loughborough, England) in the ratio of 1 : 20 (w/v) for 72 hours at room temperature. The supernatant was filtered using a steel filter, cotton wool, and Whatman Number 1 filter paper. The residue underwent the same soaking procedures twice. The supernatant collected from each extraction was pooled and evaporated using a vacuum rotary evaporator (Hei-VAP Value; Heidolph, Schwabach, Germany) at 40°C under reduced pressure. These processes yielded approximately 53 g of dried MECN (yield was 21.2% (w/w)), which was then stored at 4°C until it was used.

2.2. Phytochemical Screening of MECN. The phytochemical screening of fractions was performed according to the conventional protocols as described by Ikhiri et al. [25].

2.3. Chemicals Used in the UHPLC Analysis of MECN. Formic acid, methanol, and LCMS grade acetonitrile were purchased from Merck (Darmstadt, Germany). HPLC grade water was prepared from distilled water using a Milli-Q-system (Millipore, MA, USA) and was used during analytical HPLC analysis. Various pure flavonoid-based standards (HPLC grade) were purchased from Extrasynthese (Lyon, France). All of the other solvents and chemicals used in this study were of analytical grade. Stock and working standards were prepared by dissolving these analytes in 100% methanol. The standard solutions stored at 4°C were stable for at least 3 months.

2.4. UHPLC-ESI Profiling of MECN. The UHPLC system was performed on a Dionex 3000 UHPLC system acquired from Thermo Fisher Scientific (USA) that consists of an autosampler equipped with a column oven, a tray compartment cooler, and a binary pump with built-in solvent degasser. Samples (10 μL) were injected and the chromatographic separation was performed on a BEH C18 UHPLC column, 100 mm × 2.5 μm, 1.7 μm (WATERS) at a flow rate of 0.3 mL/min. The mobile phases used were (A) 0.1% formic acid in water and (B) 0.1% formic acid in acetonitrile. The separation was conducted using the following multistep gradient: initial conditions ($t = 0$ min) were 90% A and 10% B with a linear gradient reaching 15% B at $t = 3$ min. The gradient was then increased to 50% B in the next 7 min ($t = 10$ min) and further increased to 90% B for the next 2 min ($t = 12$ min). Finally, the programme was returned to the initial solvent composition at $t = 17$ min for the next analysis.

The UHPLC system was coupled to a Linear Ion Trap Orbitrap mass spectrometer (Q Exactive) from Thermo Fisher Scientific (USA) equipped with an electrospray ionization (ESI) source. The mass detection was performed in a range of 150–1500 m/z. The ESI source was operated in negative ion mode under the following specific conditions: source voltage: 3.2 kV; sheath gas: 35 arbitrary units; auxiliary gas: 15 arbitrary units; sweep gas: 10 arbitrary units; and capillary temperature: 320°C. Nitrogen (>99.98%) was employed as sheath, auxiliary, and sweep gas. Instrument control and data acquisition were performed with Chameleon 6.8 software and Xcalibur 2.2 software (Thermo Fisher Scientific).

2.5. GC-MS Analysis of MECN. GC-MS analysis of MECN was performed using Agilent 7890A (Agilent Technologies) coupled with MSD quadrupole detector 5975 C (Agilent Technologies). Separation of analytes by gas chromatography was carried out using a Hewlett Packard HP-5MS silica capillary column (30 m × 0.25 mm × 0.25 mm). For GC-MS detection, an electron ionization system with ionizing energy of 70 eV was used. Helium gas (99.999%) was used as the carrier gas at constant flow rate 1 mL/min and an injection volume of 1 μL was employed (split ratio of 1:10), injector temperature was 250°C, and ion-source temperature was 280°C. The oven temperature was programmed from 100°C (isothermal for 2 min), with an increase of 10°C/min, to 200°C and then 12°C/min to 280°C, ending with a 17 min isothermal at 280°C. Mass spectra were taken at 70 eV, a scan interval of 0.5 sec, and fragments from 45 to 450 Da. Total GC running time was 35.50 min. The relative % amount of each component was calculated by comparing its average peak area to the total areas; software adopted to handle mass spectra and chromatograms was a Turbomass. Interpretation on mass spectrum GC-MS was conducted using the database of National Institute Standard and Technology (NIST) having more than 62,000 patterns. The spectrum of the unknown components were compared with the spectrum of the known components stored in the NIST library.

2.6. Experimental Animals. The antinociceptive studies were carried out using either the adult male ICR mice (25–30 g) or Sprague-Dawley rats (150–180 g), which were obtained from the Animal Source Unit, Faculty of Veterinary Medicine, Universiti Putra Malaysia (UPM), Serdang, Malaysia. The animals were kept at room temperature (27 ± 2°C; 70–80% humidity; 12 h light/dark cycle) in the Animal Holding Unit, Faculty of Medicine and Health Science, UPM, for at least 48 h prior to the procedure. Commercial food pellets (Gold Coin Feedmills, Port Klang, Malaysia) and water were supplied *ad libitum*. The animal experimental protocols were in accordance with the current guidelines for the care of laboratory animals and the ethical guidelines for investigations of experimental pain in conscious animals as adopted from Zimmermann [26] and have been approved by the UPM Institutional Animal Care and Use Committee (Ref. Number UPM/IACUC/AUP-R032/2013). The number of animals and intensities of noxious stimuli used were the minimum necessary to demonstrate the consistent effects of the treatments. Experiments were conducted between 0930 and 1830 h to minimize the effects of environmental changes.

2.7. Drugs and Chemicals. Acetylsalicylic acid (ASA), morphine hydrochloride, naloxone hydrochloride, L-arginine (L-arg), Nω-nitro-L-arginine methyl ester hydrochloride (L-NAME), and 1H-[1,2,4]oxadiazole[4,3-a]quinoxalin-1-one (ODQ) were purchased from Sigma-Aldrich (St. Louis, MO, USA). Formaldehyde was purchased from R & M Chemicals (Essex, England). Acetic acid, dimethyl sulfoxide (DMSO), and methanol were purchased from Fisher Scientific (England). Drugs were dissolved in physiological saline (0.9% (w/v) NaCl). Morphine and ASA were prepared by dissolving in distilled water; MECN was dissolved in 10% DMSO (v/v) in distilled water. Control animals received only solvent vehicle. All drugs, chemicals, and MECN solutions were administered in the volume of 10 mL/kg and were freshly prepared just before use. The MECN doses (100, 250, and 500 mg/kg) used were based on our recent acute and subchronic toxicity studies of MECN (personal communication), which were further supported by the previous oral toxicity studies that reported no toxic or sedative effects at the stated doses [22, 27].

2.8. Nociceptive Tests

2.8.1. Acetic Acid-Induced Abdominal Constriction Test. The procedure was conducted as previously described [28]. Mice ($n = 6$) were treated with vehicle (10% DMSO; 10 mL/kg; per os (p.o.); negative control), ASA (100 mg/kg; p.o.; positive control), or MECN (100, 250, and 500 mg/kg; p.o.) for 60 min before the administration of phlogistic agent (0.6% acetic acid; 10 mL/kg; intraperitoneal (i.p.)). The animals were then immediately placed individually in glass cages and 5 min later abdominal constriction resulting from acetic acid injection involving contraction of the abdomen and stretching of at least one hind limb was measured. The number of abdominal constrictions produced was counted cumulatively for 25 min. Antinociceptive activity was expressed as the reduction of the mean number of abdominal constrictions in test groups compared to the control group, calculated as the percentage inhibition of abdominal constrictions (percentage of inhibition) using the following formula: (mean [(control − test group)/control group] × 100%).

2.9. Hot Plate Test. The hot plate test was carried out according to the method previously described [29]. Mice ($n = 6$) were placed on a hot plate (Model 7280; Ugo Basile, Milan, Italy) heated to 50 ± 0.2°C, and the latency to a discomfort reaction was recorded when the animals licked their forepaws or hind paws or jumped. Animals were selected a day prior to the test based on their reactivity: only animals with response latencies of 5–7 sec were used. The discomfort reaction time was recorded before and at 60, 90, 120, 150, 180, and 210 min following the administration of vehicle (10 mL/kg; p.o.; positive control), morphine (5 mg/kg; i.p.), or MECN (100, 250, and 500 mg/kg; p.o.) 60 min before the test. A cut-off time of 20 sec was set to prevent tissue injury. Prolongation of the latency times of the test groups compared with that of the controls, which indicates antinociceptive activity, was used for statistical comparison.

2.10. Formalin-Induced Paw Licking Test. The formalin-induced paw licking test was performed as previously described [30]. Rats ($n = 6$) received vehicle (10 mL/kg; p.o.), ASA (100 mg/kg; p.o.), morphine (5 mg/kg; i.p.), or MECN (100, 250, and 500 mg/kg; p.o.) 60 min before the formalin injection. Nociception was induced by injecting 50 μL formalin (5% v/v) in the intraplantar (i.pl.) region of the right hind paw. Following injection of the phlogistic agent formalin, the animals were immediately placed individually in a transparent observation glass chamber. The duration the animal spent licking the injected paw (considered an indicator of pain) was recorded. The nociceptive response develops in two phases: 0–5 min after formalin injection (early phase, neurogenic pain response) and 15–30 min after formalin injection (late phase, inflammatory pain response), which were recorded.

2.11. Involvement of Opioidergic System. The protocol used was similar to the method previously described [31]. To evaluate the involvement of opioidergic system in the antinociceptive properties of MECN, separate groups of animals ($n = 6$) were treated with the nonselective opioid receptor antagonist naloxone (5 mg/kg; i.p.) 15 min before the administration of vehicle (10 mL/kg; p.o.) or MECN (500 mg/kg; p.o.). The antinociceptive effect was evaluated using the acetic acid-induced abdominal writhing test, hot plate test, and formalin-induced paw licking test as described above.

2.12. Involvement of L-Arg/Nitric Oxide/Cyclic Guanosine Monophosphate Pathway. To investigate the possible contribution of L-arg/nitric oxide/cyclic guanosine monophosphate (L-arg/NO/cGMP) pathway to the antinociceptive effect of MECN, the previously described method was adopted [28]. Mice ($n = 6$) were pretreated with the NO precursor, L-arg (20 mg/kg; i.p.), the NO inhibitor, L-NAME (20 mg/kg; i.p.), the nonspecific guanylyl cyclase inhibitor, ODQ (2 mg/kg; i.p.), or combinations thereof (L-arg + L-NAME or L-arg + ODQ) 5 min before the administration of vehicle (10 mL/kg; p.o.) or MECN (500 mg/kg; p.o.). Sixty minutes after the administration of test solutions, mice were subjected to the acetic acid-induced abdominal writhing test as described earlier.

2.13. Statistical Analysis. Statistical analysis was performed using GraphPad Prism version 6.04 for Windows (GraphPad Software, San Diego, CA, USA). Data are expressed as the mean ± standard error of the mean (SEM). Mean differences between the control and treatment groups were determined using one-way analysis of variance (ANOVA) followed by Tukey's *post hoc* test. In all cases, differences were considered significant if $p < 0.05$.

3. Results

3.1. Phytochemicals Constituents of MECN. Except for alkaloids and tannins, the phytochemicals screening of MECN showed the presence of flavonoids, saponins, steroids, and triterpenes.

3.2. UHPLC Profile of MECN

3.2.1. Identification of Phenolic Compounds in MECN. C. nutans extract was analyzed based on the accurate mass data of the molecular ions, in which ions detected were tentatively identified by their generated molecular formula using the data analysis software (Xcalibur) that provided list of possible elemental formulas. These findings were compared together with the standard flavonoids available in the laboratory and further supported by the thorough survey of the literature (Figure 1). The widely accepted accuracy threshold for confirmation of elemental compositions was established at 5 ppm.

In the present study, major flavonoid compounds found in MECN belonged to the family of flavone *C*-glycoside. The UHPLC-ESI analysis of MECN revealed the presence of 16 phenolic compounds (Table 1). The compounds detected were gallic acid, 4-hydroxybenzoic acid, caffeic acid, coumaric acid, ferulic acid, schaftoside, vitexin, orientin, isoorientin, isovitexin, luteolin, apigenin, forsythosides H, forsythosides I, diosmetin glycoside, and diosmetin.

3.3. GC-MS Profile of MECN. The GC-MS profile of MECN is shown in Figure 2. A total of 39 peaks were identified from MECN with the major compounds constituted of (i) 2-ethyl-oxetane (16.6%), (ii) 9,12,15-octadecatrienoic

TABLE 1: Phenolic compounds tentatively identified in *C. nutans* extract.

Peak number	t_R (min)	$[M\text{-}H]^-$ (m/z)	Error (ppm)	Molecule formula	Proposed compound
1	0.63	169.01270	−2.661	$C_7H_5O_5$	Gallic acid
2	1.22	137.02347	1.091	$C_7H_5O_3$	4-Hydroxybenzoic acid
3	1.51	179.03314	−4.162	$C_9H_7O_4$	Caffeic acid
4	2.55	163.0387	−1.598	$C_9H_7O_3$	Coumaric acid
5	3.06	563.13776	−3.253	$C_{26}H_{27}O_{14}$	Schaftoside
6	3.51	193.04881	−3.757	$C_{10}H_9O_4$	Ferulic acid
7	4.04	431.09622	−2.443	$C_{21}H_{19}O_{10}$	Vitexin
8	4.52	447.09158	−1.359	$C_{21}H_{19}O_{11}$	Orientin
9	5.11	623.19568	−2.193	$C_{29}H_{35}O_{15}$	Forsythoside H
10	5.37	447.09152	−1.158	$C_{21}H_{19}O_{11}$	Isoorientin
11	5.50	623.19604	−2.193	$C_{29}H_{35}O_{15}$	Forsythoside I
12	5.55	431.09644	−1.933	$C_{21}H_{19}O_{10}$	Isovitexin
13	5.70	503.11783	−1.138	$C_{24}H_{24}O_{12}$	Diosmetin glycoside
14	6.85	285.03860	−2.682	$C_{15}H_9O_6$	Luteolin
15	7.66	269.04404	−1.523	$C_{15}H_9O_5$	Apigenin

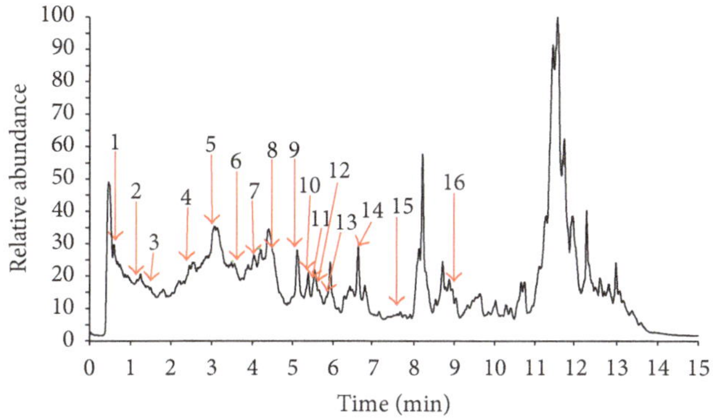

FIGURE 1: TIC (Total Ion Chromatography) profile of UHPLC-ESI of *C. nutans* extract. The numbering peaks correspond to those listed in Table 1.

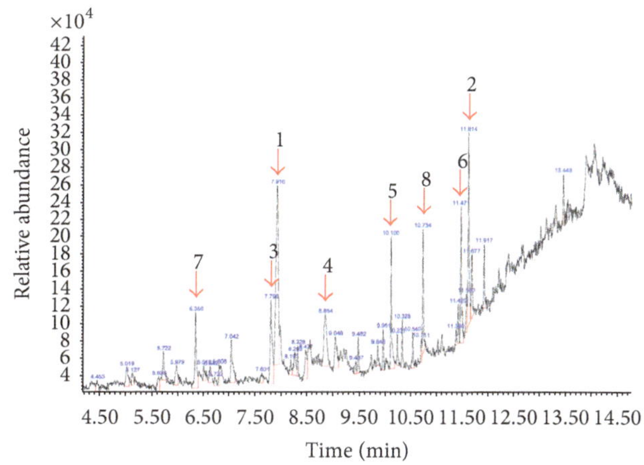

FIGURE 2: GC-MS profile of MECN showing approximately 39 detected peaks with major peaks representing (i) 2-ethyl-oxetane (16.6%), (ii) 9,12,15-octadecatrienoic acid (7.6%), (iii) 2,3-dimethylpyridine (6.4%), (iv) 3-deoxy-D-mannoic lactone (5.7%), (v) neophytadiene (5.4%), (vi) phytol (5.3%), (vii) 2,3-dihydrobenzofuran (4.5%), and (viii) *n*-hexadecanoic acid (4.6%).

acid (7.6%), (iii) 2,3-dimethylpyridine (6.4%), (iv) 3-deoxy-D-mannoic lactone (5.7%), (v) neophytadiene (5.4%), (vi) phytol (5.3%), (vii) 2,3-dihydrobenzofuran (4.5%), and (viii) *n*-hexadecanoic acid (4.6%).

3.4. Acetic Acid-Induced Abdominal Writhing Test. Figure 3 depicts the effect of MECN on acetic acid-induced abdominal writhing in mice. Administration of MECN (100, 250, and 500 mg/kg) *per os* produced significant ($p < 0.001$) and dose-related inhibition in the number of acetic acid-induced abdominal writhing responses. At the tested doses, MECN produced 32.43, 51.35, and 70.26% inhibition of constrictions, respectively, in comparison to the control group. The ED_{50} value recorded for the abdominal constriction test was 279.3 mg/kg. ASA, a standard nonsteroidal anti-inflammatory drug (NSAID), also caused a significant inhibition (46.78%) of acetic acid-induced abdominal writhing, which is equal in strength to the 250 mg/kg MECN.

3.5. Hot Plate Test. The antinociceptive effect of orally administered MECN against thermal-induced nociception is described in Table 2. At 100 and 250 mg/kg, MECN caused no significant changes in response latency to thermal-induced nociception when compared to the control group. In contrast, 500 mg/kg MECN significantly ($p < 0.05$) delayed response latency at the interval of 60 to 210 min after its administration as compared to the control group. Moreover, the opioid agonist, morphine, caused dose-dependent prolongation of latency response time at the interval of 60 to 210 min as compared to the control group (Table 2).

3.6. Formalin-Induced Paw Licking Test. Figure 4 shows the antinociceptive activity of orally administered MECN when assessed using the formalin-induced paw licking test. The extract, at 250 and 500 mg/kg, caused a significant ($p < 0.05$) decrease in the formalin-induced licking time in the first phase (neurogenic phase; 0–5 min; Figure 4(a)) of the

Table 2: Effects of MECN on the hot plate test in mice.

Group	Dose (mg/kg)	Latency of discomfort(s) at respective time interval (min)						
		0 min	60 min	90 min	120 min	150 min	180 min	210 min
10% DMSO		6.29 ± 0.15	6.88 ± 0.29	6.89 ± 0.31	6.28 ± 0.12	6.76 ± 0.43	6.67 ± 0.33	6.46 ± 0.12
Nalox	5	6.55 ± 0.33	6.02 ± 0.34	5.50 ± 0.29	5.53 ± 0.37	5.63 ± 0.09	5.35 ± 0.15	5.20 ± 0.39
	100	6.52 ± 0.24	6.50 ± 0.33	6.23 ± 0.25	6.25 ± 0.21	6.32 ± 0.27	5.99 ± 0.26	6.17 ± 0.22
MECN	250	6.08 ± 0.11	6.28 ± 0.28	6.68 ± 0.22	6.78 ± 0.19	6.59 ± 0.32	6.17 ± 0.18	6.39 ± 0.20
	500	6.65 ± 0.35	10.28 ± 0.81***	9.92 ± 0.55**	9.52 ± 1.08***	9.14 ± 0.51*	9.14 ± 0.36*	8.78 ± 0.81*
Nalox + MECN	5 + 500	6.60 ± 0.38	5.98 ± 0.38#	5.52 ± 0.57#	5.79 ± 0.27#	5.54 ± 0.30#	5.56 ± 0.32#	5.59 ± 0.32#
Morphine	5	6.02 ± 0.15	17.00 ± 0.90***	18.42 ± 0.47***	17.25 ± 0.93***	13.47 ± 1.31***	11.87 ± 1.04***	11.15 ± 0.71***
Morphine + Nalox	5 + 5	6.58 ± 0.24	7.08 ± 0.24#	7.40 ± 0.21#	7.58 ± 0.40#	7.03 ± 0.36#	7.33 ± 0.40#	7.23 ± 0.40#

Mice were treated with vehicle (10 mL/kg, p.o.), MECN (100, 250, and 500 mg/kg, p.o.), or morphine (5 mg/kg, p.o.) 60 min before the test. Naloxone (Nalox, 5 mg/kg, i.p.) was administered 15 min before MECN (500 mg/kg, p.o.), morphine (5 mg/kg, p.o.), or vehicle (10 mL/kg, p.o.). Data expressed are the mean ± SEM of reaction time (sec) of six mice. Statistical analysis was performed using 2-way ANOVA followed by Tukey's *post hoc* test. *$p < 0.05$, **$p < 0.001$, and ***$p < 0.0001$ compared to control; #$p < 0.0001$ compared to 500 mg/kg MECN or morphine-treated group.

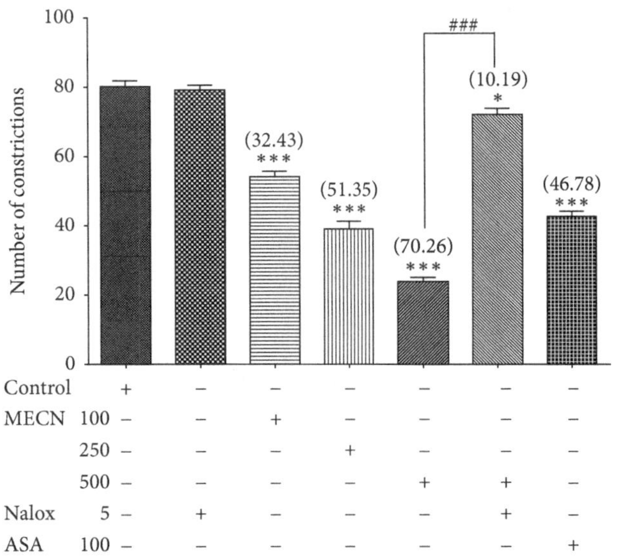

Figure 3: Effect of MECN on acetic acid-induced abdominal constriction in mice. Animals were treated with vehicle (10 mL/kg, p.o.), ASA (100 mg/kg, p.o.), or MECN (100, 250, and 500 mg/kg, p.o.) 60 min before acetic acid (0.6%, 10 mL/kg, i.p.) treatment. Naloxone (Nalox, 5 mg/kg, i.p.) was administered 15 min before MECN (500 mg/kg, p.o.) or vehicle (10 mL/kg, p.o.). Each column represents the mean ± SEM of six mice. Statistical analyses were performed using 1-way ANOVA followed by Tukey's *post hoc* test. *$p < 0.05$, ***$p < 0.001$ compared to control group; ###$p < 0.001$ compared to 500 mg/kg MECN-treated group. Values in parentheses denote percentage of inhibition.

test with the recorded percentage of nociceptive inhibition of 27.03% and 39.64%, respectively. In the second phase (inflammatory phase; 15–30 min; Figure 4(b)) of the test, all doses of MECN decreased the formalin-induced licking time significantly ($p < 0.05$) with the recorded percentage of antinociception ranging between 40 and 74% when compared to the control group. Thus, the recorded ED_{50} value for the early and late phases was >500 mg/kg or 227.7 mg/kg, respectively. Standard drugs, ASA, decreased the licking time significantly ($p < 0.05$) (60.75%) only in the second phase while morphine caused significant ($p < 0.05$) inhibition of the pain response in both phases of formalin test (77.46% and 96.47%, resp.).

3.7. Opioidergic System Involvement. Figure 3, Table 2, and Figures 4(a) and 4(b) depict the involvement of opioid receptors in the antinociceptive effect of MECN assessed using the abdominal constriction-, hot plate-, and formalin-induced paw licking test, respectively. The extract was prechallenged with a nonselective opioid antagonist, naloxone, prior to assessment using various nociceptive models. Used alone, naloxone did not affect acetic acid-induced nociception, whereas pretreatment with naloxone significantly reversed ($p < 0.001$) the antinociceptive effect of MECN.

In the hot plate test, naloxone alone also did not cause any significant changes in the response latency at 60, 90, 120, 150, 180, or 210 min whereas pretreatment with naloxone significantly ($p < 0.05$) blocked the antinociceptive effect of MECN at 60, 90, 120, 150, 180, and 210 min. Naloxone also reversed the antinociceptive effect of opioid agonist, morphine, significantly ($p < 0.05$) at 60, 90, 120, 150, 180, and 210 min.

Moreover, the antinociceptive effect of MECN and morphine in both phases of the formalin test was significantly antagonized at the early phase ($p < 0.01$) and late phase ($p < 0.001$) after pretreatment with naloxone.

3.8. L-Arg/NO/cGMP Pathway Involvement. Figures 5(a) and 5(b) show the effect of L-arg, L-NAME, ODQ, or combinations thereof on antinociceptive activity of MECN assessed using the acetic acid-induced abdominal constriction test. L-arg did not affect the acetic acid-induced nociception in 10% DMSO-treated group but significantly ($p < 0.05$) reversed the antinociceptive activity of MECN. Conversely, L-NAME caused significant ($p < 0.05$) reduction in the acetic acid-induced nociception in 10% DMSO-treated group and significantly ($p < 0.05$) reversed the antinociceptive activity of MECN. On the other hand, pretreatment of a combination between L-arg and L-NAME (as L-arg + L-NAME) exerted significant ($p < 0.05$) antinociceptive activity in the 10%

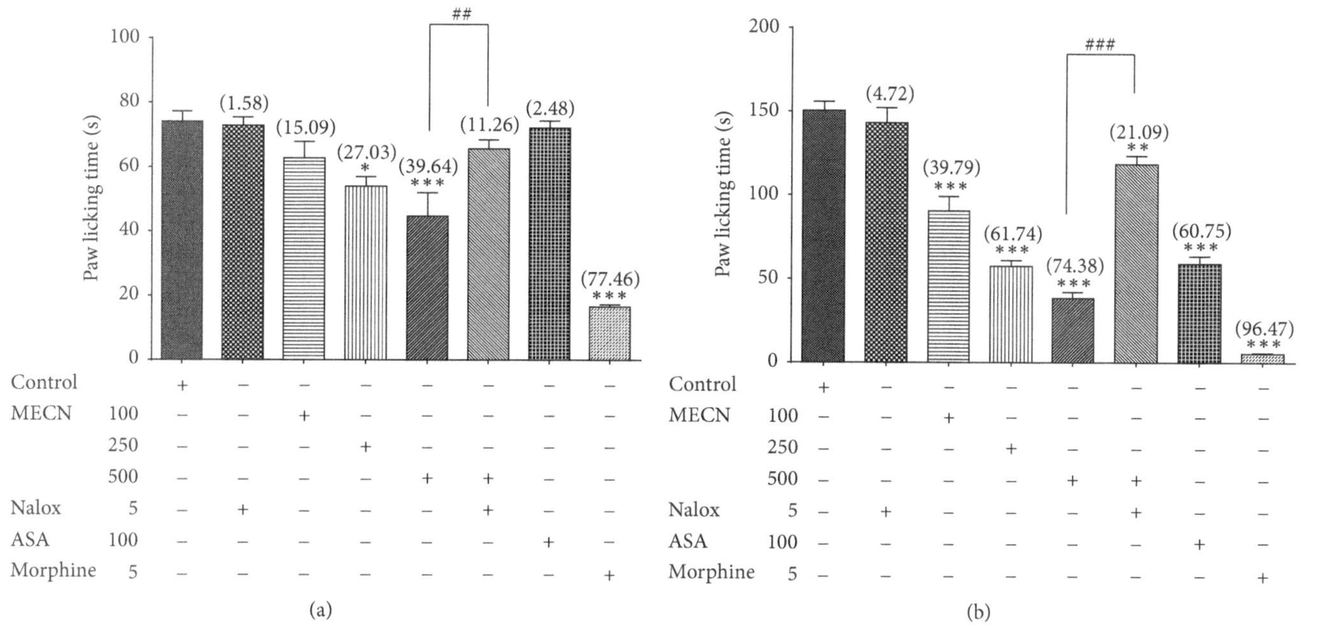

FIGURE 4: Effect of MECN on formalin-induced paw licking in rats. (a) Early phase; (b) late phase. Rats were treated with vehicle (10 mL/kg, p.o.), ASA (100 mg/kg, p.o.), MECN (100, 250, and 500 mg/kg, p.o.), or morphine (5 mg/kg, p.o.) 60 min before intraplantar administration of 5% formalin (50 μL in distilled water) into the right hind paw. Naloxone (Nalox, 5 mg/kg, i.p.) was administered 15 min before MECN (500 mg/kg, p.o.) or vehicle (10 mL/kg, p.o.). Each column represents the mean ± SEM of six rats. Statistical analyses were performed using 1-way ANOVA followed by Tukey's *post hoc* test. $^{*}p < 0.05$, $^{**}p < 0.01$, and $^{***}p < 0.001$ compared to control group; $^{\#\#}p < 0.01$, $^{\#\#\#}p < 0.001$ compared to 500 mg/kg MECN-treated group. Values in parentheses denote percentage of inhibition.

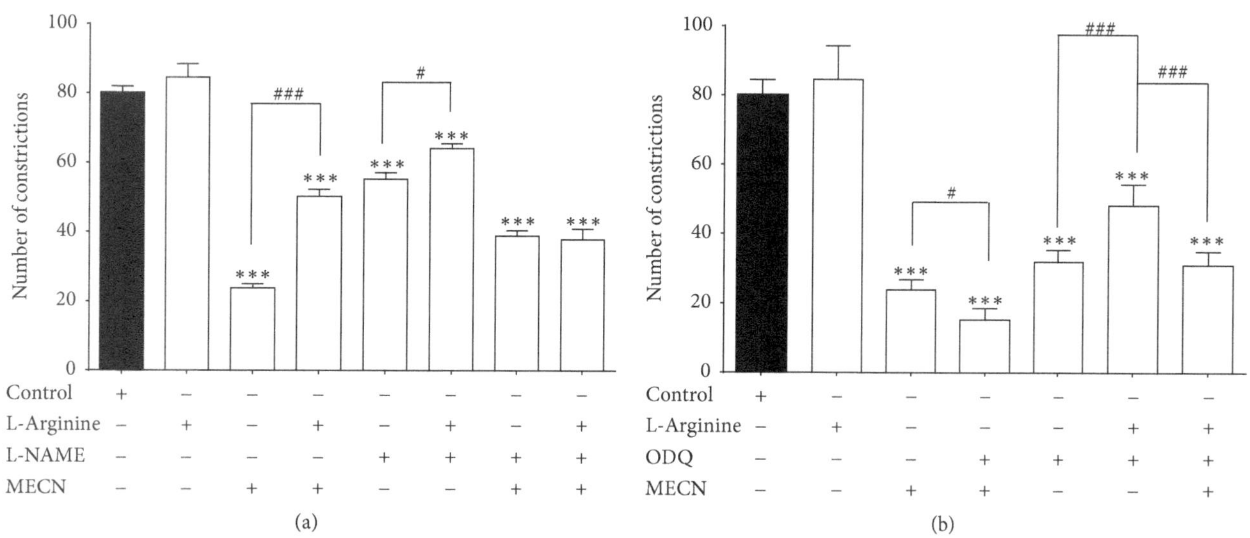

FIGURE 5: The involvement of L-arg/NO/cGMP pathway in the modulation of MECN antinociception as assessed using the abdominal constriction test. (a) Effects of pretreating animals with L-arg, L-NAME, or their combination on the antinociceptive activity of MECN. (b) Effects of L-arg, ODQ, or their combination on the antinociceptive activity of MECN. Animals were treated with MECN (500 mg/kg, p.o.) or vehicle (10 mL/kg, p.o.) 60 min before acetic acid (0.6%, 10 mL/kg, i.p.) treatment. L-arg (20 mg/kg, i.p.), L-NAME (20 mg/kg, i.p.), ODQ (2 mg/kg, i.p.), or combinations thereof (L-arg + L-NAME or L-arg + ODQ) were administered 5 min before MECN (500 mg/kg, p.o.) or vehicle (10 mL/kg, p.o.). Each column represents the mean ± SEM of six mice. Statistical analyses were performed using 1-way ANOVA followed by Tukey's *post hoc* test. $^{***}p < 0.001$ compared to control group; $^{\#}p < 0.05$, $^{\#\#\#}p < 0.001$ compared to 500 mg/kg MECN, L-NAME, L-arg, L-arg + L-NAME, or L-arg + ODQ group.

DMSO-treated group but significantly ($p < 0.05$) reversed the antinociceptive activity of MECN.

Pretreatment with ODQ or a combination between L-arg and ODQ (as L-arg + ODQ) significantly ($p < 0.05$) attenuated the acetic acid-induced nociception in 10% DMSO-treated group but failed to significantly affect the antinociceptive activity of MECN.

4. Discussion

The extract (MECN) demonstrated a wide safety margin and is safe for oral consumption up to the dose of 5000 mg/kg while for the chronic oral consumption the dose is up to 2500 mg/kg, all of which did not cause any toxicity, mortality, or body weight changes. From the acute and subchronic toxicities study, the dose range (100, 250, and 500 mg/kg) for antinociceptive study was determined and decided to be 10-, 20-, and 50-fold reduction of the dose used in acute toxicity study (5000 mg/kg) [32].

Phytochemical screening of MECN revealed the presence of flavonoids, saponins, triterpenes, and steroids, which is in line with previous reports [11, 19, 23, 33]. The UHPLC profiling of MECN demonstrated the presence of several flavonoid-based compounds that belong to the family of flavone *C*-glycoside as reported previously by Chelyn et al. [34]. Sixteen compounds were detected in MECN, namely, gallic acid, 4-hydroxybenzoic acid, caffeic acid, coumaric acid, ferulic acid, schaftoside, vitexin, orientin, isoorientin, danisovitexin, luteolin, apigenin, forsythosides H, forsythosides I, diosmetinacetylglycoside, and diosmetin. Although MECN as a crude extract contains various types of bioactive compounds, flavonoid-based compounds, in part, have been reported to demonstrate antinociceptive activity. Of those detected compounds, at least gallic acid [35], caffeic acid [36], ferulic acid [37], vitexin [38], and apigenin [39] have been reported to exert antinociceptive activity when given orally. These compounds are suggested to work synergistically to exert the observed antinociceptive activity in MECN.

Following the antinociceptive studies, MECN attenuated the chemical-induced (i.e., acetic acid- and formalin-induced) and thermal-induced (i.e., hot plate model) nociceptive models suggesting that the antinociceptive profile of MECN includes peripheral and central mechanisms of action. This suggestion was based on previous claims that any substances that can attenuate the abdominal constriction and hot plate tests [40] or reversed the response latency to formalin-induced nociception in both the early and late phases of formalin test [41] possess peripheral and central antinociceptive activity.

Further postulations could also be made regarding the mechanisms of antinociception exerted by MECN based on the extract ability to attenuate the respective nociceptive model. The abdominal constriction test is a characteristic model for inflammatory pain and is frequently used to investigate the antinociceptive potential of any extracts or natural/synthetic compounds [31]. Positive results obtained from this model also, if not supported by other models, could suggest that the tested extract/compound possesses peripherally mediated antinociceptive activity [42]. According to Ikeda et al. [43], increased level of inflammatory mediators (i.e., cyclooxygenase (COX), prostaglandins (PGs), histamine, serotonin, bradykinin, etc.) upon the administration of acetic acid leads to the excitation of peripheral nociceptive neurons entering dorsal horn of the central nervous system. Therefore, the ability of MECN to attenuate acetic acid-induced nociception indicates the peripheral antinociceptive action partly via the attenuation of several inflammatory mediators' action that lead to impediment of pain transduction at the primary afferent nociceptors. Although considered a sensitive nociception model, this test is also believed to be a nonspecific test as muscle relaxants and other drugs might give false positive results [44].

To avoid misinterpretation of results obtained from the abdominal constriction model, additional experiments using other models of nociception are warranted. The hot plate test is aimed at studying the spinal antinociceptive potential of any tested substances by measuring the animal nociceptive response latencies to thermal stimulus following treatment with the substances. The principal response of thermal-induced nociception occurs predominantly at the supraspinal level [41]. The hot plate test is specifically used to investigate the central antinociceptive potential of any extract/compound and is specifically affected only by the centrally acting drugs (i.e., opioids) [44]. The ability of MECN to reverse the painful thermal stimulus suggests the involvement of central antinociceptive mechanism. However, the fact that highest dose of MECN is required to attenuate thermal-induced nociception indicates that MECN was not a strong agent at the central thermal-stimulated nociceptive pathway.

To further support the suggested involvement of peripheral and central mechanisms in the modulation of antinociceptive activity of MECN, the formalin-induced paw licking test (or formalin test) was adopted. This model can be used to investigate the ability of new extract/compound to affect the peripheral or central nociceptive pathways due to its characteristic biphasic nociception, known as early phase and late phase [24]. The former corresponds to neurogenic pain, is observed immediately after the administration of formalin, and persists for 5 min (0–5 min) as a response to the direct action of formalin on nociceptors in the subplantar region. The late phase corresponds to inflammatory-mediated pain resulting from a tonic response due to the release of inflammatory mediators [24]. The late phase occurs between 15 and 30 min after the administration of formalin. Moreover, the ability to reverse the early phase suggests the extract/compound ability to inhibit the non-inflammatory-mediated nociception while the ability to reverse the late phase suggests the extract potential to inhibit the inflammatory-mediated nociception. From the results obtained from the three models of nociception, MECN is suggested (i) to have peripheral and central antinociceptive action; (ii) to possess antinociceptive activity against both the non-inflammatory-mediated and inflammatory-mediated nociception; and (iii) to exert opioids' characteristic due to its ability to attenuate the peripheral and central models of nociception.

Being the standard drugs for the treatment of pain, opioids effectiveness has been overshadowed by various side effects including dependence and tolerance. In an attempt to find better pain-relieving agents with possibly no or less side effects, the potential of MECN to exert its antinociceptive activity via the opioid receptors was also investigated using the three nociceptive models. From the results obtained, the peripheral and central antinociceptive activities of MECN were blocked by naloxone, a nonselective opioid antagonist, suggesting the involvement of opioid receptor system.

Further study on the involvement of L-arg/NO/cGMP pathway in the MECN-induced antinociceptive effect was also carried out based on previous reports that standard analgesics like morphine also utilized this pathway to exert its analgesic effect. To the best of our knowledge, there has been no attempt to determine the role of L-arg/NO/cGMP pathway in the modulation of antinociceptive activity of MECN. NO production in the body leads to the activation of soluble guanylate cyclase (sGC) and elevation in the cGMP level within the target cells [45]. Despite the various roles played by NO, its involvement in the mechanisms of pain modulation, either as an antinociceptive or as a pronociceptive agent, is well acknowledged and has been attributed to the NO capability to manipulate nociception processing in both the peripheral and central nervous systems [45, 46]. The L-arg/NO/cGMP pathway has been reported to play significant role in the modulation of antinociceptive activity of morphine [46, 47]. Since MECN was shown to possess characteristics of morphine, there is a need to also determine the role of L-arg/NO/cGMP pathway in the antinociceptive activity of MECN. From the results obtained, the presence of NO from the conversion of L-arg did not affect nociception threshold at the respective dose of L-arg used but reduced the antinociceptive intensity of MECN indicating the importance of NO presence. While reduction of NO level due to the administration of L-NAME alone, at the respective dose used, triggered antinociceptive action, it also reversed the antinociceptive activity of MECN. The observations following the administration of L-NAME as described above plausibly suggest that although decrease in NO level triggered antinociception as previously reported, reduced NO did not synergistically enhance or maintain, but reduced, the antinociceptive intensity of MECN. The reason for this observation was not clearly understood, but it is suggested that, at certain concentration of NO reduction, MECN tends to reduce, but not lose, its activity. The ability to maintain the antinociceptive activity also possibly suggested that MECN, which contains several bioactive compounds that exert antinociceptive activity, triggered several antinociceptive mechanisms other than the NO-mediated pathway. NO also increases cGMP levels by activating soluble guanylyl cyclase (sGC), which affects pain and analgesia. The ability of cGMP pathway to affect nociceptive process [48] can be seen when ODQ, which inhibits the cGMP pathway, induced antinociceptive activity when given alone. However, ODQ failed to affect the antinociceptive activity of MECN suggesting that MECN might have triggered an NO-mediated, cGMP-independent pathway. The role of NO-dependent, cGMP-independent pathway in the modulation of antinociceptive activity has been reported elsewhere [49] and might support the present observations. Overall, these observations suggest that the antinociceptive activity of MECN involves the modulation of, partly, L-arg/NO-mediated, but cGMP-independent, pathway. Moreover, based on these observations, the antinociceptive activity of MECN is suggested to involve modulation of different subsets of nociceptive primary sensory neurons.

5. Conclusions

This is the first demonstration that oral systemic administration of MECN has both central and peripheral antinociceptive activities, which occur via the activation of opioid receptors and modulation of the L-arg/NO-mediated, but cGMP-independent, pathway.

Competing Interests

The authors declare no potential competing interests with respect to the research, authorship, and/or publication of this paper.

Acknowledgments

This research was supported by the Fundamental Research Grant Scheme (FRGS; Reference no. R/FRGS/107.00/00290A/001/2014/000175) awarded by the Ministry of Higher Education (MOHE), Malaysia, and the Research Acculturation Collaborative Effort (RACE; Reference no. R/RACE/A07.00/00290A/002/2015/000234) from the Universiti Putra Malaysia, Malaysia. The authors thank the Faculty of Medicine and Health Sciences, Universiti Putra Malaysia, Malaysia, for providing the facilities while doing this research.

References

[1] M. O. Sofidiya, E. Imeh, C. Ezeani, F. R. Aigbe, and A. J. Akindele, "Antinociceptive and anti-inflammatory activities of ethanolic extract of *Alafia barteri*," *Revista Brasileira de Farmacognosia*, vol. 24, no. 3, pp. 348–354, 2014.

[2] K. Pandima Devi, M. Sreepriya, T. Devaki, and K. Balakrishna, "Antinociceptive and hypnotic effects of *Premna tomentosa* L. (Verbenaceae) in experimental animals," *Pharmacology Biochemistry and Behavior*, vol. 75, no. 2, pp. 261–264, 2003.

[3] E. Elisabetsky, T. A. Amador, R. R. Albuquerque, D. S. Nunes, and A. D. C. T. Carvalho, "Analgesic activity of *Psychotria colorata* (Willd. ex R. & S.) Muell. Arg. alkaloids," *Journal of Ethnopharmacology*, vol. 48, no. 2, pp. 77–83, 1995.

[4] H. O. Vongtau, J. Abbah, O. Mosugu et al., "Antinociceptive profile of the methanolic extract of *Neorautanenia mitis* root in rats and mice," *Journal of Ethnopharmacology*, vol. 92, no. 2-3, pp. 317–324, 2004.

[5] M. Khatta, "A complementary approach to pain management," November 2015, http://www.medscape.com/viewarticle/556408.

[6] Y. D'Arcy, "Pain in the older adult: pain assessment," *The Nurse Practitioner*, vol. 33, no. 3, pp. 18–25, 2008.

[7] N. M. Dhanani, T. J. Caruso, and A. J. Carinci, "Complementary and alternative medicine for pain: an evidence-based review,"

Current Pain and Headache Reports, vol. 15, no. 1, pp. 39–46, 2011.

[8] J. H. Wirth, J. C. Hudgins, and J. A. Paice, "Use of herbal therapies to relieve pain: a review of efficacy and adverse effects," *Pain Management Nursing*, vol. 6, no. 4, pp. 145–167, 2005.

[9] N. G. Cuellar, B. Cahill, J. Ford, and T. Aycock, "The development of an educational workshop on complementary and alternative medicine: what every nurse should know," *Journal of Continuing Education in Nursing*, vol. 34, no. 3, pp. 128–135, 2003.

[10] J. M. Wilkinson and P. Tinley, "Knowledge, beliefs, and use of complementary and alternative medicine by Australian podiatric physicians," *Journal of the American Podiatric Medical Association*, vol. 99, no. 2, pp. 121–128, 2009.

[11] S. Y. Shim, I. Aziana, and B. Y. Khoo, "Perspective and insight on *Clinacanthus nutans* Lindau in traditional medicine," *International Journal of Integrative Biology*, vol. 14, no. 1, pp. 7–9, 2013.

[12] D. Huang, W. Guo, J. Gao, J. Chen, and J. Olatunji, "*Clinacanthus nutans* (Burm. f.) Lindau ethanol extract inhibits hepatoma in mice through upregulation of the immune response," *Molecules*, vol. 20, no. 9, pp. 17405–17428, 2015.

[13] S. Y. Ho, W. P. Tiew, M. Priya, S. A. S. Mohamed, and A. A. Gabriel, "Phytochemical analysis and antibacterial activity of methanolic extract of *Clinacanthus nutans* leaf," *International Journal of Drug Development and Research*, vol. 5, no. 3, pp. 349–355, 2013.

[14] P. Wanikiat, A. Panthong, P. Sujayanon, C. Yoosook, A. G. Rossi, and V. Reutrakul, "The anti-inflammatory effects and the inhibition of neutrophil responsiveness by *Barleria lupulina* and *Clinacanthus nutans* extracts," *Journal of Ethnopharmacology*, vol. 116, no. 2, pp. 234–244, 2008.

[15] P. Kunsorn, N. Ruangrungsi, V. Lipipun, A. Khanboon, and K. Rungsihirunrat, "The identities and anti-herpes simplex virus activity of *Clinacanthus nutans* and *Clinacanthus siamensis*," *Asian Pacific Journal of Tropical Biomedicine*, vol. 3, no. 4, pp. 284–290, 2013.

[16] S. Sangkitporn, S. Chaiwat, K. Balachandra, T. D. Na-Ayudhaya, M. Bunjob, and C. Jayavasu, "Treatment of herpes zoster with *Clinacanthus nutans* (bi phaya yaw) extract," *Journal of the Medical Association of Thailand*, vol. 78, no. 11, pp. 624–627, 1995.

[17] B. Sriwanthana, P. Chavalittumrong, and L. Chompuk, "Effect of *Clinacanthus nutans* on human cell-mediated immune response *in vitro*," *The Thai Journal of Pharmaceutical Sciences*, vol. 20, no. 4, pp. 261–267, 1996.

[18] P. Pannangpetch, P. Laupattarakasem, V. Kukongviriyapan, U. Kukongviriyapan, B. Kongyingyoes, and C. Aromdee, "Antioxidant activity and protective effect against oxidative hemolysis of *Clinacanthus nutans* (Burm.f) Lindau," *Songklanakarin Journal of Science and Technology*, vol. 29, no. 1, pp. 1–9, 2007.

[19] Y. K. Yong, J. J. Tan, S. S. Teh et al., "*Clinacanthus nutans* extracts are antioxidant with antiproliferative effect on cultured human cancer cell lines," *Evidence-Based Complementary and Alternative Medicine*, vol. 2013, Article ID 462751, 8 pages, 2013.

[20] S. Rathnasamy, K. B. Mohamed, S. F. Sulaiman, and A. Akinboro, "Evaluation of cytotoxic, mutagenic and antimutagenic potential of leaf extracts of three medicinal plants using *Allium cepa* chromosome assay," *International Current Pharmaceutical Journal*, vol. 2, no. 8, pp. 131–140, 2013.

[21] S. Timpawat and L. Vijrabhava, "Clinical evaluation of *Clinacanthus nutans* Lindau in orabase in the treatment of recurrent *aphthous stomatitis*," *Mahidol Dental Journal*, vol. 14, no. 1, pp. 10–16, 1994.

[22] X. W. P'ng, G. A. Akowuah, and J. H. Chin, "Acute oral toxicity study of *Clinacanthus nutans* in mice," *International Journal of Pharmaceutical Sciences and Research*, vol. 3, no. 11, pp. 4202–4205, 2012.

[23] S. Sakdarat, A. Shuyprom, C. Pientong, T. Ekalaksananan, and S. Thongchai, "Bioactive constituents from the leaves of *Clinacanthus nutans* Lindau," *Bioorganic & Medicinal Chemistry*, vol. 17, no. 5, pp. 1857–1860, 2009.

[24] M. I. Mohamad Yusof, M. Z. Salleh, T. Lay Kek, N. Ahmat, N. F. Nik Azmin, and Z. A. Zakaria, "Activity-guided isolation of bioactive constituents with antinociceptive activity from *Muntingia calabura* L. leaves using the formalin test," *Evidence-Based Complementary and Alternative Medicine*, vol. 2013, Article ID 715074, 9 pages, 2013.

[25] K. Ikhiri, D. Boureima, and D.-D. Dan-Koulodo, "Chemical screening of medicinal plants used in the traditional pharmacopoeia of Niger," *International Journal of Pharmacognosy*, vol. 30, no. 4, pp. 251–262, 1992.

[26] M. Zimmermann, "Ethical guidelines for investigations of experimental pain in conscious animals," *Pain*, vol. 16, no. 2, pp. 109–110, 1983.

[27] X. W. P'ng, G. A. Akowuah, and J. H. Chin, "Evaluation of the sub-acute oral toxic effect of methanol extract of *Clinacanthus nutans* leaves in rats," *Journal of Acute Disease*, vol. 2, no. 1, pp. 29–32, 2013.

[28] N. Abacioğlu, B. Tunçtan, E. Akbulut, and I. Çakici, "Participation of the components of l-arginine/nitric oxide/cGMP cascade by chemical-induced abdominal constriction in the mouse," *Life Sciences*, vol. 67, no. 10, pp. 1127–1137, 2000.

[29] S. G. Wilson, C. D. Bryant, W. R. Lariviere et al., "The heritability of antinociception II: pharmacogenetic mediation of three over-the-counter analgesics in mice," *Journal of Pharmacology and Experimental Therapeutics*, vol. 305, no. 2, pp. 755–764, 2003.

[30] M. H. M. Sani, Z. A. Zakaria, T. Balan, L. K. Teh, and M. Z. Salleh, "Antinociceptive activity of methanol extract of *Muntingia calabura* leaves and the mechanisms of action involved," *Evidence-Based Complementary and Alternative Medicine*, vol. 2012, Article ID 890361, 10 pages, 2012.

[31] Z. A. Zakaria, S. Mustapha, M. R. Sulaiman, A. M. Mat Jais, M. N. Somchit, and F. C. Abdullah, "The antinociceptive action of aqueous extract from *Muntingia calabura* leaves: the role of opioid receptors," *Medical Principles and Practice*, vol. 16, no. 2, pp. 130–136, 2007.

[32] Z. A. Zakaria, M. H. Rahim, N. Mohtarrudin et al., "Acute and sub-chronic oral toxicity studies of methanol extract of *Clinacanthus nutans* in mice," *African Journal of Traditional, Complementary and Alternative Medicines*, vol. 13, no. 2, p. 210, 2016.

[33] P. Tuntiwachwuttikul, Y. Pootaeng-On, P. Phansa, and W. C. Taylor, "Cerebrosides and a monoacylmonogalactosylglycerol from *Clinacanthus nutans*," *Chemical and Pharmaceutical Bulletin*, vol. 52, no. 1, pp. 27–32, 2004.

[34] J. L. Chelyn, M. H. Omar, N. S. Mohd Yousof, R. Ranggasamy, M. I. Wasiman, and Z. Ismail, "Analysis of flavone *C*-glycosides in the leaves of *Clinacanthus nutans* (Burm. f.) Lindau by HPTLC and HPLC-UV/DAD," *The Scientific World Journal*, vol. 2014, Article ID 724267, 6 pages, 2014.

[35] G. Trevisan, M. F. Rossato, R. Tonello et al., "Gallic acid functions as a TRPA1 antagonist with relevant antinociceptive and antiedematogenic effects in mice," *Naunyn-Schmiedeberg's Archives of Pharmacology*, vol. 387, no. 7, pp. 679–689, 2014.

[36] A. Mehrotra, R. Shanbhag, M. R. Chamallamudi, V. P. Singh, and J. Mudgal, "Ameliorative effect of caffeic acid against inflammatory pain in rodents," *European Journal of Pharmacology*, vol. 666, no. 1–3, pp. 80–86, 2011.

[37] W.-H. Lv, L. Zhang, S.-J. Wu, S.-Z. Chen, X.-B. Zhu, and J.-C. Pan, "Analgesic effect of ferulic acid on CCI mice: behavior and neurobiological analysis," *Zhongguo Zhong Yao Za Zhi*, vol. 38, no. 21, pp. 3736–3741, 2013.

[38] S. M. Borghi, T. T. Carvalho, L. Staurengo-Ferrari et al., "Vitexin inhibits inflammatory pain in mice by targeting TRPV1, oxidative stress, and cytokines," *Journal of Natural Products*, vol. 76, no. 6, pp. 1141–1149, 2013.

[39] M. M. G. Pinheiro, F. Boylan, and P. D. Fernandes, "Antinociceptive effect of the *Orbignya speciosa* Mart. (Babassu) leaves: evidence for the involvement of apigenin," *Life Sciences*, vol. 91, no. 9-10, pp. 293–300, 2012.

[40] A. Khatun, M. Z. Imam, and M. S. Rana, "Antinociceptive effect of methanol extract of leaves of *Persicaria hydropiper* in mice," *BMC Complementary & Alternative Medicine*, vol. 15, article 63, 2015.

[41] M. Rezaee-Asl, M. Sabour, V. Nikoui, S. Ostadhadi, and A. Bakhtiarian, "The study of analgesic effects of *Leonurus cardiaca* L. in mice by formalin, tail flick and hot plate tests," *International Scholarly Research Notices*, vol. 2014, Article ID 687697, 5 pages, 2014.

[42] S. Trongsakul, A. Panthong, D. Kanjanapothi, and T. Taesotikul, "The analgesic, antipyretic and anti-inflammatory activity of *Diospyros variegata* Kruz.," *Journal of Ethnopharmacology*, vol. 85, no. 2-3, pp. 221–225, 2003.

[43] Y. Ikeda, A. Ueno, H. Naraba, and S. Oh-Ishi, "Involvement of vanilloid receptor VR1 and prostanoids in the acid-induced writhing responses of mice," *Life Sciences*, vol. 69, no. 24, pp. 2911–2919, 2001.

[44] D. Le Bars, M. Gozariu, and S. W. Cadden, "Animal models of nociception," *Pharmacological Reviews*, vol. 53, no. 4, pp. 597–652, 2001.

[45] Z. A. Zakaria, M. R. Sulaiman, M. N. Somchit, A. M. M. Jais, and D. I. Ali, "The effects of l-arginine, d-arginine, l-name and methylene blue on *Channa striatus*-induced peripheral antinociception in mice," *Journal of Pharmacy and Pharmaceutical Sciences*, vol. 8, no. 2, pp. 199–206, 2005.

[46] Y. Cury, G. Picolo, V. P. Gutierrez, and S. H. Ferreira, "Pain and analgesia: the dual effect of nitric oxide in the nociceptive system," *Nitric Oxide*, vol. 25, no. 3, pp. 243–254, 2011.

[47] V. Granados-Soto, M. D. O. Rufino, L. D. Gomes Lopes, and S. H. Ferreira, "Evidence for the involvement of the nitric oxide-cGMP pathway in the antinociception of morphine in the formalin tests," *European Journal of Pharmacology*, vol. 340, no. 2-3, pp. 177–180, 1997.

[48] D. Sachs, F. Q. Cunha, and S. H. Ferreira, "Peripheral analgesic blockade of hypernociception: activation of arginine/NO/cGMP/protein kinase G/ATP-sensitive K^+ channel pathway," *Proceedings of the National Academy of Sciences of the United States of America*, vol. 101, no. 10, pp. 3680–3685, 2004.

[49] N. Morioka, A. Inoue, T. Hanada et al., "Nitric oxide synergistically potentiates interleukin-1β-induced increase of cyclooxygenase-2 mRNA levels, resulting in the facilitation of substance P release from primary afferent neurons: involvement of cGMP-independent mechanisms," *Neuropharmacology*, vol. 43, no. 5, pp. 868–876, 2002.

7

A Meta-Analysis of Randomized Controlled Trials of Yiqi Yangyin Huoxue Method in Treating Diabetic Nephropathy

Jiao Ying Ou,[1,2,3,4] Di Huang,[1,2,3] Yan Sheng Wu,[1,2,3] Lin Xu,[1,2,3] Fei He,[1,2,3] Hui Ling Wang,[1,2,3] Li Qiang Shi,[1,2,3] Qiang Wan,[1,2,3] Li Qun He,[1,2,3] and Jian Dong Gao[1,2,3]

[1] *Department of Nephrology, Shuguang Hospital, Shanghai University of Traditional Chinese Medicine, No. 528 Zhang Heng Road, Shanghai 201203, China*
[2] *TCM Institute of Kidney Disease, Shanghai University of Traditional Chinese Medicine, No. 528 Zhang Heng Road, Shanghai 201203, China*
[3] *Shanghai Key Laboratory of Traditional Chinese Clinical Medicine, No. 528 Zhang Heng Road, Shanghai 201203, China*
[4] *Department of Internal Medicine, Shanghai TCM-Integrated Hospital of Shanghai University of Traditional Chinese Medicine, No. 184 Baoding Road, Shanghai 200082, China*

Correspondence should be addressed to Jian Dong Gao; gaojiandong@hotmail.com

Academic Editor: Kieran Cooley

Objective. The purpose of this systematic review is to evaluate the evidence of Yiqi Yangyin Huoxue Method for diabetic nephropathy. *Methods.* 11 electronic databases, through September 2015, were searched to identify randomized controlled trials of Yiqi Yangyin Huoxue Method for diabetic nephropathy. The quality of the included trials was assessed using the Jadad scale. *Results.* 26 randomized controlled trials were included in our review. Of all the included trials, most of them were considered as high quality. The aggregated results suggested that Yiqi Yangyin Huoxue Method is beneficial to diabetic nephropathy in bringing down the microalbuminuria (SMD = −0.98, 95% CI −1.22 to −0.74), serum creatinine (SMD = −0.56, 95% CI −0.93 to −0.20), beta-2 microglobulin (MD = 0.06, 95% CI 0.01 to 0.12), fasting plasma glucose (MD = −0.35, 95% CI −0.62 to −0.08), and 2-hour postprandial blood glucose (MD = 1.13, 95% CI 0.07 to 2.20), but not in decreasing blood urea nitrogen (SMD = −0.72, 95% CI −1.47 to 0.02) or 2-hour postprandial blood glucose (SMD = −0.48, 95% CI −1.01 to 0.04). *Conclusions.* Yiqi Yangyin Huoxue Method should be a valid complementary and alternative therapy in the management of diabetic nephropathy, especially in improving UAER, serum creatinine, fasting blood glucose, and beta-2 microglobulin. However, more studies with long follow-up are warrant to confirm the current findings.

1. Introduction

Diabetic nephropathy (DN) is one of the common complications of diabetes. Due to the increase in the global prevalence of diabetes, the incidence of diabetic nephropathy is rising year by year, the data has shown that there are 30–40% type 1 diabetes mellitus (T1DM) and type 2 diabetes mellitus (T2DM) for the development of DN [1]. In Western countries the ratio is higher, about 37%–40% of the patients with DN ESRD, which is currently the primary cause of end-stage renal disease [2]. In China, about 30% of type 1 diabetes and 20% of type 2 diabetes developed into DN, of which about 53% of the patients died of renal failure caused by diabetic nephropathy [3]. For hundreds of years, Chinese clinicians have accumulated rich clinical experience in the treatment of chronic kidney disease (CKD) and DN.

It has been recorded that Chinese medicine had been used to treat CKD and DN for at least two thousand years. Nowadays, Chinese herbal medicine is still widely used in the treatment of chronic kidney disease and DN. Herbs that act to tonify qi and yin and invigorate blood (Yiqi Yangyin Huoxue) were beneficial for DN in many clinical trials. The studies of Yiqi Yangyin Huoxue Method for diabetic nephropathy have been conducted; however, owing to the low quality of the reported trials, the effect of Yiqi Yangyin Huoxue Method for diabetic nephropathy remains less defined. Therefore, the purpose of this review is to evaluate the evidence of Yiqi Yangyin Huoxue Method for diabetic nephropathy by investigating related trials. To our knowledge, this is a comprehensive review summarizing the efficacy of Yiqi Yangyin Huoxue Method for diabetic nephropathy focusing on the urinary albumin excretion rate (UAER), serum creatinine (SCr), urine beta-2 microglobulin, fasting plasma glucose (FBG), and so forth. Based on our findings, scientific evaluation on the efficacy of Yiqi Yangyin Huoxue Method for diabetic nephropathy will be offered.

2. Methods

2.1. Search Strategy. The following electronic databases through September 2015 were searched: China Knowledge Resource Integrated (CNKI), Wanfang Data, VIP, Social Science Journal, Sinomed, PubMed, EMBASE, Cochrane Library, Sciverse science direc, Springer, and OVID. The following key words were used in combination, Yiqi Yangyin Huoxue, Supplementing qi, nourishing yin, activating blood circulation, diabetic nephropathy, diabetes, kidney disease, renal disease, and random. The reference lists of selected reviews were also screened. In order to identify unpublished studies, dissertations and trial registrations were searched. And we contacted experts in the field.

2.2. Study Selection

2.2.1. Inclusion Criteria. The studies that met the following criteria were included: (1) study design included randomized controlled trials (RCTs) or quasirandomized controlled trials; (2) the target population was patients diagnosed with diabetic nephropathy (Mogensen I–IV) [4]; (3) the main intervention should be Yiqi Yangyin Huoxue herbs plus routine treatment compared with control group with only routine treatment (diabetic diet plus exercise plus hypoglycemic drugs or insulin); (4) the outcomes included the microalbuminuria excretion, serum creatinine, urine beta-2 microglobulin, and fasting plasma glucose; (5) the study was available in either English or Chinese.

2.2.2. Exclusion Criteria. The trials that met the following criteria were excluded: (1) Yiqi Yangyin Huoxue herbs were used as an adjuvant treatment; (2) the target population was incongruent with diagnostic criteria of DN; (3) the main intervention was mixed with too many measures; (4) the study was not allocated with appropriate comparator or without randomization; (5) the studies with data unavailable or duplicate publication were excluded.

2.2.3. Intervention. The treatment group and control group were all given the routine treatment for diabetic nephropathy (diabetic diet plus exercise plus hypoglycemic drugs or insulin), while the treatment was intervened by Yiqi Yangyin Huoxue herbs on the basis of routine treatment.

2.3. Literature Screening. Literature screening was performed by two authors (Di Huang and Jian Dong Gao) independently. They screened literature on the inclusion criteria. All identified abstracts and full texts of potentially relevant abstracts were screened independently by two authors. The corresponding author was contacted when relevant information was not reported. And disagreements were resolved by consensus among authors.

2.4. Methodological Quality Assessment. The quality of the eligible studies was assessed by Jadad scale [5]. It assesses the quality of published clinical trials based Methods relevant to random assignment, double blinding, and the flow of patients. There are 11 items. The range of possible scores is 0 (bad) to 5 (good) (the trial that attracts 1-2 scores was considered as low quality, while that with 3–5 means high quality) [6, 7]: (1) was the Method used to generate the sequence of randomization described? (2) Was the Method used to generate the sequence of randomization described as computer-generated? (+2 Points); (3) the study was described as randomized, but the Method used to generate the sequence of randomization was not described (+1 Point); (4) the study was described as quasirandomized (+0 Points); (5) was the study described as double blind? (+1 Point); (6) was the Method of double blinding described and appropriate (identical placebo, active placebo, dummy, etc.)? (+2 Points); (7) the Method of double blinding was described only (+1 Point); (8) the Method of double blinding was described, but inappropriate (+0 Points); (9) was there a description of withdrawals and dropouts? (10) the withdrawals and dropouts were described in detail (+1 Point); and (11) the withdrawals and dropouts were not mentioned (+0 Points). The corresponding author was contacted when relevant information was not reported.

2.5. Data Abstraction. Three reviewers independently extracted data onto predefined criteria in Table 1. The information extracted from the participants was gender, age, nation, diagnosis Method, and course of disease. The outcome measures extracted from the trial were microalbuminuria, serum creatinine, urine beta-2 microglobulin, fasting plasma glucose, and so forth.

2.6. Data Synthesis and Analysis. We employed the Cochrane Collaboration software (Review Manager Version 5.3 for Windows; Copenhagen: The Nordic Cochrane Centre) for meta-analysis. The heterogeneity was assessed with chi-square test. If the heterogeneity test results were $p > 0.05$, then there is homogeneity in multiple independent trials and fixed effect model was adopted. If heterogeneity test results were $p \leq 0.05$, then there is heterogeneity in multiple independent studies and the random effect model was used. The mean differences and 95% confidence interval were adopted as the effect of expression. The effect size was tested with hypothesis test—z test. If $p \leq 0.05$, there is a statistical significance in the research of multiple combined statistics; if $p > 0.05$, there is no statistical significance in the merged statistic. When the experimental effect index value is equal to

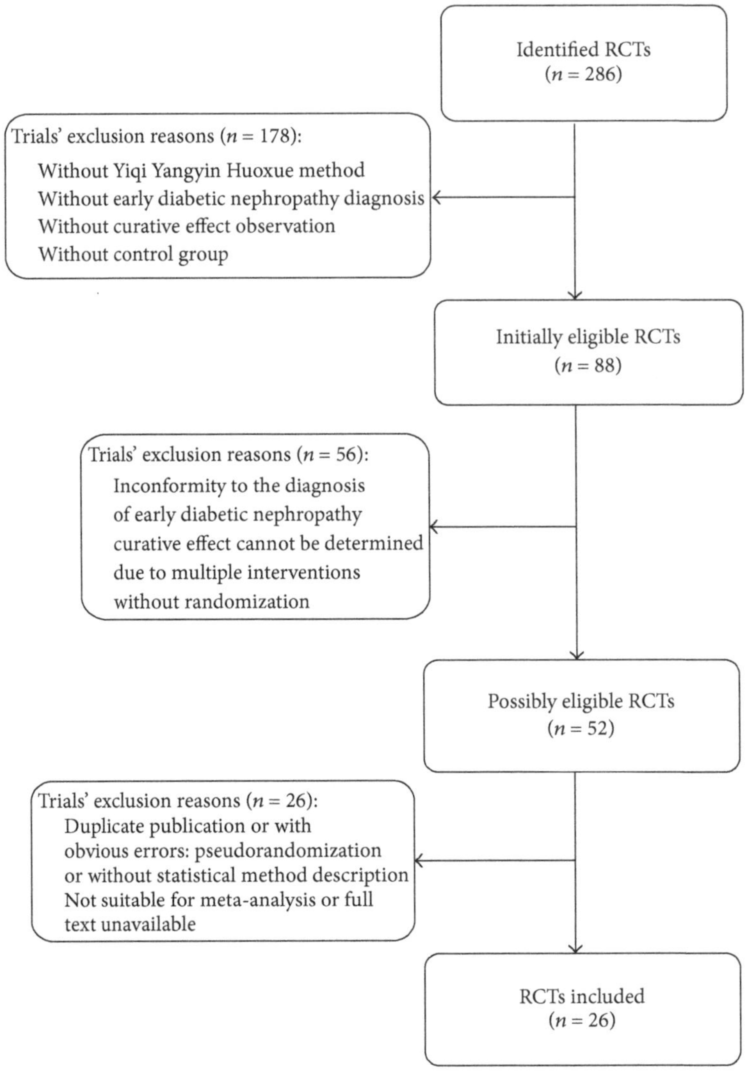

FIGURE 1: Flow diagram.

0, the MD experiment effect is invalid, which means its 95% CI contains 0 and it is equivalent to $p > 0.05$; namely, there is no statistical significance, if the upper and lower limits do not contain 0 (were greater than 0 or less than 0), which means being equivalent to $p < 0.05$ and it is statistically significant. The confidence of estimates of effect was assessed based on GRADE Working Group grades of evidence, high quality: further research is very unlikely to change our confidence in the estimate of effect; moderate quality: further research is likely to have an important impact on our confidence in the estimate of effect and may change the estimate; low quality: further research is very likely to have an important impact on our confidence in the estimate of effect and is likely to change the estimate; and very low quality: we are very uncertain about the estimate.

3. Results

3.1. Literature Search. 286 records were identified from 11 English and Chinese databases (Figure 1). After removing duplicates, 108 potentially relevant abstracts were initially screened, and 178 were excluded for failing to meet the inclusion criteria. We retrieved and reviewed 52 full-text articles. 26 [8–33] studies were excluded due to nonrandomized, duplicate publications, suspicion of counterfeit, and failure to get available data. 26 RCTs of them were eligible [34–59]. No dissertations and trial registrations were obtained. The characteristic of selected studies was shown in Table 1.

3.2. Study Characteristics. 17 out of the 26 RCTs were high quality trials, one for 5 points, eight for 4 points, and eight for 3 points and the rest of the 9 were relatively low, only 2 points. Randomization was conducted in all articles, of which there are 2 with allocation concealment; 7 mentioned the blinding and the withdrawals and dropouts or resign were mentioned in 4 trials. We were not able to perform a sensitivity analysis on the quality of the trials due to the shortage of single-end report (Table 2).

Table 1: The characteristics of the eligible studies.

Year	First author	Nation	Course of disease (month)	Case (T/C)	Intervention group	Control group	Course of treatment (week)	Outcome measures	Follow-up (month)
2000	Fang [34]	China	103.2	50/50	Yiqi Yangyin Huoxue + routine treatment	Routine treatment	8	Symptom score, FBG, UAER, and urine beta-2 microglobulin	NMT
2002	Lan [35]	China	60~120	40/30	Yiqi Yangyin Huoxue + routine treatment	Routine treatment + pancreatic kininogenase enteric-coated tablets	4	UAER, Symptom score	NMT
2002	Fan [36]	China	69.36 ± 24.08	34/31	Yiqi Yangyin Huoxue + routine treatment	Routine treatment	8	Symptom score, UAER, and FBG	NMT
2007	Wu [37]	China	NMT	26/24	Yiqi Yangyin Huoxue + routine treatment	Routine treatment	8	Symptoms, FBG, 2hPBG, and UAER	NMT
2008	Si [38]	China	220.8	34/32	Yiqi Yangyin Huoxue + routine treatment	Routine treatment	3~4	UAER, FBG, and PBG	NMT
2009	Xiaochao [39]	China	111.6	50/46	Yiqi Yangyin Huoxue + routine treatment	Routine treatment	8	Symptom score, UAER, and blood sugar	NMT
2010	Jin [40]	China	120	46/42	Yiqi Yangyin Huoxue + routine treatment	Routine treatment	8	Symptom score, UAER, FBG, and creatinine	NMT
2010	Xiaozhou [41]	China	158.4	35/34	Yiqi Yangyin Huoxue + routine treatment	Routine treatment	12	UAER, FBG, and creatinine	NMT
2011	Hui [42]	China	48~114	20/20	Yiqi Yangyin Huoxue + routine treatment	Routine treatment	4	UAER	NMT
2011	Fang [43]	China	134.4	32/32	Yiqi Yangyin Huoxue + routine treatment	Routine treatment	8	FBG, 2hPBG, and UAER	NMT
2011	Xiu [44]	China	122.16~171	30/30	Yiqi Yangyin Huoxue + routine treatment	Routine treatment	12	UAER, urea nitrogen, and creatinine	NMT
2012	Xianyu [45]	China	NMT	32/28	Yiqi Yangyin Huoxue + routine treatment	Routine treatment	8	FBG, 2hPBG, and UAER	NMT
2012	Sheng [46]	China	82.8~97.2	32/32	Yiqi Yangyin Huoxue + routine treatment	Routine treatment	8	UAER, urea nitrogen, creatinine, and FBG	NMT
2012	Guiying [47]	China	100.2	28/27	Yiqi Yangyin Huoxue + routine treatment	Routine treatment	8	Symptom score, UAER	NMT
2012	Gengliang [48]	China	72~94	40/40	Yiqi Yangyin Huoxue + routine treatment	Routine treatment	8	UAER	NMT
2012	Baowen [49]	China	18~96	60/60	Yiqi Yangyin Huoxue + routine treatment	Routine treatment	12	FBG, UAER, urea nitrogen, and creatinine	NMT
2013	Enli [50]	China	14.75~20.06	30/30	Yiqi Yangyin Huoxue + routine treatment	Routine treatment	8	FBG, 2hPBG, and UAER	NMT
2013	Xiaomin [51]	China	15.6~291.6	60/60	Yiqi Yangyin Huoxue + routine treatment	Routine treatment + benazepril	8	FBG, UAER	NMT
2013	Jing [52]	China	NMT	27/13	Yiqi Yangyin Huoxue + routine treatment	Routine treatment +placebo	12	UAER	NMT
2013	Jie [53]	China	68.4~108	60/60	Yiqi Yangyin Huoxue + routine treatment	Routine treatment + benazepril	8	FBG, 2hPBG	NMT
2013	Xiao [54]	China	59.04~136.68	34/34	Yiqi Yangyin Huoxue + routine treatment	Routine treatment	8	FBG, UAER, urea nitrogen, and creatinine	NMT
2013	Shijing [55]	China	8~180	41/41	Yiqi Yangyin Huoxue + routine treatment	Routine treatment	8	FBG, 2hPBG, UAER, urea nitrogen, and creatinine	NMT

Table 1: Continued.

Year	First author	Nation	Course of disease (month)	Case (T/C)	Intervention group	Control group	Course of treatment (week)	Outcome measures	Follow-up (month)
2013	Wu [56]	China	36~204	32/32	Yiqi Yangyin Huoxue + routine treatment	Routine treatment	12	FBG, UAER, and creatinine	NMT
2013	Rui [57]	China	1~156	30/30	Yiqi Yangyin Huoxue + routine treatment	Routine treatment	12	FBG, UAER	NMT
2014	Liucun [58]	China	31.02~134.4	44/42	Yiqi Yangyin Huoxue + routine treatment	Routine treatment	8	UAER, urea nitrogen, and creatinine	NMT
2015	Maoqing [59]	China	12~180	39/39	Yiqi Yangyin Huoxue + routine treatment	Routine treatment	24	FBG, UAER, and urea nitrogen	2015

NMT: not mentioned; FBG: fasting blood-glucose; UAER: urinary albumin excretion rate; PBG: postmeal blood glucose.

Table 2: Methodological quality assessment.

Year	First author	Randomization	Blinding	Allocation concealment	Withdrawals and dropouts	Reason of dropouts and withdrawals	Jadad score
2000	Fang [34]	Yes	Yes	NMT	NMT	No	3
2002	Lan [35]	Yes	No	NMT	NMT	No	2
2002	Fan [36]	Yes	No	NMT	NMT	No	2
2007	Wu [37]	Yes	No	NMT	NMT	No	2
2008	Si [38]	Yes	No	NMT	NMT	No	2
2009	Xiaochao [39]	Yes	No	NMT	NMT	No	2
2010	Jin [40]	Yes	No	NMT	NMT	No	2
2010	Xiaozhou [41]	Yes	Yes	NMT	MT	Yes	4
2011	Hui [42]	Yes	No	NMT	NMT	No	2
2011	Fang [43]	Yes	Yes	NMT	NMT	No	3
2011	Xiu [44]	Yes	Yes	MT	NMT	No	4
2012	Xianyu [45]	Yes	No	NMT	NMT	No	2
2012	Sheng [46]	Yes	No	NMT	NMT	No	2
2012	Guiying [47]	Yes	Yes	NMT	MT	Yes	4
2012	Gengliang [48]	Yes	Yes	NMT	MT	Yes	4
2012	Baowen [49]	Yes	Yes	MT	MT	Yes	5
2013	Enli [50]	Yes	No	NMT	NMT	No	2
2013	Xiaomin [51]	Yes	No	NMT	NMT	No	2
2013	Jing [52]	Yes	No	NMT	NMT	No	2
2013	Jie [53]	Yes	No	NMT	NMT	No	2
2013	Xiao [54]	Yes	No	NMT	NMT	No	2
2013	Shijing [55]	Yes	No	NMT	NMT	No	2
2013	Wu [56]	Yes	No	NMT	NMT	No	2
2013	Wu [57]	Yes	No	NMT	NMT	No	2
2014	Liucun [58]	Yes	No	NMT	NMT	No	2
2015	Maoqing [59]	Yes	No	NMT	NMT	No	2

MT: mentioned; NMT: not mentioned.

3.3. Quantitative Data Synthesis

3.3.1. Microalbuminuria (UAER). According to the urine microprotein changes in forest plot, the effect size of the 22 selected trials [35–37, 39–44, 46–52, 54–59] was SMD = −0.98 and 95% CI −1.22 to −0.74; test of the effect size was $z = 8.02$ and $p < 0.00001$; and the heterogeneity analysis ($p < 0.05$) suggests that there is heterogeneity in 22 articles; therefore random effect model was used. The aggregated results of 21 RCTs [35, 36, 39–44, 46–52, 54–59] suggested that Yiqi Yangyin Huoxue Method showed favorable effects for decreasing microalbuminuria of diabetic nephropathy, while one trial failed to prove the effect [34]. There was moderate quality of evidence on improving UAER based on GRADE.

3.3.2. Blood Urea Nitrogen. According to the blood urea nitrogen changes in forest plot, the effect size of the 6 selected trials [44, 49, 54, 55, 58, 59] was SMD = −0.72, 95% CI −1.47 to 0.02; test of the effect size was $z = 1.90$, $p = 0.06$; and the heterogeneity analysis ($p < 0.05$) suggests that there is heterogeneity in 6 articles. The aggregated results of 6 RCTs suggested that Yiqi Yangyin Huoxue Method did not show favorable effects for lowering blood urea nitrogen level of diabetic nephropathy. There was moderate quality of evidence on improving blood urea nitrogen based on GRADE (Figure 2).

3.3.3. Serum Creatinine. According to the serum creatinine changes in forest plot, the effect size of the 6 selected trials [37, 40, 44, 49, 56, 58] was SMD = −0.56, 95% CI −0.93 to −0.20; test of the effect size was $z = 3.02$, $p = 0.003$; the heterogeneity analysis ($p = 0.002$) suggests that there is heterogeneity in 6 articles. The aggregated results of 4 RCTs [44, 49, 56, 58] suggested that Yiqi Yangyin Huoxue Method showed favorable effects for decreasing serum creatinine of diabetic nephropathy while the other 2 trials [37, 40] failed to show this effect. There was moderate quality of evidence on improving serum creatinine based on GRADE (Figure 2).

3.3.4. Beta-2 Microglobulin. According to the blood urea nitrogen changes in forest plot, the effect size of the 2 selected trials [36, 37] was MD = 0.06, 95% CI 0.01 to 0.12; test of the effect size was $z = 2.32$, $p = 0.02$; the heterogeneity analysis ($p > 0.05$) suggests that there is homogeneity in 2 articles.

Study or subgroup	Experimental Mean	Experimental SD	Experimental Total	Control Mean	Control SD	Control Total	Weight	Std. mean difference IV, random, 95% CI	Year
1.1.1 UAER									
Lan and Lijia, 2002	−72.4	21.8	40	−44.7	20.62	30	4.6%	−1.29 [−1.81, −0.76]	2002
Fan et al., 2002	−88.5	29.23	34	−15.4	32.58	31	4.1%	−2.34 [−2.98, −1.70]	2002
Wu et al., 2007	−45.32	42.22	26	−25.52	46.41	24	4.4%	−0.44 [−1.00, 0.12]	2007
Xiaochao et al., 2009	−39.7	43.05	50	−1.97	55.4	46	5.0%	−0.76 [−1.17, −0.34]	2009
Xiaozhou et al., 2010	−72.55	37.23	35	−54.1	38.41	34	4.8%	−0.48 [−0.96, −0.00]	2010
Jin et al., 2010	−33.79	44.52	46	−16.32	44.05	42	5.0%	−0.39 [−0.81, 0.03]	2010
Xiu, 2011	−101.44	24.34	30	−43.95	23.9	30	4.0%	−2.35 [−3.02, −1.68]	2011
Hui et al., 2011	−51.53	26.08	20	−10.04	23.53	20	3.8%	−1.64 [−2.36, −0.91]	2011
Fang et al., 2011	−109.59	32.87	32	−78.57	34.56	32	4.6%	−0.91 [−1.42, −0.39]	2011
Gengliang, 2012	−29.5	7.65	40	−16.8	7.05	40	4.6%	−1.71 [−2.23, −1.19]	2012
Baowen et al., 2012	−70	50.57	60	−47	49.1	60	5.2%	−0.46 [−0.82, −0.10]	2012
Guiying and Dengyu, 2012	−51.98	29.19	28	−35.81	30.28	27	4.5%	−0.54 [−1.07, 0.00]	2012
Sheng, 2012	−39.8	29.99	32	−20.1	28.91	32	4.7%	−0.66 [−1.16, −0.16]	2012
Shijing, 2013	−148.64	135.59	41	−46.1	148.48	41	4.9%	−0.71 [−1.16, −0.27]	2013
Xiaomin, 2013	−82.1	65.4	56	−48.44	68.91	57	5.1%	−0.50 [−0.87, −0.12]	2013
Enli et al., 2013	−80.7	29.75	30	−14.6	32.41	30	4.1%	−2.10 [−2.74, −1.46]	2013
Rui and Wenwang, 2013	−104.67	35.4	30	−76.15	38.77	30	4.6%	−0.76 [−1.28, −0.23]	2013
Wu, 2013	−153.4	128.31	32	−47.1	140.54	32	4.6%	−0.78 [−1.29, −0.27]	2013
Jing et al., 2013	−13.81	8.73	15	10.45	15.93	8	2.7%	−2.01 [−3.08, −0.94]	2013
Xiao, 2013	−70.7	29.75	34	−44.6	32.41	34	4.7%	−0.83 [−1.33, −0.33]	2013
Liucun, 2014	−627	685.44	44	−389	807.34	42	5.0%	−0.32 [−0.74, 0.11]	2014
Maoqing, 2015	−89.11	41.74	39	−49.47	57.24	39	4.8%	−0.78 [−1.24, −0.32]	2015
Subtotal (95% CI)			**794**			**761**	**100.0%**	**−0.98 [−1.22, −0.74]**	
Heterogeneity: $\tau^2 = 0.25$; $\chi^2 = 102.86$, df = 21 ($p < 0.00001$); $I^2 = 80\%$									
Test for overall effect: $z = 8.02$ ($p < 0.00001$)									
1.1.2 SCr									
Wu et al., 2007	−1.77	19.72	26	0.36	22.42	24	15.1%	−0.10 [−0.65, 0.46]	2007
Jin et al., 2010	−2.97	11.04	46	−3.62	12.99	42	17.7%	0.05 [−0.36, 0.47]	2010
Xiu, 2011	−21.39	34.54	30	1.34	42.52	30	15.8%	−0.58 [−1.10, −0.06]	2011
Baowen et al., 2012	−28	20.8	60	−10	24.56	60	18.6%	−0.79 [−1.16, −0.41]	2012
Wu, 2013	−36.6	24.73	32	−6.9	25.25	32	15.5%	−1.17 [−1.71, −0.64]	2013
Liucun, 2014	−79.9	65.51	44	−26.3	66.72	42	17.3%	−0.80 [−1.24, −0.36]	2014
Subtotal (95% CI)			**238**			**230**	**100.0%**	**−0.56 [−0.93, −0.20]**	
Heterogeneity: $\tau^2 = 0.15$; $\chi^2 = 18.60$, df = 5 ($p = 0.002$); $I^2 = 73\%$									
Test for overall effect: $z = 3.02$ ($p = 0.003$)									
1.1.3 BUN									
Xiu, 2011	−6.34	1.55	30	−2.25	1.74	30	15.6%	−2.45 [−3.13, −1.77]	2011
Baowen et al., 2012	−0.2	2.03	60	0.2	1.92	60	17.2%	−0.20 [−0.56, 0.16]	2012
Xiao, 2013	−4.5	3.53	34	−1.4	4.18	34	16.6%	−0.79 [−1.29, −0.30]	2013
Shijing, 2013	−7.16	4.22	41	4.17	3.61	41	16.9%	0.75 [0.31, 1.20]	2013
Liucun, 2014	−4.07	2.56	44	−1.08	1.97	42	16.8%	−1.29 [−1.76, −0.83]	2014
Maoqing, 2015	−11.98	13.29	39	−5.12	13.56	39	16.8%	−0.51 [−0.96, −0.05]	2015
Subtotal (95% CI)			**248**			**246**	**100.0%**	**−0.72 [−1.47, 0.02]**	
Heterogeneity: $\tau^2 = 0.81$; $\chi^2 = 76.70$, df = 5 ($p < 0.00001$); $I^2 = 93\%$									
Test for overall effect: $z = 1.90$ ($p = 0.06$)									
Test for subgroup differences: $\chi^2 = 3.56$, df = 2 ($p = 0.17$), $I^2 = 43.8\%$									

Std. mean difference IV, random, 95% CI

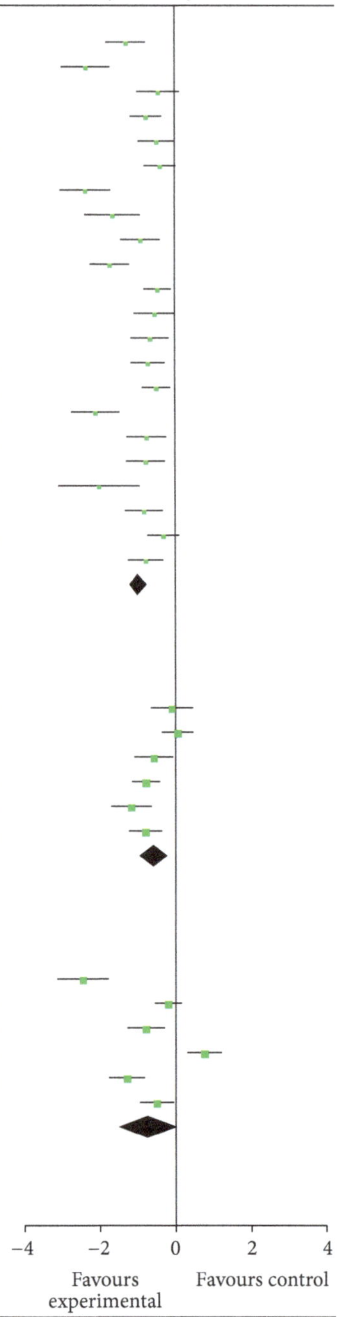

FIGURE 2: Forest plot showing the effect of Yiqi Yangyin Huoxue Method for diabetic nephropathy. UAER: urinary albumin excretion rate, SCr: serum creatinine, and BUN: blood urea nitrogen.

The aggregated results of 2 RCTs suggested that Yiqi Yangyin Huoxue Method showed favorable effects for bringing down beta-2 microglobulin of diabetic nephropathy. There was moderate quality of evidence on improving beta-2 microglobulin based on GRADE (Figure 3).

3.3.5. Fasting Blood Glucose. According to the fasting blood glucose changes in forest plot, the effect size of the 17 selected trials [34, 36–40, 43, 45, 49–54, 56, 57, 59] was MD = −0.35, 95% CI −0.62 to −0.08; test of the effect size was $z = 2.50$, $p = 0.01$; the heterogeneity analysis ($p < 0.05$) suggests that there is heterogeneity in 17 articles. The aggregated results of 17 RCTs suggested that Yiqi Yangyin Huoxue Method showed favorable effects for decreasing fasting blood glucose of diabetic nephropathy. There was moderate quality of evidence on improving fasting blood glucose based on GRADE (Figure 4).

Study or subgroup	Experimental Mean	Experimental SD	Experimental Total	Control Mean	Control SD	Control Total	Weight	Mean difference IV, fixed, 95% CI
Fang et al., 2000	0.07	0.095	20	0.01	0.085	20	92.7%	0.06 [0.00, 0.12]
Wu et al., 2007	0.16	0.43	26	0.05	0.275	24	7.3%	0.11 [−0.09, 0.31]
Total (95% CI)			**46**			**44**	**100.0%**	**0.06 [0.01, 0.12]**

Heterogeneity: $\chi^2 = 0.23$, df $= 1$ ($p = 0.63$); $I^2 = 0\%$
Test for overall effect: $z = 2.32$ ($p = 0.02$)

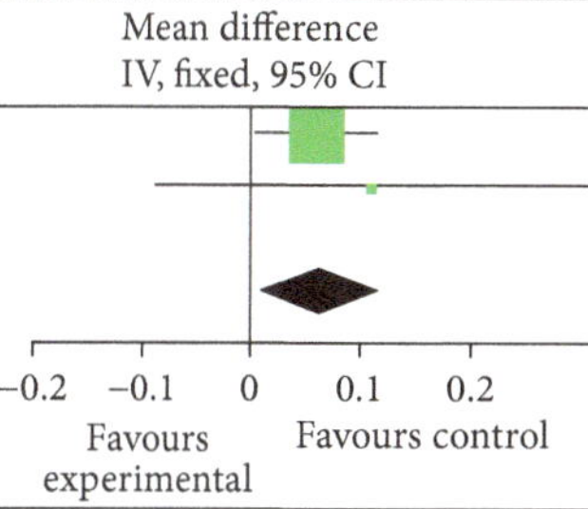

FIGURE 3: Forest plot showing the effect of Yiqi Yangyin Huoxue Method for diabetic nephropathy in beta-2 microglobulin.

Study or subgroup	Experimental Mean	Experimental SD	Experimental Total	Control Mean	Control SD	Control Total	Weight	Std. mean difference IV, random, 95% CI	Year
1.1.1 FBG									
Fang et al., 2000	−1.86	1.76	50	−0.78	1.71	50	6.2%	−0.62 [−1.02, −0.22]	2000
Fan et al., 2002	−0.97	2.9	34	−1.33	2.92	31	5.8%	0.12 [−0.36, 0.61]	2002
Wu et al., 2007	−1.1	1.64	26	−1.06	1.98	24	5.5%	−0.02 [−0.58, 0.53]	2007
Donghui, 2008	−1.39	2.64	34	−0.71	2.02	32	5.8%	−0.28 [−0.77, 0.20]	2008
Xiaochao et al., 2009	−2.3	1.1	50	−0.2	0.9	46	5.7%	−2.06 [−2.56, −1.56]	2009
Jin et al., 2010	−1.79	1.28	46	−2.08	1.37	42	6.1%	0.22 [−0.20, 0.64]	2010
Fang et al., 2011	−1.5	0.82	32	−0.79	1.04	32	5.7%	−0.75 [−1.26, −0.24]	2011
Xianyu and Huoxue, 2012	−2.69	1.55	32	−1.91	2.07	28	5.7%	−0.43 [−0.94, 0.09]	2012
Baowen et al., 2012	−0.6	2.36	60	−0.7	2.31	60	6.3%	0.04 [−0.32, 0.40]	2012
Shijing, 2013	−2.69	1.75	41	−0.81	2.22	41	5.9%	−0.93 [−1.39, −0.47]	2013
Xiao, 2013	−2.8	3.07	34	−2.4	3.87	34	5.9%	−0.11 [−0.59, 0.36]	2013
Rui and Wenwang, 2013	−0.73	1.41	30	−0.98	1.54	30	5.7%	0.17 [−0.34, 0.67]	2013
Xiaomin, 2013	−2.81	2.99	56	−2.68	2.76	57	6.3%	−0.04 [−0.41, 0.32]	2013
Wu, 2013	−3.5	1.65	32	−1.2	1.61	23	5.3%	−1.39 [−1.99, −0.79]	2013
Jie et al., 2013	−0.3	1.05	60	−0.29	1	60	6.3%	−0.01 [−0.37, 0.35]	2013
Enli et al., 2013	−0.97	2.9	30	−1.33	2.9	30	5.7%	0.12 [−0.38, 0.63]	2013
Maoqing, 2015	−1.11	1.55	39	−0.88	1.44	39	6.0%	−0.15 [−0.60, 0.29]	2015
Subtotal (95% CI)			**686**			**659**	**100.0%**	**−0.35 [−0.62, −0.08]**	
Heterogeneity: $\tau^2 = 0.28$; $\chi^2 = 98.12$, df $= 16$ ($p < 0.00001$); $I^2 = 84\%$									
Test for overall effect: $z = 2.50$ ($p = 0.01$)									
1.1.3 PBG									
Wu et al., 2007	−1.76	3.75	26	−2.02	2.95	24	13.9%	0.08 [−0.48, 0.63]	2007
Donghui, 2008	−3.93	3.91	34	−0.92	3.02	32	14.2%	−0.85 [−1.35, −0.34]	2008
Fang et al., 2011	−3.79	1.86	32	−3.09	1.61	32	14.3%	−0.40 [−0.89, 0.10]	2011
Xianyu and Huoxue, 2012	−3.88	2.39	32	−2.65	2.83	28	14.2%	−0.47 [−0.98, 0.05]	2012
Jie et al., 2013	−0.21	1.59	60	0.17	1.53	60	15.2%	−0.24 [−0.60, 0.12]	2013
Enli et al., 2013	−3.7	1.33	30	−4.27	1.35	30	14.2%	0.42 [−0.09, 0.93]	2013
Shijing, 2013	−2.33	0.7	41	−0.94	0.71	41	14.0%	−1.95 [−2.48, −1.42]	2013
Subtotal (95% CI)			**255**			**247**	**100.0%**	**−0.48 [−1.01, 0.04]**	
Heterogeneity: $\tau^2 = 0.44$; $\chi^2 = 49.11$, df $= 6$ ($p < 0.00001$); $I^2 = 88\%$									
Test for overall effect: $z = 1.80$ ($p = 0.07$)									

Test for subgroup differences: $\chi^2 = 0.20$, df $= 1$ ($p = 0.66$), $I^2 = 0\%$

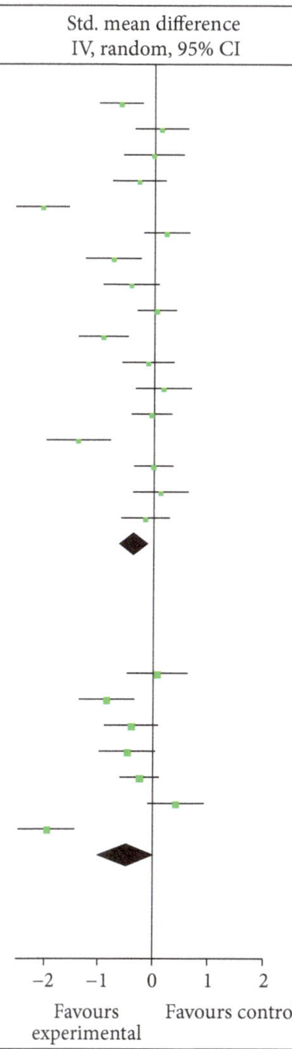

FIGURE 4: Forest plot showing the effect of Yiqi Yangyin Huoxue Method for diabetic nephropathy. FBG: fasting blood glucose; PBG: postprandial blood glucose.

3.3.6. Two-Hour Postprandial Blood Glucose. According to the 2-hour postprandial blood glucose (2hPBG) changes in forest plot, the effect size of the 7 selected trials [37, 38, 43, 45, 50, 53, 55] was SMD = −0.48, 95% CI −1.01 to 0.04; test of the effect size was $z = 1.80$, $p = 0.07$; the heterogeneity analysis ($p < 0.05$) suggests that there is heterogeneity in 7 articles. The aggregated results of 7 RCTs suggested that Yiqi Yangyin Huoxue Method did not show favorable effects for decreasing 2-hour postprandial blood glucose of diabetic nephropathy (Figure 4). There was moderate quality of evidence on improving 2-hour postprandial blood glucose based on GRADE.

3.4. Efficiency Analysis. In the end of the course of treatment, the aggregated results of 22 RCTs [35–37, 39–44, 46–52, 54–59] (SMD = −0.98, 95% CI −1.22 to −0.74) and test of the effect size ($z = 8.02$, $p < 0.00001$) suggested that Yiqi Yangyin Huoxue Method showed favorable effects for decreasing microalbuminuria of diabetic nephropathy; the aggregated results of 6 RCTs [44, 49, 54, 55, 58, 59] (SMD = −0.72, 95% CI −1.47 to 0.02) and test of the effect size ($z = 1.90$, $p = 0.06$) suggested that Yiqi Yangyin Huoxue Method did not show favorable effects for decreasing blood urea nitrogen; the aggregated results of 6 RCTs [37, 40, 44, 49, 56, 58] (SMD = −0.56, 95% CI −0.93 to −0.20) and test of the effect size ($z = 3.02$, $p = 0.003$) suggested that Yiqi Yangyin Huoxue Method showed favorable effects for decreasing serum creatinine; the aggregated results of 2 RCTs [36, 37] (MD = 0.06, 95% CI 0.01 to 0.12) and test of the effect size ($z = 2.32$, $p = 0.02$) suggested that Yiqi Yangyin Huoxue Method showed favorable effects for decreasing beta-2 microglobulin; the aggregated results of 17 RCTs [34, 36–40, 43, 45, 49–54, 56, 57, 59] (SMD = −0.35, 95% CI −0.62 to −0.08) and test of the effect size ($z = 2.50$, $p = 0.01$) suggested that Yiqi Yangyin Huoxue Method showed favorable effects for decreasing fasting blood glucose; and the aggregated results of 7 RCTs [37, 38, 43, 45, 50, 53, 55] (SMD = −0.48, 95% CI −1.01 to 0.04) and test of the effect size ($z = 1.80$, $p = 0.07$) suggested that Yiqi Yangyin Huoxue Method showed favorable effects for decreasing 2-hour postprandial blood glucose of diabetic nephropathy.

3.5. Heterogeneity Analysis. The heterogeneity analysis on the 22 trials of microalbuminuria suggests that there is heterogeneity ($p < 0.00001$, $p < 0.05$). The heterogeneity analysis on the 6 trials of blood urea nitrogen indicates that there is heterogeneity ($p < 0.00001$, $p < 0.05$). The heterogeneity analysis on the 6 trials of serum creatinine suggests that there is heterogeneity ($p < 0.00001$, $p < 0.05$). The heterogeneity analysis on the 2 trials of beta-2 microglobulin suggests that there is homogeneity ($p = 0.63$, $p > 0.05$). The heterogeneity analysis on the 17 trials of fasting blood glucose suggests that there is heterogeneity ($p = 0.02$, $p < 0.05$). The heterogeneity analysis on the 7 trials of 2-hour postprandial blood glucose suggests that there is heterogeneity ($p = 0.02$, $p < 0.05$).

4. Discussion

Current systematic review suggested that Yiqi Yangyin Huoxue Method showed positive effects for diabetic nephropathy on improving UAER, serum creatinine, fasting blood glucose, and beta-2 microglobulin, but not for blood urea nitrogen or PBG. However, there was heterogeneity in UAER, serum creatinine, fasting blood glucose, blood urea nitrogen, and PBG in the meta-analysis. Methodological quality of some studies was relatively low (only 2 points), but there was moderate quality of evidence on improving these outcomes based on GRADE.

Diabetic nephropathy (DN) is one of the most common chronic complications of diabetes. Severe microvascular pathological changes are common in diabetic patients with a history of more than 10 years. It is a major cause of death in patients with type 1 diabetes and its severity is second only to heart, cerebrovascular diseases in patients with type 2 diabetes. In TCM, the pathogenesis of diabetic nephropathy is deficiency of qi and yin and qi failing to circulate blood [60]. So the principle of treatment is to nourish qi and yin and promote blood circulation to resolve blood stasis. Drugs that function to tonify the kidney, nourish yin, reinforce spleen qi, and circulate blood (to resolve stasis) were often included in the formulas. The patients with edema were usually associated with drugs that function to resolve swelling. The outcome measures are UAER, urine beta-2 microglobulin, blood sugar, and so forth. In recent years, there are more and more randomized controlled trials on Yiqi Yangyin Huoxue Method for the treatment of diabetic nephropathy, which bring about opportunities for objective and comprehensive evaluation of the effect of this method, so this study conducted a meta-analysis to investigate its efficacy by the way of evidence-based medicine [61, 62].

This systematic review found that the present trials of Yiqi Yangyin Huoxue Method for the treatment of diabetic nephropathy were poor in methodology, blinding, allocation concealment, and randomization. In our study, all eligible trials included were Chinese. The course of the disease ranged from 18 months to 220.8 months and that of treatment from 3 to 12 weeks. 17 out of the 26 RCTs were high quality trials (3–5 points), and the rest were relatively low (only 2 points). Randomization was conducted in all articles, of which there are 2 with allocation concealment and 7 mentioning the blinding, and the withdrawals and dropouts or resign were mentioned in 4 trials. Though the quality of the included trials was relatively low, our review still provides stronger evidence of Yiqi Yangyin Huoxue Method for the treatment of diabetic nephropathy. Our systematic review showed the positive evidence that Yiqi Yangyin Huoxue Method had favorable effects for lowering the urine trace albumin excretion, serum creatinine, urine beta-2 microglobulin, fasting plasma glucose, and 2-hour postprandial blood glucose.

Our results are different from previous systematic reviews. Yan's [63] systematic review suggested that Yiqi Huoxue Qingre (invigorating qi and yin and activating blood) Method seemed to be an effective intervention in diabetic nephropathy. However, it did not meet the recognized pathogenesis for DN. The onset and process of DN are both deficiency of qi and yin and blood stasis, and Yiqi Huoxue Qingre therapeutic principle should be to tonify qi and yin and activate blood. In addition, the outcome measures were more considerate compared with Li's [64] review. Two-hour postprandial blood glucose was employed as an outcome because it is an important factor in the treatment of diabetic nephropathy. With more detailed subgroup analyses and comprehensive outcome measures, our update provides stronger evidence of Yiqi Yangyin Huoxue Method for diabetic nephropathy.

In our review, heterogeneity was found in the microalbuminuria excretion, serum creatinine, urine beta-2 microglobulin, fasting plasma glucose, and so forth of the included trials. The heterogeneity may be possibly from the risk of bias because effect estimate from studies that have low risk of bias might be different comparing to studies having high risk of bias. The reasons of the heterogeneity may be as follows: (1) the course of disease ranged from 18 to 220.8 months; (2) the course of treatment ranged from 3 to 12 weeks; (3) the outcome measures were different in the eligible trials; (4) the age and complications were different; and (5) the drugs used in Yiqi Yangyin Huoxue Method were also different. Firstly, antidiabetics and insulin were used in routine treatment of different trials. Secondly, the drugs used in the formula of Yiqi Yangyin Huoxue Method were different. Usually, drugs that were characterized with blood activating include *Salvia miltiorrhiza*, rhubarb, angelica, motherwort, red peony root, rhizoma ligustici wallichii, peach kernel, and cortex moutan; drugs that were characterized with invigorating qi include *Astragalus*, yam, *Atractylodes*, radix pseudostellariae, and dangshen; and drugs that were characterized with enriching yin include raw radix rehmanniae, cooked rehmannia, wolfberry fruit, radix scrophulariae, rhizoma polygonati, dogwood, and fructus ligustri lucidi. The drugs in each prescription therapeutic principle in the study of the trials were the same, but the type, dose, and origin were not identical.

Our study found that Yiqi Yangyin Huoxue Method had favorable effects for diabetic nephropathy; however, there is a major limitation for the included trials, that is, a small sample, and the quality of the trials was relatively low in methodology. Few studies observed the side effects of the treatment; thus the conclusions on the effect and safety should be interpreted with caution. More studies of Yiqi Yangyin Huoxue Method for diabetic nephropathy with large scale, high quality, and long follow-up are warrant to confirm the current findings.

5. Conclusion

Yiqi Yangyin Huoxue Method should be a valid complementary and alternative therapy in the management of diabetic nephropathy, especially on improving UAER, serum creatinine, fasting blood glucose, and beta-2 microglobulin. However, more studies with long follow-up are warrant to confirm the current findings.

Competing Interests

The authors declare that there is no conflict of interests regarding the publication of this paper.

Authors' Contributions

Jiao Ying Ou and Di Huang contributed equally to this work.

Acknowledgments

This work is supported by Shanghai Three-Year Project of Traditional Chinese Medicine (ZYSNXD-CCYJXYY).

References

[1] D. Zhang, S. Efendic, K. Brismar, and H. F. Gu, "Effects of MCF2L2, ADIPOQ and SOX2 genetic polymorphisms on the development of nephropathy in type 1 Diabetes Mellitus," *BMC Medical Genetics*, vol. 11, article 116, 2010.

[2] W. J. C. De Grauw, E. H. van de Lisdonk, W. H. E. M. van Gerwen et al., "Microalbuminuria in patients with Type 2 diabetes mellitus from general practice: course and predictive value," *Diabetic Medicine*, vol. 18, no. 2, pp. 139–143, 2001.

[3] Z. T. Bloomgarden, "American diabetes association annual meeting, 1997, and the Teczem Consultant Meeting. Diabetic nephropathy," *Diabetes Care*, vol. 21, no. 2, pp. 315–319, 1998.

[4] C. E. Mogensen, A. Schmitz, and C. K. Christensen, "Comparative renal pathophysiology relevant to IDDM and NIDDM patients," *Diabetes/Metabolism Reviews*, vol. 4, no. 5, pp. 453–483, 1988.

[5] A. R. Jadad, R. A. Moore, D. Carroll et al., "Assessing the quality of reports of randomized clinical trials: is blinding necessary?" *Controlled Clinical Trials*, vol. 17, no. 1, pp. 1–12, 1996.

[6] D. Moher, B. Pham, A. Jones et al., "Does quality of reports of randomised trials affect estimates of intervention efficacy reported in meta-analyses?" *The Lancet*, vol. 352, no. 9128, pp. 609–613, 1998.

[7] L. L. Kjaergard, J. Villuumsen, and C. Gluud, "Quality of randomised clinical trials affects estimates of intervention efficacy," in *Proceedings of the 7th Cochrane Colloquium*, p. 57, Universita STommaso D'Aquino, Rome, Italy, 1999.

[8] W. C. Jun, "Qi and nourishing Yin, activating blood change chaotic method for the treatment of chronic renal failure: a 22-case of clinical observation," *Journal of Beijing Chinese Medicine*, vol. 13, no. 3, pp. 18–20, 1997.

[9] C. Jingrong, "Taohongshenqi yin with western medicine forthe treatment of early diabetic nephropathy in 48 patients," *Journal of Shaanxi TCM*, vol. 30, no. 4, pp. 408–409, 2009.

[10] Z. Ting, "Yiqi Yangyin Huoxue Method for diabetic nephropathy: 28 cases," *Journal of Shanxi Traditional Chinese Medicine*, vol. 1, pp. 11–12, 2002.

[11] N. Shenghong, "Clinical observation on treatment of diabetic nephropathy with Yiqi Yangyin Huoxuedecoction," *Modern Combine Traditional Chinese and Western Medicine Journal*, no. 33, pp. 4278–4279, 2010.

[12] T. Lou, "Combined treatment of traditional Chinese and western medicine for early diabetic nephropathy: 45 cases," *Journal of Shandong Traditional Chinese Medicine*, vol. 29, no. 9, pp. 628–629, 2010.

[13] S. Feng, "Combined treatment of traditional Chinese and western medicine for early diabetic nephropathy: 36 cases," *Journal of Practical Internal Medicine of Traditional Chinese Medicine*, vol. 24, no. 7, pp. 71–72, 2010.

[14] X. XiaoJun, "Yiqi Yangyin Huoxue method for the treatment of diabetic nephropathy: a clinical curative effect analysis," *Chinese and Foreign Medicine*, vol. 29, no. 6, p. 76, 2010.

[15] Y. Yifu, "Clinical observation of Yiqi Yangyin Huoxueherbs for the treatment of 36 cases of early diabetic nephropathy," *Journal of Fujian University of Traditional Chinese Medicine*, vol. 20, no. 6, pp. 51–52, 2010.

[16] J. Chen, X. Ni, Z. Wei et al., "Combined treatment of traditional Chinese and western medicine for early diabetic nephropathy: 36 cases," *Chinese Medical Emergency*, no. 8, pp. 1406–1407, 2010.

[17] C. Rui, "Clinical observation of Yiqi Yangyin Huoxueherbs for the treatment of 60 cases of early type 2 diabetic nephropathy," *The Journal of Neuroscience*, vol. 14, pp. 1211–1212, 2010.

[18] X. Haojie, Y. Meihua, Z. Le et al., "A systematic review of Yiqi Yangyin Huoxue method for the treatment of early type 2 diabetic nephropathy," *Journal of Tropical Medicine*, vol. 11, no. 10, pp. 1147–1150, 2011.

[19] Y. Nizhi and L. Fang, "Yiqi Yangyin Huoxue method for the treatment of diabetic nephropathy: 40 cases," *Journal of Liaoning Traditional Chinese Medicine Journal*, vol. 12, no. 1, pp. 16–17, 1999.

[20] F. Hailing, "Yiqi Yangyin Huoxue Method for the treatment of diabetic nephropathy: 40 cases," *Journal of Henan Traditional Chinese Medicine*, vol. 31, no. 4, pp. 389–390, 2011.

[21] Y. Wang and H. Guo, "Clinical observation of Yiqi Yangyin Huoxue herbs for the treatment of 30 cases of early diabetic nephropathy," *Journal of Hebei Traditional Chinese Medicine*, no. 8, pp. 1132–1133, 2011.

[22] H. Yin, L. Kong, X. Lu et al., "Yiqi Yangyin Huoxue herbs for the treatment of elderly patients with diabetic nephropathy and its influence on serum inhibition-C," *Chinese Journal of Gerontology*, vol. 32, no. 13, pp. 2893–2894, 2012.

[23] Y. Xiang and C. Ming, "Curative effect observation of combined treatment of traditional Chinese and western medicine for diabetic nephropathy," *Modern Combine Traditional Chinese and Western Medicine Journal*, vol. 28, no. 9, pp. 3107–3108, 2012.

[24] H. Xie, M. H. Yan, L. Zhang et al., "A system review for Yiqi Yangyin Huoxue method combined ACEI or ARB drugs the treatment of early type 2 diabetic nephropathy," *Journal of Chinese Medicine*, vol. 11, no. 10, pp. 1147–1150, 2011.

[25] L. Wei, C. Xinlian, W. Guofang, and Y. Li, "Yiqi Yangyin Huoxue Method for the treatment of diabetic nephropathy: 46 cases," *Journal of Medical Frontier*, vol. 2, no. 6, pp. 8–9, 2012.

[26] G. Baowen, R. X. Qing, Z. Yanping et al., "clinical research of blood rheology and blood lipid of Yiqi Yangyin Huoxue Method treatment of early diabetic nephropathy," *The Light of Traditional Chinese Medicine*, vol. 27, no. 4, pp. 689–691, 2012.

[27] L. Yuling, "Ginseng and astragalus decoction for the treatment of diabetic nephropathy: 30 cases," *Journal of Shaanxi TCM Journal*, vol. 28, no. 8, pp. 981–982, 2007.

[28] W. Xiuling, L. Fang, Y. Haiqiang, D. Su, and J. M. Li, "The traditional Chinese medicine with tripterygiumwilfordii glycoside in treatment of diabetic nephropathy proteinuria: 1 case," *Traditional Chinese Medicine in Sichuan*, vol. 9, no. 6, pp. 38–39, 2013.

[29] J. Shi and H. Wang, "Experimental research of Yi-Qi Yang-Yin and Qing-Li Huo-Xue treatment in preventing MCNS rats," *Journal of Zhejiang College of TCM*, vol. 32, no. 6, pp. 876–882, 2004.

[30] L. Zhihong, L. Guangzhen, W. Jianjun, Z. Yirui, and X. Xue, "Experimental study of Yishenkang on minimal lesion nephrotic syndrome," *World Journal of Integrated Traditional and Western Medicine*, vol. 13, no. 4, pp. 67–70, 2008.

[31] S. W. Lee, "Study on traditional Chinese and western medicine treatment of primary nephrotic syndrome," *Tianjin Journal of Traditional Chinese Medicine*, vol. 36, no. 2, pp. 113–118, 2012.

[32] Y. Hui, L. Qing, K. Lingyu, Y. Fang, and P. Liu, "Yiqi Yangyin Huoxue Method for serum inhibition in patients with diabetic nephropathy C and the effect of the urine trace albumin," *Journal of Hebei Traditional Chinese Medicine*, no. 3, pp. 339–341, 2012.

[33] X. Lihui, "Clinical observation of Yiqi Yangyin Huoxue herbs for the treatment of early diabetic nephropathy," *Journal of Liaoning Traditional Chinese Medicine Journal*, vol. 29, no. 3, p. 154, 2002.

[34] B. Fang, Z. Peimin, Z. Qingmei et al., "Clinical observation of combined traditional Chinese and western medicine treatment of early diabetic nephropathy," *Chinese Journal of Combining Traditional Chinese and Western Medicine*, vol. 20, no. 5, pp. 335–357, 2000.

[35] Z. Lan and W. M. M. Lijia, "Yiqi Yangyin Huoxue Bushen method for the treatment of diabetic nephropathy: a clinical curative effect analysis," *Chinese Journal of Chinese Medicine Information*, vol. 9, no. 11, pp. 13–14, 2002.

[36] G. Fan, T. Xianyu, T. Aihua et al., "Yiqi Yangyin Huoxue Bushen Method for the treatment of diabetic nephropathy: a clinical curative effect analysis," *Journal of New Traditional Chinese Medicine*, no. 9, pp. 39–40, 2002.

[37] C. Wu, X. Chen, G. Kong, M. Wei, and P. Fan, "Clinical observation of Yiqi Yangyin Huoxue herbs for the treatment of elderly diabetic nephropathy: 26 cases," *Journal of Shaanxi Traditional Chinese Medicine*, vol. 28, no. 8, pp. 977–980, 2007.

[38] D. Si, "Clinical observation on treatment of early diabetic nephropathy Qi and activating blood method," *Journal of Shandong Traditional Chinese Medicine*, vol. 27, no. 12, pp. 807–808, 2008.

[39] W. Xiaochao, L. Kemian, D. GongJie et al., "The curative effect of Heavy dose of treatment on early diabetic nephropathy with activating blood circulation," *The Light of Traditional Chinese Medicine*, vol. 24, no. 11, pp. 2060–2061, 2009.

[40] H. Jin, W. Yiqi, and Y. Huoxue, "Method in the treatment of 46 cases of early diabetic nephropathy," *Journal of Fujian Traditional Chinese Medicine*, vol. 9, no. 1, pp. 17–18, 2010.

[41] G. Xiaozhou, L. Lan, N. Qing et al., "Yiqi Yangyin Huoxue method in the treatment of early diabetic nephropathy," *Journal of New Traditional Chinese Medicine*, no. 3, pp. 35–36, 2010.

[42] Z. Hui, M. Wei, G. J. Gong et al., "Clinical research of Yiqi Yangyin Huoxue Method for the treatment of early diabetic nephropathy," *Journal of New Traditional Chinese Medicine*, vol. 43, no. 3, pp. 25–26, 2011.

[43] G. Fang, L. Y. Long, and H. Y. Hua, "Clinical observation of Qi huoxue fang on treatment of early diabetic nephropathy," *Journal of Fujian University of Traditional Chinese Medicine*, vol. 6, pp. 15–17, 2011.

[44] Z. Xiu, "Clinical observation of Qi huoxue fang on treatment of 30 cases of diabetic nephropathy," *China Medical Guide*, vol. 20, no. 9, pp. 147–149, 2011.

[45] X. Xianyu and Y. Y. Huoxue, "Method in the treatment of 32 cases of early diabetic nephropathy," *Journal of Jilin Medical*, vol. 5, pp. 930–931, 2012.

[46] S. Sheng, "Clinical observation on treatment of diabetic nephropathy with Yiqi Yangyin Huoxue Method and western medicine," *Chinese Medicine Clinical Journal*, vol. 24, no. 2, pp. 121–122, 2012.

[47] P. Guiying and L. Dengyu, "A Clinical observation of combined traditional Chinese and western medicine for the treatment of early diabetic nephropathy," *World Magazine which Combines Traditional Chinese Medicine with Western Medicine*, vol. 7, no. 4, pp. 332–357, 2012.

[48] Z. Gengliang, "Yiqi Yangyin Huoxue method for the treatment of diabetic nephropathy: 40 cases," *Journal of Hebei Traditional Chinese Medicine*, no. 6, pp. 829–830, 2012.

[49] G. Baowen, J. Y. Liang, H. Mingfei, L. Wei, and L. Wang, "Clinical observation of Yiqi Yangyin Huoxue herbs for the treatment of 60 cases of early diabetic nephropathy," *Journal of Traditional Chinese Medicine*, no. 12, pp. 1032–1050, 2012.

[50] C. Enli, W. Yuming, L. Mingxing et al., "Yiqi Yangyin Huoxue method for the treatment of diabetic nephropathy: a 60-case clinical curative effect analysis," *Journal of Yunnan Traditional Chinese Medicine*, no. 6, pp. 26–27, 2013.

[51] D. Xiaomin, "Yiqi huoxue fang for the treatment of qi and Yin deficiency and blood stasisof early diabetic nephropathy clinical research," *Journal of Global Chinese Medicine*, vol. 6, no. 9, pp. 661–664, 2013.

[52] G. Jing, L. Jing, M. S. An, and Z. Jie, "Method of nourishing Qi and Yin, promoting blood circulation to remove blood stasis in the treatment of type 2 diabetic nephropathy III, two virtual IV period of qi and Yin and blood stasis: 40 cases of clinical research," *The World of Traditional Chinese Medicine*, vol. 12, pp. 530–534, 2013.

[53] L. Jie, H.-T. Yang, Y. Bo et al., "Activating blood Method on diabetic nephropathy (III), focusing on the effects of TCM syndrome and urinary protein," *Chinese Journal of Traditional Chinese and Western Medicine Combined with Kidney Disease*, vol. 1, pp. 230–232, 2013.

[54] L. Xiao, "Yiqi Huoxue decoction in the treatment of Qi and Yin deficiency of diabetic nephropathy: an effect observation," *Journal of Contemporary Chinese Medicine*, vol. 8, pp. 138–140, 2013.

[55] W. Shijing, "Yiqi Yangyin Huoxue method for the treatment of diabetic nephropathy: a clinical curative effect analysis," *Journal of Chinese Medicine Science*, vol. 98, pp. 98–99, 2013.

[56] W.-L. Wu, "The clinical effect of Yiqi Yangyin Huoxue Method for the treatment of diabetic nephropathy," *China Medical Guide*, vol. 32, pp. 193–194, 2013.

[57] W. Rui and C. Wenwang, "Yiqi huoxue fang for treatment of 30-cases early diabetic nephropathy," *Journal of Henan Traditional Chinese Medicine*, vol. 11, pp. 1923–1924, 2013.

[58] M. Liucun, "Observation on the Method of nourishing qi and Yin, promoting blood circulation to remove blood stasis in the treatment of diabetic nephropathy," *The World's Latest Medical Information Abstract*, vol. 14, no. 2, pp. 163–164, 2014.

[59] Y. Maoqing, "Yiqi Yangyin Huoxue Method for the treatment of early diabetic nephropathy: a clinical curative effect analysis," *Journal of Yanbian Medicine*, vol. 13, no. 5, pp. 116–117, 2015.

[60] X. D. Guo, X. Wang, X. Wei et al., "Combined traditional Chinese and western medicine for treatment of early diabetic nephropathy: 33 cases observation," *Journal of Practical Medicine Magazine*, vol. 24, no. 1, pp. 24–25, 2008.

[61] H. Shilin and C. Xiu, *An Introduction to Medical Research Method*, People's Medical Publishing, Beijing, China, 2008.

[62] L. Guo and S. Fumin, *Modern Clinical Epidemiology*, Shanghai Medical University Press, Shanghai, China, 2000.

[63] Z. Yan, S. Wei, H. Quan, H. Yan-li, and Y. Xue-Feng, "The efficacy of chinese herbal medicine supplementing qi, clearing heat and activating blood circulation inthe management of urine protein in diabetic nephropathy: a meta—analysis," *Liaoning Journal of Traditional Chinese Medicine* , vol. 38, no. 1, pp. 97–101, 2011.

[64] M. Li, W. Wang, J. Xue, Y. Gu, and S. Lin, "Meta-analysis of the clinical value of Astragalus membranaceus in diabetic nephropathy," *Journal of Ethnopharmacology*, vol. 133, no. 2, pp. 412–419, 2011.

8

Analysis of Advantages and Disadvantages of the Location Methods of International Auricular Acupuncture Points

Pei-Jing Rong,[1] Jing-Jun Zhao,[1] Lei Wang,[2] and Li-Qun Zhou[3]

[1] *Institute of Acupuncture and Moxibustion, China Academy of Chinese Medical Sciences, Beijing 100700, China*
[2] *School of Acupuncture-Moxibustion and Tuina, Beijing University of Chinese Medicine, Beijing 100029, China*
[3] *School of Basic Medical Science, Beijing University of Chinese Medicine, Beijing 100029, China*

Correspondence should be addressed to Li-Qun Zhou; zhouliqun6080@126.com

Academic Editor: Morry Silberstein

The international standardization of auricular acupuncture points (AAPs) is an important basis for auricular therapy or auricular diagnosis and treatment. The study on the international standardization of AAPs has gone through a long process, in which the location method is one of the key research projects. There are different points of view in the field of AAPs among experts from different countries or regions. By only analyzing the nine representative location methods, this paper tried to offer a proper location method to locate AAPs. Through analysis of the pros and cons of each location method, the location method applied in the WFAS international standard of AAPs is thoroughly considered as an appropriate method. It is important to keep the right direction during developing an International Organization for Standardization (ISO) international standard of auricular acupuncture points and to improve the research quality of international standardization for AAPs.

1. Introduction

The third regional conference of the working group of the standardization of acupuncture points was held in Seoul, South Korea, in 1987 [1]. In this conference, the China Association of Acupuncture-Moxibustion put forward a draft of international standard of auricular acupuncture points (AAPs) including ninety points. The draft was seriously discussed and the board set up three criteria of selection: (1) points which use international and common names; (2) points whose therapeutic values are well proven; (3) points whose location in the auricular area appears to be generally well-defined. Forty-three points that fulfilled all three criteria were classified with an alphanumeric code (a two-letter abbreviation and one number), pinyin, Han character, and English name. Thirty-six points that fulfilled the first and second criteria were not attributed a code, but only pinyin, Han character, and English nomenclature. Eleven points that failed to fulfill all three of the criteria were excluded. After a last inconclusive 1990 WHO meeting [2] in Lyon, Chinese researchers continued the standardization work and mainly continued due to the contribution of the publication of Chinese National Standard in 1993 [3]. This document was updated in 2008 [4] by a second document.

An international standard of AAPs is an inevitable requirement when the auricular diagnosis and treatment medicine develops for a long period and goes to a high level. Through more than 30 years of effort, great progress and achievements have been made in researches on the international standard of AAPs. Up to now, an international standard has been formulated and issued by the World Federation of Acupuncture-Moxibustion Societies. An International Organization for Standardization (ISO) international standard is also in development. Nevertheless, there are still debates on the location methods for locating AAPs, including location based on "points," "subzones," "coordinate," and other methods.

The corresponding author of this paper has been engaged in the study on the international standardization of AAPs since 1986 and had the honor to participate in the whole process of research work on the Chinese national standard of AAPs and international standard of AAPs. As the chief

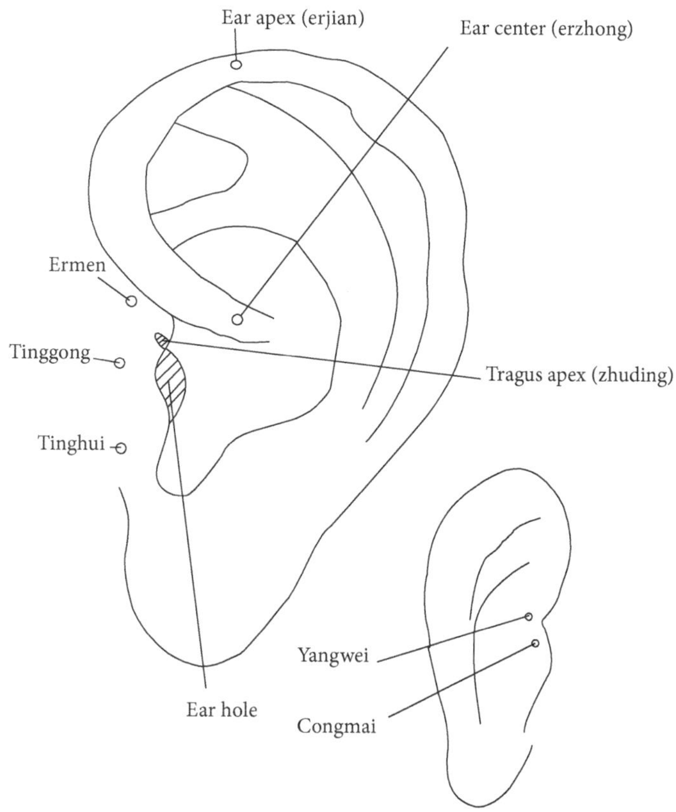

FIGURE 1: AAPs described by Chinese experts before the 18th century, recorded in Professor Huang Li-Chun's book, Auricular Diagnosis and Treatment.

expert of the project, he finished the international standard for auricular acupuncture point [5], which was issued by the World Federation of Acupuncture-Moxibustion Societies. Therefore, he had a comprehensive understanding on the background, content, advantages, and disadvantages of different location methods during developing this international standard. This paper aimed to analyze these location methods and provide a reference for the formulation of an ISO standard of AAPs in the future.

2. Methods

From perspectives of historical context of AAPs, clinical inheritance, and practice of AAPs, the understanding of the essence of points, advantages, and disadvantages of the following nine location methods for locating AAPs were analyzed, including (1) the location method based on points for the anterior of the auricle, (2) the location method based on subzones for the anterior of the auricle, (3) the location method based on the divided subzones according to anatomy of the anterior of the auricle, (4) the location method based on Nogier's Point Zero for the anterior of the auricle, (5) the location method based on the facial ties of the knee of the helix and lobe, (6) the location method based on both points and subzones of the anterior of the auricle, (7) the location method based on smaller subzones of the anterior of the auricle, (8) the location method based on subzones, points, and lines for the anterior and posterior of the auricle, and (9) the location method based on subzones, points, and lines for full cover of the anterior and posterior of the auricle. The analysis is described in detail with pictures so that readers can understand easily.

3. Results and Discussion

3.1. The Location Method Based on Points for the Anterior of the Auricle. No specific illustration of the location of AAPs can be found in Chinese ancient medical books [6] (Figure 1 [7]), except the posterior auricular map [8] (Figure 2) with the theory, where each of the five areas of the posterior of the auricle corresponded to each of the five Zang-organs, including heart, liver, spleen, lung, and kidney. Therefore, it is difficult to identify whether there was the thought of location of AAPs based on points at the old time. The ear reflex map of French physician, Paul Nogier, was introduced to China in 1958 by Dr. Ye Xiao-Lin. And this map was the earliest representative systematic auricular map in modern time [9–11] (Figure 3(a) [9] and Figure 3(b) [12]). The location method based on points and subzones is adopted in his two maps. The location method based on points is applied to represent the somatic structures of the body. Although the thought of location method of subzones to represent viscera and organs of the body was used, Figure 3(b) is only a sketch map. The location method based on points has three advantages. Firstly,

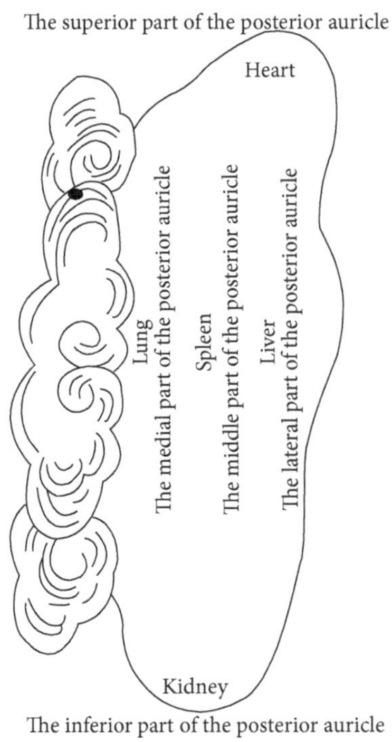

Figure 2: The posterior auricular map in 1888.

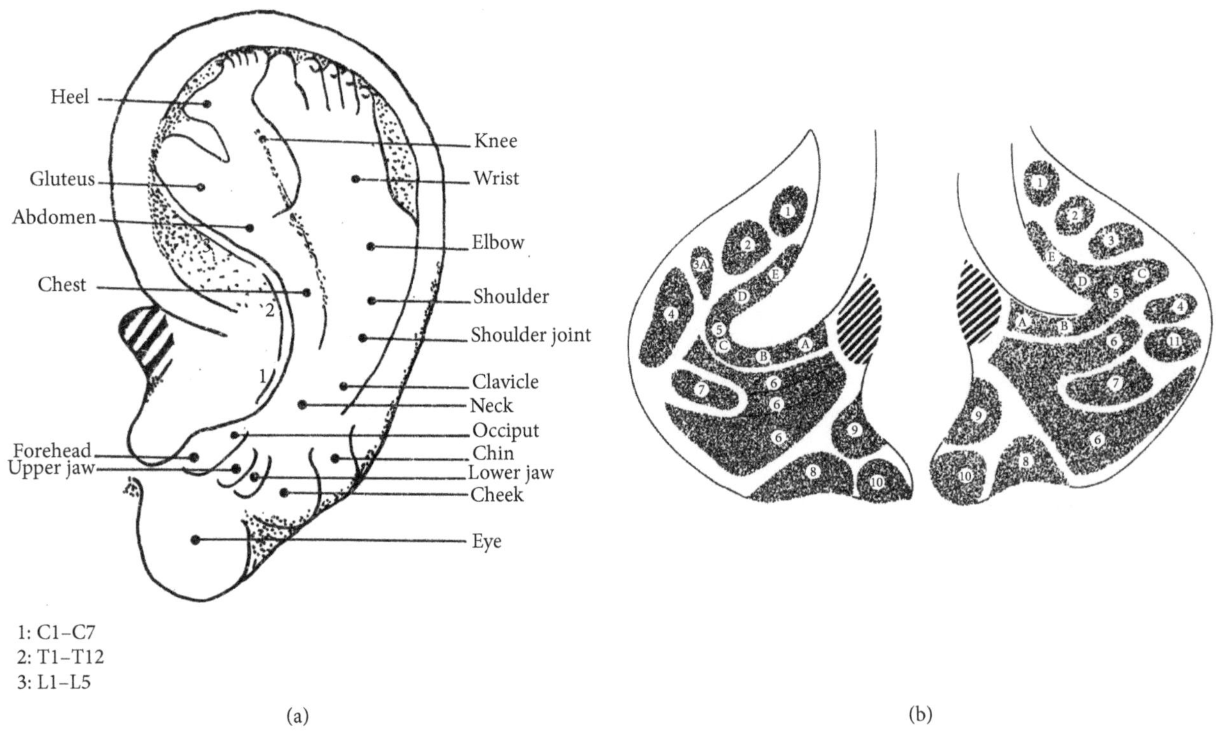

Figure 3: (a) Paul Nogier's findings of inverted fetus on the auricle representing the somatic structures in 1957. (b) Paul Nogier's findings of inverted fetus on the auricle representing viscera and organs in 1957. (1) Bladder; (2) kidney; (3) pancreas; (3A) gallbladder; (4) liver; (5A) oesophagus; (5B) cardia; (5C) stomach; (5D) small intestine; (5E) large intestine; (6) lung; (7) heart; (8) subcortex; (9) internal nose; (10) endocrine; (11) spleen.

the original is respected and it can comprehensively reflect the historic appearance of the development of auricular therapy in China and France. Secondly, it is visualized and it can effectively guide the clinical application of AAPs. Thirdly, those points which are marked at tips of the different zones of the auricle (e.g., the tip of the tragus) or notches (e.g., the intertragic notch) are easy to describe the location accurately with auricular anatomical terms. With the above advantages, this location method was adopted in the earliest draft of the international standard of AAPs. However, it has also some limitations. At first, it cannot accurately reflect the corresponding somatic structures, viscera, and organs reflexed on the auricle. Then, those points that are not located at the tips of the different zones of the auricle or notches cannot be accurately marked and described with auricular anatomical terms. Thirdly, it cannot cover the whole auricle. As a result, this location method was not the only location method in the later drafts.

Figure 2 is from Zhang Zhen-Jun's (Zhang Di-Shan's) book, *Essential Techniques for Massage*. The superior part of the posterior auricle corresponds to heart, the inferior part corresponds to kidney, the middle part corresponds to spleen, the lateral side corresponds to liver, and the medial side corresponds to lung.

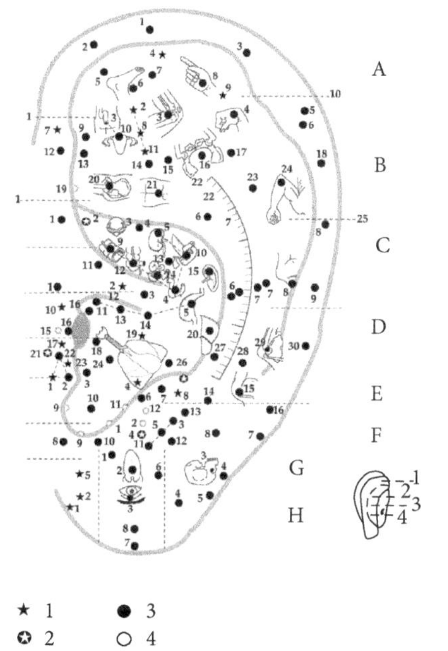

FIGURE 4: Dr. Jarricot's auricular map in 1973.

3.2. The Location Method Based on Subzones for the Anterior of the Auricle. With awareness of the limitations of the location method based purely on points, the Chinese academic circle in the late 1980s tried to locate AAPs according to the subzones. There were different zones on the auricle according to the anatomical structures of the auricle. Each zone was further divided into different subzones. The work began with the aim to locate AAPs at the ear lobe and concha where it was difficult to use points to locate these AAPs. The subdivision in vertical and horizontal lines of the ear lobe was published by Jarricot and Wong [13], who divided the whole outer auricle in horizontal stripes ((A) to (H), from top to bottom) which was called "the Great Ear of the School of Chen-Yang" (Figure 4). A Chinese physician, Dr. Wang, made also the exploration to locate AAPs by subzones in his book [14] (Figure 5), Auricular Acupuncture. According to the Chinese history of acupuncture, auricular acupuncture, and Nogier's auricular maps introduced into China in 1958, the location method based only on points is used to name acupuncture points, or AAPs. As a breakthrough of the thinking inertia, auricular point is just a point, and this location method based on subzones not only walked a significant step forward from perspectives of the clinical application of AAPs and description of the location of AAPs, but also provided an innovative idea for future study on the location of AAPs. The shortcoming of this method is that the division of zones is not comprehensive and standardized and lacks anatomical basis. Most of the AAPs are located by the location method based on points. The location method based on subzones is only applied to locate AAPs on the lobe, the inferior concha. There is not a general principle to specify the subzones, which makes it difficult to duplicate on different people. There is no description of anatomical borders, which can divide the auricle into zones and subzones.

3.3. The Location Method Based on the Divided Subzones according to Anatomy of the Anterior of the Auricle. In 1990, Oleson and Kroening, scholars from University of California, Los Angeles, the United States of America, first located all AAPs at the visible surface of the anterior auricle according to the anatomy of the auricle in his article [15] (Figure 6). Each subzone was coded by the initials of its corresponding anatomical structure and a number. For example, the first subzone of triangular fossa is short for TF1 and the second subzone of triangular fossa is short for TF2. His original intention was to ease the dispute over the problem-one name with different positions, or one auricular acupuncture point (AAP) with different names in Chinese and French auricular acupuncture systems, and to advocate neglecting the traditional names of AAPs but to name them with codes. Innovations of this location method are as follows. Firstly, location of AAPs is completely based on subzones instead of points, breaking through the limitations of the location method based on points. Secondly, the location method based on the divided subzones according to anatomy of the auricle has been proved to be the right direction to locate AAPs. Thirdly, the coding system, the name of the anatomical structure and a number, is simple and clear. Fourthly, according to the theory of bioholographic law, AAPs are the projections of the body parts on the auricle and therefore the location method based on the divided subzones can objectively reflect the correspondence between AAPs and the body parts. The shortcomings are as follows. Firstly, tips of the different zones of the auricle or notches are not proper to be marked as subzones. Secondly, the academic value of the historical evolution and clinical significance of AAPs are neglected. Thirdly, those AAPs at the junction of the neighboring anatomical structures of the auricle cannot be straight forwardly and accurately marked. Fourthly, the

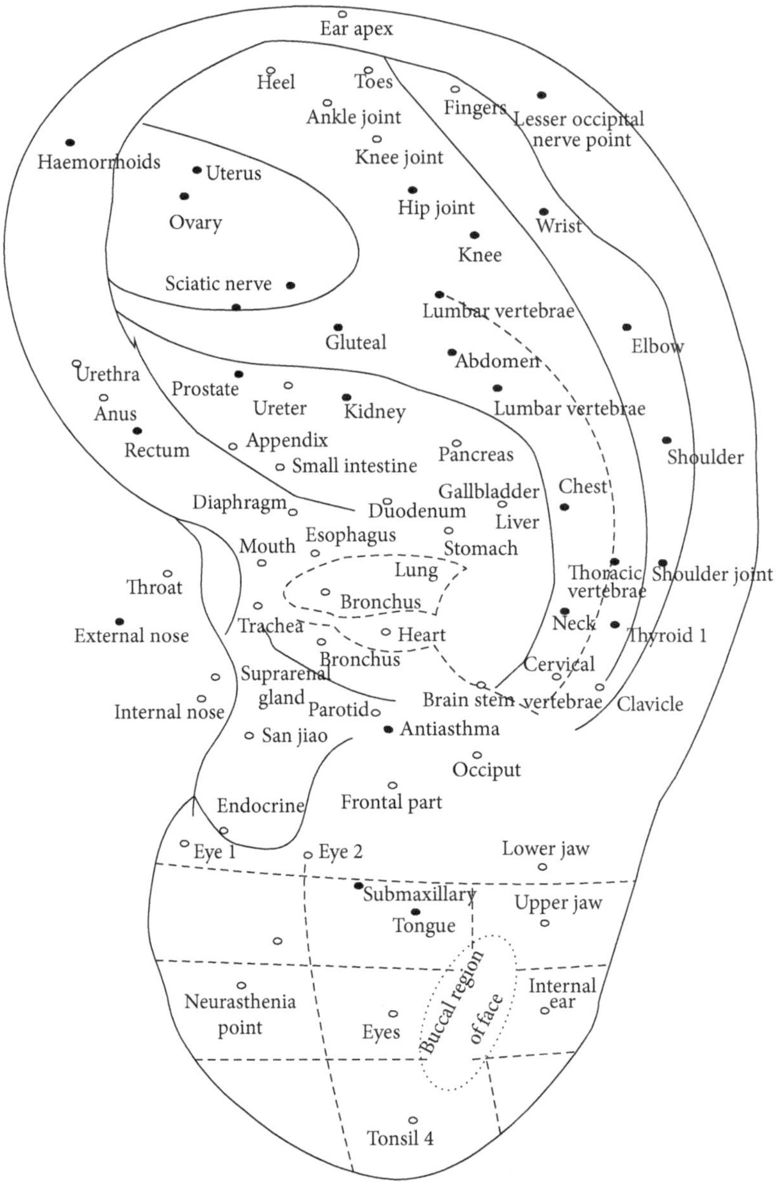

FIGURE 5: Dr. Wang Zhong's auricular map in 1984.

border of the neighboring anatomical structures of the auricle, such as scapha and antihelix, cannot be clarified and lacks detailed anatomical evidence. Finally, the posterior of the auricle is not divided into zones and further subzones.

3.4. The Location Method Based on Nogier's Point Zero for the Anterior of the Auricle. This method was proposed in 1990 by Dr. Bossy at the international conference on AAPs held by the WHO Regional Office for the Western Pacific in Lyon, France, to solve the long-troubling problem of international standardization of AAPs. The zero point was set at the helix crus notch and the auricle is divided into four quadrants by the horizontal and vertical axis. AAPs were marked by the intersections of the latitude and longitude lines in each quadrant. Dr. Rouxeville [16] further divided each quadrant into three equal sectors (Figure 7). Three other authors, the Russian Durinyan [17] and Romoli and Mazzoni [18] from Italy, also developed a grid with a variable number of sectors centered in Point Zero. The sectogram was obtained by subdividing the auricle into three semiaxes (A), (B), and (C) going, respectively, through the visual intersection point of the posterior edge of the raising branch of the helix with the lower branch of the antihelix (A) and through the antitragus-antihelix groove (B) and tangent to the posterior edge of the tragus (C). The resulting main sectors (A)-(B), (A)-(C), and (B)-(C) were subdivided, respectively, into 16 sectors, (A)-(B) and (A)-(C), and into 8 sectors, (B)-(C) (Figure 8). The location method based on Nogier's Point Zero for the anterior of the auricle has the thought of locating AAPs with subzones. The advantage of this method is that it could accurately locate every point with no controversy about the nomenclature and locations of AAPs. However, as the saying goes, "no leaves are

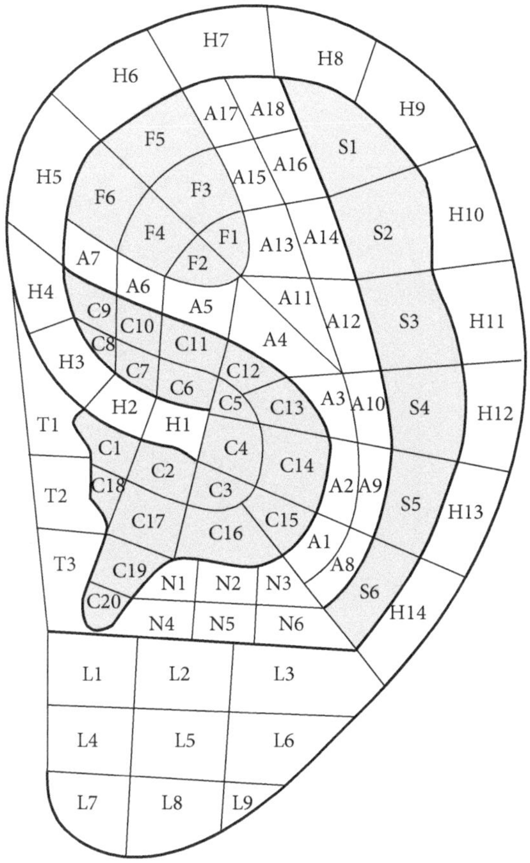

FIGURE 6: Oleson's nomenclature of subzones in 1983.

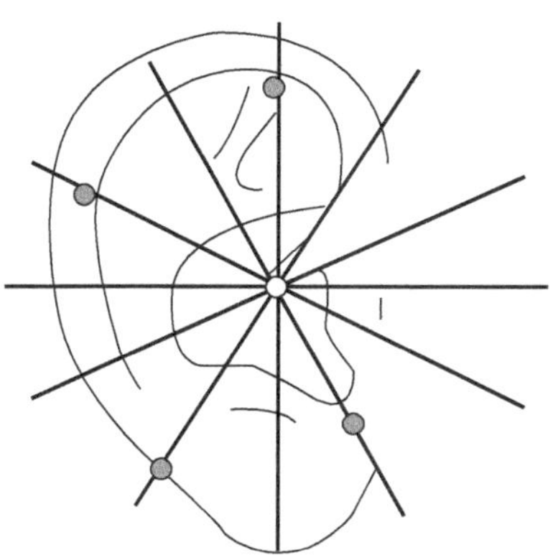

FIGURE 7: Dr. Rouxeville's location method of auricular acupuncture points in 1980.

exactly the same in the world," no ears have exactly the same shape. The latitude and longitude coordinates hardly match the actual positions of AAPs based on anatomical structures, which therefore is difficult to serve as a repeatable, standard location method. Up to now, this location method is not applied extensively enough.

3.5. The Location Method Based on the Facial Ties of the Knee of the Helix and Lobe. This location method (Figures 9(a) and 9(b)), proposed by Dr. David Alimi, took for base the anatomical structures of the ear as the ties which were constant at all humans: namely, the facial ties of the knee of the helix and lobule. These ties (their epicenter) were always aligned on a perfect right which always passed by the corpus callosum [19]. The corpus callosum connects the left and right cerebral hemispheres and facilitates interhemispheric communication. The point was considered to represent the corpus callosum, called 0 premium by the largest number, pulled tangents in these ties. A semicircle of an angular value of 180 degrees was divided into 20 equal angles, with 9 degrees for each sector. The group was a segmentogram recovering the totality of the anterior and posterior surfaces of the auricle. This location method is based on the division of subzones. However, this location method is not based on the anatomical structures of the auricle, and it is more complicated than Oleson's location method in 1983 and Chinese location method based on points and subzones when applied in clinical practice [20].

3.6. The Location Method Based on Both Points and Subzones of the Anterior of the Auricle. This method was proposed in 1988 by an article entitled "The Project of the Standardization of AAPs" by the China Association of Acupuncture-Moxibustion in the Journal of Traditional Chinese Medicine [21] (Figure 10). The article put forward for the first time a new location method, in which AAPs were named mainly by the divided auricular subzones and by supplementing

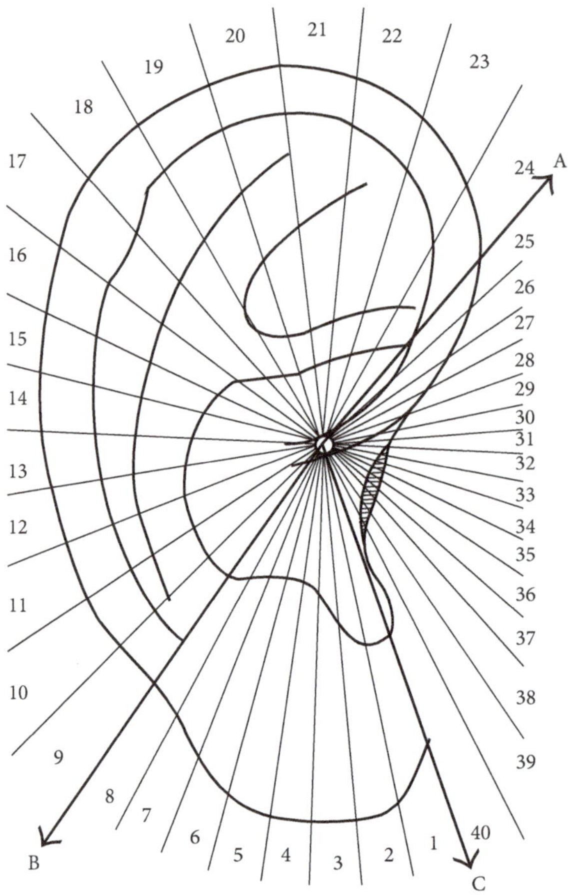

Figure 8: Professor Romoli's location method of auricular acupuncture points in 2009. Auricular sectogram, centered on Nogier's Point Zero, with the three half-lines (A), (B), and (C) subdividing the auricle.

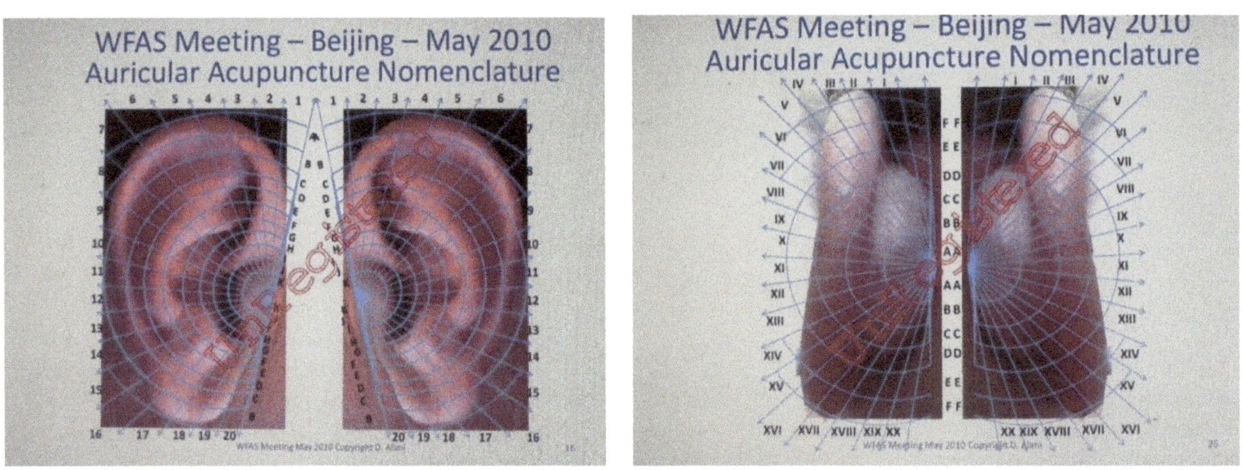

(a) (b)

Figure 9: (a) Dr. Alimi's location method for the anterior of the auricle in 2010. (b) Dr. Alimi's location method for the posterior of the auricle in 2010.

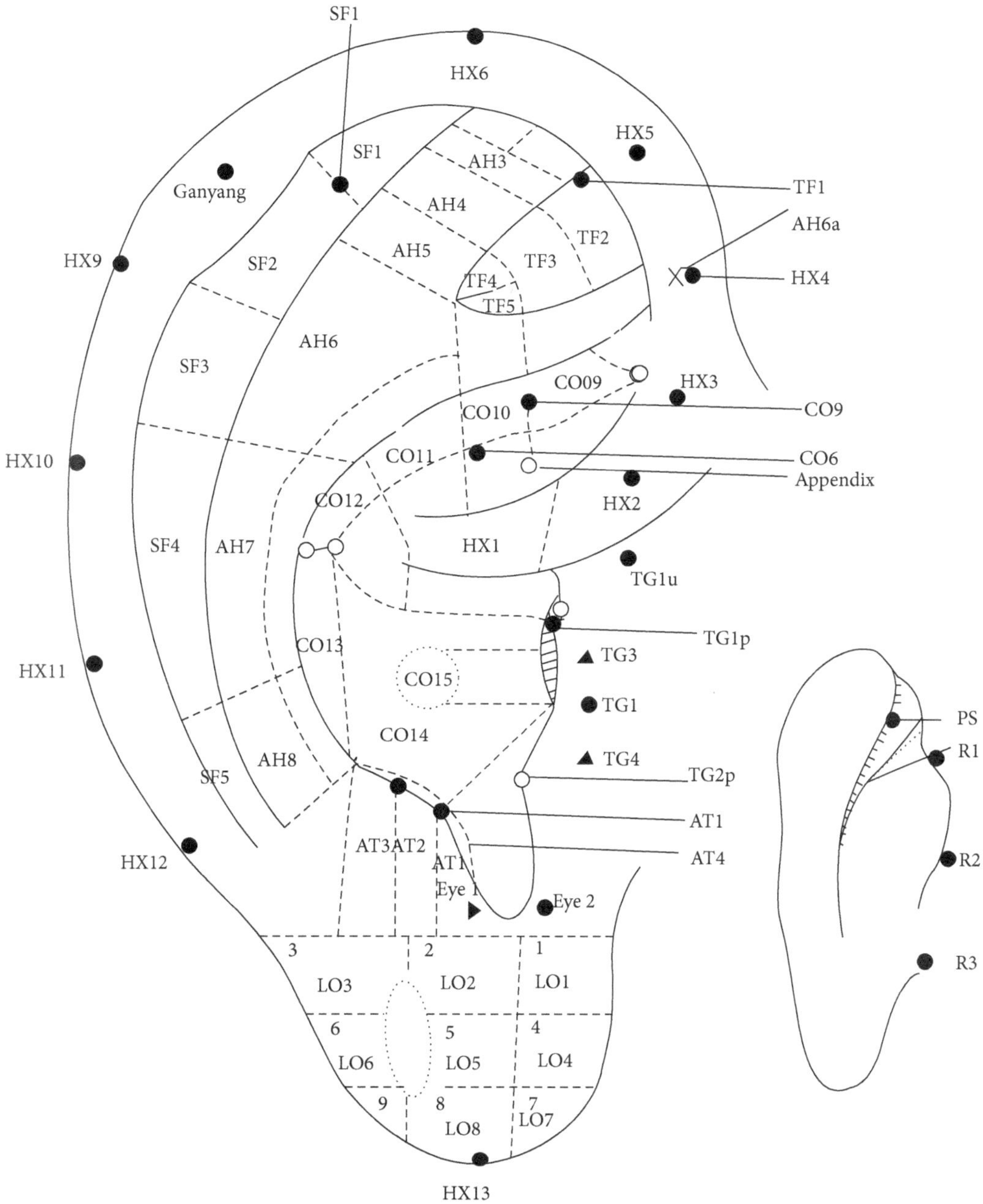

FIGURE 10: Standard project of auricular acupuncture points by the China Association of Acupuncture-Moxibustion in 1988.

with the location method based on points, and also basically covered the anterior of the auricle. Advantages of this method are as follows. Firstly, it is based on the anatomy of the auricle, taking into account the complicated structure of the surface of the auricle. For AAPs at relatively flat area, the location method is based on subzones. For AAPs at tips of the different zones of the auricle or notches, the location method is based on points. It opens up a new thought of locating AAPs by different location methods according to the actual situation. Secondly, it is of great importance to create the location method which integrates auxiliary lines to locate AAPs according to the anatomical structures of the auricle, for example, at the ear lobe. The disadvantages are as follows. Firstly, a complete location principle was not formed. The application of the location method based on both points and subzones of the anterior of the auricle is not normative enough. For example, the location method based on points is still used for AAPs at the flat helix. Secondly, a considerable part of the anterior of auricle is still unmarked. Thirdly, there was no specification on how to locate AAPs on the posterior of the auricle.

3.7. The Location Method Based on Smaller Subzones of the Anterior of the Auricle. The book, *Practical Auricular Acupuncture Therapy*, was published by Shanxi Science and Technology Press of China in 1988 which further divided the previous subzones into a number of even smaller subzones to improve the accuracy of the location of AAPs [22] (Figure 11).

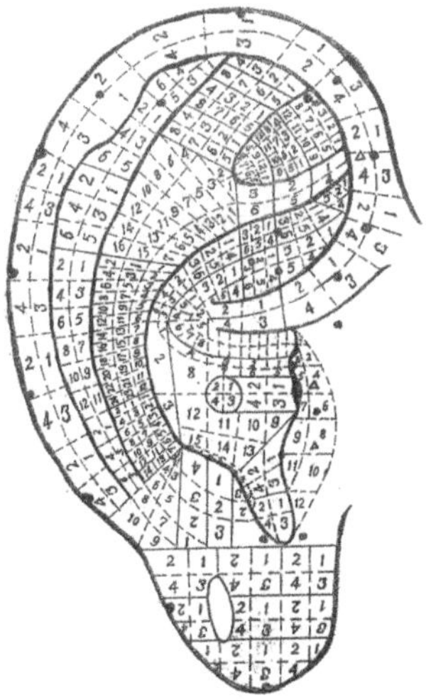

FIGURE 11: The location method based on smaller subzones of the anterior of the auricle in 1988.

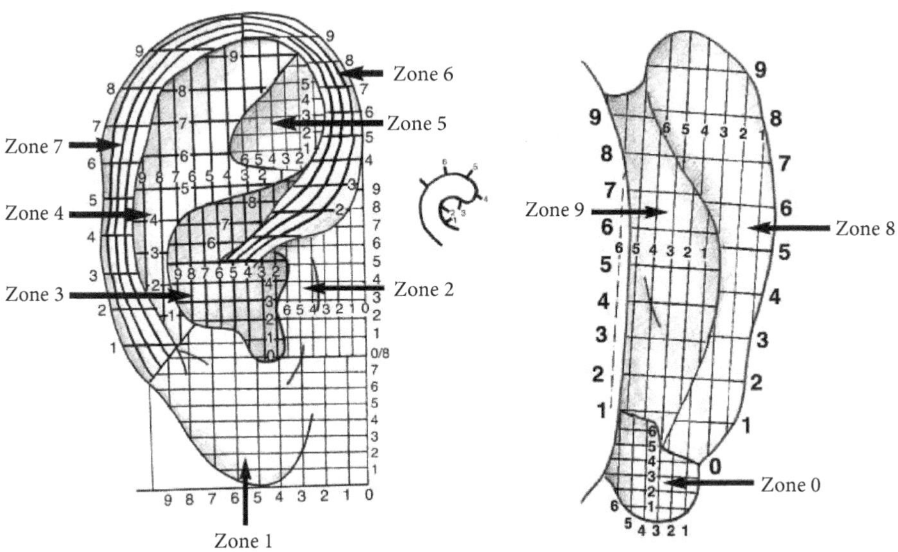

(a) (b)

FIGURE 12: (a) Dr. Wojak's location method for the anterior of the auricle in 2010. (b) Dr. Wojak's location method for the posterior of the auricle in 2010.

One similar location method [19], proposed by Dr. Winfred Wojak from Germany, divided the anterior auricle into 7 zones/areas and the posterior auricle into three zones/areas (Figures 12(a) and 12(b)). The anterior 7 zones included Zone 1, Zone 2, Zone 3, Zone 4, Zone 5, Zone 6, and Zone 7. The posterior 3 zones included Zone 8, Zone 9, and Zone 0. Each zone/area, except the helix, was divided into 9 vertical lines and 9 or 6 horizontal lines, which depended on the sizes of the zones/areas. For example, Zone 5 (the triangular fossa) and Zone 0 (the posterior of the lobe) were divided into 6 horizontal lines. The advantages of this method are as follows. Firstly, the location method inherits the objectivity and normativeness of the previous location method based on the anatomical structures of the auricle. Secondly, it considers the demand for an accurate description of the location of the point where the needle is inserted in the clinical practice of AAPs. It is helpful to choose the right point under the condition of the application of the location method based on subzones. Thirdly, this location method encompasses the idea, and subzones can be further divided into smaller subzones, which can be also further divided into even points. This idea unifies the location method based on points and the location method based on subzones according to the clinical demand. The shortcomings of this method are as follows. Firstly, the divided smaller subzones are even more complicated than the previous location method based on subzones, which brings difficulty in getting popular. Secondly, due to the complexity of the structures of the

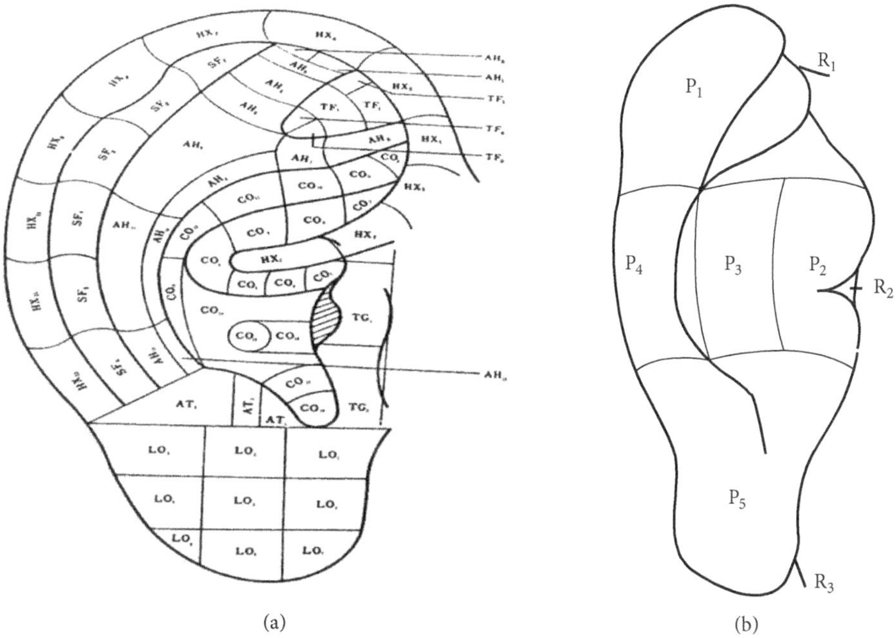

FIGURE 13: (a) The subzones of the anterior of the auricle [3, 4] and the international standard of auricular acupuncture points, issued by the World Federation of Acupuncture-Moxibustion Societies in 2013. (b) The subzones of the posterior of the auricle [3, 4] and the international standard of auricular acupuncture points, issued by the World Federation of Acupuncture-Moxibustion Societies in 2013.

auricle, it is difficult to make further division of auricular zones according to the anatomical structures of the auricle. Therefore, this method does not become the mainstream location method for locating AAPs, though it is a helpful thought for the location of AAPs.

3.8. The Location Method Based on Subzones, Points, and Lines for the Anterior and Posterior of the Auricle. After retaining the advantages and discarding the disadvantages of the above location methods, a new location method based on subzones, points, and lines for the anterior and posterior of the auricle was formed and applied in the clinical practice of AAPs. The Chinese National Standard, The Nomenclature and Location of AAPs, was issued in 1993. This standard systematically adopted this location method for the first time [3] (Figures 13(a) and 13(b)). The advantages of this new location method are as follows. Firstly, it keeps as many traditional locations of AAPs whose clinical therapeutic effects are proved as possible, which ensures the consistency of the nomenclature and location of auricular points. Secondly, it absorbs the advantages of all of the above location methods and also integrates the location method based on the natural auricular groove at the posterior of the auricle, making the location of AAPs more systematic. Thirdly, the idea of imaginary marking points and lines (Figures 14 and 15) proposed by the corresponding author, Professor Zhou [23], is adopted in this standard. Imaginary Point (A) is located at the medial edge of the helix at the junction between the middle and upper one-third of the line from the notch of helix crus and the inferior edge of the inferior antihelix crus. Imaginary Point (D) is located where a level line drawn from the end of the helix crus crosses the concha edge of the antihelix. Imaginary Point (B) is located at the junction of the middle and posterior one-third of the line extending from the end of the helix crus to Point (D). Imaginary Point (C) is located at the junction of the upper one-quarter and lower three-quarters of the posterior edge of the orifices of the external auditory meatus. Line (AB) is a curved line that extends from Point (A) to Point (B) and mirrors the concha edge of the antihelix. Line (BC) is a curved line extending from Point (B) to Point (C) that mirrors the inferior edge of the helix crus. In this way Z. Liqun makes it possible to describe accurately the locations of all AAPs according to the anatomical structures of the auricle and thus promotes the development of the standardization of localization of AAPs. Finally, it is helpful for the publication, research, teaching, and clinical application of AAPs. The limitation of this method is that there are still a small number of subzones unnamed, such as the anterior part of the helix and the two subzones at the anterior and posterior of the ear apex.

3.9. The Location Method Based on Subzones, Points, and Lines for Full Cover of the Anterior and Posterior of the Auricle. The method based on subzones according to the anatomical structures of the auricle, points, and lines for full cover of the anterior and posterior of the auricle was adopted by the new Chinese National Standard, Nomenclature and Locations of AAPs (GB/T13734-2008) [4] (Figures 13(a) and 13(b)) and also by the International Standard, Auricular acupuncture point (Figures 13(a) and 13(b)), issued by the World Federation of Acupuncture-Moxibustion Societies [5]. This location method marks the increasing maturity of the

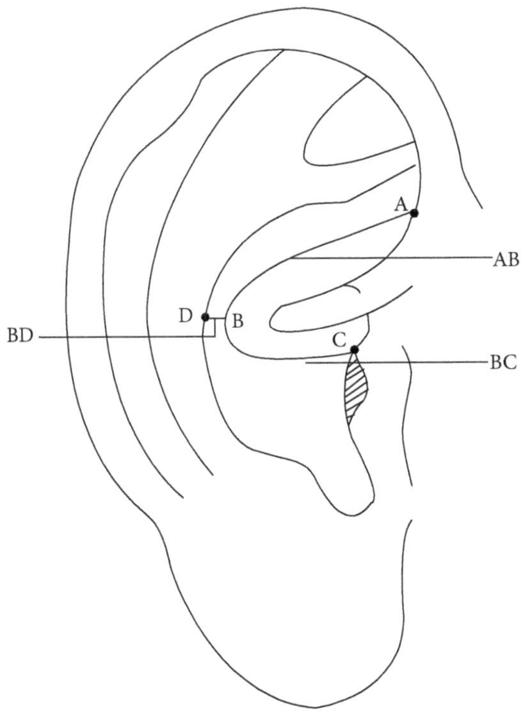

FIGURE 14: Marking points and lines in 1992.

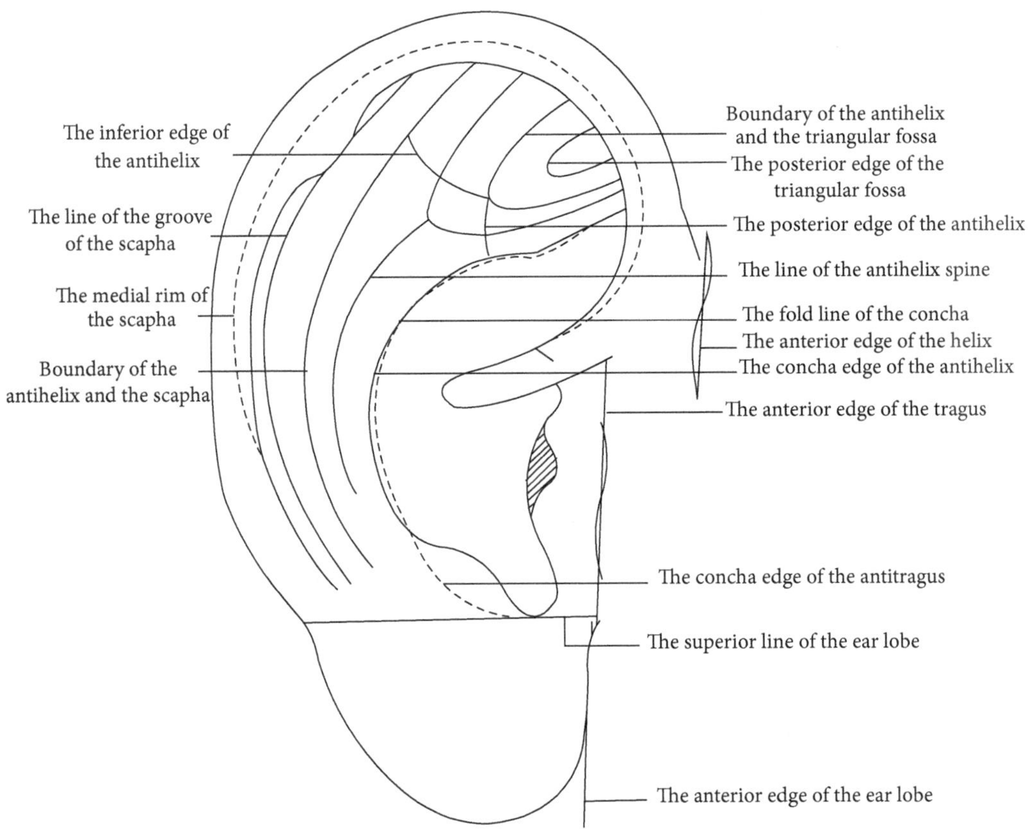

FIGURE 15: Marking lines in 1992.

location of international standard of AAPs. Firstly, it accumulates the successful experience from the research work on international standardization of AAPs in the past 20 years and avoids the disadvantages of the above-mentioned location methods. Secondly, it names the two unnamed subzones in the former Chinese national standard in 1993 so that all subzones, points, and lines can be matched to a name, covering all areas of the auricle. However, this method still has some limitations. Firstly, there are some disagreements on the names of certain subzones or points between China and Europe. Secondly, some zones or subzones, especially the zones of the posterior of the auricle, are too big to insert the needle on the posterior of the auricle. The location method for the posterior of the auricle needs to be further improved.

4. Conclusion

The research on history, mechanism, and clinical application of auricular therapy has experienced a long process [24]. The nomenclature, location method, and consistency between name and location are three topics in the research field of international standardization of AAPs. Through analyzing the advantages and disadvantages of these nine representative location methods, we tried to offer a proper location method to locate AAPs.

The location method based on subzones according to the anatomical structures of the auricle, points, and lines for full cover of the anterior and posterior of the auricle is an appropriate method and is adopted by the WFAS international standard of AAPs. It is important to keep the right direction during developing an ISO international standard of auricular acupuncture points and to improve the research quality of international standardization for AAPs and of auricular diagnosis and treatment.

Competing Interests

The authors declare that they have no competing interests.

Acknowledgments

This work was supported by National Basic Research Program of China (to Pei-Jing Rong), no. 2012CB518503, and National Science & Technology Pillar Program during the Twelfth Five-Year Plan Period (to Pei-Jing Rong), no. 2012BAF14B10; National Science & Technology Program (to Li-Qun Zhou), 2006BAK04A20; and the World Federation of Acupuncture and Moxibustion Societies Program (to Li-Qun Zhou), WFAS-2009 b26-3.

References

[1] D. S. Wang, "The draft of nomenclature of auricular acupuncture points approved by the region of west pacific of WHO," *Foreign Medical Sciences*, vol. 10, no. 1, p. 64, 1988 (Chinese).

[2] WHO, "Report of the working group on auricularacupuncture nomenclature," Tech. Rep., WHO, Lyon, France, 1990, http://whqlibdoc.who.int/hq/1991/WHO_TRM_91.2.pdf.

[3] Chinese Committee of Diagnosis and Treatment of Auricular Acupuncture Points Affiliated to the China Association of Acupuncture-Moxibustion, *Nomenclature and Location of Auricular Acupuncture Points (GB/T13734-92) of the National Standard of the People's Republic of China*, China Standard Press, Beijing, China, 1993 (Chinese).

[4] Chinese Committee of Diagnosis and Treatment of Auricular Acupuncture Points affiliated to the China Association of Acupuncture-Moxibustion, *Nomenclature and Location of Auricular Acupuncture Points (GB/T13734-2008) of the National Standard of the People's Republic of China*, China Standard Press, Beijing, China, 2008 (Chinese).

[5] The World Federation of Acupuncture-Moxibustion Societies (WFAS), "Auricular acupuncture point (WFAS STANDARD-002: 2012)," *World Journal of Acupuncture—Moxibustion*, vol. 23, no. 3, pp. 12–21, 2013.

[6] L. Q. Zhou, "The origin and development of auricular diagnosis and treatment," in *Proceedings of the International Symposium on Auricular Acupuncture Diagnosis and Treatment with Auricular Points*, pp. 87–88, Beijing, China, 1998 (Chinese).

[7] L. C. Huang, *Auricular Diagnosis and Treatment*, Scientific and Technical Documentation Press, 1991 (Chinese).

[8] Z. J. Zhang, *Essential Techniques for Massage (Wangzhenzunjing)*, Beijing People's Medical Publishing House, 1955 (Chinese).

[9] X. L. Ye, "The new discovery of acupuncture abroad-the introduction to auricular acupuncture therapy," *Shanghai Journal of Traditional Chinese Medicine*, no. 12, pp. 45–48, 1958 (Chinese).

[10] P. F. M. Nogier, R. J. Bourdiol, and F. Bahr, *Loci Auriculomedicinae*, Maisonneuve, Moulins-les-Metz, France, 1975 (French).

[11] F. Bahr and B. Strittmatter, *Ear Acupuncture: A Precise Pocket Atlas Based on the Works of Nogier/Bahr*, People's Military Medical Press, Beijing, Peoples, 2014 (Chinese).

[12] P. F. M. Nogier, "On the auricular acupuncture (Über die Akupunktur der Ohrmuschel)," *German Journal of Acupuncture and Related Techniques (DZA)*, vol. 3-4, pp. 25–33, 1957 (German).

[13] H. Jarricot and M. Wong, "De l'auriculothérapie," *Méridiens*, vol. 21-22, pp. 85–137, 1973.

[14] Z. Wang, *Auricular Acupuncture*, Shanghai Science and Technology Press, Shanghai, China, 1984 (Chinese).

[15] T. D. Oleson and R. J. Kroening, "A new nomenclature for identifying Chinese and Nogier auricular acupuncture points," *American Journal of Acupuncture*, vol. 11, no. 4, pp. 325–344, 1983.

[16] Y. Rouxeville, *Éléments D'auriculothérapie*, Maisionneuver, Sainte-Ruffine, France, 1980 (French).

[17] R. A. Durinyan, "Anatomy and physiology of auricular reflex therapy," *Scandinavian Journal of Acupuncture and Electrotherapy*, no. 3-4, pp. 83–91, 1986 (Russian).

[18] M. Romoli and R. Mazzoni, "The validation of a new system of transcription of acupuncture points on the ear: the auricular sectogram," *German Journal of Acupuncture and Related Techniques*, vol. 52, no. 3, pp. 7–10, 2009.

[19] L. Wang, "Status and strategies analysis on international standardization of auricular acupuncture points," Beijing University of Chinese Medicine, pp. 45–46, January 2016, http://cdmd.cnki.com.cn/Article/CDMD-10026-1012363203.htm.

[20] L. Wang, B. X. Zhao, and L. Q. Zhou, "Status and strategies analysis on international standardization of auricular acupuncture points," *Journal of Traditional Chinese Medicine*, vol. 33, no. 3, pp. 408–412, 2013.

[21] China Association of Acupuncture and Moxibustion, "The project of the standardization of auricular acupuncture points," *Journal of Traditional Chinese Medicine*, no. 6, pp. 75–77, 1988 (Chinese).

[22] L. Gu and L. Q. Zhou, *Practical Handbook of Auricular Diagnosis and Treatment*, Shanxi Science Education Press, Taiyuan, China, 1988 (Chinese).

[23] L. Q. Zhou, "Some supplementary ideas on the standardization of auricular acupuncture points," *Journal of Traditional Chinese Medicine*, vol. 33, no. 10, pp. 48–49, 1992 (Chinese).

[24] P. W. Hou, H. C. Hsu, Y. W. Lin, N. Tang, C. Y. Cheng, and C. L. Hsieh, "The history, mechanism, and clinical application of auricular therapy in traditional Chinese medicine," *Evidence-Based Complementary and Alternative Medicine*, vol. 2015, Article ID 495684, 13 pages, 2015.

9

Chinese Herbal Medicine as Adjunctive Therapy to Chemotherapy for Breast Cancer

Xu Sun,[1] Xing Zhang,[1,2] Jia-Yun Nian,[1,2] Jiao Guo,[1,2] Yi Yin,[3] Gan-Lin Zhang,[1] Ming-Wei Yu,[1] Yi Zhang,[1] Xiao-Min Wang,[1] Guo-Wang Yang,[1] Lin Yang,[1] Pei-Yu Cheng,[1] and Jin-Ping Li[1,4]

[1]*Department of Oncology, Beijing Hospital of Traditional Chinese Medicine, Capital Medical University, Beijing 100010, China*
[2]*Beijing University of Chinese Medicine, Beijing 100029, China*
[3]*Department of Oncology, Third Affiliated Hospital of Henan College of Traditional Chinese Medicine, Zhengzhou 450000, China*
[4]*Department of Medical Biochemistry and Microbiology, Uppsala University, 75123 Uppsala, Sweden*

Correspondence should be addressed to Xiao-Min Wang; wangxiaomin_bhtcm@126.com

Academic Editor: Kamal D. Moudgil

Chinese herbal medicine (CHM) has been increasingly employed during therapy for breast cancer, but its efficacy remains a matter of debate. This systematic review examined randomized controlled trials to provide a critical evaluation of this treatment. The results demonstrated that the combined use of CHM with chemotherapy may improve the immediate tumor response and reduce chemotherapy-associated adverse events. Our findings highlight the poor quality of Chinese studies, and additional well-designed randomized controlled trials addressing the role of CHM are warranted. The lack of molecular-based evidence for CHM and Zheng has resulted in a limited understanding and acceptance of CHM and traditional Chinese medicine in Western countries. We believe that researchers should immediately explore a CHM-based cure, and CHM should be applied to routine care as soon as conclusive data are available.

1. Introduction

Breast cancer is the leading cause of cancer-related deaths in women worldwide [1]. Breast cancer has been one of the fastest growing cancers in China over the past 30 years, with an incidence approaching approximately 96%, which is only slightly lower than that of lung cancer [2].

Chemotherapy plays a key role in the systemic treatment of breast cancer, and it is the cornerstone of therapy for patients who are not candidates for endocrine therapy [3]. Adjuvant chemotherapy can increase the pathological complete response (CR) rate and improve survival in most patients with early stage breast cancer [4–6]. The primary objectives of treatment are palliation and improved survival for the vast majority of metastatic breast cancers, which are incurable.

The chemical agents used in chemotherapy are selectively destructive to malignant tissues, but these agents also damage healthy tissue, which results in adverse side effects that negatively impact compliance with cancer treatment. Therefore, there is a clinical need to find an intervention to manage the adverse side effects of chemotherapy and increase patient tolerance and well-being.

Many breast cancer patients take complementary and alternative medicine (CAM), usually in combination with anticancer treatments, and the global use of CAM continues to increase dramatically [7–9]. The application of CAM in Western countries ranges from 9% to 69% [7, 8, 10–15]. Notably, these studies highlighted the use of traditional Chinese herbal medicine (CHM) for breast cancer.

Traditional Chinese medicine (TCM) was developed thousands of years ago, long before the advent of modern science. The use of TCM-based CHM for breast cancer has been described in Chinese medical texts for more than 2000 years [16, 17]. CHM, including botanical, animal, and mineral agents, used by TCM physicians aims to control the side effects and toxicities of cancer therapies, which improves the patient's quality of life (QoL), prevents recurrence, and prolongs survival [18].

Most studies on the clinical efficacy of CHM are based on either personal experience or case reports. Therefore, it is difficult to reach evidence-based conclusions. We conducted this systematic review to evaluate the efficacy of CHM as an adjunctive therapy to chemotherapy for the treatment of breast cancer compared with the use of chemotherapy alone because of the high prevalence of breast cancer in women and the frequent use of chemotherapy in women who present to TCM practitioners.

2. Methods

This systematic review was conducted using the PRISMA statement [19]. We developed a protocol prior to conducting the review.

2.1. Databases. Two authors independently searched for publications dated as late as August 30, 2014, in the following electronic databases: MEDLINE via OvidSP, EMBASE via OvidSP (as shown in the list below), CINAHL via OvidSP, AMED via OvidSP, PubMed, CENTRAL via OvidSP, Chinese BioMedical Literature Database (CBM), the Chinese database CNKI, Wan Fang, and VIP. The following terms were used in the search: breast cancer, breast neoplasm, breast tumor, mammary cancer, mammary neoplasm, human mammary carcinomas, chemotherapy, Chinese herbals, Chinese herbal drugs, Chinese medicine, traditional Chinese medicine, CHM, TCM, herbals, Kampo, herbal therapy, complementary medicine, alternative medicine, plants, and botany. A manual review of the reference lists of all accepted papers was also conducted.

Search Strategy for EMBASE via OvidSP to Identify Potential Articles

(1) Clinical trial/
(2) Randomized controlled trial/
(3) Randomization/
(4) Single blind procedure/
(5) Double blind procedure/
(6) Crossover procedure/
(7) Placebo/
(8) Randomized controlled trial$.tw.
(9) Rct.tw.
(10) Random allocation.tw.
(11) Randomly allocated.tw.
(12) Allocated randomly.tw.
(13) (allocated adj2 random).tw.
(14) Single blind$.tw.
(15) Double blind$.tw.
(16) ((treble or triple) adj (blind$)).tw.
(17) Placebo$.tw.
(18) Prospective study/
(19) Or/1–18
(20) Case study/
(21) Case report.tw.
(22) Abstract report/or letter/
(23) Or/20–22
(24) 19 not 23
(25) exp breast neoplasms/
(26) (breast adj5 neoplasm$).ti,ab.
(27) (breast adj5 cancer$).ti,ab.
(28) (breast adj5 tumo$).ti,ab.
(29) (breast adj5 carcinoma$).ti,ab.
(30) (breast adj5 adenocarcinoma$).ti,ab.
(31) (breast adj5 dcis).ti,ab.
(32) (breast adj5 ductsl).ti,ab.
(33) (breast adj5 sarcoma$).ti,ab.
(34) (breast adj5 infiltrating).ti,ab.
(35) (breast adj5 intraductal).ti,ab.
(36) (breast adj5 lobular).ti,ab.
(37) (breast adj5 medullary).ti,ab.
(38) Or/25–37
(39) exp chinese medicine/
(40) exp medicine, east asian traditional/or exp medicine, chinese traditional/or exp medicine, kampo/or exp medicine, korean traditional/or exp medicine, mongolian traditional/
(41) exp complementary medicine/
(42) exp traditional chinese medicine/
(43) Or/39–42
(44) 38 and 43
(45) 24 and 44

2.2. Inclusion Criteria. The inclusion criteria were as follows. (1) *Types of Studies.* There were randomized controlled trials (RCTs) with two arms, without blinding or language restrictions. (2) *Types of Participants.* They were female breast cancer patients who were diagnosed using pathological sections and treated with chemotherapy. (3) *Types of Interventions.* They included chemotherapy protocols of experimental and control groups that were the same or comparable; CHM was used in experimental groups as adjunctive therapy to chemotherapy; placebo or blank controls were eligible; and other treatment was identical in both groups. (4) *Type of Outcome.* The following primary outcomes were included: survival;

immediate tumor response, defined as CR or partial response (PR) using the World Health Organization scale; control of nausea and vomiting; and improvement in myelosuppression. The following secondary outcomes were included: performance status evaluated using the Karnofsky performance score (KPS); immune system response, including percent change in T lymphocytes and natural killer (NK) cell activity; QoL; and other side effects, such as alopecia, chemotherapy-related cardiotoxicity, and cognitive dysfunction.

2.3. Exclusion Criteria. The exclusion criteria were studies of breast cancer patients with other primary cancer; sample size < 30; CHM used in both groups other than experimental medicine and placebo; studies with > 20% withdrawal and/or dropout rates; nonoriginal studies; or duplicate studies.

2.4. Study Selection. Two authors independently screened the trials by first scanning abstracts, titles, and key words to select potential studies based on the inclusion and exclusion criteria. Full articles of the potential studies were obtained for a final determination. If a disagreement occurred, the two authors reviewed the study again, and a third reviewer resolved any disagreement.

2.5. Quality Assessment. Methodological quality was assessed using the 5-point Jadad scale [20]. The Jadad scale includes three domains: randomization, blinding, and withdrawals and dropouts. Only studies with a Jadad score of 3, 4, or 5 were included.

2.6. Assessment of the Risk of Bias. The risk of bias was assessed using the method recommended by the *Cochrane Handbook* [21]. This tool is a domain-based evaluation in which critical assessments are made separately for the following concepts: randomization, blinding, outcome reporting, and other issues.

2.7. Data Management. Two authors independently extracted the following variables: article title; author(s); journal title; year of publication; study design; sample size; sampling and diagnostic procedures; loss to follow-up; exclusions and reasons; baseline characteristics of patients (e.g., age, breast cancer stage); intervention characteristics (e.g., chemotherapy drugs, CHM patterns, CHM type, duration, and dosage); outcome(s); and conclusions. A third reviewer reviewed the extracted data and stored the original data in a secure computer to avoid changes.

2.8. Statistical Analysis. We performed a meta-analysis using RevMan 5.2 only when sufficient and suitable data were obtained. We conducted a narrative synthesis when there were too few clinically homogeneous studies for a meta-analysis. We calculated the RR and MD separately for dichotomous and continuous variables. A random effects model was used for pooling because of the clinical heterogeneity of CHM, which includes the complexity of ingredients and different therapeutic methods. We analyzed the pre- and posttreatment data separately to avoid biases from estimations of the values of change from baseline. We assessed heterogeneity using the χ^2 test, with a p value < 0.10 indicating a significant difference. Subgroup analyses were conducted to investigate the source of heterogeneity. Funnel plot asymmetry was used to investigate publication bias when there were at least 10 studies. The total effect was tested using the Z test, and $p < 0.05$ was used to identify significant effects.

3. Results

3.1. Characteristics of Included Studies. The initial search identified 2,109 studies published before October 2014 (Figure 1). Review of the titles and abstracts resulted in the inclusion of 243 studies. Of these, 211 studies were excluded after review of the full text because the studies were duplicates and animal experiments, had a small sample size, had a Jadad score < 3, or did not report the clinical stage. Notably, 90 Chinese studies were excluded because of a low Jadad score, which suggests that Chinese studies in this field are of poor quality. A total of 31 studies were finally included in the meta-analysis, of which 28 were retrieved from Chinese databases and 3 from English databases.

Of the total 2,805 patients who were enrolled in these studies, 1,391 received CTC therapy and 1,319 received chemotherapy alone. Ninety-five patients withdrew or dropped out (Table 1).

All trials were described as randomized and had two parallel groups. Concealment of allocation was not reported in any of the Chinese studies. The blinding process was described in the 3 English studies and in only 1 Chinese study. Eight studies reported withdrawals and dropouts. The risk of bias, as assessed using the tool from the Cochrane Collaboration, is shown in Figures 2 and 3.

All recruited patients in the 31 studies were diagnosed using pathological sections, and all studies had a Jadad score of 3, 4, or 5, indicating that the baseline characteristics were comparable among studies (Table 1).

3.2. Survival. One study reported 2-year survival with better survival in the CTC group than in the chemotherapy group, but the difference was not significant (RR = 1.15, 95% CI = 0.86–1.53) [26]. However, the median survival time differed significantly between these groups in another study (WMD = 1.90, 95% CI = 0.77–3.03) [25]. However, neither trial was of high quality.

3.3. Immediate Tumor Response. The immediate tumor response was investigated in 20 studies (1,282 patients). CTC therapy was associated with a significantly higher rate of CR or PR (RR = 1.15, 95% CI = 1.06–1.25, and $p = 0.0006$) (Figure 4) [22, 24–26, 28–35, 37, 40, 43–47, 51]. The exclusion of any one study did not influence the estimated treatment effect. The funnel plot indicated publication bias (Figure 5).

3.4. Decrease in Chemotherapy Toxicity. Chemotherapy-induced nausea and vomiting (CINV) is one of the most serious and unwanted side effects of chemotherapy [53–55].

Table 1: Characteristics of the included studies for the use of CHM as an adjunct for chemotherapy in breast cancer patients.

Study	Number of participants/dropouts	TNM stage	Duration (weeks)	Control group interventions	CHM interventions	Outcome(s)	Jadad scale score
Dang and Wang 2010 [22]	48/0	I–III	9	CTF	Aidi injection	Tumor response, cardiotoxicity, KPS, and chemotoxicity	3
Barton et al. 2013 [23]	210/44	I–IV	52	TE/TEC	Ginkgo Biloba	Cognitive dysfunction	5
Fang 2009 [24]	60/0	III/IV	3	CTF	Shenqi Wuweizi pill	Tumor response, KPS, and chemotoxicity	3
Fu and Kou 2007 [25]	88/0	IV	8	NP	Aidi injection	Tumor response, KPS, chemotoxicity, and median survival	3
Hong et al. 2014 [26]	91/7	II–IV	18	TEC	Xihuang pill	Tumor response, KPS, and overall survival	3
Huang et al. 2003 [27]	66/0	II–IV	4	CMF	Bazhen decoction	KPS and chemotoxicity	3
Huang et al. 2007 [28]	60/0	IV	6	CTF	Jianpi Xiaoji decoction	Tumor response, KPS, and immune system	3
Huang et al. 2008 [29]	60/0	III/IV	6	CTF	Shenqi Fuzheng injection	Tumor response, KPS, and chemotoxicity	3
Huang et al. 2013 [30]	60/0	IV	18–24	CEF	Huangqi injection	Tumor response, KPS, chemotoxicity, and median survival	3
Li et al. 2003 [31]	101/0	I–III	6~9	CMF	Rukang I prescription	Tumor response, KPS, and chemotoxicity	3
Li and Gong 2006 [32]	52/0	I–III	9	CEF	Aidi injection	Tumor response and chemotoxicity	3
Lu 2010 [33]	60/0	III/IV	6	CAF	Huangqi injection	Tumor response	3
Lv et al. 2014 [34]	54/0	IV	12–16	FAC	Yiqi Huoxue Huayu decoction	Tumor response, KPS, chemotoxicity, and immune system	3
Ni 2006 [35]	57/0	IV	13	Docetaxel + THP	Gaolisheng injection	Tumor response and chemotoxicity	3
Pérol et al. 2012 [36]	430/27	I–IV	8–12	FAC	Cocculine	Chemotherapy-induced emesis	5
Qi 2010 [37]	40/0	II–IV	6	TE	Yiqi Yangxue Shugan decoction	Tumor response, KPS, quality of life, and chemotoxicity	3
Qin 2013 [38]	78/0	I–IV	21	CAF	Fuzheng Qiqi Jiedu decoction	KPS	3
Semiglazov et al. 2006 [39]	352/21	I–III	16–24	CMF	Mistletoe extract	Quality of life	5
Shen 2007 [40]	100/0	IV	6	NVB + THP	Aiyishu injection	Tumor response and KPS	3
Sun et al. 2010 [41]	86/0	II–IV	3	CAF/AC	Zaofan pill	Chemotoxicity	3
Wang 2007 [42]	60/0	II-III	9	CEF	Taohong Siwu decoction	Quality of life and chemotoxicity	3
Wang 2010 [43]	40/0	II–IV	8	TE	Yiqijianpi Huayujiedu decoction	Tumor response, quality of life, and chemotoxicity	3
Wen et al. 2010 [44]	60/0	IV	3	TA	Fuzheng Xiaoyan prescription	Tumor response, quality of life, chemotoxicity, and immune system	3
Xiong 2012 [45]	48/0	IV	6	NVB + CAP	Fuzhengxiaoji decoction	Tumor response and KPS	3
Yang 2004 [46]	59/0	IV	6	NVB + THP	Aidi injection	Tumor response, KPS, and immune system	3
Yang et al. 2008 [47]	59/4	III B-IV	6–8	NP	Guben Yiliu II decoction	Tumor response and KPS	3
Yi et al. 2008 [48]	60/0	IV	12	DOX	Ginkgo Biloba	Cardiotoxicity	3
Zhang et al. 2010 [49]	80/0	I/II/III	18	CEF	Huangqi Taohong decoction	Immune system	3
Zhang et al. 2011 [50]	45/0	III-IV	6	CTF	Fuzheng Quyu Jiedu prescription	Immune system and quality of life	3
Zhang and Li 2013 [51]	96/0	II-III	3-4	CTF	Tiaogan Jianpi prescription	Tumor response	3
Zhong 2009 [52]	40/0	I–IV	6	TE	Shugan Tiaoli Chongren decoction	Quality of life, KPS, and chemotoxicity	3

KPS: Karnofsky performance score.

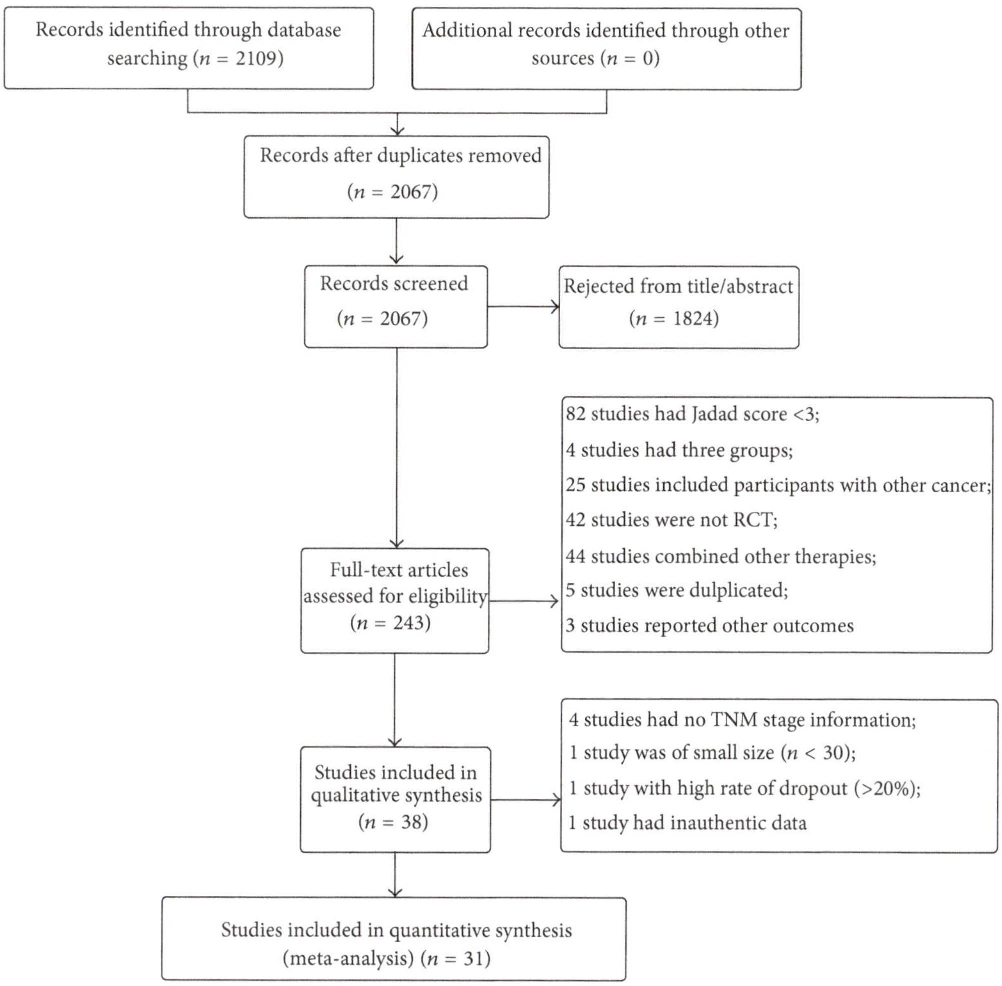

FIGURE 1: Study flow diagram of the selection process.

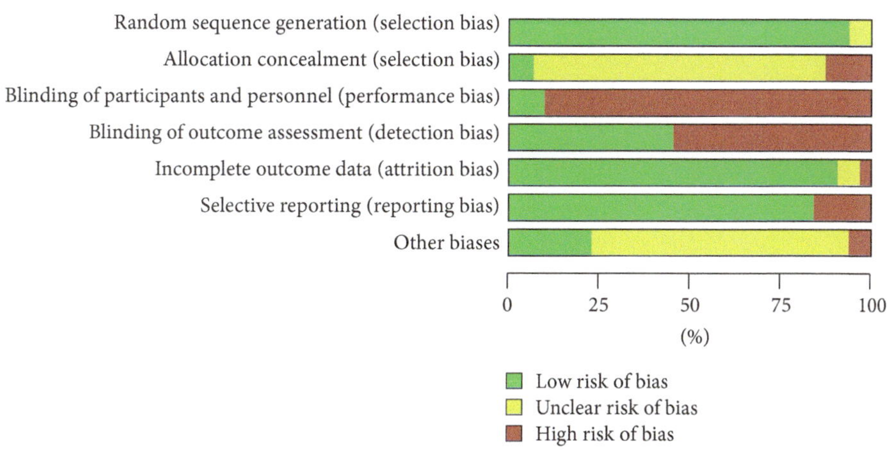

FIGURE 2: Risk of bias in included studies.

The frequency of grade II–IV CINV was significantly lower in the CTC group than in the chemotherapy group (RR = 0.53, 95% CI = 0.37–0.77, and $p = 0.0009$, 8 studies, 428 patients) (Figure 6) [22, 27, 30, 34, 42–44, 52]. The frequency of grade III-IV CINV was significantly lower in patients undergoing CTC therapy (RR = 0.23, 95% CI = 0.13–0.42, and $p < 0.00001$, 10 studies, 581 patients) (Figures 7 and 8) [22, 27, 30–32, 34, 42–44, 52]. However, one study, conducted in France, reported no differences in scores for nausea, vomiting, or global emesis on the Functional Living Index-Emesis tool

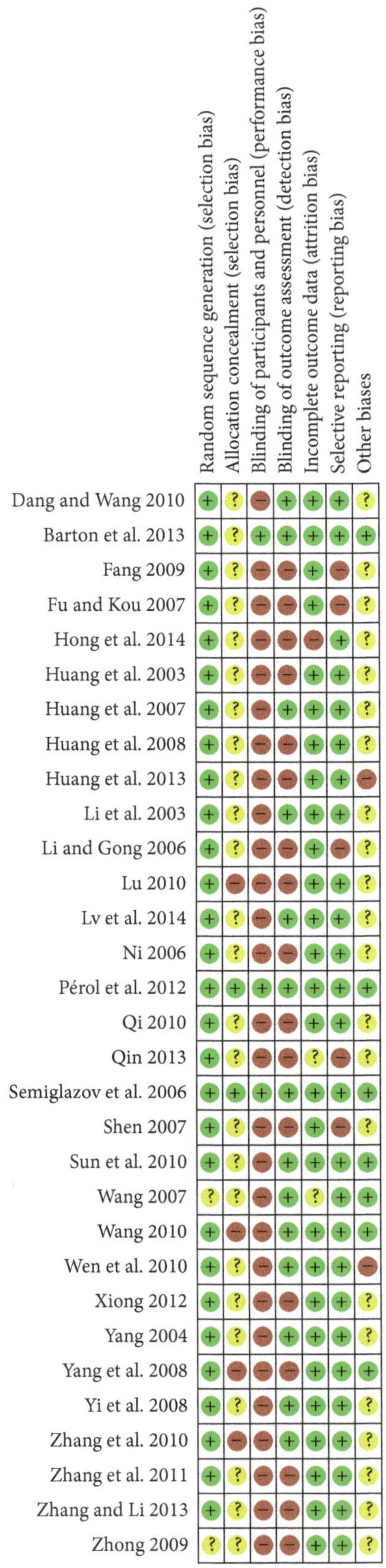

FIGURE 3: Summary of the risk of bias in included studies.

Study or subgroup	CTC Events	CTC Total	CT Events	CT Total	Weight	Risk ratio M-H, random, 95% CI
Dang and Wang 2010	26	28	18	20	20.7%	1.03 [0.86, 1.23]
Fang 2009	15	30	13	30	2.2%	1.15 [0.67, 1.99]
Fu and Kou 2007	26	44	27	44	5.7%	0.96 [0.69, 1.35]
Hong et al. 2014	10	42	8	42	1.0%	1.25 [0.55, 2.85]
Huang et al. 2007	21	30	18	30	4.7%	1.17 [0.80, 1.70]
Huang et al. 2008	15	30	13	30	2.2%	1.15 [0.67, 1.99]
Huang et al. 2013	17	30	12	30	2.3%	1.42 [0.83, 2.43]
Li et al. 2003	56	61	30	40	17.6%	1.22 [1.01, 1.49]
Li and Gong 2006	29	32	15	20	8.6%	1.21 [0.92, 1.59]
Lu 2010	17	30	15	30	2.9%	1.13 [0.70, 1.82]
Lv 2014	19	27	11	27	2.5%	1.73 [1.03, 2.90]
Ni 2006	11	30	5	27	0.8%	1.98 [0.79, 4.97]
Qi 2010	2	20	1	20	0.1%	2.00 [0.20, 20.33]
Shen 2007	35	51	34	49	9.6%	0.99 [0.76, 1.29]
Wang 2010	5	20	4	20	0.5%	1.25 [0.39, 3.99]
Wen et al. 2010	21	30	18	30	4.7%	1.17 [0.80, 1.70]
Xiong 2012	12	24	10	24	1.7%	1.20 [0.65, 2.23]
Yang 2004	22	31	19	28	5.7%	1.05 [0.74, 1.47]
Yang et al. 2008	14	28	11	27	1.9%	1.23 [0.68, 2.21]
Zhang and Li 2013	33	48	20	48	4.5%	1.65 [1.12, 2.43]
Total (95% CI)		**666**		**616**	**100.0%**	**1.15 [1.06, 1.25]**
Total events	406		302			

Heterogeneity: $\tau^2 = 0.00$; $\chi^2 = 13.56$, df = 19 ($p = 0.81$); $I^2 = 0\%$
Test for overall effect: $Z = 3.44$ ($p = 0.0006$)

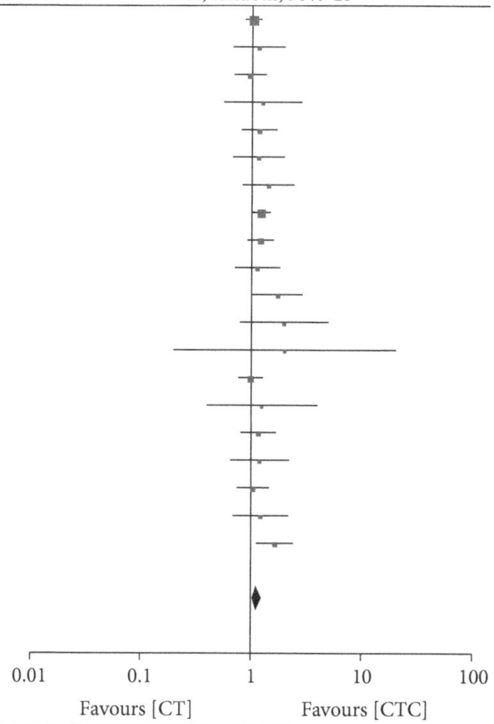

FIGURE 4: Immediate tumor response in breast cancer (CR + PR).

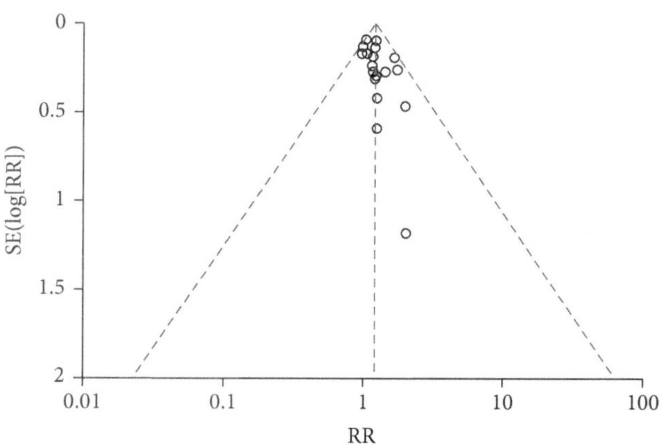

FIGURE 5: Funnel plot of immediate tumor response in breast cancer (CR + PR).

between the two arms (WMD = 0.02, 95% CI = −0.29–0.33) [36], and another study reported a significant difference [41]. These two studies were not pooled for analysis because of the different data types.

Grade III-IV-induced reductions in white blood cell (WBC) counts were significantly less frequent in the CTC group (RR = 0.68, 95% CI = 0.58–0.78, and $p < 0.00001$, 11 studies, 653 patients) (Figures 9 and 10) [24, 27, 29–32, 34, 42–44, 52]. Grade III-IV-induced reductions in WBC counts were also significantly less frequent in the CTC group (RR = 0.29, 95% CI = 0.17–0.47, and $p < 0.00001$, 9 studies, 530 patients) (Figure 11) [27, 30–32, 34, 42–44, 52].

Figure 12 shows that grade I–IV-induced reductions in platelets decreased in the CTC group (RR = 0.52, 95% CI = 0.33–0.80, and $p = 0.003$, 6 studies, 314 patients) [30, 34, 42–44, 52].

Grade I–IV-induced reductions in hemoglobin were significantly less frequent in participants undergoing combined treatment (RR = 0.63, 95% CI = 0.44–0.90, and $p = 0.001$, 3 studies, 154 patients) (Figure 13) [34, 42, 52].

3.5. Performance Status. Different types of KPS data were calculated in the studies. The first type was the improvement or stabilization of the KPS using a cutoff value of a 10-point change. The second type was the pre- and posttreatment KPS values. KPS improvement (≥10-point increase) was significantly better in the CTC group (RR = 1.81, 95% CI = 1.49–2.19, and $p < 0.00001$, 13 studies, 850 patients) (Figures 14 and 15) [24, 25, 27–30, 34, 35, 38, 40, 44–46]. The rate of improvement and stabilization (change in KPS of >0) was also significantly higher in participants receiving CTC (RR = 1.36, 95% CI = 1.26–1.47, and $p < 0.00001$, 13 studies, 850 patients) (Figures 16 and 17) [24, 25, 27–30, 34, 35, 38, 40, 44–46].

Pre- and posttreatment KPSs were reported in 6 studies. The difference in pretreatment KPS was not significant between the two arms (MD = −0.24, 95% CI = −1.32–0.84, and $p = 0.67$, 6 studies, 368 patients) (Figure 18) [22, 26, 31, 37, 47, 52]. The posttreatment KPS was significantly higher in the CTC group than in the chemotherapy group

Study or subgroup	CTC Events	CTC Total	CT Events	CT Total	Weight	Risk ratio M-H, random, 95% CI
Dang and Wang 2010	16	28	17	20	26.2%	0.67 [0.46, 0.97]
Huang et al. 2003	9	37	13	29	15.8%	0.54 [0.27, 1.09]
Huang et al. 2013	6	30	14	30	13.2%	0.43 [0.19, 0.96]
Lv et al. 2014	4	27	10	27	9.5%	0.40 [0.14, 1.12]
Wang 2007	12	30	12	30	17.8%	1.00 [0.54, 1.86]
Wang 2010	4	20	9	20	9.9%	0.44 [0.16, 1.21]
Wen et al. 2010	2	30	15	30	6.0%	0.13 [0.03, 0.53]
Zhong 2009	0	20	3	20	1.6%	0.14 [0.01, 2.60]
Total (95% CI)		**222**		**206**	**100.0%**	**0.53 [0.37, 0.77]**
Total events	53		93			

Heterogeneity: $\tau^2 = 0.10$; $\chi^2 = 11.58$, df = 7 ($p = 0.12$); $I^2 = 40\%$

Test for overall effect: $Z = 3.33$ ($p = 0.0009$)

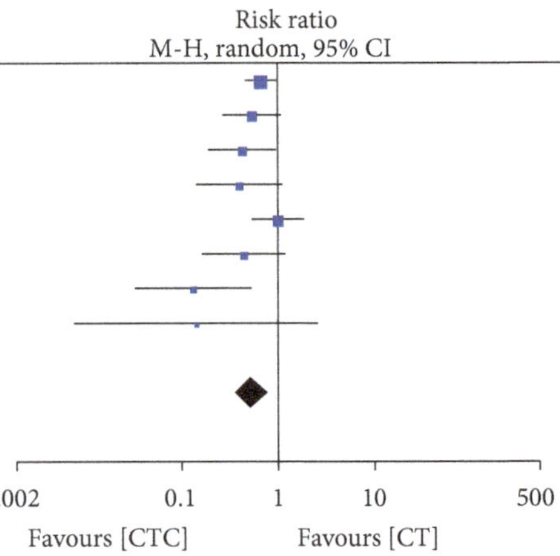

FIGURE 6: Nausea and vomiting during treatment for breast cancer (toxicity grades II–IV).

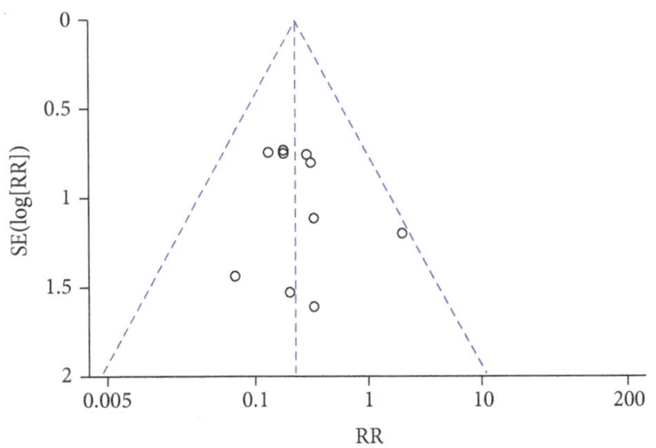

FIGURE 7: Funnel plot of nausea and vomiting during treatment for breast cancer (toxicity grades III-IV).

(MD = 6.31, 95% CI = 3.66–8.97, and $p < 0.00001$, 6 studies, 368 patients) (Figure 19).

3.6. Immunostimulation. Figures 20–24 show that, in the pooled studies, the differences in pretreatment T lymphocytes ($CD3^+$, $CD4^+$, $CD8^+$, and $CD4^+/CD8^+$) and NK cell levels between the two arms were not significant ($CD3^+$, MD = −1.09, 95% CI = −2.34–0.17, $p = 0.09$, and $I^2 = 0\%$; $CD4^+$, MD = −0.28, 95% CI = −1.08–0.52, $p = 0.50$, and $I^2 = 0\%$; $CD8^+$, MD = −0.12, 95% CI = −0.10–0.76, $p = 0.79$, and $I^2 = 0\%$; $CD4^+/CD8^+$, MD = −0.02, 95% CI = −0.11–0.08, $p = 0.71$, and $I^2 = 0\%$; NK cells, MD = −0.71, 95% CI = −2.36–0.94, $p = 0.40$, and $I^2 = 0\%$).

CTC therapy showed an advantage for $CD3^+$ and $CD4^+/CD8^+$ cells posttreatment (MD = 7.56, 95% CI = 6.28–8.85, $p < 0.00001$, and $I^2 = 5\%$, 6 studies, 358 patients, and MD = 0.26, 95% CI = 0.16–0.37, and $p < 0.00001$, 6 studies, 358 patients, resp.) (Figures 25 and 26) [28, 34, 44, 46, 49, 50]. However, the result indicates that the posttreatment NK cell level was not significantly different between the CTC and chemotherapy groups (MD = 2.30, 95% CI = −0.18–4.78, and $p = 0.07$, 2 studies, 134 patients) (Figure 27) [34, 49]. Heterogeneity existed among the included studies in terms of $CD4^+$ and $CD8^+$ cells posttreatment.

CTC therapy also resulted in significantly better posttreatment $CD4^+$ levels (MD = 7.30, 95% CI = 3.67–10.93, $p < 0.0001$, and $I^2 = 94\%$, 6 studies, 358 patients) (Figure 28). A subgroup analysis indicated that TNM stage may have affected the homogeneity. In the pooled studies, there were no significant differences in posttreatment $CD8^+$ levels between the two arms (MD = 1.41, 95% CI = −3.31–6.13, $p = 0.56$, and $I^2 = 96\%$, 6 studies, 356 patients) (Figure 29). The differences in sample size may have contributed to the heterogeneity of the studies.

3.7. QoL. Six studies reported on QoL, but we were not able to pool these results because each study used a different scale and data type. The study by Semiglazov et al. was of high quality and low risk, and the QoL was assessed using 3 FACT-G subscales (physical, emotional, and functional well-being) [39]. The intervention group exhibited improvements in the FACT-G total score and in the physical, emotional, and functional well-being scores, and the placebo group had poorer scores. Four studies that reported significantly improved QoL using combined therapy, as assessed using the Chinese version of the FACT-G, were of mixed quality [37, 42, 50, 52]. Two studies reported QoL as assessed using the Chinese version of the EORTC QLQ C-30. Zhong observed improvements in the physical and emotional subscales and the overall health QoL score with CTC therapy [52]. Wang reported significant within-group improvements in some subscales in both groups, but there were no details of comparisons between groups [43].

3.8. Other Outcomes. One high-quality study evaluated CTC therapy for the prevention of chemotherapy-related cognitive dysfunction and reported no significant difference between the two arms [23]. Two studies that reported chemotherapy-related cardiotoxicity had significant heterogeneity, and CTC

Study or subgroup	CTC Events	CTC Total	CT Events	CT Total	Weight	Risk ratio M-H, random, 95% CI
Dang and Wang 2010	2	28	8	20	16.1%	0.18 [0.04, 0.75]
Huang et al. 2003	2	37	5	29	13.6%	0.31 [0.07, 1.50]
Huang et al. 2013	2	30	7	30	15.0%	0.29 [0.06, 1.26]
Li et al. 2003	2	61	10	40	15.5%	0.13 [0.03, 0.57]
Li and Gong 2006	2	32	7	20	15.4%	0.18 [0.04, 0.78]
Lv et al. 2014	0	27	2	27	3.7%	0.20 [0.01, 3.98]
Wang 2007	2	30	1	30	6.0%	2.00 [0.19, 20.90]
Wang 2010	1	20	3	20	7.0%	0.33 [0.04, 2.94]
Wen et al. 2010	0	30	7	30	4.2%	0.07 [0.00, 1.12]
Zhong 2009	0	20	1	20	3.4%	0.33 [0.01, 7.72]
Total (95% CI)		**315**		**266**	**100.0%**	**0.23 [0.13, 0.42]**
Total events	13		51			

Heterogeneity: $\tau^2 = 0.00$; $\chi^2 = 5.23$, df = 9 ($p = 0.81$); $I^2 = 0\%$

Test for overall effect: $Z = 4.92$ ($p < 0.00001$)

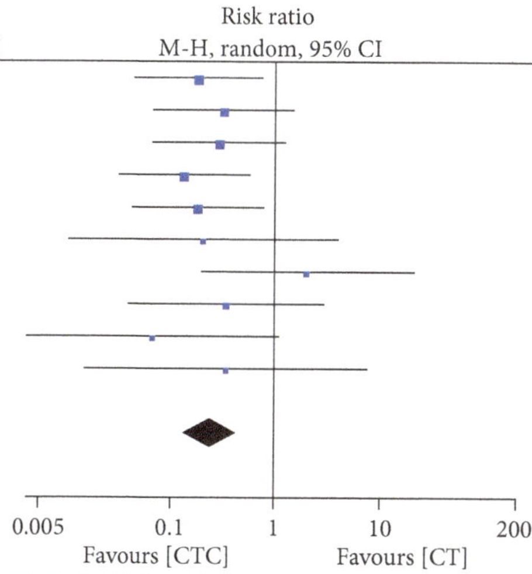

FIGURE 8: Nausea and vomiting during treatment for breast cancer (toxicity grades III-IV).

Study or subgroup	CTC Events	CTC Total	CT Events	CT Total	Weight	Risk ratio M-H, random, 95% CI
Fang 2009	9	30	17	30	4.7%	0.53 [0.28, 0.99]
Huang et al. 2003	15	37	23	29	8.8%	0.51 [0.33, 0.79]
Huang et al. 2008	9	30	17	30	4.7%	0.53 [0.28, 0.99]
Huang et al. 2013	9	30	18	30	4.8%	0.50 [0.27, 0.93]
Li et al. 2003	42	61	31	40	19.1%	0.89 [0.70, 1.13]
Li et al. 2006	22	32	18	20	16.3%	0.76 [0.58, 1.01]
Lv et al. 2014	16	27	22	27	11.5%	0.73 [0.51, 1.04]
Wang 2007	16	30	22	30	9.9%	0.73 [0.49, 1.08]
Wang 2010	13	20	19	20	12.6%	0.68 [0.49, 0.96]
Wen et al. 2010	8	30	18	30	4.3%	0.44 [0.23, 0.86]
Zhong 2009	6	20	12	20	3.3%	0.50 [0.23, 1.07]
Total (95% CI)		**347**		**306**	**100.0%**	**0.68 [0.58, 0.78]**
Total events	165		217			

Heterogeneity: $\tau^2 = 0.01$; $\chi^2 = 13.27$, df = 10 ($p = 0.21$); $I^2 = 25\%$

Test for overall effect: $Z = 5.29$ ($p < 0.00001$)

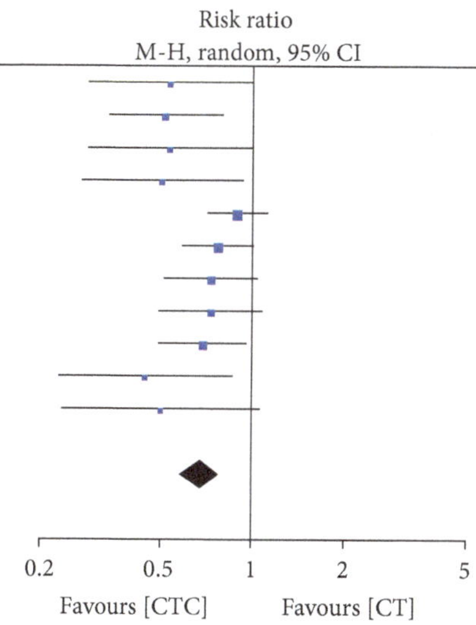

FIGURE 9: Reductions in WBCs during breast cancer treatment (toxicity grades I–IV).

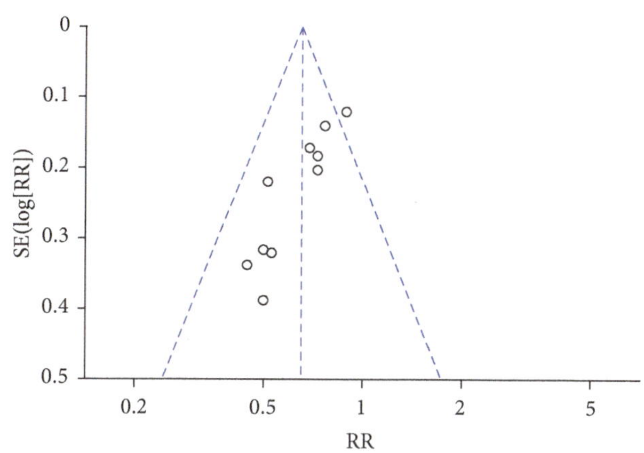

FIGURE 10: Funnel plot of the reduction in WBCs during breast cancer treatment (toxicity grades I–IV).

did not have a significant advantage in the prevention of creatinine kinase-MB isoenzyme (WMD = −21.11, 95% CI = −52.65–10.42, and $p = 0.19$) (Figure 30) [22, 48].

4. Discussion

Treatment of breast cancer using CHM has been described in Chinese medical texts for more than 2,000 years. Accepting TCM as science rather than myth remains a challenge in Western countries despite the recent increase in the use of CHM.

This review has several limitations. First, we did not identify studies in languages other than Chinese and English. CAM use is reportedly high in East Asia, where CHM originated, with use rates of 29–83% in South Korea and 50% in one study in Japan [56, 57]. Therefore, additional studies

Study or subgroup	CTC Events	CTC Total	CT Events	CT Total	Weight	Risk ratio M-H, random, 95% CI
Huang et al. 2003	0	37	3	29	3.0%	0.11 [0.01, 2.10]
Huang et al. 2013	1	30	4	30	5.6%	0.25 [0.03, 2.11]
Li et al. 2003	2	61	8	40	11.4%	0.16 [0.04, 0.73]
Li and Gong 2006	2	32	5	20	10.7%	0.25 [0.05, 1.17]
Lv et al. 2014	3	27	7	27	16.5%	0.43 [0.12, 1.49]
Ni 2006	6	30	16	27	41.8%	0.34 [0.15, 0.74]
Wang 2007	1	20	3	20	5.4%	0.33 [0.04, 2.94]
Wang 2010	0	30	5	30	3.1%	0.09 [0.01, 1.57]
Wen et al. 2010	0	20	1	20	2.6%	0.33 [0.01, 7.72]
Total (95% CI)		**287**		**243**	**100.0%**	**0.29 [0.17, 0.47]**
Total events	15		52			

Heterogeneity: $\tau^2 = 0.00$; $\chi^2 = 2.28$, df = 8 ($p = 0.97$); $I^2 = 0\%$
Test for overall effect: $Z = 4.86$ ($p < 0.00001$)

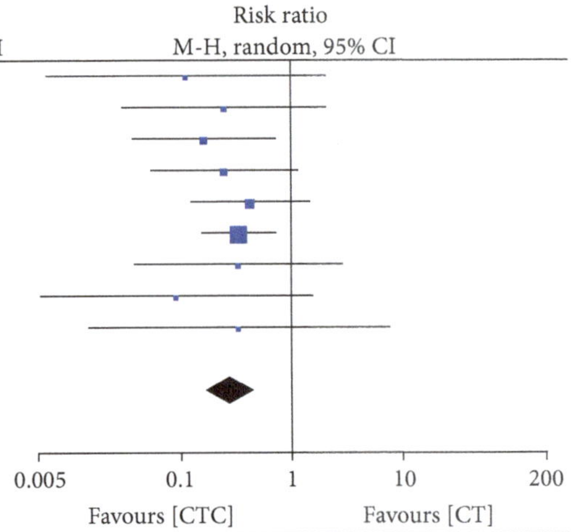

Figure 11: Reduction in WBCs during breast cancer treatment (toxicity grades III-IV).

Study or subgroup	CTC Events	CTC Total	CT Events	CT Total	Weight	Risk ratio M-H, random, 95% CI
Huang et al. 2013	10	30	14	30	22.7%	0.71 [0.38, 1.35]
Lv et al. 2014	11	27	21	27	27.9%	0.52 [0.32, 0.86]
Wang 2007	3	30	10	30	10.4%	0.30 [0.09, 0.98]
Wang 2010	11	20	15	20	29.0%	0.73 [0.46, 1.17]
Wen et al. 2010	2	30	16	30	8.2%	0.13 [0.03, 0.50]
Zhong 2009	0	20	1	20	1.9%	0.33 [0.01, 7.72]
Total (95% CI)		**157**		**157**	**100.0%**	**0.52 [0.33, 0.80]**
Total events	37		77			

Heterogeneity: $\tau^2 = 0.12$; $\chi^2 = 8.92$, df = 5 ($p = 0.11$); $I^2 = 44\%$
Test for overall effect: $Z = 2.96$ ($p = 0.003$)

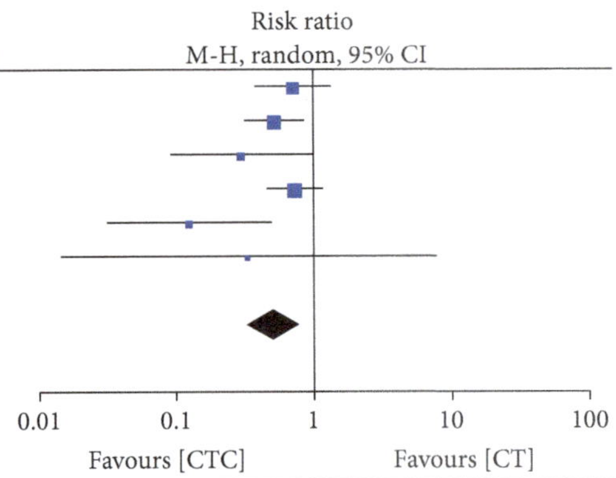

Figure 12: Reduction in platelets during breast cancer treatment (toxicity grades I–IV).

Study or subgroup	CTC Events	CTC Total	CT Events	CT Total	Weight	Risk ratio M-H, random, 95% CI
Lv et al. 2014	14	27	22	27	69.6%	0.64 [0.42, 0.95]
Wang 2007	5	30	13	30	16.0%	0.38 [0.16, 0.94]
Zhong 2009	6	20	6	20	14.4%	1.00 [0.39, 2.58]
Total (95% CI)		**77**		**77**	**100.0%**	**0.63 [0.44, 0.90]**
Total events	25		41			

Heterogeneity: $\tau^2 = 0.01$; $\chi^2 = 2.10$, df = 2 ($p = 0.35$); $I^2 = 5\%$
Test for overall effect: $Z = 2.51$ ($p = 0.01$)

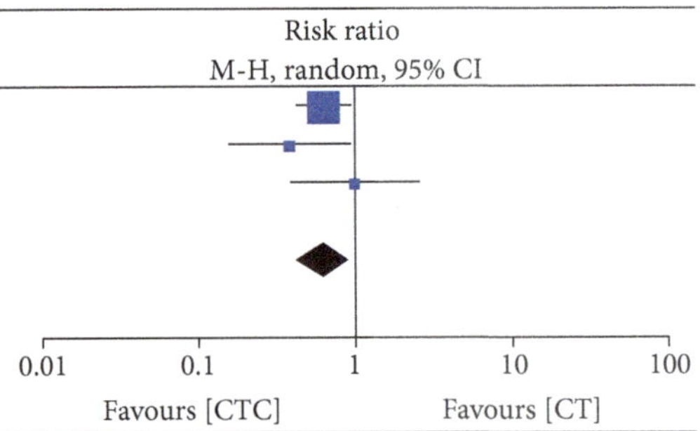

Figure 13: Reduction in hemoglobin during breast cancer treatment (toxicity grades I–IV).

should be identified from or conducted in these areas to further investigate the efficacy of CHM. Second, all of the included Chinese studies had relatively small sample sizes, ranging from 40 to 101 participants. None of these studies reported the details of sample size calculation. Third, the Chinese trials did not clearly report allocation concealment or blinding, and none of the Chinese studies were placebo controlled or double blinded, which could have resulted in bias and an overestimation of CTC efficacy [58]. Publication bias may also have existed. The asymmetry of the funnel plot may be the result of an insufficient number of trials and significant statistical heterogeneity (Figures 5, 7, 15, and 17). There were also different data types and assessment methods for outcomes, which may have resulted in statistical heterogeneity.

We also cannot ignore the low quality of the included trials; however, that may not be a sound reason to exclude a systematic review. A systematic review embraces the features of

Study or subgroup	CTC Events	CTC Total	CT Events	CT Total	Weight	Risk ratio M-H, random, 95% CI
Fang 2009	9	30	5	30	4.0%	1.80 [0.68, 4.74]
Fu and Kou 2007	15	44	13	44	10.0%	1.15 [0.62, 2.13]
Huang et al. 2003	12	37	3	29	2.8%	3.14 [0.97, 10.08]
Huang et al. 2007	15	30	8	30	7.8%	1.88 [0.94, 3.75]
Huang et al. 2008	9	30	5	30	4.0%	1.80 [0.68, 4.74]
Huang et al. 2013	14	30	7	30	6.6%	2.00 [0.94, 4.25]
Lv et al. 2014	15	27	8	27	8.3%	1.88 [0.96, 3.67]
Ni 2006	11	30	2	27	1.9%	4.95 [1.20, 20.36]
Qin 2013	27	39	11	39	12.8%	2.45 [1.43, 4.22]
Shen 2007	26	51	19	49	19.2%	1.31 [0.84, 2.05]
Wen et al. 2010	16	30	6	30	6.0%	2.67 [1.21, 5.88]
Xiong 2012	13	24	8	24	8.2%	1.63 [0.83, 3.19]
Yang 2004	17	31	8	28	8.4%	1.92 [0.98, 3.74]
Total (95% CI)		**433**		**417**	**100.0%**	**1.81 [1.49, 2.19]**
Total events	199		103			

Heterogeneity: $\tau^2 = 0.00$; $\chi^2 = 9.36$, df = 12 ($p = 0.67$); $I^2 = 0\%$
Test for overall effect: $Z = 5.98$ ($p < 0.00001$)

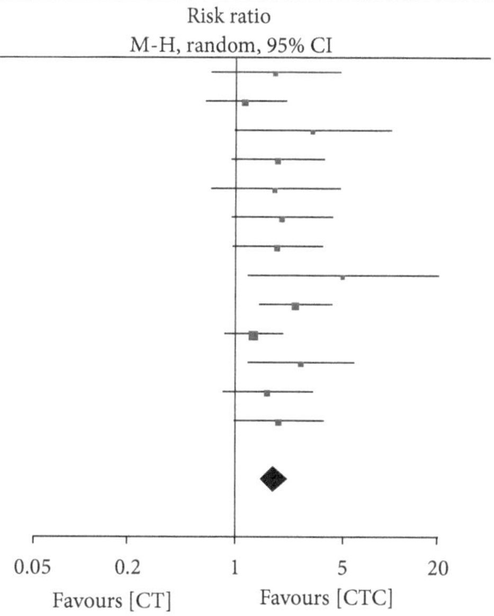

FIGURE 14: Improvement in KPS during breast cancer treatment.

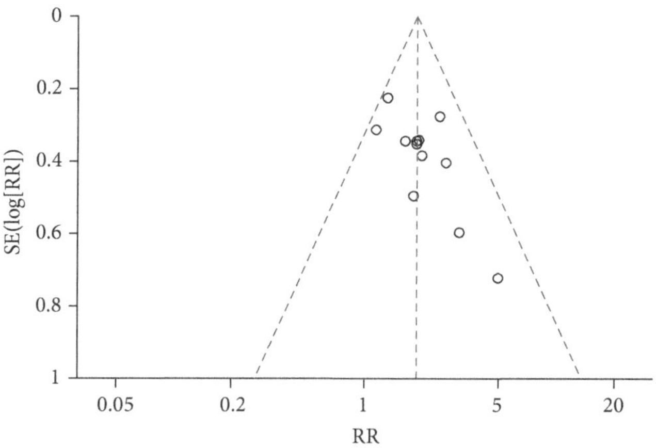

FIGURE 15: Funnel plot of improvement in KPS during breast cancer treatment.

systematization and comprehensiveness, which differentiate it from a normal review. In addition, the CHM used differed significantly among trials. Inevitably, the pharmacological actions of these treatments would not be the same. A random effects model was used for pooling because of the clinical heterogeneity. Because of this limitation, we cannot draw a convincing conclusion. Nevertheless, the problems with the current studies identified in this review are significant, and a great deal of work needs to be done to evaluate the efficacy of CAM using a modern and rigorous methodology.

Only 3 studies evaluated the Zheng TCM pattern, which is another key limitation of the included studies [37, 42, 52]. Zheng, also known as syndrome or pattern, is the core concept in TCM, and it describes the entire physiological and/or pathological pattern of the patient [59]. Zheng is usually evaluated through a comprehensive analysis of clinical signs and symptoms. TCM practitioners collect the signs by inspection, auscultation, olfaction, inquiry, pulse, and palpation. TCM practitioners in clinical practice prescribe CHM based on Zheng.

CHM therapy is more efficacious when based on the correct judgment of the Zheng classification according to the Chinese medical system. One clinical study found that the therapeutic effect of CHM for the treatment of irritable bowel syndrome was more sustainable when based on the TCM pattern than on standard treatment [60]. The key role of Zheng in TCM should not be ignored despite the controversial results reported by other clinical studies, which indicate that the efficacy of Zheng-based treatment is not advantageous over standard treatment [61–63]. Patients are not administered the same CHM for a long period of time in real practice, and the treatments reported in clinical trials did not follow a pattern that is commonly used in actual clinical practice because Zheng is dynamic during the treatment course. The biggest challenge in the exploration of Zheng-based CHM therapy using an RCT is the standardization of Zheng. Currently, the process of Zheng is highly subjective, and a nationwide and objective process is needed to improve its use. Randomized, multicenter trials should be conducted for this purpose. Analyses of Zheng at the molecular level may also enable acceptance of TCM on a scientific basis for the West.

Table 2 lists the herbal medicines that were commonly used for the treatment of breast cancer in the identified studies in this review. The pooled data in this review demonstrated that the adjunctive use of CHM with chemotherapy may improve immediate tumor response and performance status and reduce the occurrence of adverse events associated with chemotherapy. We were unable to verify whether CHM helped stimulate the immune system, as measured using $CD3^+$, $CD4^+$, $CD8^+$, and $CD4^+/CD8^+$ cells, because of the mixed quality and significance of the included studies. The evidence is too limited to make any confident conclusions.

Study or subgroup	CTC Events	CTC Total	CT Events	CT Total	Weight	Risk ratio M-H, random, 95% CI
Fang 2009	23	30	15	30	3.7%	1.53 [1.02, 2.31]
Fu and Kou 2007	39	44	31	44	12.8%	1.26 [1.01, 1.57]
Huang et al. 2003	31	37	18	29	6.0%	1.35 [0.98, 1.85]
Huang et al. 2007	25	30	18	30	5.5%	1.39 [1.00, 1.94]
Huang et al. 2008	23	30	15	30	3.7%	1.53 [1.02, 2.31]
Huang et al. 2013	26	30	18	30	5.8%	1.44 [1.04, 2.00]
Lv et al. 2014	25	27	18	27	7.4%	1.39 [1.04, 1.85]
Ni 2006	28	30	16	27	5.7%	1.57 [1.14, 2.18]
Qin 2013	38	39	24	39	9.5%	1.58 [1.23, 2.04]
Shen 2007	48	51	40	49	27.3%	1.15 [0.99, 1.34]
Wen et al. 2010	26	30	16	30	4.6%	1.63 [1.13, 2.34]
Xiong 2012	21	24	13	24	3.9%	1.62 [1.09, 2.40]
Yang 2004	25	31	15	28	4.1%	1.51 [1.02, 2.21]
Total (95% CI)		**433**		**417**	**100.0%**	**1.36 [1.26, 1.47]**
Total events	378		257			

Heterogeneity: $\tau^2 = 0.00$; $\chi^2 = 11.05$, df = 12 ($p = 0.52$); $I^2 = 0\%$
Test for overall effect: $Z = 7.75$ ($p < 0.00001$)

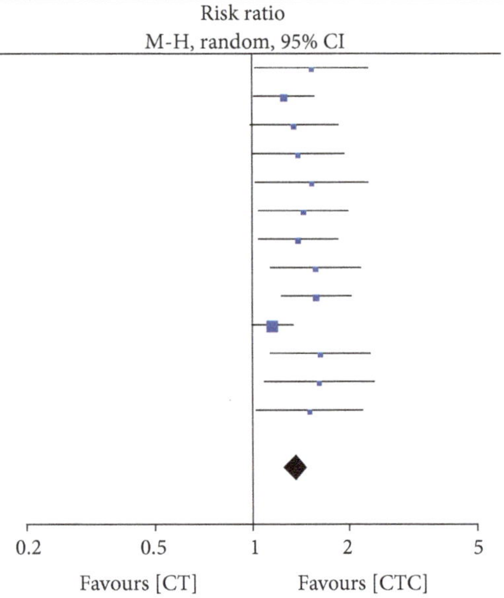

FIGURE 16: Improvement and stabilization of performance status during breast cancer treatment.

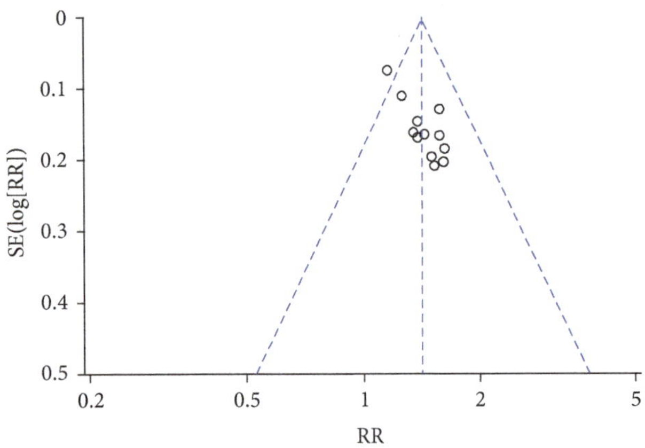

FIGURE 17: Funnel plot of improvement and stabilization of performance status during breast cancer treatment.

TABLE 2: Herbal medicines commonly used in the treatment of breast cancer.

Chinese herbal medicine	Frequency Count	%
Radix Astragalus	20	9.22
Rhizoma Atractylodis Macrocephalae	12	5.53
Poria	10	4.61
Angelica	8	3.69
Codonopsis pilosula	8	3.69
Radix Glycyrrhizae	7	3.23
Ligustrum lucidum	7	3.23
Oldenlandia diffusa	6	2.76
Pericarpium Citri Reticulatae	6	2.76
Panax	6	2.76
Pseudobulbus Cremastrae seu Pleiones	6	2.76

These results suggest that combined therapy has potential benefits for breast cancer patients. The finding of CHM efficacy as an adjunctive therapy for breast cancer is similar to the findings of other reviews for hepatocellular carcinoma, non-small-cell lung cancer, colorectal cancer, and nasopharyngeal carcinoma [58, 64–66]. A recent systematic review involving 8 RCTs showed that CHM combined with conventional therapy for breast cancer was efficacious in improving QoL and decreasing hot flashes, but this study did not identify as many clinical trials as it could have [67]. Breast cancer patients undergoing chemotherapy and/or endocrine therapy were included in that review, and the effect of CHM for breast cancer should have been examined separately in those two groups. In addition, the review focused on the effects on QoL and hot flashes but did not evaluate other cancer-related symptoms. Finally, the reviewers only presented a narrative synthesis without a meta-analysis, which made the conclusion unconvincing.

GRADE should be applied to judge the evidence and make recommendations regarding the application of CHM in the treatment of breast cancer. The present study suggests that recommendations for CHM combined with chemotherapy could be made for breast cancer, but TCM may be too complex to be immediately adopted by physicians in Western countries. The most fundamental and often-overlooked challenge is the lack of a 1 : 1 correlation between modern allopathic and Chinese holistic medical approaches [68]. We cannot make specific recommendations despite the rapid increase in the use of CHM and reported potential benefits because of the complexity of this system and the variable data.

Current evidence on the use of CHM as an adjunctive treatment with chemotherapy for breast cancer remains equivocal. Our findings highlight the poor quality of Chinese

Study or subgroup	CTC Mean	CTC SD	CTC Total	CT Mean	CT SD	CT Total	Weight	Mean difference IV, random, 95% CI
Dang and Wang 2010	72.87	4.69	28	71.89	5.03	20	14.9%	0.98 [−1.83, 3.79]
Hong et al. 2014	56.98	6.35	42	55.4	6.12	42	16.5%	1.58 [−1.09, 4.25]
Li et al. 2003	70.78	4.4	61	71.19	4.53	40	36.7%	−0.41 [−2.20, 1.38]
Qi 2010	79.49	4.5	20	81.27	3.67	20	18.1%	−1.78 [−4.32, 0.76]
Yang et al. 2008	74.64	7.44	28	74.81	8.02	20	5.9%	−0.17 [−4.64, 4.30]
Zhong 2009	77.5	6.38	20	79.5	6.86	27	8.1%	−2.00 [−5.81, 1.81]
Total (95% CI)			**199**			**169**	**100.0%**	**−0.24 [−1.32, 0.84]**

Heterogeneity: $\tau^2 = 0.00$; $\chi^2 = 4.78$, df $= 5$ ($p = 0.44$); $I^2 = 0\%$
Test for overall effect: $Z = 0.43$ ($p = 0.67$)

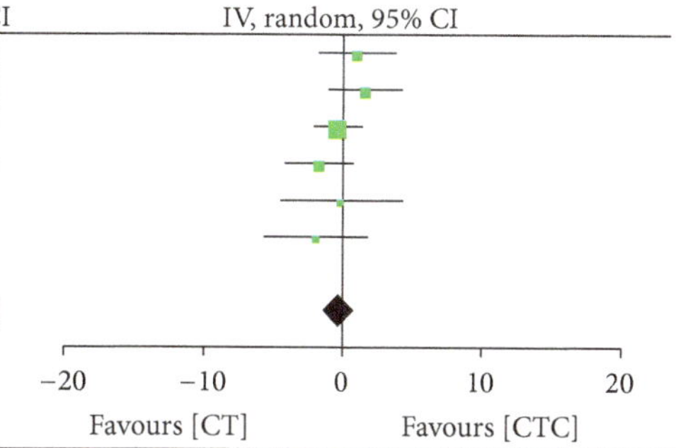

FIGURE 18: KPS before breast cancer treatment.

Study or subgroup	CTC Mean	CTC SD	CTC Total	CT Mean	CT SD	CT Total	Weight	Mean difference IV, random, 95% CI
Dang and Wang 2010	71.55	4.47	28	68.37	4.96	20	17.2%	3.18 [0.45, 5.91]
Hong et al. 2014	69.7	7.2	42	56.72	6.55	42	16.7%	12.98 [10.04, 15.92]
Li et al. 2003	77.35	4.17	61	70.95	4.95	40	19.0%	6.40 [4.54, 8.26]
Qi 2010	84.9	4.47	20	79.88	4.78	20	16.9%	5.02 [2.15, 7.89]
Yang et al. 2008	73.2	6.69	28	68.5	5.57	27	16.0%	4.70 [1.45, 7.95]
Zhong 2009	86	5.03	20	80.5	7.59	20	14.2%	5.50 [1.51, 9.49]
Total (95% CI)			**199**			**169**	**100.0%**	**6.31 [3.66, 8.97]**

Heterogeneity: $\tau^2 = 8.76$; $\chi^2 = 26.65$, df $= 5$ ($p < 0.0001$); $I^2 = 81\%$
Test for overall effect: $Z = 4.66$ ($p < 0.00001$)

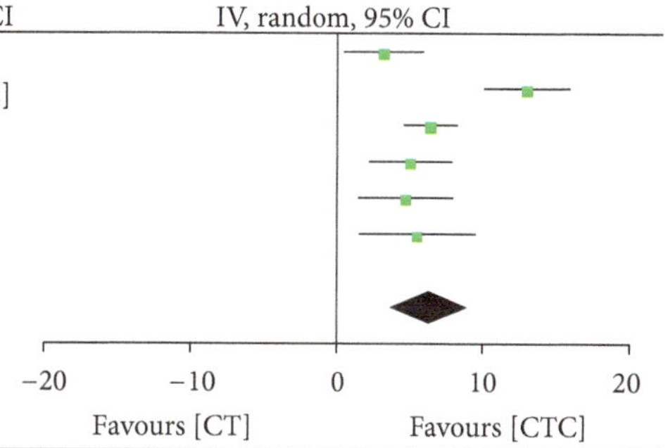

FIGURE 19: KPS after breast cancer treatment.

Study or subgroup	CTC Mean	CTC SD	CTC Total	CT Mean	CT SD	CT Total	Weight	Mean difference IV, random, 95% CI
Huang et al. 2007	51.9	8.7	30	52.7	9.1	30	7.8%	−0.80 [−5.31, 3.71]
Lv et al. 2014	55.9	7.3	27	56.8	6.3	27	11.9%	−0.90 [−4.54, 2.74]
Wen et al. 2010	51.9	8.7	30	52.7	9.1	30	7.8%	−0.80 [−5.31, 3.71]
Yang 2004	51.3	7.1	31	52.4	7	28	12.2%	−1.10 [−4.70, 2.50]
Zhang et al. 2010	70.85	7.56	40	70.48	8.49	40	12.7%	0.37 [−3.15, 3.89]
Zhang et al. 2011	55.33	3.41	23	56.94	2.8	22	47.6%	−1.61 [−3.43, 0.21]
Total (95% CI)			**181**			**177**	**100.0%**	**−1.09 [−2.34, 0.17]**

Heterogeneity: $\tau^2 = 0.00$; $\chi^2 = 1.02$, df $= 5$ ($p = 0.96$); $I^2 = 0\%$
Test for overall effect: $Z = 1.69$ ($p = 0.09$)

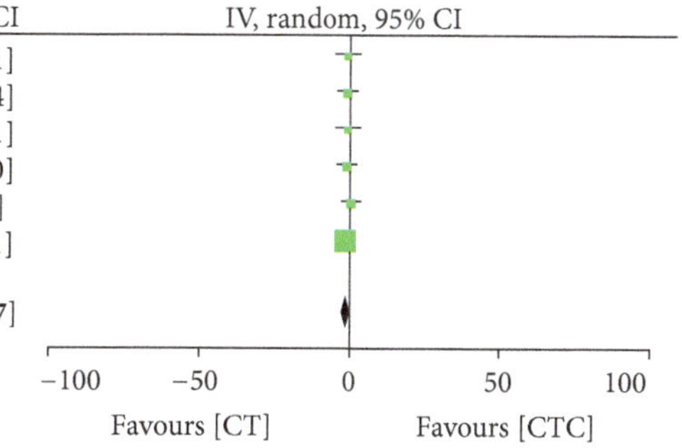

FIGURE 20: $CD3^+$ before treatment.

Study or subgroup	CTC Mean	CTC SD	CTC Total	CT Mean	CT SD	CT Total	Weight	Mean difference IV, random, 95% CI
Huang et al. 2007	47.7	8.5	30	46.8	9	30	3.3%	0.90 [−3.53, 5.33]
Lv et al. 2014	41.5	6.5	27	42.8	6.8	27	5.1%	−1.30 [−4.85, 2.25]
Wen et al. 2010	47.7	8.5	30	46.8	9	30	3.3%	0.90 [−3.53, 5.33]
Yang 2004	47.6	6.5	31	46.3	6.3	28	6.0%	1.30 [−1.97, 4.57]
Zhang et al. 2010	43.5	7.53	40	41.94	5.26	40	7.9%	1.56 [−1.29, 4.41]
Zhang et al. 2011	36.28	1.9	23	36.91	1.21	22	74.5%	−0.63 [−1.56, 0.30]
Total (95% CI)			**181**			**177**	**100.0%**	**−0.28 [−1.08, 0.52]**

Heterogeneity: $\tau^2 = 0.00$; $\chi^2 = 3.91$, df $= 5$ ($p = 0.56$); $I^2 = 0\%$
Test for overall effect: $Z = 0.68$ ($p = 0.50$)

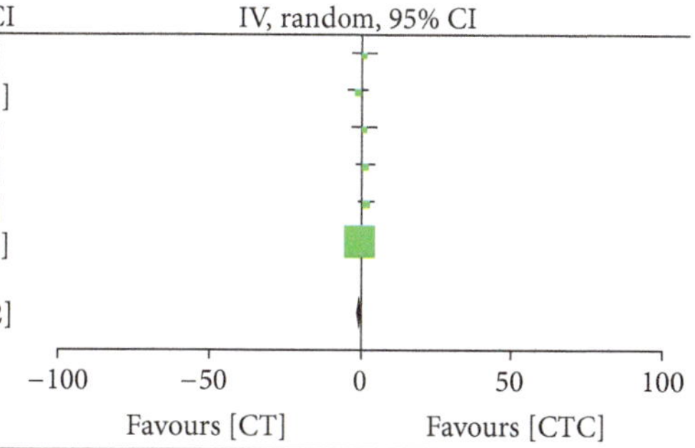

FIGURE 21: $CD4^+$ before treatment.

Study or subgroup	CTC Mean	CTC SD	CTC Total	CT Mean	CT SD	CT Total	Weight	Mean difference IV, random, 95% CI
Huang et al. 2007	29.6	7.6	30	29.5	2.7	30	9.3%	0.10 [−2.79, 2.99]
Lv et al. 2014	30.5	7.3	27	30.8	6.3	27	5.9%	−0.30 [−3.94, 3.34]
Wen et al. 2010	29.6	7.6	30	29.5	2.7	30	9.3%	0.10 [−2.79, 2.99]
Yang 2004	28.9	3.8	31	29.3	3.7	28	21.1%	−0.40 [−2.32, 1.52]
Zhang et al. 2010	28.84	5.83	40	30.66	7.29	40	9.3%	−1.82 [−4.71, 1.07]
Zhang et al. 2011	28.4	2.48	23	28.1	1.99	22	45.1%	0.30 [−1.01, 1.61]
Total (95% CI)			**181**			**177**	**100.0%**	**−0.12 [−1.00, 0.76]**

Heterogeneity: $\tau^2 = 0.00$; $\chi^2 = 1.86$, df = 5 ($p = 0.87$); $I^2 = 0\%$
Test for overall effect: $Z = 0.26$ ($p = 0.79$)

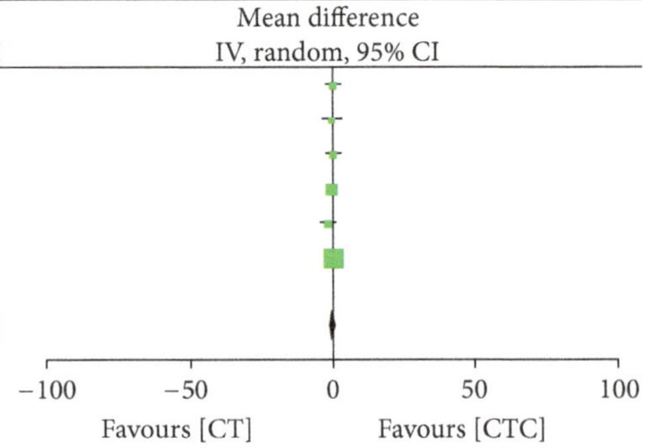

FIGURE 22: CD8$^+$ before treatment.

Study or subgroup	CTC Mean	CTC SD	CTC Total	CT Mean	CT SD	CT Total	Weight	Mean difference IV, random, 95% CI
Huang et al. 2007	1.8	0.4	30	1.8	0.5	30	17.7%	0.00 [−0.23, 0.23]
Lv et al. 2014	1.51	0.37	27	1.62	0.41	27	21.4%	−0.11 [−0.32, 0.10]
Wen et al. 2010	1.8	0.4	30	1.8	0.5	30	17.7%	0.00 [−0.23, 0.23]
Yang 2004	1.5	0.5	31	1.5	0.4	28	17.6%	0.00 [−0.23, 0.23]
Zhang et al. 2010	1.61	0.48	40	1.57	0.51	40	19.8%	0.04 [−0.18, 0.26]
Zhang et al. 2011	1.27	0.76	23	1.31	0.61	22	5.8%	−0.04 [−0.44, 0.36]
Total (95% CI)			**181**			**177**	**100.0%**	**−0.02 [−0.11, 0.08]**

Heterogeneity: $\tau^2 = 0.00$; $\chi^2 = 1.11$, df = 5 ($p = 0.95$); $I^2 = 0\%$
Test for overall effect: $Z = 0.37$ ($p = 0.71$)

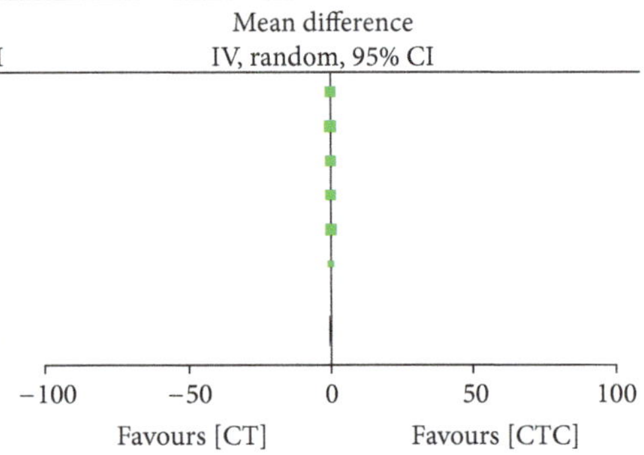

FIGURE 23: CD4$^+$/CD8$^+$ before treatment.

Study or subgroup	CTC Mean	CTC SD	CTC Total	CT Mean	CT SD	CT Total	Weight	Mean difference IV, random, 95% CI
Lv et al. 2014	13.5	4.77	27	13.8	5.22	27	38.2%	−0.30 [−2.97, 2.37]
Zhang et al. 2010	11.52	4.58	40	12.48	4.98	40	61.8%	−0.96 [−3.06, 1.14]
Total (95% CI)			**67**			**67**	**100.0%**	**−0.71 [−2.36, 0.94]**

Heterogeneity: $\tau^2 = 0.00$; $\chi^2 = 0.15$, df = 1 ($p = 0.70$); $I^2 = 0\%$
Test for overall effect: $Z = 0.84$ ($p = 0.40$)

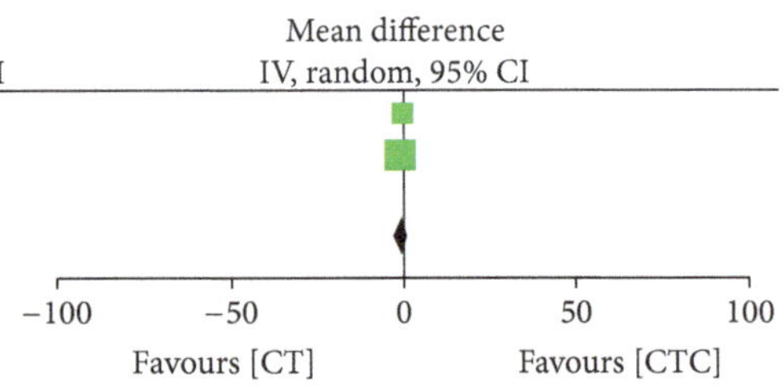

FIGURE 24: Natural killer cell level before treatment.

Study or subgroup	CTC Mean	CTC SD	CTC Total	CT Mean	CT SD	CT Total	Weight	Mean difference IV, random, 95% CI
Huang et al. 2007	52.1	4.9	30	43.8	9	30	11.8%	8.30 [4.63, 11.97]
Lv et al. 2014	60.9	6.7	27	52.9	7.3	27	11.4%	8.00 [4.26, 11.74]
Wen et al. 2010	52.1	4.9	30	43.8	9	30	11.8%	8.30 [4.63, 11.97]
Yang 2004	52.4	6.9	31	42.2	5.9	28	14.8%	10.20 [6.93, 13.47]
Zhang et al. 2010	79.36	8.42	40	72.03	7.94	40	12.3%	7.33 [3.74, 10.92]
Zhang et al. 2011	56.93	3.03	23	50.91	3.66	22	37.9%	6.02 [4.05, 7.99]
Total (95% CI)			**181**			**177**	**100.0%**	**7.56 [6.28, 8.85]**

Heterogeneity: $\tau^2 = 0.12$; $\chi^2 = 5.24$, df = 5 ($p = 0.39$); $I^2 = 5\%$
Test for overall effect: $Z = 11.55$ ($p < 0.00001$)

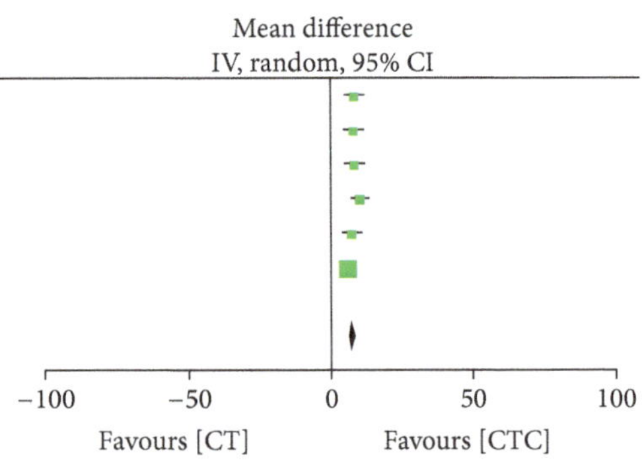

FIGURE 25: CD3$^+$ after breast cancer treatment.

Study or subgroup	CTC Mean	CTC SD	CTC Total	CT Mean	CT SD	CT Total	Weight	Mean difference IV, random, 95% CI
Huang et al. 2007	1.9	0.6	30	1.6	0.4	30	15.8%	0.30 [0.04, 0.56]
Lv et al. 2014	1.75	0.58	27	1.55	0.47	27	13.3%	0.20 [−0.08, 0.48]
Wen et al. 2010	1.9	0.6	30	1.6	0.4	30	15.8%	0.30 [0.04, 0.56]
Yang 2004	1.6	0.5	31	1.4	0.3	28	24.3%	0.20 [−0.01, 0.41]
Zhang et al. 2010	1.78	0.56	40	1.49	0.4	40	23.1%	0.29 [0.08, 0.50]
Zhang et al. 2011	1.53	0.15	23	1.18	0.87	22	7.7%	0.35 [−0.02, 0.72]
Total (95% CI)			**181**			**177**	**100.0%**	**0.26 [0.16, 0.37]**

Heterogeneity: $\tau^2 = 0.00$; $\chi^2 = 0.98$, df = 5 ($p = 0.96$); $I^2 = 0\%$
Test for overall effect: $Z = 5.05$ ($p < 0.00001$)

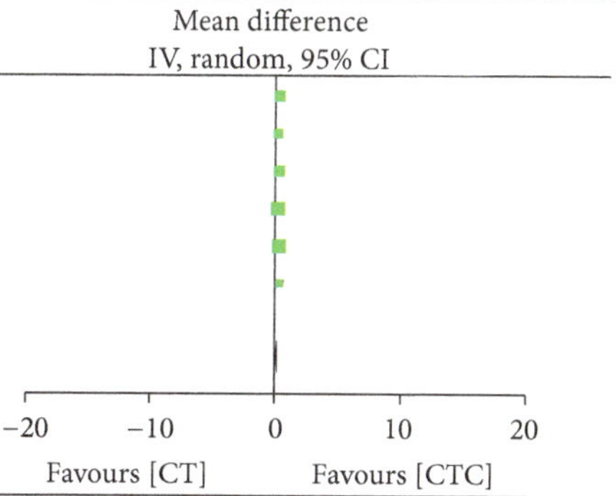

FIGURE 26: $CD4^+/CD8^+$ after breast cancer treatment.

Study or subgroup	CTC Mean	CTC SD	CTC Total	CT Mean	CT SD	CT Total	Weight	Mean difference IV, random, 95% CI
Lv et al. 2014	15.9	3.25	27	12.5	4.13	27	57.0%	3.40 [1.42, 5.38]
Zhang et al. 2010	13.46	5.46	40	12.62	6.92	40	43.0%	0.84 [−1.89, 3.57]
Total (95% CI)			**67**			**67**	**100.0%**	**2.30 [−0.18, 4.78]**

Heterogeneity: $\tau^2 = 1.79$; $\chi^2 = 2.21$, df = 1 ($p = 0.14$); $I^2 = 55\%$
Test for overall effect: $Z = 1.81$ ($p = 0.07$)

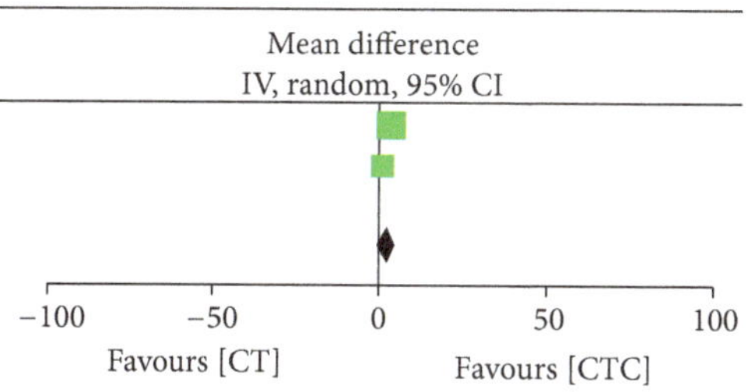

FIGURE 27: Natural killer cell level after breast cancer treatment.

Study or subgroup	Experimental Mean	Experimental SD	Experimental Total	Control Mean	Control SD	Control Total	Weight	Mean difference IV, random, 95% CI
13.1.1 TNM stage IV								
Huang et al. 2007	45.3	2.8	30	35.6	4.8	30	17.2%	9.70 [7.71, 11.69]
Lv et al. 2014	46.9	7.1	27	39.4	4.1	27	16.0%	7.50 [4.41, 10.59]
Wen et al. 2010	45.3	2.8	30	35.5	4.8	30	17.2%	9.80 [7.81, 11.79]
Yang 2004	46.7	6.5	31	35.1	5.4	28	16.1%	11.60 [8.56, 14.64]
Subtotal (95% CI)			**118**			**115**	**66.4%**	**9.70 [8.41, 10.98]**
Heterogeneity: $\tau^2 = 0.23$; $\chi^2 = 3.46$, df = 3 ($p = 0.33$); $I^2 = 13\%$								
Test for overall effect: $Z = 14.80$ ($p < 0.00001$)								
13.1.2 TNM stage (I–IV)								
Zhang et al. 2010	46.14	7.51	40	42.88	6.95	40	15.9%	3.26 [0.09, 6.43]
Zhang et al. 2011	37.26	2.06	23	35.16	2.09	22	17.7%	2.10 [0.89, 3.31]
Subtotal (95% CI)			**63**			**62**	**33.6%**	**2.25 [1.12, 3.38]**
Heterogeneity: $\tau^2 = 0.00$; $\chi^2 = 0.45$, df = 1 ($p = 0.50$); $I^2 = 0\%$								
Test for overall effect: $Z = 3.89$ ($p = 0.0001$)								
Total (95% CI)			**181**			**177**	**100.0%**	**7.30 [3.67, 10.93]**

Heterogeneity: $\tau^2 = 18.93$; $\chi^2 = 83.67$, df = 5 ($p < 0.00001$); $I^2 = 94\%$
Test for overall effect: $Z = 3.94$ ($p < 0.0001$)
Test for subgroup differences: $\chi^2 = 72.70$, df = 1 ($P < 0.00001$); $I^2 = 98.6\%$

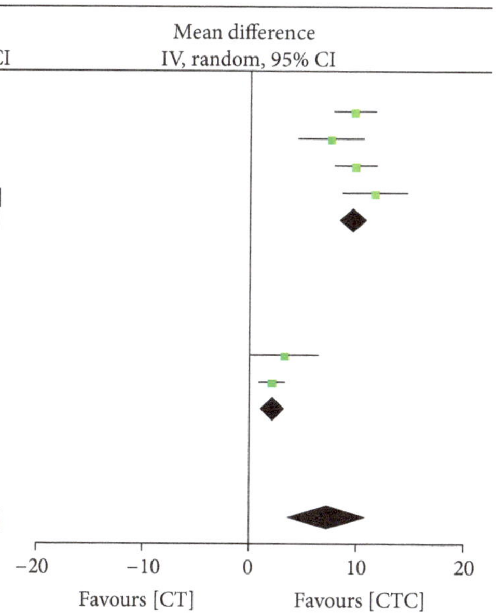

FIGURE 28: $CD4^+$ after breast cancer treatment.

studies, and additional well-designed RCTs addressing the role of CHM are warranted. The lack of molecular-based evidence for CHM and Zheng has resulted in a limited understanding and acceptance of CHM and TCM in Western countries. We believe that researchers should immediately explore a CHM-based cure, and CHM should be applied to routine care as soon as conclusive data are available [69]. For researchers devoted to the promotion of TCM or CHM, numerous barriers need to be addressed, including the standardizations of the Zheng classification and herbal agents, appropriate study designs, and the identification of the mechanisms of CHM at the molecular level.

Study or subgroup	CTC Mean	CTC SD	CTC Total	CT Mean	CT SD	CT Total	Weight	Mean difference IV, random, 95% CI
11.8.1 Sample size < 60								
Lv et al. 2014	25.5	9.3	27	28.5	7.1	27	15.5%	−3.00 [−7.41, 1.41]
Zhang et al. 2011	25.17	1.85	23	29.83	2.41	22	17.7%	−4.66 [−5.92, −3.40]
Subtotal (95% CI)			**50**			**49**	**33.1%**	**−4.54 [−5.75, −3.32]**
Heterogeneity: $\tau^2 = 0.00$; $\chi^2 = 0.50$, df = 1 ($p = 0.48$); $I^2 = 0\%$								
Test for overall effect: $Z = 7.34$ ($p < 0.00001$)								
11.8.2 Sample size = 60								
Huang et al. 2007	27.5	9	30	22.5	1.6	30	16.5%	5.00 [1.73, 8.27]
Wen et al. 2010	27.5	9	30	22.5	1.6	30	16.5%	5.00 [1.73, 8.27]
Yang 2004	27.1	3.5	31	21.4	3.1	28	17.5%	5.70 [4.02, 7.38]
Subtotal (95% CI)			**91**			**88**	**50.4%**	**5.46 [4.10, 6.82]**
Heterogeneity: $\tau^2 = 0.00$; $\chi^2 = 0.23$, df = 2 ($p = 0.89$); $I^2 = 0\%$								
Test for overall effect: $Z = 7.86$ ($p < 0.00001$)								
11.8.3 Sample size > 60								
Zhang et al. 2010	29.55	6.17	40	29.23	8.76	40	16.4%	0.32 [−3.00, 3.64]
Subtotal (95% CI)			**40**			**40**	**16.4%**	**0.32 [−3.00, 3.64]**
Heterogeneity: not applicable								
Test for overall effect: $Z = 0.19$ ($p = 0.85$)								
Total (95% CI)			**181**			**177**	**100.0%**	**1.41 [−3.31, 6.13]**
Heterogeneity: $\tau^2 = 32.46$; $\chi^2 = 116.33$, df = 5 ($p < 0.00001$); $I^2 = 96\%$								
Test for overall effect: $Z = 0.58$ ($p = 0.56$)								
Test for subgroup differences: $\chi^2 = 115.59$, df = 2 ($p < 0.00001$); $I^2 = 98.3\%$								

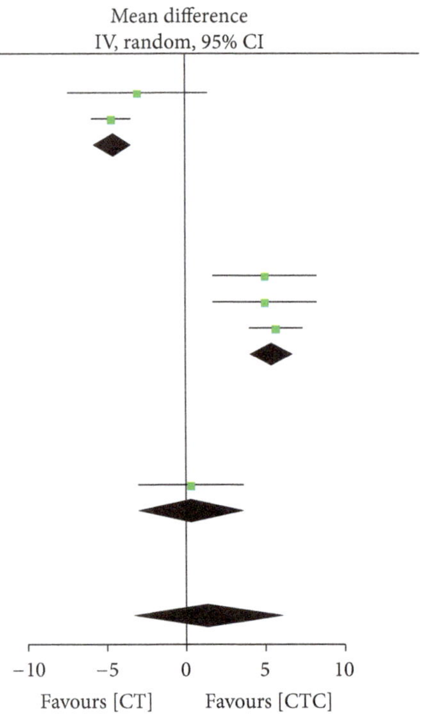

FIGURE 29: $CD8^+/CD8^+$ after breast cancer treatment.

Study or subgroup	Experimental Mean	Experimental SD	Experimental Total	Control Mean	Control SD	Control Total	Weight	Mean difference IV, random, 95% CI
Dang and Wang 2010	20.38	4.21	20	25.5	6.51	20	50.3%	−5.12 [−8.52, −1.72]
Yi et al. 2008	29.4	2.85	30	66.7	16.5	30	49.7%	−37.30 [−43.29, −31.31]
Total (95% CI)			**50**			**50**	**100.0%**	**−21.11 [−52.65, 10.42]**
Heterogeneity: $\tau^2 = 511.60$; $\chi^2 = 83.84$, df = 1 ($p < 0.00001$); $I^2 = 99\%$								
Test for overall effect: $Z = 1.31$ ($p = 0.19$)								

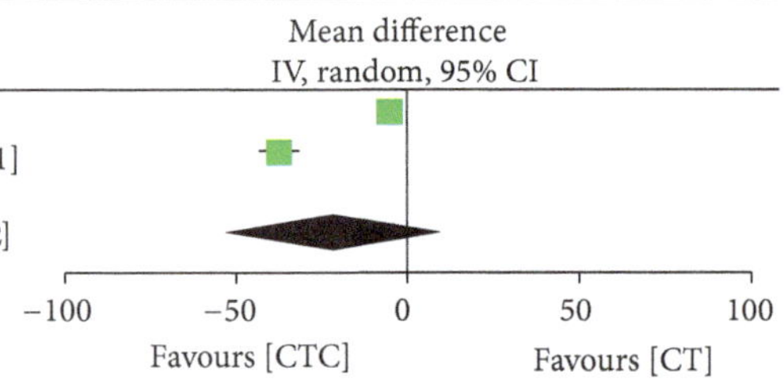

FIGURE 30: CK-MB (U/L) after breast cancer treatment.

Disclosure

The authors were not employed or contracted by the funder. The funder did not play a role in study design, data collection, or analysis.

Competing Interests

The authors declare that they have no competing interests.

Authors' Contributions

Xu Sun, Xing Zhang, Jia-Yun Nian, Jiao Guo, and Yi Yin contributed equally to this work. Xu Sun, Xiao-Min Wang, and Yi Yin drafted the protocol (unpublished). Xing Zhang, Jia-Yun Nian, and Jiao Guo developed and ran the search strategy. Xing Zhang, Jia-Yun Nian, and Jiao Guo obtained copies of studies. Xu Sun, Xing Zhang, and Jia-Yun Nian selected which studies to include. Gan-Lin Zhang, Ming-Wei Yu, and Yi Zhang extracted data from studies. Gan-Lin Zhang, Pei-Yu Cheng, and Lin Yang entered data into RevMan. Xu Sun, Guo-Wang Yang, and Jin-Ping Li conducted the analysis. Xu Sun, Xiao-Min Wang, and Yi Yin interpreted the analysis. Xu Sun, Gan-Lin Zhang, and Ming-Wei Yu drafted the final review.

Acknowledgments

This study was funded by the Beijing Municipal Science and Technology Commission (D161100005116001), National Natural Science Foundation of China (nos. 81173239; 81373815; 81202840), Specialized Research Fund for the Doctoral Program of Higher Education of China (20131107110014), and Beijing Municipal Administration of Hospitals (XMLX201410).

References

[1] L. A. Torre, F. Bray, R. L. Siegel, J. Ferlay, J. Lortet-Tieulent, and A. Jemal, "Global cancer statistics, 2012," *CA Cancer Journal for Clinicians*, vol. 65, no. 2, pp. 87–108, 2015.

[2] L. You, R. An, K. Liang, and X. Wang, "Anti-breast cancer agents from Chinese herbal medicines," *Mini-Reviews in Medicinal Chemistry*, vol. 13, no. 1, pp. 101–105, 2013.

[3] L. Del Mastro, A. Fabi, M. Mansutti et al., "Randomised phase 3 open-label trial of first-line treatment with gemcitabine in association with docetaxel or paclitaxel in women with metastatic breast cancer: a comparison of different schedules and treatments," *BMC Cancer*, vol. 13, article 164, 2013.

[4] D. Amadori, O. Nanni, M. Marangolo et al., "Disease-free survival advantage of adjuvant cyclophosphamide, methotrexate, and fluorouracil in patients with node-negative, rapidly proliferating breast cancer: a randomized multicenter study," *Journal of Clinical Oncology*, vol. 18, no. 17, pp. 3125–3134, 2000.

[5] P. Rastogi, S. J. Anderson, H. D. Bear et al., "Preoperative chemotherapy: updates of National Surgical Adjuvant Breast and Bowel Project Protocols B-18 and B-27," *Journal of Clinical Oncology*, vol. 26, no. 5, pp. 778–785, 2008.

[6] K. Boér, I. Láng, E. Juhos, T. Pintér, and J. Szántó, "Adjuvant therapy of breast cancer with docetaxel-containing combination (TAC)," *Pathology & Oncology Research*, vol. 9, no. 3, pp. 166–169, 2003.

[7] P. Harris and R. Rees, "The prevalence of complementary and alternative medicine use among the general population: a systematic review of the literature," *Complementary Therapies in Medicine*, vol. 8, no. 2, pp. 88–96, 2000.

[8] E. Ernst, "Prevalence of use of complementary/alternative medicine: a systematic review," *Bulletin of the World Health Organization*, vol. 78, no. 2, pp. 252–257, 2000.

[9] H. A. Tindle, R. B. Davis, R. S. Phillips, and D. M. Eisenberg, "Trends in use of complementary and alternative medicine by us adults: 1997–2002," *Alternative Therapies in Health and Medicine*, vol. 11, no. 1, pp. 42–49, 2005.

[10] C. C. L. Xue, A. L. Zhang, V. Lin, C. Da Costa, and D. F. Story, "Complementary and alternative medicine use in Australia: a national population-based survey," *Journal of Alternative and Complementary Medicine*, vol. 13, no. 6, pp. 643–650, 2007.

[11] E. Ernst and A. White, "The BBC survey of complementary medicine use in the UK," *Complementary Therapies in Medicine*, vol. 8, no. 1, pp. 32–36, 2000.

[12] W. J. Millar, "Use of alternative health care practitioners by Canadians," *Canadian Journal of Public Health*, vol. 88, no. 3, pp. 154–158, 1997.

[13] U. Wolf, S. Maxion-Bergemann, G. Bornhöft, P. F. Matthiessen, and M. Wolf, "Use of complementary medicine in Switzerland," *Forschende Komplementarmedizin*, vol. 13, no. 2, pp. 4–6, 2006.

[14] B. Hanssen, S. Grimsgaard, L. Launsø, V. Fønnebø, T. Falkenberg, and N. K. Rasmussen, "Use of complementary and alternative medicine in the Scandinavian countries," *Scandinavian Journal of Primary Health Care*, vol. 23, no. 1, pp. 57–62, 2005.

[15] K. Thomas and P. Coleman, "Use of complementary or alternative medicine in a general population in Great Britain. Results from the National Omnibus survey," *Journal of Public Health*, vol. 26, no. 2, pp. 152–157, 2004.

[16] B. Wang, *The Yellow Emperor's Classic of Internal Medicine—Simple Questions*, People's Health Publishing House, Beijing, China, 1979.

[17] D. Tian, *Spiritual Axis*, People's Health Publishing House, Beijing, China, 2005.

[18] I. Cohen, M. Tagliaferri, and D. Tripathy, "Traditional Chinese medicine in the treatment of breast cancer," *Seminars in Oncology*, vol. 29, no. 6, pp. 563–574, 2002.

[19] D. Moher, A. Liberati, J. Tetzlaff, and D. G. Altman, "Preferred reporting items for systematic reviews and meta-analyses: the PRISMA statement," *Open Medicine*, vol. 3, no. 3, pp. e123–e130, 2009.

[20] A. R. Jadad, R. A. Moore, D. Carroll et al., "Assessing the quality of reports of randomized clinical trials: is blinding necessary?" *Controlled Clinical Trials*, vol. 17, no. 1, pp. 1–12, 1996.

[21] J. P. T. Higgins, D. G. Altman, P. C. Gøtzsche et al., "The Cochrane Collaboration's tool for assessing risk of bias in randomised trials," *The British Medical Journal*, vol. 343, no. 7829, Article ID d5928, 2011.

[22] X. G. Dang and L. Wang, "Evaluation of efficacy on breast cancer treated by Aidi injection plus CTF program of neoadjuvant chemotherapy and the impacts on serum sFas," *World Journal of Integrated Traditional and Western Medicine*, vol. 5, no. 1, pp. 54–56, 2010.

[23] D. L. Barton, K. Burger, P. J. Novotny et al., "The use of *Ginkgo biloba* for the prevention of chemotherapy-related cognitive dysfunction in women receiving adjuvant treatment for breast cancer, N00C9," *Supportive Care in Cancer*, vol. 21, no. 4, pp. 1185–1192, 2013.

[24] X. D. Fang, "Clinical observation on Jianpi Yiqi formula combined with chemotherapy in the treatment of 30 cases with advanced breast cancer," *Journal of Traditional Chinese Medicine*, vol. 50, supplement 1, pp. 174–176.

[25] L. Fu and X. G. Kou, "Clinical observation on Aidi injection combined with chemotherapy in the treatment of 44 cases with breast cancer," *Journal of Practical Traditional Chinese Medicine*, vol. 23, no. 8, p. 517.

[26] R. Hong, Y. Q. Wu, and Y. Wu, "Effects of Xihuangwan in assistanr treatment of patients with advanced breast cancer," *Zhong Guo Zhong Yao Za Zhi*, vol. 39, no. 6, pp. 1120–1123, 2014.

[27] Z. F. Huang, J. S. Wei, Z. Y. Shi, and K. Zhong, "Study of Bazhen decoction and chemotherapy on mammary cancer in metaphase or later period," *Xian Dai Zhong Xi Yi Jie He Za Zhi*, vol. 12, no. 11, pp. 1123–1126, 2003.

[28] Z. F. Huang, J. B. Liu, Q. S. Chen, H. Z. Li, Z. J. Zhang, and C. J. Huang, "The influence of Jianpi Xiaoji Tang combined with chemotherapy on life quality and immunologic function in late stage of mammary cancer," *Journal of New Chinese Medicine*, vol. 39, no. 5, pp. 88–89.

[29] Z. F. Huang, J. S. Wei, H. Z. Li, Z. Q. Tan, Z. J. Zhang, and C. Chen, "Effect of Shenqi Fuzheng injection combined with chemotherapy on thirty patients with advanced breast cancer," *Chinese Journal of Integrated Traditional and Western Medicine*, vol. 28, no. 2, pp. 152–154, 2008.

[30] C. J. Huang, J. B. Liu, and T. H. Liao, "Effect of Astragalus injection combined chemotherapy on life quality and immune function in advanced breast cancer," *Nei Mongol Journal of Traditional Chinese Medicine*, vol. 32, no. 32, pp. 66–67.

[31] X. Q. Li, Y. Wang, S. T. Zhao, X. H. Ni, and S. Q. Ma, "Clinical observation on no. 1 decoction of Rukang affecting breast cancer matastasis of 61 cases," *Chinese Journal of Traditional Medical Science and Technology*, vol. 10, no. 5, pp. 305–306.

[32] X. Q. Li and S. B. Gong, "Effect of Aidi injection combined with CEF regimn chemotherapy in the treatment of breast cancer,"

Pharmacology and Clinics of Chinese Materia Medica, vol. 3, no. 22, pp. 176–177.

[33] X. A. Lu, "Effect of Astragalus Injection on the Quality of breast cancer patients," *Zhong Guo Zhong Yi Yao Xian Dai Yuan Cheng Jiao Yu*, vol. 8, no. 11, pp. 36–37.

[34] Y. Lv, L. Z. Huang, D. Mao, X. J. Dai, J. Yang, and S. Q. Zhang, "Clinical research on treatment of advanced breast cancer based on Yiqi Huoxue method combined with chemotherapy," *Acta Chinese Medicine and Pharmacology*, vol. 42, no. 3, pp. 93–96.

[35] X. L. Ni, "Clinical study of gaolishen injection combined with chemotherapy for the advanced breast cancer," *China Practical Medical*, vol. 1, no. 4, pp. 64–65.

[36] D. Pérol, J. Provençal, A.-C. Hardy-Bessard et al., "Can treatment with Cocculine improve the control of chemotherapy-induced emesis in early breast cancer patients? A randomized, multi-centered, double-blind, placebo-controlled Phase III trial," *BMC Cancer*, vol. 12, article 603, 2012.

[37] M. H. Qi, *Clinical Research of Breast Cancer Treatments by Yiqi Yangxue Shugan Decotion Assisting TE Chemotherapy*, The First Clinical Medical College, Nanjing University of Chinese Medicine, 2010.

[38] L. Qin, "Effect of Fuzheng Yiqi Jiedu decoction in the treatment of 39 breast cancer cases after surgery," *Traditional Chinese Medicine Rearch*, vol. 26, no. 7, pp. 19–21.

[39] V. F. Semiglazov, V. V. Stepula, A. Dudov, J. Schnitker, and U. Mengs, "Quality of life is improved in breast cancer patients by standardised mistletoe extract PS76A2 during chemotherapy and follow-up: a randomised, placebo-controlled, double-blind, multicentre clinical trial," *Anticancer Research*, vol. 26, no. 2, pp. 1519–1529, 2006.

[40] T. Shen, "Clinical observation of Aiyishu injection combined with chemotherapy in advanced stage breast cancer," *China Medicine Guides*, vol. 4, no. 26, pp. 44–45.

[41] W. H. Sun, M. Y. Luo, and J. Yu, "Preventive effect of Zanfan pill on the myelosupression of breast cancer patients receiving chemotherapy," *Strait Pharmaceutical Journal*, vol. 22, no. 5, pp. 100–102.

[42] Y. H. Wang, *Effect on Quality of Life about Paients with Breast Cancer Received Neoadjuvant Chemotherapy and Taohong Siwu Tang*, Guangzhou University of Chinese Medicine, 2007.

[43] L. F. Wang, *Impact on QOL of Patients with Advanced Breast Cancer Treated by YiQiJianPi and HuaYuJieDu Method Combined with TE Regiment Chemotherapy*, The First Clinical Medical College, Nanjing University of Chinese Medicine, 2010.

[44] H. Y. Wen, Y. L. Ma, and C. X. Wang, "Effect on QOL and immunity of patients with advanced breast cancer treated by fuzheng xiaoyan decoction combined with chemotherapy," *Jiang Su Zhong Yi Yao*, vol. 42, no. 8, pp. 23–24.

[45] L. G. Xiong, "Study on the effect of Fuzheng Xiaoji recipe combined with chemotherapy on the life quality and serum tumor markers of late breast cancer patients," *Yunnan Journal of Traditional Chinese Medicine and Materia Medica*, vol. 33, no. 4, pp. 14–15, 2012.

[46] L. Yang, "Clinical study of Aidi injection combined with chemotherapy on advanced breast cancer," *Chinese Journal of Integrated Traditional and Western Medicine*, vol. 24, no. 8, pp. 755–756, 2004.

[47] G. W. Yang, Y. M. Xu, Q. Fu et al., "Clinical observation on Gubne Yiliu II combined with chemotherapy in the treatment of 28 cases of advanced breast cancer," *Journal of Traditional Chinese Medicine*, vol. 49, no. 12, pp. 1081–1083.

[48] S.-Y. Yi, K.-J. Nan, S.-J. Chen et al., "Effect of extract of Ginkgo biloba on doxorubicin-associated cardiotoxicity in patients with breast cancer," *Chinese Journal of Integrated Traditional and Western Medicine*, vol. 28, no. 1, pp. 68–70, 2008.

[49] W. H. Zhang, C. Y. Zhao, X. F. Zhang et al., "Effect of radix astragali taohong decoction on dellular immune function in breast cancer patients with postoperative chemotherapy," *Chinese Journal of Breast Disease*, vol. 2, no. 4, pp. 137–143.

[50] Y. C. Zhang, X. J. Li, Y. J. Jia, J. Chen, and Y. Y. Sun, "Clinical observation of "Fuzheng Quyu Jiedu Prescription" combining with chemotherapy in treating postoperative breast cancer," *Shanghai Journal of Traditional Chinese Medicine*, vol. 45, no. 11, pp. 64–66, 2011.

[51] X. Y. Zhang and G. C. Li, "Clinical study of Tiaogan Lipi method combined with Neoadjuvan chemotherapy for the treatment of breast cancer," *Modern Practical Medicine*, vol. 25, no. 10, pp. 1145–1146.

[52] R. Zhong, *Clinical Rearch of Shu Gan Tiao Li Chong Ren Decoction with the Chemotherapy in the Treatment of Breast Cancer's QOL*, The First Clinical Medical College, Nanjing University of Chinese Medicine, 2009.

[53] M. P. Coleman, "Trends in breast cancer incidence, survival, and mortality," *The Lancet*, vol. 356, no. 9229, pp. 590–593, 2000.

[54] A. Glaus, B. Fäh, R. Hornung, H. Senn, and F. Stiefel, "Breast cancer prevention behaviour: a perspective of women from three language regions of Switzerland," *Pflege*, vol. 17, no. 6, pp. 385–394, 2004.

[55] L. Lohr, "Chemotherapy-induced nausea and vomiting," *Cancer Journal*, vol. 14, no. 2, pp. 85–93, 2008.

[56] S. Hori, I. Mihaylov, J. C. Vasconcelos, and M. McCoubrie, "Patterns of complementary and alternative medicine use amongst outpatients in Tokyo, Japan," *BMC Complementary and Alternative Medicine*, vol. 8, article 14, 2008.

[57] H.-J. Seo, S.-M. Baek, S. G. Kim, T.-H. Kim, and S. M. Choi, "Prevalence of complementary and alternative medicine use in a community-based population in South Korea: a systematic review," *Complementary Therapies in Medicine*, vol. 21, no. 3, pp. 260–271, 2013.

[58] L. L. D. Zhong, H.-Y. Chen, W. C. S. Cho, X.-M. Meng, and Y. Tong, "The efficacy of Chinese herbal medicine as an adjunctive therapy for colorectal cancer: a systematic review and meta-analysis," *Complementary Therapies in Medicine*, vol. 20, no. 4, pp. 240–252, 2012.

[59] F. Cheung, "TCM: made in China," *Nature*, vol. 480, no. 7378, pp. S82–S83, 2011.

[60] A. Bensoussan, N. J. Talley, M. Hing, R. Menzies, A. Guo, and M. Ngu, "Treatment of irritable bowel syndrome with Chinese herbal medicine: a randomized controlled trial," *The Journal of the American Medical Association*, vol. 280, no. 18, pp. 1585–1589, 1998.

[61] D. C. Cherkin, K. J. Sherman, A. L. Avins et al., "A randomized trial comparing acupuncture, simulated acupuncture, and usual care for chronic low back pain," *Archives of Internal Medicine*, vol. 169, no. 9, pp. 858–866, 2009.

[62] A. T. Lathia, S. M. Jung, and L. X. Chen, "Efficacy of acupuncture as a treatment for chronic shoulder pain," *Journal of Alternative and Complementary Medicine*, vol. 15, no. 6, pp. 613–618, 2009.

[63] E. A. Macklin, P. M. Wayne, L. A. Kalish et al., "Stop Hypertension with the Acupuncture Research Program (SHARP): results of a randomized, controlled clinical trial," *Hypertension*, vol. 48, no. 5, pp. 838–845, 2006.

[64] W. C. S. Cho and H.-Y. Chen, "Clinical efficacy of traditional chinese medicine as a concomitant therapy for nasopharyngeal carcinoma: a systematic review and meta-analysis," *Cancer Investigation*, vol. 27, no. 3, pp. 334–344, 2009.

[65] S. G. Li, H. Y. Chen, C. S. Ou-Yang et al., "The efficacy of chinese herbal medicine as an adjunctive therapy for advanced non-small cell lung cancer: a systematic review and meta-analysis," *PLoS ONE*, vol. 8, no. 2, Article ID e57604, 2013.

[66] P. Wu, J. J. Dugoua, O. Eyawo, and E. J. Mills, "Traditional Chinese medicines in the treatment of hepatocellular cancers: a systematic review and meta-analysis," *Journal of Experimental and Clinical Cancer Research*, vol. 28, article 112, 2009.

[67] W. Kim, W.-B. Lee, J.-W. Lee et al., "Traditional herbal medicine as adjunctive therapy for breast cancer: a systematic review," *Complementary Therapies in Medicine*, vol. 23, no. 4, pp. 626–6232, 2015.

[68] N. E. Haddad and O. Palesh, "Acupuncture in the treatment of cancer-related psychological symptoms," *Integrative Cancer Therapies*, vol. 13, no. 5, pp. 371–385, 2014.

[69] E. Ernst, K. Schmidt, and M. Baum, "Complementary/alternative therapies for the treatment of breast cancer. A systematic review of randomized clinical trials and a critique of current terminology," *Breast Journal*, vol. 12, no. 6, pp. 526–530, 2006.

10

Antioxidant and Anti-Inflammatory Effects of Rhei Rhizoma and Coptidis Rhizoma Mixture on Reflux Esophagitis in Rats

O Jun Kwon,[1] Min Yeong Kim,[2] Sung Ho Shin,[2] Ah Reum Lee,[2] Joo Young Lee,[2] Bu-il Seo,[2] Mi-Rae Shin,[2] Hyun Gyu Choi,[3] Jeong Ah Kim,[3] Byung Sun Min,[4] Gyo-Nam Kim,[5] Jeong Sook Noh,[6] Man Hee Rhee,[7] and Seong-Soo Roh[2]

[1]*Kyeoungbuk Institute for Regional Program Evaluation, Gyeongbuk TP, 27 Sampoong-ro, Gyeongsan, Gyeongsangbuk-do 38542, Republic of Korea*
[2]*College of Korean Medicine, Daegu Haany University, Gyeongsan 38610, Republic of Korea*
[3]*College of Pharmacy, Research Institute of Pharmaceutical Sciences, Kyungpook National University, Daegu 41566, Republic of Korea*
[4]*College of Pharmacy, Catholic University of Daegu, Gyeongsangbuk-do 38430, Republic of Korea*
[5]*Department of Food Science and Biotechnology, Kyungnam University, Gyeongsangnam-do 51767, Republic of Korea*
[6]*Department of Food Science & Nutrition, Tongmyong University, Busan 48520, Republic of Korea*
[7]*College of Veterinary Medicine, Kyungpook National University, Daegu 41566, Republic of Korea*

Correspondence should be addressed to Man Hee Rhee; rheemh@knu.ac.kr and Seong-Soo Roh; ddede@dhu.ac.kr

Academic Editor: Filippo Maggi

The purpose of this study was to investigate the antioxidant and anti-inflammatory effects of the combined extract of Rhei rhizoma and Coptidis rhizoma (RC-mix) in experimental model of acute reflux esophagitis. The antioxidant activity was assessed by *in vitro* 2,2-diphenyl-1-picrylhydrazyl (DPPH) and 2,2′-azino-bis(3-ethylbenzothiazoline-6-sulfonic acid) (ABTS) assays. RC-mix was given at 100, 200, and 400 mg/kg body weight 2 h prior to induction of reflux esophagitis (RE). After 5 h, the effects of RC-mix treated rats were compared with those of normal and control rats. The representative flavonoid contents of RC-mix, such as sennoside A, epiberberine, coptisine, palmatine, and berberine, were detected using HPLC. The elevated esophageal mucosa damage was markedly ameliorated by RC-mix treatment in a dose-dependent manner. Furthermore, the administration of RC-mix reduced the increase of serum reactive oxygen species (ROS) and peroxynitrite ($ONOO^-$). The improvement of superoxide dismutase (SOD) and heme oxygenase-1 (HO-1) levels were marked in the group given RC-mix. Moreover, the elevation of inflammatory mediators and cytokines by nuclear factor-kappa B (NF-κB) activation in control rats decreased by RC-mix pretreatment. These results indicate that RC-mix treatment reduces the pathological states of esophagitis *via* regulating NF-κB mediated inflammation related to oxidative stress.

1. Introduction

Gastroesophageal reflux disease (GERD) includes a wide range of reflux disease, from intermittent symptoms like acid regurgitation or heartburn to endoscopic reflux esophagitis and Barrett's esophagus [1]. In 2005, the percentage of GERD prevalence in Eastern Asia was 2.5%–4.8%, whereas, in the Western world, it was much higher, about 10%–20% [2]. Thereafter, from 2005 to 2010, it reached the prevalence of 5.2%–8.5% in Eastern Asia and of 6.3%–18.3% in Southeast and Western Asia [3]. The epidemiology of GERD has shown that it is caused by an excessive exposure to gastric contents such as gastric acid, pepsin, trypsin, and bile acids in earlier days [4]. So, a management of GERD requires lifestyle modification, medical therapy like antacids, histamine-receptor antagonists, or proton-pump inhibitors, and surgical therapy [5]. However, despite their well-known healthy effects, these therapies could determine relapse, incomplete mucosal healing, the development of severe complications, and various adverse effects because of the long-term use [6, 7]. Recent studies have reported that oxidative stress has a more important role than acids in the pathogenesis of reflux esophagitis (RE) [8, 9]. The esophageal mucosa is formed by stratified squamous epithelium that consists of 20 to 30 layers of cells. The esophageal mucosa is in a state of continuous exposure to potentially damaging endogenous and exogenous factors. For instance, the gastric acid combined with even small amounts of pepsin causes a potent damage of the mucosal barrier, resulting in increased hydrogen ion permeability, mucosal morphologic changes, and local hemorrhage [10]. The development of reflux esophagitis too, at a cellular level, is due to hydrogen ion diffusion into mucosa, leading to tissue acidification and necrotic damage [11]. All these injuries trigger a series of cellular infiltrations and cytokine release that result in an inflammatory response and damage in the esophageal tissue. Various inflammatory and immune cells including macrophages, neutrophils, dendritic cells, and lymphocytes are activated and generated reactive oxygen species (ROS). Overproduction of ROS can contribute to the immediate development of inflammatory process. Administration of antioxidants acting as free radical scavengers has been found to prevent esophageal mucosal damage by blocking the free radicals [12].

At present, natural products from plant with antioxidant activities have been highlighted as promising sources for treating the inflammation. Rhei rhizoma (RR, Dahuang in Korean medicine) is one of the traditional herbal medicines widely cited in Chinese, Korean, and Japanese pharmacopoeias for its several biological effects, such as purgative, antipyretic, anti-inflammatory, antiangiogenic, and antineoplasmic activities [13]. It has been reported that sennoside A represents one of the more important components of RR and it becomes rheinanthrone, when transformed into its active metabolite. It exerts a protective effect against oxidative stress-related endothelial cell injury [14]. *Coptis chinensis* too is a widely used herb in traditional Korean medicine that have attracted much attention because of its multiple pharmacological effects, such as antibacterial, antiviral, anticancer, and antioxidative effects [15, 16]. Berberine, a primary component of Coptidis rhizoma, exerts a potent anti-inflammatory action in various disease [17, 18]. According to these reports, RC-mix may regulate effectively the inflammation of RE against oxidative stress. However, virtually no studies have investigated its chemical profiling and pharmacological activity in reflux-induced esophagitis. Therefore, we investigated the effects of RC-mix on rats with reflux esophagitis to examine its preventive effect against oxidative stress-related inflammation.

2. Materials and Methods

2.1. Materials. The protease inhibitor mixture solution and ethylenediaminetetraacetic acid (EDTA) were purchased from Wako Pure Chemical Industries, Ltd. (Osaka, Japan). Phenylmethylsulfonyl fluoride (PMSF) was purchased from Sigma Chemical Co. (St. Louis, MO, USA). 2′,7′-Dichlorofluorescein diacetate (DCF-DA) was obtained from Molecular Probes (Eugene, OR, USA). The pierce bicinchoninic acid (BCA) protein assay kit was obtained from Thermo Scientific (Rockford, IL, USA). ECL Western Blotting Detection Reagents and pure nitrocellulose membranes were supplied by GE Healthcare (Piscataway, NJ, USA). Rabbit polyclonal antibodies against nuclear factor-kappa B p65 (NF-κBp65; 1:1,000, SC-372), nuclear factor-erythroid 2-related factor 2 (Nrf-2; 1:1,000, SC-7228), heme oxygenase-1 (HO-1; 1:1,000, SC-10789), superoxide dismutase (SOD; 1:1,000, SC-11407), and catalase (1:1,000, SC-50508); goat polyclonal antibodies against tumor necrosis factor-α (TNF-α; 1:1,000, SC-1351) and interleukin-6 (IL-6; 1:1,000, SC-1266); mouse monoclonal antibodies against cyclooxygenase-2 (COX-2; 1:1,000, SC-19999), inducible nitric oxide synthase (iNOS, 1:1,000, SC-7271), phosphor-inhibitory kappa B alpha (p-IκBα; 1:1,000, SC-8404) histone (1:1,000, SC-8030), and β-actin (1:1,000, SC-4778) were purchased from Santa Cruz Biotechnology, Inc. (Santa Cruz, CA, USA). Rabbit anti-goat (1:3,000, SC-2774), goat anti-rabbit (1:5,000, SC-2004), and goat anti-mouse (1:5,000, SC-2005) immunoglobulin G (IgG) horseradish peroxidase- (HRP-) conjugated secondary antibodies were acquired from Santa Cruz Biotechnology, Inc. (Santa Cruz, CA, USA). All other chemicals and reagents used were of the analytical grade commercially available (Sigma Aldrich Co., Ltd., USA).

2.2. Plant Materials. Rhei rhizoma (roots of *Rheum tanguticum* Maxim.) and Coptidis rhizoma (roots of *Coptis chinensis* Franch.) were purchased from Ominherb Co. (Yeongcheon, Korea). A voucher herbarium specimen has been deposited at the Herbarium of Daegu Haany University and was identified by Professor S. S. Roh, the herbarium leader of Daegu Haany University. Dried slices of Rhei rhizoma (15 g) and Coptidis rhizoma (15 g) mixture (RC-mix) boiled with distilled water (300 mL) at room temperature for 2 h and the solvent was evaporated *in vacuo* to obtain powder with a yield of 14.2%, by weight, of the original RC-mix.

2.3. Analysis of Rhei Rhizoma and Coptidis Rhizoma Mixture by HPLC Chromatogram. The water extract of Rhei rhizoma and Coptidis rhizoma mixture (1 mg) was dissolved in 1 mL of 50% methanol with multi-vortexing. We injected 50 μL of the sample into a reverse-phase HPLC using a ZORBAX Eclipse XDB-C18, analytical 4.6 × 150 mm, 5 microns, with a column temperature of 25°C. Mobile phase component A is methanol and B is water (10 mM 1-hexanesulfonic acid sodium). The gradient conditions were as follows: 15% A, 0 min, 50% A, 15 min, and 30% A, 30 min. The flow rate was 2.0 mL/min. The UV absorbance from 254 nm was monitored using an Agilent 1200 series with an 2998 Photodiode Array Detector from Waters Co. (Manchester, UK). All peaks were assigned by carrying out coinjection tests with authentic samples and comparing them with the UV spectral data. The major components of Rhei rhizoma and Coptidis rhizoma were sennoside A, epiberberine, coptisine, palmatine, and berberine. Sennoside A was detected from Rhei rhizoma and epiberberine, coptisine, palmatine, and berberine were detected from Coptidis rhizoma. The measurement was

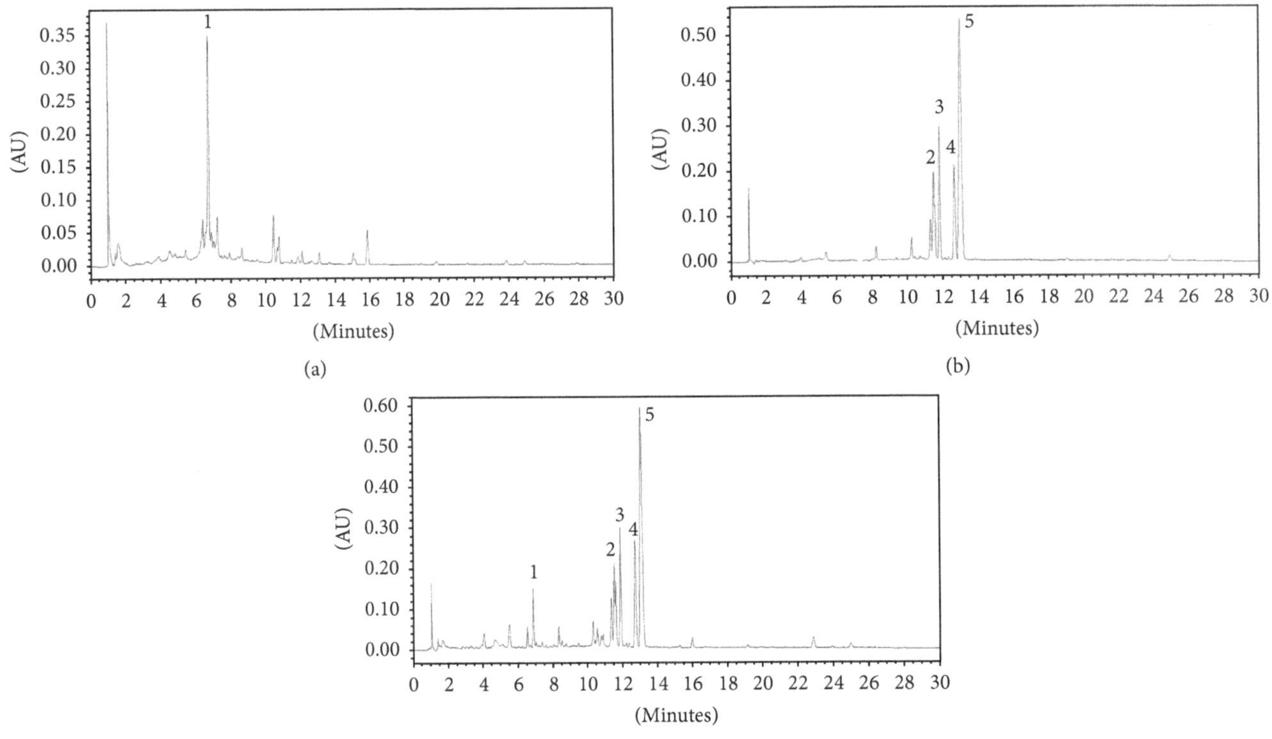

Figure 1: HPLC chromatogram of RC-mix extract (1 mg/mL) detected 254 nm. Signals 1–5 identified to be sennoside A, epiberberine, coptisine, palmatine, and berberine in regular sequence. RC-mix, a water extract of Rhei rhizoma and Coptis rhizoma mixture.

repeated three times. Representative HPLC results are illustrated in Figure 1.

2.4. Experimental Animals and Treatment. Animal experiments were carried out according to the "Guidelines for Animal Experimentation" approved by the Ethics Committee of the Daegu Haany University (Approval number 2015-055). Six-week-old male Sprague-Dawley rats were purchased from Samtako (Osan, Korea). Rats were maintained under a 12 h light/dark cycle and housed at a controlled temperature (23 ± 1°C) and humidity (about 55%). After adaptation (1 week), a total of 30 SD rats were randomly divided into 5 groups ($n = 6$ per group). The rats were fasted for 18 h prior to surgical procedures and kept in raised mesh-bottom cages to prevent coprophagy but were provided free access to water. The rats were anaesthetized with an injection of Zoletil 0.75 mg/kg (Virbac S. A. France). A midline laparotomy was performed to expose the stomach; both the pylorus and the transitional junction between the forestomach and the corpus were exposed and then ligated with a 2-0 silk thread without a pyloric ring, employing the method originally proposed by Omura et al. [19]. The vagus nerves were left intact. Group one included the normal rats (N). Group two included the RE control rats (Veh). Group three included the RC-mix 100 mg/kg (RC100). Group four included the RC-mix 200 mg/kg (RC200). Group five included the RC-mix 400 mg/kg (RC400). The normal and RE control rat groups were given water, while the other groups were orally given RC-mix at a dose of 100, 200, and 400 mg/kg body weight. Based on our previous experiment, the maximum concentration of RC-mix was determined as 400 mg/kg [20]. The administration of water or RC-mix extract in rats was provided using a stomach tube only one time 2 h before abdominal surgery. The rats in all groups were sacrificed 5 h after the surgery. The entire esophagus was removed immediately and examined for gross mucosal injury. The esophageal tissue was immediately frozen in liquid nitrogen, and blood samples were collected by a vena cava puncture from anesthetized rats. Subsequently, the esophagus and serum were kept at −80°C until analysis.

2.5. DPPH Radical Scavenging Activity of RC-Mix Extract. Antioxidant activity determination of RC-mix extract was performed by the DPPH radical scavenging according to the method of Hatano et al. [21]. The reduction of the stable purple free radical DPPH to the yellow hydrazine is achieved by trapping the unpaired electrons, and the degree of discoloration indicates the scavenging activity of samples [22]. 100 μL of an ethanolic solution of RC-mix extract (blank: 100 μL of ethanol) was added to 100 μL of an ethanolic solution of DPPH (60 μM) using 96-well microtitre plate. The ascorbic acid (standard sample) and RC-mix extract were prepared for eight concentrations (1, 2.5, 5, 10, 25, 50, 100, and 200 μg/mL). After mixing gently and leaving to stand for 30 min at room temperature, the optical density was determined using a Microplate Reader, model infinite M200 PRO (Tecan, Austria). The mixture was measured spectrophotometrically at 540 nm. The antioxidant activity of each sample was expressed in terms of the IC_{50} (micromolar concentration required to inhibit DPPH radical formation by 50%, calculated from the log-dose inhibition curve). The radical scavenging activity was calculated as a percentage using the following equation:

$$\text{DPPH radical scavenging activity (\%)} = \left[1 - \left(\frac{A_{\text{sample}}}{A_{\text{blank}}}\right)\right] \times 100. \tag{1}$$

2.6. ABTS Radical Scavenging Activity of RC-Mix Extract. ABTS radical scavenging activity of the different extracts was measured according to the modified method of Re et al. [23]. ABTS stock solution was dissolved in water to a 7.4 mM concentration. The ABTS radical cation (ABTS) was produced by reacting ABTS stock solution with 2.45 mM potassium persulfate and allowing the mixture to stand for 14 h at room temperature in the dark. The ABTS solution was diluted with ethanol to obtain an absorbance of 0.70 ± 0.02 at 750 nm. After adding 95 μL of diluted ABTS solution ($A_{750\,\text{nm}} = 0.70 \pm 0.02$) to 5 μL of sample, the mixture was left at room temperature for 15 min in the dark. The absorbance at 750 nm was measured using a Microplate Reader, model infinite M200 PRO (Tecan, Austria). The blank was prepared in the same manner, except distilled water was used instead of the sample. The radical scavenging activity was calculated as a percentage using the following equation:

$$\text{ABTS radical scavenging activity (\%)} = \left[1 - \left(\frac{A_{\text{sample}}}{A_{\text{blank}}}\right)\right] \times 100. \tag{2}$$

2.7. Esophageal Lesion Score. The rat esophagus was cut with scissors in longitudinal direction from the gastroesophageal junction to the pharynx after sacrifice. The inner mucus was washed away with 0.9% NaCl and laid out on paper. Thereafter, the dissected esophagus was photographed with an optical digital camera (Sony, Tokyo, Japan) and analyzed using the i-Solution Lite software program. The gross mucosal damage ratio was calculated as follows:

$$\text{The gross mucosal damage ratio (\%)} = \left[\frac{\text{width of area with esophageal mucosal damage}\left(\text{mm}^2\right)}{\text{width of total area of esophagus}\left(\text{mm}^2\right)}\right] \times 100. \tag{3}$$

2.8. Measurement of ROS Level in the Serum. The ROS levels were measured by employing the method of Ali et al. [24]. 25 mM DCF-DA was added to the serum. After incubation for 30 min, the changes in fluorescence values were determined at an excitation wavelength of 486 nm and emission wavelength of 530 nm.

2.9. Measurement of Peroxynitrite Level in the Serum. The peroxynitrite ($ONOO^-$) level was assessed by a modified Kooy's method with minor modifications [25], which involves the monitoring of highly fluorescent rhodamine 123, which is rapidly produced from nonfluorescent dihydrorhodamine (DHR) 123 in the presence of $ONOO^-$. And its final fluorescent intensities remained unchanged over time. Serum was added to the rhodamine buffer. In brief, the rhodamine buffer (pH 7.4) consisted of 50 mM sodium phosphate dibasic, 50 mM sodium phosphate monobasic, 90 mM sodium chloride, 5 mM potassium chloride, and 5 mM diethylenetriamine penta-acetic acid. The final DHR 123 concentration was 5.0 μM. Five minutes after treating with or without the addition of authentic $ONOO^-$, the background and final fluorescent intensities of the samples were measured. The assay buffer was prepared prior to use and placed on ice. The fluorescence intensity of the oxidized DHR 123 was measured with a microplate fluorescence reader, model infinite M200 PRO (Tecan, Austria), at 485 nm excitation and 535 nm emission. The results were expressed as the inhibition level of oxidation of DHR 123 and calculated from the final fluorescence intensity minus background fluorescence intensity.

2.10. Preparation of Cytosol and Nuclear Fractions. Protein extraction was performed according to the method of Komatsu with minor modifications [26]. Esophageal tissues for cytosol fraction were homogenized with ice-cold lysis buffer A (250 mL) containing 10 mM HEPES (pH 7.8), 10 mM KCl, 2 mM $MgCl_2$, 1 mM DTT, 0.1 mM EDTA, 0.1 mM PMSF, and 1,250 μL protease inhibitor mixture solution. The homogenate incubated at 4°C for 20 min. And then 10% NP-40 was added and mixed well. After centrifugation (13,400 ×g for 2 min at 4°C) using Eppendorf 5415R (Hamburg, Germany), the supernatant liquid (cytosol fraction) was separated by new e-tube. The left pellets were washed twice by buffer A and the supernatant was discarded. Next, the pellets were suspended with lysis buffer C (20 mL) containing 50 mM HEPES (pH 7.8), 50 mM KCl, 300 mM NaCl, 1 mM DTT, 0.1 mM EDTA, 0.1 mM PMSF, 1% (v/v) glycerol, and 100 μL protease inhibitor mixture solution suspended and incubated at 4°C for 30 min. After centrifugation (13,400 ×g for 10 min at 4°C), the nuclear fraction was prepared to collect the supernatant. Both cytosol and nuclear fractions were kept at −80°C before the analysis.

2.11. Immunoblotting Analyses. For the estimation of Nrf-2, NF-κBp65, and histone, 10 μg of protein from each nuclear fraction was electrophoresed through 8–10% sodium dodecyl sulfate polyacrylamide gel (SDS-PAGE). Separated proteins were transferred to a nitrocellulose membrane, blocked with 5% (w/v) skim milk solution for 1 h, and then incubated with primary antibodies (Nrf-2, NF-κBp65, and histone) and overnight at 4°C. After the blots were washed, they were incubated with anti-rabbit or anti-mouse IgG HRP-conjugated secondary antibody for 1 h at room temperature. In addition, 10–15 μg protein of each postnuclear fraction of SOD, catalase, HO-1, p-IκBα, COX-2, iNOS, TNF-α, IL-6, and β-actin was electrophoresed through 8–15% SDS-PAGE. Each antigen-antibody complex was visualized using ECL Western Blotting Detection Reagents and detected by chemiluminescence with Sensi-Q 2000 Chemidoc (Lugen Sci Co.,

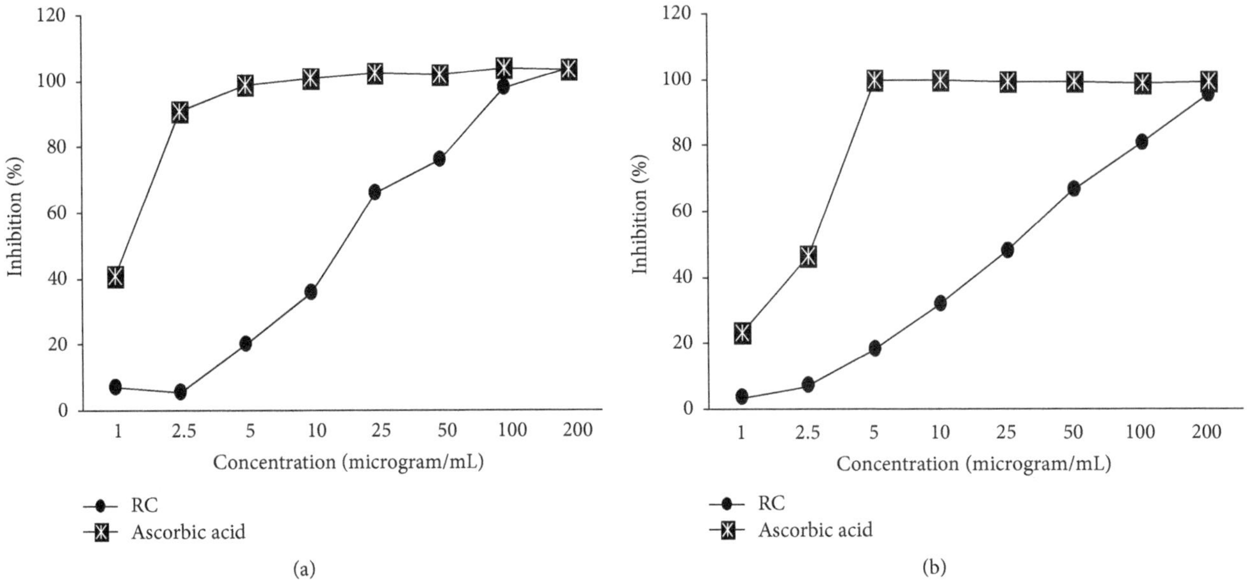

FIGURE 2: DPPH radical scavenging activity (a) and ABTS radical scavenging activity (b) of RC-mix, water extract of Rhei rhizoma and Coptis rhizoma mixture. Each experiment was run in triplicate.

Ltd., Gyeonggi-do, Korea). Band densities were measured using ATTO Densitograph Software (ATTO Corporation, Tokyo, Japan) and quantified as the ratio to histone or β-actin. The protein levels of the groups are expressed relative to those of the normal rat (represented as 1).

2.12. Statistical Analysis. The data are expressed as the mean ± SEM. Significance was assessed by one-way analysis of variance (ANOVA) followed by Dunnett's multiple comparison test using SPSS version 22.0 software (SPSS Inc., Chicago, IL, USA). Values of $p < 0.05$ were considered significant. Also, simple regression analysis was performed to investigate the correlation between DPPH radical scavenging and ABTS radical scavenging using the Microsoft Excel 2010 statistical package.

3. Results

3.1. Compositional Contents Analysis of RC-Mix Extract Using HPLC Chromatogram. Representative HPLC results are illustrated in Figure 1. The ratio of each flavonoid was as follows: Rhei rhizoma and Coptidis rhizoma mixture: 3.14% sennoside A, 8.08% epiberberine, 7.92% coptisine, palmatine 8.89%, and berberine 28.96%. The data showed that the alkaloid present at the highest amount of RC-mix was berberine. The next most abundant ones were palmatine and coptisine.

3.2. DPPH Radical Scavenging Activity and ABTS Radical Scavenging Activity. In this study, *DPPH* and *ABTS radical scavenging activity* were performed to determine and confirm antioxidant activity of RC-mix. IC_{50} (μg/mL) represents half maximal concentration of tested compounds to scavenge DPPH and ABTS radical. As shown in Figure 2(a), the IC_{50} of DPPH radical scavenging activity of RC-mix was found at 17.74 ± 2.14 μg/mL and the IC_{50} value of ascorbic acid (positive control) as a positive control was 1.28 ± 0.04 μg/mL. The calculated IC_{50} value of RC-mix against the $ABTS^+$ radical was determined to be 27.60 ± 0.94 μg/mL and the IC_{50} value of ascorbic acid (positive control) as a positive control was 2.20 ± 0.02 μg/mL (Figure 2(b)).

3.3. Gross Mucosal Damage in the Esophagus . Figure 3(a) shows the results of the morphological examination of the esophagus. Morphological changes such as hyperemia and multiple erosions were observed in the rats with reflux esophagitis and damage to the normal rats was not apparent. The oral administration of RC-mix led to a marked decrease of gross mucosal damage in a dose-dependent manner. Accordingly, gross mucosal injury ratio in RE rats significantly increased compared with normal rats, but RC200 and RC400 pretreatment led to a significant decrease ($p < 0.01$, $p < 0.001$, resp.) (Figure 3(b)).

3.4. The ROS and $ONOO^-$ Levels in the Serum. As shown in Figure 4, the levels of ROS and $ONOO^-$ in the serum in RE control rats were markedly higher than those of normal rats, whereas these enhanced levels were significantly inhibited by the administration of RC-mix. The reduced ROS level both RC200 and RC400 recovered nearly to those of normal (Figure 4(a)). The $ONOO^-$ level in RC-mix treated experimental rats in comparison with RE control rats significantly decreased (Figure 4(b)). RC200 and RC400 treatment were superior to that of RC100. However, RC200 and RC400 showed a similar inhibitory effect.

3.5. Esophageal Nrf-2, HO-1, SOD, and Catalase Protein Expressions. Figures 5(a) and 5(b) showed that esophageal

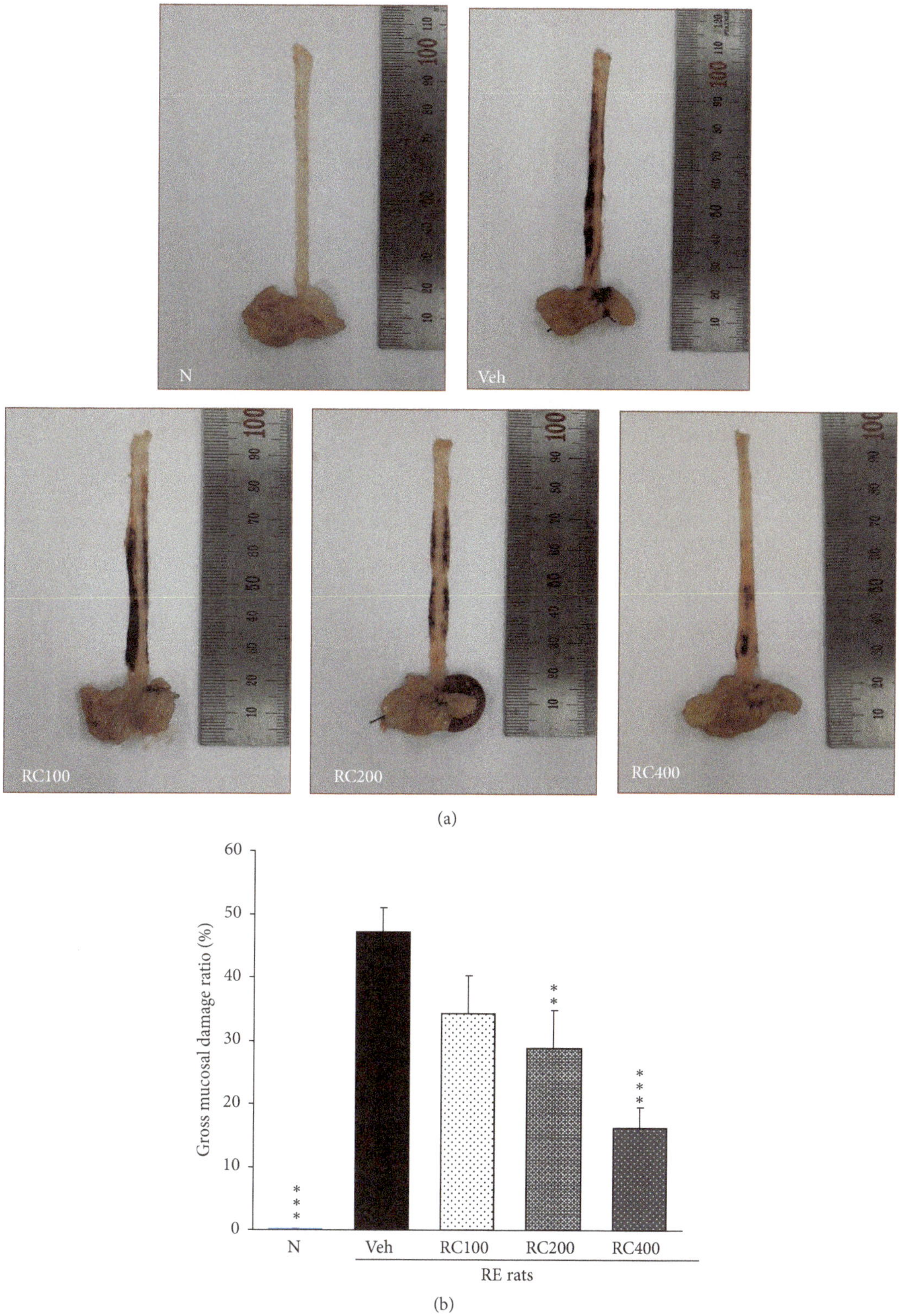

Figure 3: Gross evaluation of the esophageal mucosal damage. (a) Representative microphotographs of the esophagus. Esophageal lesion observed in rats with induced reflux esophagitis (RE) was ameliorated by RC-mix (100, 200, and 400 mg/kg body weight/day, p.o.) administration. (b) Gross mucosal injury ratio at the end of experiment. The gross mucosal injury was increased in RE rats compared with normal rats, but RC-mix administration led to a significant decrease (RC200, $p < 0.01$; RC400, $p < 0.001$). N, normal rats; Veh, positive control rats with reflux esophagitis (RE); RC100, RC200, and RC400 RE rats, animals treated with RC-mix 100 mg/kg, RC-mix 200 mg/kg, and RC-mix 400 mg/kg body weight, respectively. Data are the means ± SEM. Significance: $^{*}p < 0.05$, $^{**}p < 0.01$, and $^{***}p < 0.001$ versus RE control rat values. $n = 6$ in each group.

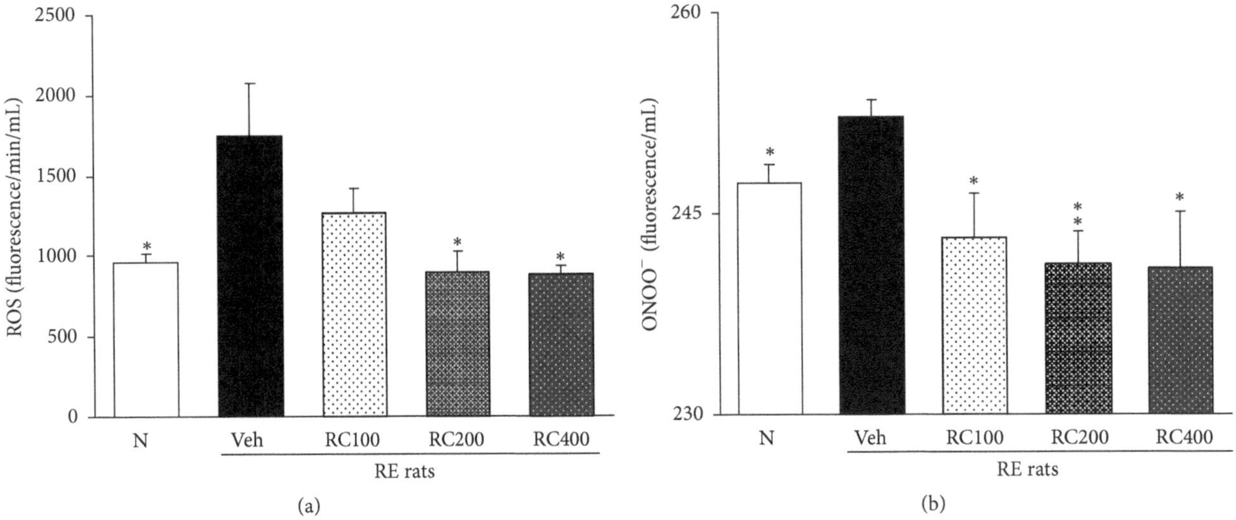

FIGURE 4: Effect of RC-mix on serum ROS and $ONOO^-$ production in rats with induced reflux esophagitis (RE). N, normal rats; Veh, positive control rats with reflux esophagitis (RE); RC100, RC200, and RC400 RE rats, animals treated with RC-mix 100 mg/kg, RC-mix 200 mg/kg, and RC-mix 400 mg/kg body weight, respectively. Data are the means ± SEM. Significance: $^*p < 0.05$, $^{**}p < 0.01$ versus RE control rat values. $n = 6$ in each group.

expressions of Nrf-2 and HO-1 in RE control rats had tendency to decrease compared with those of normal rats. However, RC400 administration significantly regulated the nuclear Nrf-2 and cytosolic HO-1 expressions in the esophagus of reflux-induced esophagitis rats ($p < 0.01$, $p < 0.05$, resp.). These results suggest that induction of HO-1 may be through Nrf-2 activation. The protein expressions of SOD-1 and catalase were decreased in RE control rats compared with normal rats; however, RC-mix treatment led to upregulations of SOD and catalase (Figures 5(c) and 5(d)). Herein, SOD and HO-1 protein expressions in RC400-treated rats were increased significantly, whereas catalase showed a tendency to increase (without significance) in the esophagus.

3.6. Esophageal p-IκBα and NF-κBp65 Protein Expressions. As shown in Figure 6, the expression of p-IκBα and NF-κBp65 proteins was analyzed by Western blot. The protein levels of p-IκBα(Figure 6(a)) and NF-κBp65 (Figure 6(b)) increased in the esophagus of RE control rats, whereas these elevated levels significantly reduced in RC-mix treated rats with reflux-induced esophagitis. Particularly, p-IκBα level was lowered nearly to that of normal rats by RC-mix 400 mg/kg treatment.

3.7. Esophageal COX-2, iNOS, TNF-α, and IL-6 Protein Expressions. The quantified COX-2, iNOS, TNF-α, and IL-6 protein expressions are shown in Figures 7(a), 7(b), 7(c), and 7(d), respectively. The inflammation-related protein expressions in the RE control rats were significantly augmented in the esophagus compared with normal rats. However, treatment with RC-mix suppressed these proteins in the esophagus. Moreover, COX-2 and IL-6 decreased significantly in all RC experimental rats and, above all, the administration of RC400 reduced nearly to normal levels or below in the esophagus. iNOS and TNF-α protein expression exhibited no significant changes in RC100 and RC200 but RC400 reduced significantly.

4. Discussion

Despite noticeable advances in modern medicine, reflux esophagitis (RE) remains one of worldwide problems with a considerable impact on quality of life and healthcare costs [27]. The etiology of RE is complex and various rather than a single cause, including hypersensitivity of the esophageal mucosa to physiological reflux, reduced mucosal defense mechanisms, and gastric motility disturbances [28]. It is generally shown that refluxate containing acid, pepsin, and bile causes inflammation, ulceration, and destruction of the normal squamous epithelium of the esophagus [29]. Synthetic drugs used in the treatment of RE are inadequate and sometimes can have serious side effects. In view of the undesirable side effects of synthetic agents, the treatment of RE is focused on traditional herbal medicines. In the present report, we explored the potential of Rhei rhizoma and *Coptis chinensis* mixture on experimentally induced reflux esophagitis in rats.

Rhei rhizoma is a famous traditional Korean medicine and used for treating many diseases, such as liver injury, gastrointestinal disease, constipation, and ulcers. The major antigastritis and antipeptic ulcer active constituents of Rhei rhizoma were sennoside A, emodin, aloe-emodin, chrysophanol, and rhein [30, 31]. Coptidis rhizoma has various pharmacological properties, such as gastroprotective, antidiabetic, hypolipidemic, analgesic, and neuroprotective effect [32, 33]. The major active compounds are alkaloids, including berberine, coptisine, palmatine, jatrorrhizine, and their chemical structures [34]. Particularly, berberine has been widely reported to improve reflux esophagitis, gastroenteritis,

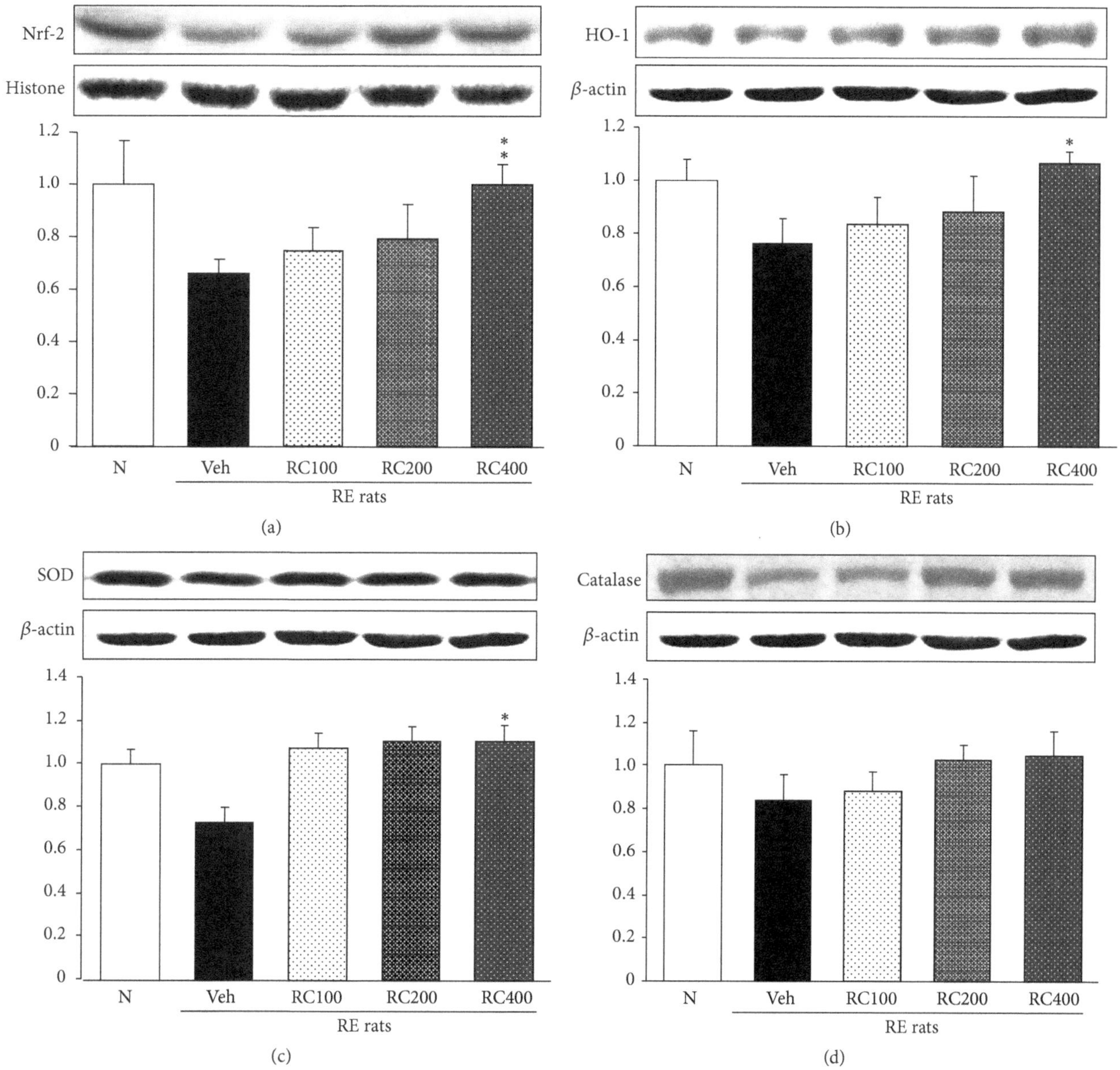

FIGURE 5: Esophageal Nrf-2 (a), HO-1 (b), SOD (c), and catalase (d) protein expressions. N, normal rats; Veh, positive control rats with reflux esophagitis (RE); RC100, RC200, and RC400 RE rats, animals treated with RC-mix 100 mg/kg, RC-mix 200 mg/kg, and RC-mix 400 mg/kg body weight, respectively. Data are the means ± SEM. Significance: $^{*}p < 0.05$, $^{**}p < 0.01$ versus RE control rat values. $n = 6$ in each group.

diarrhea, and colitis with few side effects [35, 36]. However, the mechanisms underlying the effects of Rhei rhizoma and Coptidis rhizoma mixture have yet to be investigated in an experimental model of reflux esophagitis. Therefore, the present study was conducted using an experimental reflux esophagitis model. The analyses of RC-mix have shown that berberine was the highest alkaloid present. Our previous study has reported that berberine could protect the esophageal mucosal damage in reflux-induced esophagitis by suppressing proinflammatory cytokines [37]. DPPH and ABTS radical scavenging assays, based on hydrogen atom transfer and electron transfer reaction together, have demonstrated that *in vitro* analytical methods are reliable determination of antioxidant activity of biological sample [38]. The results of the *in vitro* antioxidant assays (DPPH and ABTS, Figure 2) showed that the administration of RC-mix could improve RE-induced oxidative stress in the esophagus of rats.

The general pathophysiology of gastric disorders including RE has focused on the imbalance between offensive and defensive factors. The esophageal mucosa, through its preepithelial (mucus and bicarbonate ion), epithelial (epithelial cells), and deep postepithelial (blood vessels) mechanisms, represents one of the important defense mechanisms [39]. The preepithelial superficial defense mechanism is weak, so esophageal epithelial cells are easily exposed to

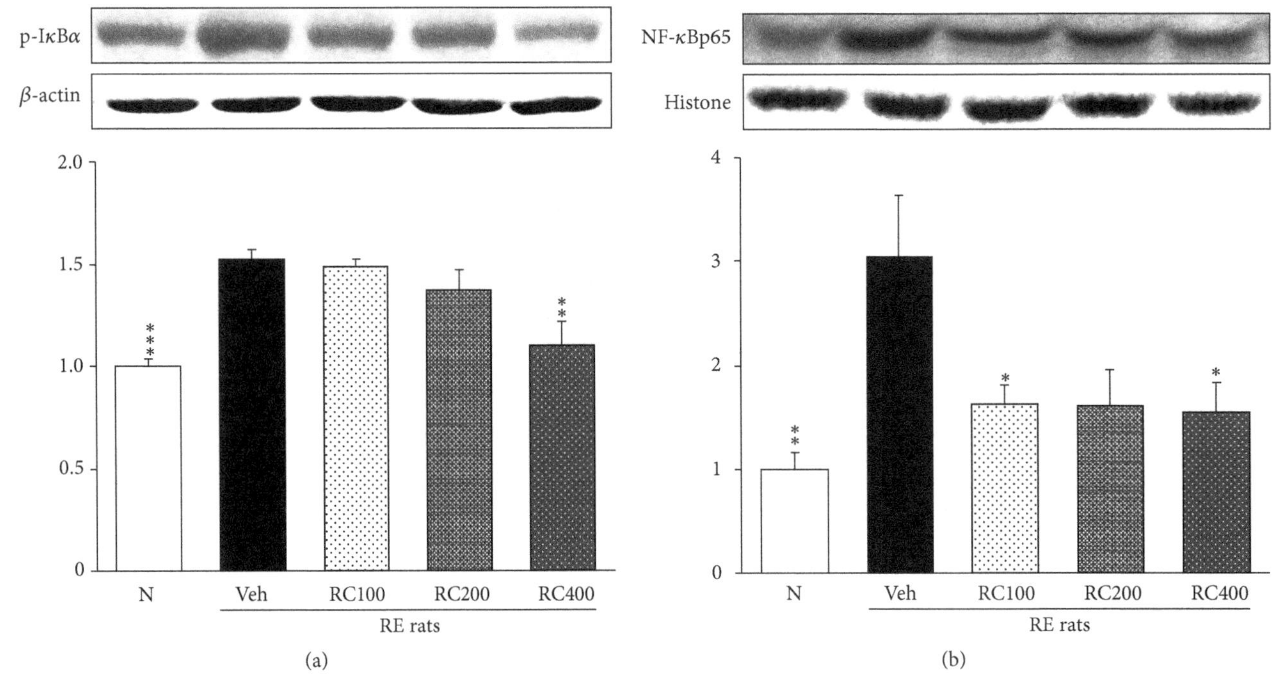

FIGURE 6: Esophageal p-IκBα (a) and NF-κBp65 (b) protein expressions. N, normal rats; Veh, positive control rats with reflux esophagitis (RE); RC100, RC200, and RC400 RE rats, animals treated with RC-mix 100 mg/kg, RC-mix 200 mg/kg, and RC-mix 400 mg/kg body weight, respectively. Data are the means ± SEM. Significance: $^{*}p < 0.05$, $^{**}p < 0.01$, and $^{***}p < 0.001$ versus RE control rat values. $n = 6$ in each group.

refluxed contents and the prolonged contact with acid and pepsin can lead to morphological changes of esophageal tissues, including dilation of intracellular spaces, extensive erosion of esophageal mucosa, detachment of epithelial layer, and mucosal degeneration [40]. In the present study, the esophageal lesion score in RE control rats was remarkably increased compared with that of normal rats as already demonstrated by other authors [7]. However, the lesion score was significantly attenuated in both RC200 and RC400 animal groups, suggesting the potential therapeutic effect of RC-mix against RE.

The action of oxidative stress in inflammation-based GI tract diseases was widely known and, in the development of RE, it also results to be more important than the injuries caused by gastric acids [8, 41]. An imbalance in the generation of free radicals like ROS and reactive nitrogen species such as $ONOO^-$ (which is highly toxic) was found to be responsible for the esophageal tissue damage; this finding was supported by the studies showing that tissue damage could be prevented with the use of antioxidant agent [42]. ROS causes oxidative damage in cellular components such as DNA, proteins, and membrane lipids. Overproduction of ROS results in oxidative stress, which leads to oxidative damage in cells by altering the structure of biomacromolecules, and this process has been implicated in a number of diseases. Therefore, the reduction of intracellular ROS may help prevent the onset and progression of diseases *via* protection of vital molecules [43]. Inducible nitric oxide synthase (iNOS) is a Ca^{2+}-dependent cytosolic enzyme that forms nitric oxide (NO) from l-arginine, and NO reacts with the free radical superoxide (O^{2-}) to form the toxic free radical peroxynitrite ($ONOO^-$). Free radicals such as $ONOO^-$ and O^{2-} damage cellular membranes and intracellular proteins, enzymes, and DNA. Elevated $ONOO^-$, a powerful oxidant, produces oxidative stress, an imbalance between oxidants and antioxidants [44]. In the present study, the induced esophageal reflux determined the esophagus tissue damage, which was combined to an increase of ROS production. However, the RC-mix treatment was able to reduce the oxidative stress by significantly reducing the ROS production.

Nrf-2 is usually present within the cytosol; however, oxidative stress induces the translocation of Nrf-2 into nucleus. Nrf-2 leads to the transcription of antioxidant enzyme including SOD, catalase, and HO-1 by binding to antioxidant response element (ARE) [45]. Nrf-2-dependent genes, including SOD, catalase, and HO-1, are very important for cellular defense against oxidative stress and proper management of free iron is increased [46]. SOD interacts with O_2^- to form H_2O_2, which is subsequently catabolised by catalase to H_2O. HO-1 degrades heme to carbon monoxide (CO), biliverdin, and iron. The cytoprotection by HO-1 is mediated by various different mechanisms, including the catabolism of prooxidant heme to the antioxidant bile pigments biliverdin and bilirubin; the coordinate induction of ferritin, which chelates free iron; and the liberation of CO, which exerts meaningful anti-inflammatory and antiapoptotic effects [47]. Moreover, recent study suggests that HO-1 plays a critical role including cytoprotective and antioxidant and antiapoptotic activities in inflammatory diseases of the upper (esophagus and stomach) and lower (intestine) gastrointestinal tract [48].

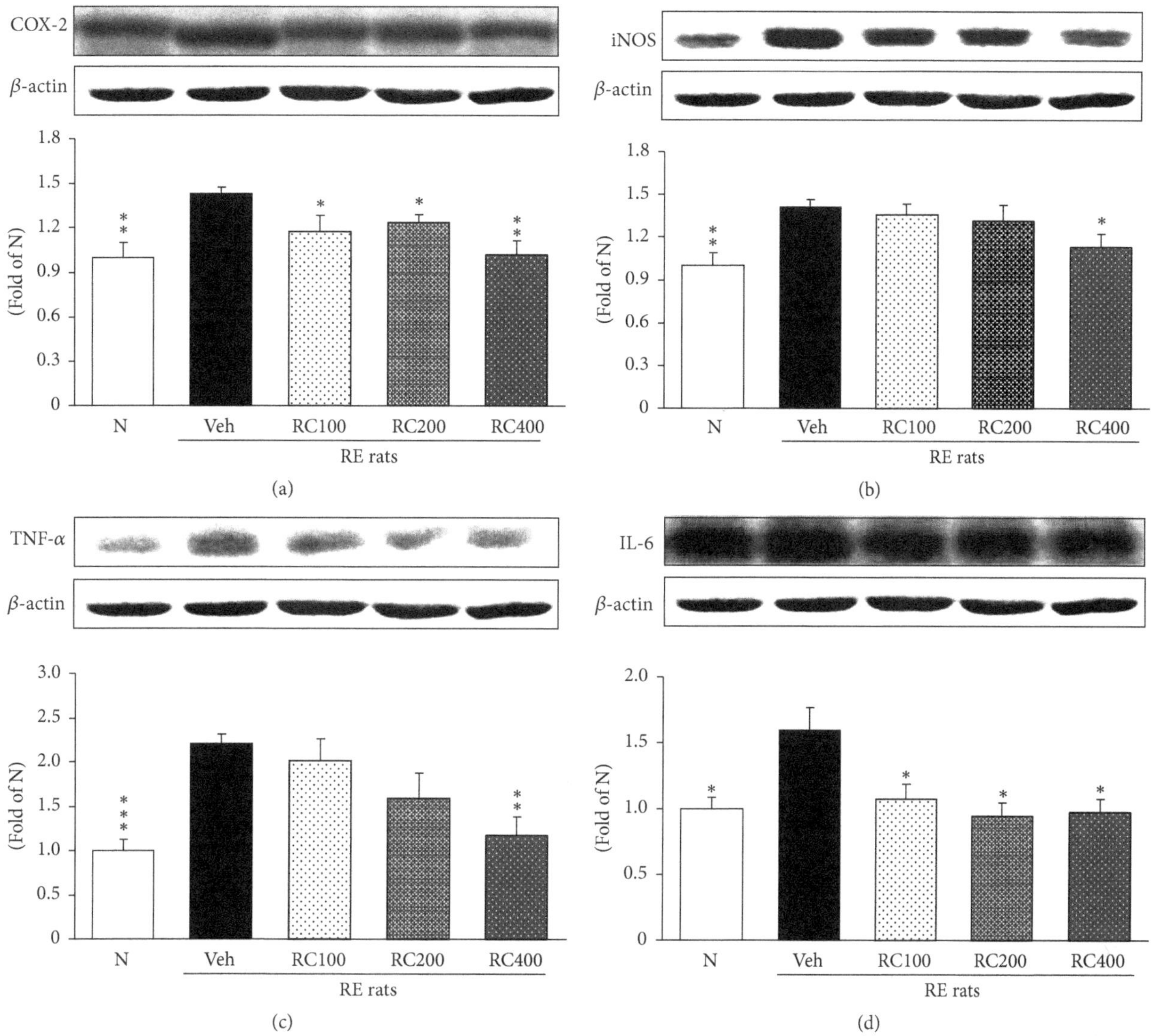

FIGURE 7: Esophageal COX-2 (a), iNOS (b), TNF-α (c), and IL-6 (d) protein expressions. N, normal rats; Veh, positive control rats with reflux esophagitis (RE); RC100, RC200, and RC400 RE rats, animals treated with RC-mix 100 mg/kg, RC-mix 200 mg/kg, and RC-mix 400 mg/kg body weight, respectively. Data are the means ± SEM. Significance: $^{*}p < 0.05$, $^{**}p < 0.01$, and $^{***}p < 0.001$ versus RE control rat values. $n = 6$ in each group.

In this study, the oral administration of RC-mix tended to increase SOD and catalase activities in a dose-dependent manner and the level of SOD became significantly higher in RC400 treated animals. In addition, the induced reflux esophagitis rats showed a decreased expression of HO-1 in esophageal tissues compared with normal rats, whereas the RC-mix administration resulted in a significant upregulation of HO-1 in RC400 rats. This suggests that the RC-mix treatment may effectively scavenge oxyradicals during the oxidative stress induced by the induced reflux esophagitis.

Our previous study [20] showed that NF-κB pathway plays a key role in impairment of esophageal barrier function due to exposure to the gastroesophageal refluxate and regulates the transcription of a wide variety of genes involved in the inflammatory and immune response [49]. The NF-κB dimer is sequestered in the cytoplasm of most cells through interaction with the inhibitory IκBα protein and the inhibition of IκBα phosphorylation leads to stabilization of NF-κB/IκBα interaction thus preventing nuclear translocation of NF-κB [50]. The phosphorylation of IκBα results in the translocation of NF-κB and it means NF-κB activation. A variety of stimuli can trigger NF-κB activation such as infections, inflammatory cytokines, ultraviolet irradiation, and oxidative stress. The results of the present study show that RC-mix at a dose of 400 mg/kg body weight seems to reduce the phosphorylation of IκBα and therefore could prevent the translocation of NF-κB in esophageal tissue. Namely, the administration of RC400 significantly suppressed NF-κB activation through the marked inhibition of IκBα phosphorylation.

NF-κB regulates the expression of inducible enzymes including COX-2 and iNOS and promotes the transcription

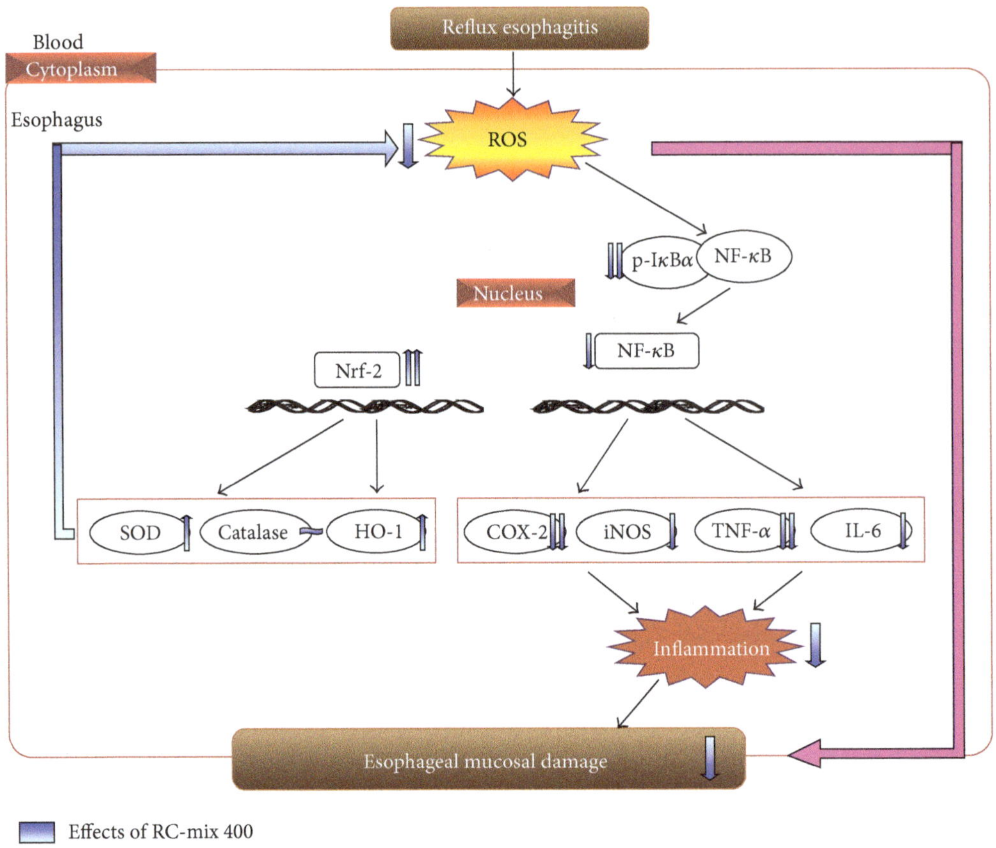

Figure 8: Predicted mechanism in esophageal tissue on administering RC400. RC400 decreased serum ROS and $ONOO^-$ production. Further, RC400 ameliorated the values of proinflammatory mediators (COX-2 and iNOS) and cytokines (TNF-α and IL-6) regulated by NF-κB and increased oxidative defense factor SOD and HO-1 proteins.

of target genes such as TNF-α and IL-6. The role of COX-2 was augmented under inflammatory conditions, such as reflux esophagitis and Barrett's esophagus [51], and iNOS, which generates nitric oxide (NO), is an important mediator of reflux-induced cell signaling in esophageal cells. The upregulation of iNOS expression results in the overproduction of NO. NO reacts with O_2^- and forms $ONOO^-$. $ONOO^-$ can directly cause DNA damage and participate in inflammation-related carcinogenesis [52]. When monocytes and macrophages are exposed to inflammatory stimuli, they secrete pleiotropic cytokines such as TNF-α and IL-6. TNF-α exerts multiple and potent proinflammatory activity, and its blockade results in profound downregulatory effects [53]. In addition, IL-6, which is a broad-spectrum cytokine with characteristics of an acute-phase reactant, has both proinflammatory and anti-inflammatory functions that affect processes ranging from immunity to tissue repair and metabolism [54]. In the present study, treatment with RC-mix in the reflux esophagitis model significantly decreased esophageal protein upregulation of NF-κB related inflammatory mediators (COX-2 and iNOS). In addition, the protein expression of IL-6 was significantly downregulated following the administration of RC-mix. Whereas RC100 and RC200 did not significantly affect the expression of TNF-α the latter was significantly reduced by RC400 treatment.

A recent study has shown that ROS are one of the potent factors in the pathogenesis of esophageal mucosal damage mediated by oxidative stress in an experimental model of reflux esophagitis [55]. In the present study, the administration of RC-mix reduced the oxidative stress biomarker and increased the activities of SOD and HO-1. Furthermore, the anti-inflammatory effects of RC-mix suggested that the inactivation of NF-κB by blocking the phosphorylation of IκBα led to the inhibition of the release of proinflammatory cytokines and mediators, reducing the inflammatory damage that is typical in the esophageal mucosa of rats with reflux esophagitis (Figure 8).

5. Conclusions

Rhei rhizoma and Coptidis rhizoma mixture includes the major flavonoids such as sennoside A, epiberberine, coptisine, palmatine, and berberine. RC-mix has a protective effect against esophageal mucosal damage in a dose-dependent manner. The RC-mix treated rats exhibited stronger anti-inflammatory activity through the elevation of antioxidant enzymes and the suppression of NF-κB activation. Thus, the antioxidative abilities of RC-mix may potentially be used for the prevention of esophageal mucosal damage.

Competing Interests

The authors declare that they have no competing interests.

Acknowledgments

This study was supported by the Traditional Korean Medicine R&D Program funded by the Ministry of Health & Welfare through the Korea Health Industry Development Institute (KHIDI; HI13C0542).

References

[1] N. Vakil, S. V. van Zanten, P. Kahrilas et al., "The Montreal definition and classification of gastroesophageal reflux disease: a global evidence-based consensus," *The American Journal of Gastroenterology*, vol. 101, no. 8, pp. 1900–1943, 2006.

[2] J. Dent, H. B. El-Serag, M.-A. Wallander, and S. Johansson, "Epidemiology of gastro-oesophageal reflux disease: a systematic review," *Gut*, vol. 54, no. 5, pp. 710–717, 2005.

[3] H.-K. Jung, "Epidemiology of gastroesophageal reflux disease in Asia: a systematic review," *Journal of Neurogastroenterology and Motility*, vol. 17, no. 1, pp. 14–27, 2011.

[4] F. Rieder, P. Biancani, K. Harnett, L. Yerian, and G. W. Falk, "Inflammatory mediators in gastroesophageal reflux disease: impact on esophageal motility, fibrosis, and carcinogenesis," *American Journal of Physiology—Gastrointestinal and Liver Physiology*, vol. 298, no. 5, pp. G571–G581, 2010.

[5] R. Badillo and D. Francis, "Diagnosis and treatment of gastroesophageal reflux disease," *World Journal of Gastrointestinal Pharmacology and Therapeutics*, vol. 5, no. 3, pp. 105–112, 2014.

[6] V. D. Corleto, S. Festa, E. Di Giulio, and B. Annibale, "Proton pump inhibitor therapy and potential long-term harm," *Current Opinion in Endocrinology, Diabetes and Obesity*, vol. 21, no. 1, pp. 3–8, 2014.

[7] J.-W. Kang and S.-M. Lee, "Protective effects of chlorogenic acid against experimental reflux esophagitis in rats," *Biomolecules and Therapeutics*, vol. 22, no. 5, pp. 420–425, 2014.

[8] Y. J. Kim, E.-H. Kim, and K. B. Hahm, "Oxidative stress in inflammation-based gastrointestinal tract diseases: challenges and opportunities," *Journal of Gastroenterology and Hepatology*, vol. 27, no. 6, pp. 1004–1010, 2012.

[9] Y. Erbil, U. Türkoglu, U. Barbaros et al., "Oxidative damage in an experimentally induced gastric and gastroduodenal reflux model," *Surgical Innovation*, vol. 12, no. 3, pp. 219–225, 2005.

[10] K. Takeuchi and K. Nagahama, "Animal model of acid-reflux esophagitis: pathogenic roles of acid/pepsin, prostaglandins, and amino acids," *BioMed Research International*, vol. 2014, Article ID 532594, 10 pages, 2014.

[11] M. W. Pawlik, S. Kwiecien, R. Pajdo et al., "Esophagoprotective activity of angiotensin-(1–7) in experimental model of acute reflux esophagitis. Evidence for the role of nitric oxide, sensory nerves, hypoxia-inducible factor-1alpha and proinflammatory cytokines," *Journal of Physiology and Pharmacology*, vol. 65, no. 6, pp. 809–822, 2014.

[12] J. S. Lee, T. Y. Oh, B. O. Ahn et al., "Involvement of oxidative stress in experimentally induced reflux esophagitis and Barrett's esophagus: clue for the chemoprevention of esophageal carcinoma by antioxidants," *Mutation Research*, vol. 480-481, pp. 189–200, 2001.

[13] Q. Huang, G. Lu, H.-M. Shen, M. C. M. Chung, and N. O. Choon, "Anti-cancer properties of anthraquinones from rhubarb," *Medicinal Research Reviews*, vol. 27, no. 5, pp. 609–630, 2007.

[14] X.-F. Zhong, G.-D. Huang, T. Luo, Z.-Y. Deng, and J.-N. Hu, "Protective effect of rhein against oxidative stress-related endothelial cell injury," *Molecular Medicine Reports*, vol. 5, no. 5, pp. 1261–1266, 2012.

[15] E. Cui, X. Zhi, Y. Chen et al., "*Coptis chinensis* and myrobalan (*Terminalia chebula*) can synergistically inhibit inflammatory response in vitro and in vivo," *Evidence-Based Complementary and Alternative Medicine*, vol. 2014, Article ID 510157, 8 pages, 2014.

[16] S. Jiang, Y. Wang, D. Ren et al., "Antidiabetic mechanism of Coptis chinensis polysaccharide through its antioxidant property involving the JNK pathway," *Pharmaceutical Biology*, vol. 53, no. 7, pp. 1022–1029, 2015.

[17] D. A. Ghareeb, S. Khalil, H. S. Hafez et al., "Berberine reduces neurotoxicity related to nonalcoholic steatohepatitis in rats," *Evidence-Based Complementary and Alternative Medicine*, vol. 2015, Article ID 361847, 13 pages, 2015.

[18] Z. Li, Y.-N. Geng, J.-D. Jiang, and W.-J. Kong, "Antioxidant and anti-inflammatory activities of Berberine in the treatment of diabetes mellitus," *Evidence-Based Complementary and Alternative Medicine*, vol. 2014, Article ID 289264, 12 pages, 2014.

[19] N. Omura, H. Kashiwagi, G. Chen, Y. Suzuki, F. Yano, and T. Aoki, "Establishment of surgically induced chronic acid reflux esophagitis in rats," *Scandinavian Journal of Gastroenterology*, vol. 34, no. 10, pp. 948–953, 1999.

[20] M. Y. Kim, Y. O. Shin, J. Y. Lee et al., "Improving effect of a combined extract of rhei rhizoma and glycyrrhizae rhizoma through anti-oxidative stress in reflux esophagitis rats," *The Korea Journal of Herbology*, vol. 30, no. 4, pp. 37–44, 2015.

[21] T. Hatano, R. Edamatsu, M. Hiramatsu et al., "Effects of the interaction of tannins with co-existing substances. VI.: effects of tannins and related polyphenols on superoxide anion radical, and on 1, 1-diphenyl-2-picrylhydrazyl radical," *Chemical and Pharmaceutical Bulletin*, vol. 37, no. 8, pp. 2016–2021, 1989.

[22] P. Kumkrai, O. Weeranantanapan, and N. Chudapongse, "Antioxidant, α-glucosidase inhibitory activity and sub-chronic toxicity of *Derris reticulata* extract: its antidiabetic potential," *BMC Complementary and Alternative Medicine*, vol. 15, article 35, 2015.

[23] R. Re, N. Pellegrini, A. Proteggente, A. Pannala, M. Yang, and C. Rice-Evans, "Antioxidant activity applying an improved ABTS radical cation decolorization assay," *Free Radical Biology and Medicine*, vol. 26, no. 9-10, pp. 1231–1237, 1999.

[24] S. F. Ali, C. P. LeBel, and S. C. Bondy, "Reactive oxygen species formation as a biomarker of methylmercury and trimethyltin neurotoxicity," *NeuroToxicology*, vol. 13, no. 3, pp. 637–648, 1992.

[25] N. W. Kooy, J. A. Royall, H. Ischiropoulos, and J. S. Beckman, "Peroxynitrite-mediated oxidation of dihydrorhodamine 123," *Free Radical Biology and Medicine*, vol. 16, no. 2, pp. 149–156, 1994.

[26] S. Komatsu, "Extraction of nuclear protein," *Methods in Molecular Biology*, vol. 355, pp. 73–77, 2007.

[27] A. Altomare, M. P. L. Guarino, S. Cocca, S. Emerenziani, and M. Cicala, "Gastroesophageal reflux disease: update on inflammation and symptom perception," *World Journal of Gastroenterology*, vol. 19, no. 39, pp. 6523–6528, 2013.

[28] P. Singh, N. Singh, S. Sengupta, and G. Palit, "Ameliorative effects of *Panax quinquefolium* on experimentally induced

reflux oesophagitis in rats," *Indian Journal of Medical Research*, vol. 135, no. 3, pp. 407–413, 2012.

[29] W. O. A. Rohof, D. P. Hirsch, and G. E. E. Boeckxstaens, "Pathophysiology and management of gastroesophageal reflux disease," *Minerva Gastroenterologica e Dietologica*, vol. 55, no. 3, pp. 289–300, 2009.

[30] Y. Ding and Z. H. Huang, "Research progress in pharmacological effects of emodin," *Pharmacology and Clinics of Chinese Materia Medica*, vol. 23, no. 5, pp. 236–238, 2007.

[31] R. X. Zhang, "Brief investigation on effects of rhubarb other than purgative effect," *Chinese Medicine Modern Distance Education of China*, vol. 6, no. 10, pp. 1217–1218, 2008.

[32] J. Jung, J. S. Choi, and C.-S. Jeong, "Inhibitory activities of palmatine from *Coptis chinensis* against *Helicobactor pylori* and gastric damage," *Toxicological Research*, vol. 30, no. 1, pp. 45–48, 2014.

[33] Y. Tjong, S. Ip, L. Lao et al., "Analgesic effect of *Coptis chinensis* rhizomes (Coptidis Rhizoma) extract on rat model of irritable bowel syndrome," *Journal of Ethnopharmacology*, vol. 135, no. 3, pp. 754–761, 2011.

[34] L. Liu and Z. Chen, "Analysis of four alkaloids of Coptis chinensis in rat plasma by high performance liquid chromatography with electrochemical detection," *Analytica Chimica Acta*, vol. 737, pp. 99–104, 2012.

[35] C. Chen, Z. Yu, Y. Li, J. Fichna, and M. Storr, "Effects of berberine in the gastrointestinal tract—a review of actions and therapeutic implications," *The American Journal of Chinese Medicine*, vol. 42, no. 5, pp. 1053–1070, 2014.

[36] Y. Zhang, X. Wang, S. Sha et al., "Berberine increases the expression of NHE3 and AQP4 in sennosideA-induced diarrhoea model," *Fitoterapia*, vol. 83, no. 6, pp. 1014–1022, 2012.

[37] B. K. Choo and S.-S. Roh, "Berberine protects against esophageal mucosal damage in reflux esophagitis by suppressing proinflammatory cytokines," *Experimental and Therapeutic Medicine*, vol. 6, no. 3, pp. 663–670, 2013.

[38] D. Lee, D. Kim, and J. Je, "Antioxidant and cytoprotective effects of lotus (Nelumbo nucifera) leaves phenolic fraction," *Preventive Nutrition and Food Science*, vol. 20, no. 1, pp. 22–28, 2015.

[39] N. Yoshida and T. Yoshikawa, "Defense mechanism of the esophageal mucosa and esophageal inflammation," *Journal of Gastroenterology*, vol. 38, supplement 15, pp. 31–34, 2003.

[40] N. Yoshida, "Inflammation and oxidative stress in gastroesophageal reflux disease," *Journal of Clinical Biochemistry and Nutrition*, vol. 40, no. 1, pp. 13–23, 2007.

[41] T. Y. Oh, J. S. Lee, B. O. Ahn et al., "Oxidative stress is more important than acid in the pathogenesis of reflux oesophagitis in rats," *Gut*, vol. 49, no. 3, pp. 364–371, 2001.

[42] M. J. Lee, H. J. Song, J. Y. Jeong, S. Y. Park, and U. D. Sohn, "Antioxidative and anti-inflammatory effects of QGC in cultured feline esophageal epithelial cells," *Korean Journal of Physiology and Pharmacology*, vol. 17, no. 1, pp. 81–87, 2013.

[43] X. Pan, L. Zhu, H. Lu, D. Wang, Q. Lu, and H. Yan, "Melatonin attenuates oxidative damage induced by acrylamide in vitro and in vivo," *Oxidative Medicine and Cellular Longevity*, vol. 2015, Article ID 703709, 12 pages, 2015.

[44] M. L. Pall, "The NO/ONOO-cycle as the central cause of heart failure," *International Journal of Molecular Sciences*, vol. 14, no. 11, pp. 22274–22330, 2013.

[45] J. A. Johnson, D. A. Johnson, A. D. Kraft et al., "The Nrf2-ARE pathway: an indicator and modulator of oxidative stress in neurodegeneration," *Annals of the New York Academy of Sciences*, vol. 1147, pp. 61–69, 2008.

[46] L. Xiong, J. Xie, C. Song et al., "The activation of Nrf2 and its downstream regulated genes mediates the antioxidative activities of xueshuan xinmaining tablet in human umbilical vein endothelial cells," *Evidence-Based Complementary and Alternative Medicine*, vol. 2015, Article ID 187265, 7 pages, 2015.

[47] M. Chang, J. Xue, V. Sharma, and A. Habtezion, "Protective role of hemeoxygenase-1 in gastrointestinal diseases," *Cellular and Molecular Life Sciences*, vol. 72, no. 6, pp. 1161–1173, 2015.

[48] H. Chen, Y. Fang, W. Li et al., "NFkB and Nrf2 in esophageal epithelial barrier function," *Tissue Barriers*, vol. 1, no. 5, Article ID e27463, 2013.

[49] T. Lawrence and C. Fong, "The resolution of inflammation: anti-inflammatory roles for NF-κB," *The International Journal of Biochemistry and Cell Biology*, vol. 42, no. 4, pp. 519–523, 2010.

[50] M. M. M. Abdel-Latif, J. O'Riordan, H. J. Windle et al., "NF-κB activation in esophageal adenocarcinoma: relationship to barrett's metaplasia, survival, and response to neoadjuvant chemoradiotherapy," *Annals of Surgery*, vol. 239, no. 4, pp. 491–500, 2004.

[51] N. S. Buttar, K. K. Wang, M. A. Anderson et al., "The effect of selective cyclooxygenase-2 inhibition in Barrett's esophagus epithelium: an in vitro study," *Journal of the National Cancer Institute*, vol. 94, no. 6, pp. 422–429, 2002.

[52] E. McAdam, H. N. Haboubi, G. Forrester et al., "Inducible nitric oxide synthase (iNOS) and nitric oxide (NO) are important mediators of reflux-induced cell signalling in esophageal cells," *Carcinogenesis*, vol. 33, no. 11, pp. 2035–2043, 2012.

[53] W. Cao, L. Cheng, J. Behar, C. Fiocchi, P. Biancani, and K. M. Harnett, "Proinflammatory cytokines alter/reduce esophageal circular muscle contraction in experimental cat esophagitis," *The American Journal of Physiology—Gastrointestinal and Liver Physiology*, vol. 287, no. 6, pp. G1131–G1139, 2004.

[54] N. Nishimoto and T. Kishimoto, "Inhibition of IL-6 for the treatment of inflammatory diseases," *Current Opinion in Pharmacology*, vol. 4, no. 4, pp. 386–391, 2004.

[55] T.-Y. Oh, J.-S. Lee, B.-O. Ahn et al., "Oxidative damages are critical in pathogenesis of reflux esophagitis: implication of antioxidants in its treatment," *Free Radical Biology and Medicine*, vol. 30, no. 8, pp. 905–915, 2001.

11

Evaluation of the Isoflavone Genistein as Reversible Human Monoamine Oxidase-A and -B Inhibitor

Najla O. Zarmouh, Samia S. Messeha, Faisel M. Elshami, and Karam F. A. Soliman

College of Pharmacy & Pharmaceutical Sciences, Florida A & M University, Tallahassee, FL 32307, USA

Correspondence should be addressed to Karam F. A. Soliman; karam.soliman@famu.edu

Academic Editor: Michele Navarra

Monoamine oxidases inhibitors (MAOIs) are effective therapeutic drugs for managing Parkinson's disease (PD) and depression. However, their irreversibility may lead to rare but serious side effects. As finding safer and reversible MAOIs is our target, we characterized the *recombinant human* (*h*) MAO-A and MAO-B inhibition potentials of two common natural isoflavones, genistein (GST) and daidzein (DZ) using luminescence assay. The results obtained showed that DZ exhibits partial to no inhibition of the isozymes examined while GST inhibited *h*MAO-B (IC_{50} of 6.81 μM), and its *h*MAO-A inhibition was more potent than the standard deprenyl. Furthermore, the reversibility, mode of inhibition kinetics, and tyramine oxidation of GST were examined. GST was a time-independent reversible and competitive *h*MAO-A and *h*MAO-B inhibitor with a lower K_i of *h*MAO-B (1.45 μM) than *h*MAO-A (4.31 μM). GST also inhibited *h*MAO-B tyramine oxidation and hydrogen peroxide production more than *h*MAO-A. Docking studies conducted indicated that the GST reversibility and *h*MAO-B selectivity of inhibition may relate to C5-OH effects on its orientation and its interactions with the threonine 201 residue of the active site. It was concluded from this study that the natural product GST has competitive and reversible MAOs inhibitions and may be recommended for further investigations as a useful therapeutic agent for Parkinson's disease.

1. Introduction

Neurological disorders such as Parkinson's disease (PD) and major depressive disorder (MDD) are associated with brain neurotransmitters depletion, particularly dopamine (DA), serotonin (5-HT), and norepinephrine (NE). MDD comorbidities may affect 72% of PD patients [1]. However, the currently available drugs for PD patients have wearing-off complications and for MDD are unsuccessful in at least 40% of the patients [2, 3]. In depressive and aging PD patients, the activity of brain monoamine oxidase (MAO) is significantly elevated compared to healthy individuals [4, 5]. Moreover, in the aging population, improving brain neurotransmitters and reducing MAO activities by using MAO inhibitors (MAOIs) were proven beneficial whereas other antidepressants mechanisms appear less effective [6].

MAO exists in two isoforms, MAO-A, and MAO-B [7]. The therapeutic value of the reversible inhibitors of MAO-A (RIMA) for depression has been firmly established [8] while MAO-B inhibitors (MAO-BIs) are used in PD. MAO-BIs maintain a higher level of DA from its precursor L-dopa in PD patients and may even benefit Alzheimer's disease (AD) [9, 10]. Deprenyl (DEP), a current MAO-BI used for PD, was recently approved as transdermal patches (Emsam®) for MDD treatment to become the most prevalent MAOI useful for the elderly [6].

In the brain, the mitochondrial bound flavin-containing amine oxidoreductase (MAO; EC 1.4.3.4) works to catalyze monoamine neurotransmitters oxidative deamination to maintain homeostasis. MAO-A catalyzes NE, DA, and 5-HT, while MAO-B catalyzes DA more specifically [11]. The abnormal elevation of MAO activity is associated with oxidative stress due to their production of hydrogen peroxide (H_2O_2) and aldehydes [12, 13]. Glutathione peroxidase and other enzymes become limited in buffering H_2O_2, and oxidative stress occurs and rises with the presence of iron, aggravating DNA and lipid membrane damage and contributing to glial and neuronal cell death. Hence, MAO inhibition provides a valuable strategy for the prevention of oxidative stress in addition to its ability in maintaining functional neurotransmitters levels.

The earlier discovered nonselective MAOIs, such as phenelzine, or the current selective MAO-BIs such as DEP have an irreversible inhibitory mechanism [14]. MAO irreversible inhibition may lead to the rare incidences of "the cheese effect" or drug interactions side effects [15]. Recent research had recognized that reversible or competitive inhibition of MAOs might be more important than isoform selectivity or high potency [16]. Therefore, reversible MAO inhibition is possibly the best strategy to prevent the cheese effect reaction caused by tyramine rich food ingestion. Therefore, the higher levels of the substrates or the withdrawal of the reversible inhibitors would allow the inhibitor substitution and, consequently, a faster recovery of the enzyme leading to fewer side effects.

Flavonoids as chromone-containing polyphenolic structures are well-known natural antioxidant agents that may affect the catecholamine synthesis [17, 18]. Apigenin, luteolin, and quercetin are examples of flavonoids with potent MAO inhibitory activities [19]. The flavonoids subclass isoflavones, in particular, were an interesting investigational class of compounds in the last two decades due to their presence in medicinal and nutritional traditional plants.

Genistein (GST) and daidzein (DZ) are two isoflavone analogs naturally found in traditionally used medicinal plants such as bakuchi, soybeans, and red clover [20–22]. Previously, both analogs showed different activities on distinct MAOs sources; DZ showed no significant rat MAO inhibition [23] while GST showed a weak bovine plasma MAO inhibition [24]. In our search for natural MAOIs, GST and DZ were investigated for *recombinant human* MAO isozymes (*h*MAO-A and *h*MAO-B) inhibition with the objective to understand the mechanism of action and structure-activity relationship. By choosing these two structurally close compounds (natural chemical analogs), any difference in their inhibitory activity can disclose the structure-activity relationship between the extra GST functional group and the MAO-A or MAO-B inhibitions. Comparing another compound (e.g., DZ metabolite s-equol) with GST will not enable us to make a clear conclusion. Ultimately, the current study investigates the possibility of identifying safer and reversible natural MAO inhibitors for the possible therapeutic use in the management of PD.

2. Materials and Methods

2.1. Materials. MAO-Glow™ Assay kit was obtained from Promega (Madison, WI, USA). Genistein (GST) (purity > 98%) and tyramine HCl were obtained from Santa Cruz Biotechnology Inc. (Dallas, TX, USA). The isozymes *h*MAO-A and *h*MAO-B derived from recombinant baculovirus and their aliquoted active units (U) were obtained from Sigma-Aldrich. Each *h*MAO-A and *h*MAO-B stock was diluted with 10 mM HEPES in cold Hank's Balanced Salt Solution (HBSS) (pH 7.4) and kept in −80°C until use. Daidzein (DZ) (purity ≥ 98%) and selective standard MAOIs including DEP and clorgyline (CLORG) and other materials were also purchased from Sigma-Aldrich (St. Louis, MO, USA).

2.2. hMAO-A and hMAO-B Assay. GST and DZ *h*MAO-A and *h*MAO-B inhibitory effects were tested by measuring the decrease in Arbitrary Light Units (ALU) using MAO-Glow Assay [25] with slight modifications. The initial velocity linearity of the isozymes was validated before the experiments at RT and in the presence and absence of standard DEP. For the assay, GST and DZ were serially diluted with buffer (pH 7.4) to a maximum final concentration of 250 μM each. Ethanol and DMSO were used (<2%) as solvents. In white opaque 96-well plates, 12.5 μL of each analog was plated with 25 μL of *h*MAO-A or *h*MAO-B for a 0.88 U/mL final concentration (0.04 U per reaction). In other wells, reaction buffer substituted each isozyme (to make the blanks) and each analog (to make negative control). After 40 min incubation, 12.5 μL luciferin derivative substrate (LDS) was added for a final concentration of 40 and 4 μM for *h*MAO-A and *h*MAO-B, respectively. After 2 h incubation, the reactions were stopped by adding 50 μL of Reporter Luciferin Detection Reagent (RLDR). Plates were incubated for 30 min to produce luminescence signal and then samples were read on Synergy HTX Multi-Reader (Bio-Tek, USA).

2.3. GST Mode of hMAO-A and hMAO-B Inhibition

2.3.1. Recovery by Dilution Assay. The recovery of both *h*MAO-A and *h*MAO-B after the inhibition by GST was measured by a previously reported preincubation and dilution method [26] with slight modifications using MAO-Glow Assay at RT [24]. Briefly, 100x isozymes (88 U/mL) or buffer (for blanks) was preincubated separately with GST or buffer (for negative controls) at concentrations of 10x IC_{50} and 100x IC_{50} for 40 min at RT (pH 7.4). For positive control, standards at 10x IC_{50} were simultaneously preincubated (0.03 μM CLORG for *h*MAO-A and 1.01 μM DEP for *h*MAO-B). Tests of GST of 4x IC_{50} with 4x of each isozyme was also simultaneously conducted for extra control. All reactions were subsequently diluted 100-fold when mixed with LDS in a 96-well plate to yield final concentrations of GST of 0.1x IC_{50} and 1x IC_{50}. The microplates were then incubated for 30, 40, 50, and 60 min. RLDR was added, and luminescence was measured as mentioned above.

2.3.2. Michaelis-Menten. The modes of MAO inhibitory effects of GST were analyzed by Michaelis-Menten kinetics using MAO-Glow Assay. Standard DEP was used to validate the method. Seven serially diluted LDS concentrations and a buffer (for a negative control) were prepared for a maximum final range from 0 to 150 μM for *h*MAO-A and 0 to 40 μM for *h*MAO-B. Three GST concentrations for a final of 5, 10, and 20 μM and a buffer (for a negative control) were mixed with each isozyme for a final concentration of 0.88 U/mL (2 : 1 ratio). After 40 min, the reactions were initiated by adding 19 μL of the enzyme and GST (or buffer) mixture to LDS in 96-well plates. After 1.5 h of incubation, RLDR was added, and the luminescence signal was detected as mentioned in the *hMAO-A and hMAO-B assay*.

2.4. Tyramine Oxidation Assay. A slightly modified continuous spectrophotometric method [27] was used to determine the selectivity of tyramine oxidation by *h*MAO-A or *h*MAO-B inhibited by GST. DEP was used as a standard control for this assay. Briefly, after optimizing tyramine used concentration for *h*MAO-A, 5x substrate and peroxidase chromogen reagent were mixed (1:1) for final of 0.5 mM tyramine HCl. In 96-well plates, 25 μL of GST serial dilutions up to 46 μM final concentrations were mixed with 50 μL isozyme for 0.7 U/mL final concentrations (0.09 U per reaction). After 40 min incubation at RT, 50 μL of the reagent/substrate mix was added to initiate the reaction and to make the final concentrations. The developing color (H_2O_2 indicator) was monitored over time at 490 nm by the μQuant Microplate Spectrophotometer (Bio-Tek, USA).

2.5. Docking Studies. GST, its analog DZ, and a selective MAO-B standard rasagiline (RAS) were docked as test ligands to the X-ray structure of *human* MAO-A and MAO-B at their Ligand Binding Domain. HYBRID of OEDocking (v3.0.1.) by OpenEye Scientific Software (Santa Fe, NM) was used as the docking method [28]. Briefly, MAO-A and MAO-B crystal structures were imported from Protein Data Bank pdf (PDB) to Sybyl-X 1.3 Modeling Suite (Tripos International, St. Louis, MO). Before docking, the conformer ensembles of all the test ligands were generated using OMEGA v2.4.6 (Open Eye Scientific Software, Santa Fe, NM) [28]. Using Structure Preparation tool, MAOs chain A was extracted; each flavin adenine dinucleotide cofactor (FAD) covalently linked to its cysteine residue (CYS: 406: A and CYS: 397: A) was retained in MAO-A and MAO-B, respectively. Hydrogen atoms were added to the isozymes, water molecules were retained, and MMFF94 and MMFF94s force fields were assigned to the atoms. The prediction method was validated by redocking the bound ligands complexes of MAO-A-harmine (PDB: 2Z5X) and MAO-B-2-BFI (PDB: 2XCG) in the crystal structures. The best ten poses retrieved were identical to the original poses of the cognate ligands with root mean square deviation (RMSD) between values <2 Å. Data were presented as HYBRID Chemgauss 4 scores.

2.6. Statistical Analysis. All analyses were performed by GraphPad Prism Software 6.02 (San Diego, CA, USA). IC_{50} values were determined by nonlinear regression best-fit model of normalized response with variable slope. The inhibitor constant (K_i) values were obtained from the competitive inhibition model. Lineweaver-Burk plot was obtained from Michaelis-Menten data. Relative selectivity (RS) folds were defined by the ratio of *h*MAO-A IC_{50} to *h*MAO-B IC_{50}. The significance of the difference between two groups was determined using an unpaired t-test, between the control and treatments using one-way ANOVA followed by Dunnett's multiple comparisons tests and between two sets of data using two-way ANOVA followed by Sidak's multiple comparisons test.

3. Results

3.1. GST MAOs Inhibition Compared with DZ. The specific inhibitory potentials of GST (Figure 1(a)) on A and B isozymes were investigated and compared to DZ (Figure 1(b)) and DEP using MAO luminescence assay (Figures 1(c) and 1(d)). The data obtained show that GST inhibited *h*MAOs superiorly more than DZ ($p < 0.0001$). DZ showed minor or partial inhibitory effect up to 250 μM of the tested concentrations ($p < 0.0001$). Meanwhile, GST had a sigmoidal inhibitory pattern and potency with an *h*MAO-B mean IC_{50} of 6.81 μM to be 1.4% of DEP potency (Figure 1(d)). However, GST *h*MAO-A inhibitory potency was more potent than DEP by 1.48-fold with mean IC_{50} of 9.7 μM (Figure 1(c)).

3.2. Mode of Inhibition of MAO-A and MAO-B Isozymes

3.2.1. Recovery of hMAO-A and hMAO-B after Inhibition. The recovery of the *h*MAO isozymes after GST inhibition was examined to determine reversibility of inhibition. The isozyme activities were determined after enzyme-inhibitor dilution with LDS (Figures 2(a) and 2(b)). At as low as 0.1x IC_{50} value concentrations, irreversible standard inhibitors expectedly reduced the isozyme activities to 6% (CLORG) and 4.3% (DEP), which indicates an unrecovered reduction of MAO activity after incubation with 10x IC_{50} concentrations. Meanwhile, preincubation of 0.1x IC_{50} GST with either *h*MAO-A or *h*MAO-B allowed a recovery of *h*MAO-A and *h*MAO-B catalytic rates to 86.8% and 86.1%, respectively. Their recovered activities measured in the presence of GST at its mean 1x IC_{50} value were 42.3% (MAO-A) and 47.1% (MAO-B). Both isozymes recoveries from GST were close to 90% or 50%, which is expected from a reversible inhibitor. No significant difference was found between the 100x IC_{50} and 4x IC_{50} or between 100x IC_{50} of both preincubated enzyme-inhibitor mixtures (data not shown). To investigate if the inhibition of activity is time-dependent, as it is known for irreversible inhibitors, we measured the postincubation time recovery in Figures 2(c) and 2(d) for *h*MAO-A and *h*MAO-B, respectively. The results obtained provide more evidence that GST is a reversible inhibitor of *h*MAO-A and *h*MAO-B up to the tested 60 min at RT and a maximum of 100x IC_{50} value.

3.2.2. Competitiveness of hMAO-A and hMAO-B Inhibition. Further investigations on the competitiveness of GST reversible inhibition on both MAOs are illustrated in Figure 3. The Michaelis-Menten kinetics for both isozymes at their predetermined initial rates of reaction are presented as Lineweaver-Burk plot (Figures 3(a) and 3(b)). The intersection of all linear regression lines at y-axis and not x-axis indicates a competitive mode of inhibition. Meanwhile, DEP linear regression crossed y-axis with hMAO-A and x-axis with MAO-B, confirming its noncompetitive *h*MAO-B mode of inhibition (data not shown). V_{max} and LDS K_m in the presence of GST were further determined and illustrated as folds of change (Figures 3(c) and 3(d)). GST showed no significant change in V_{max} values ($p = 0.10$ for *h*MAO-A and $p = 0.44$ for *h*MAO-B) while LDS K_m values increased severalfold with GST increased concentrations ($p < 0.002$ for

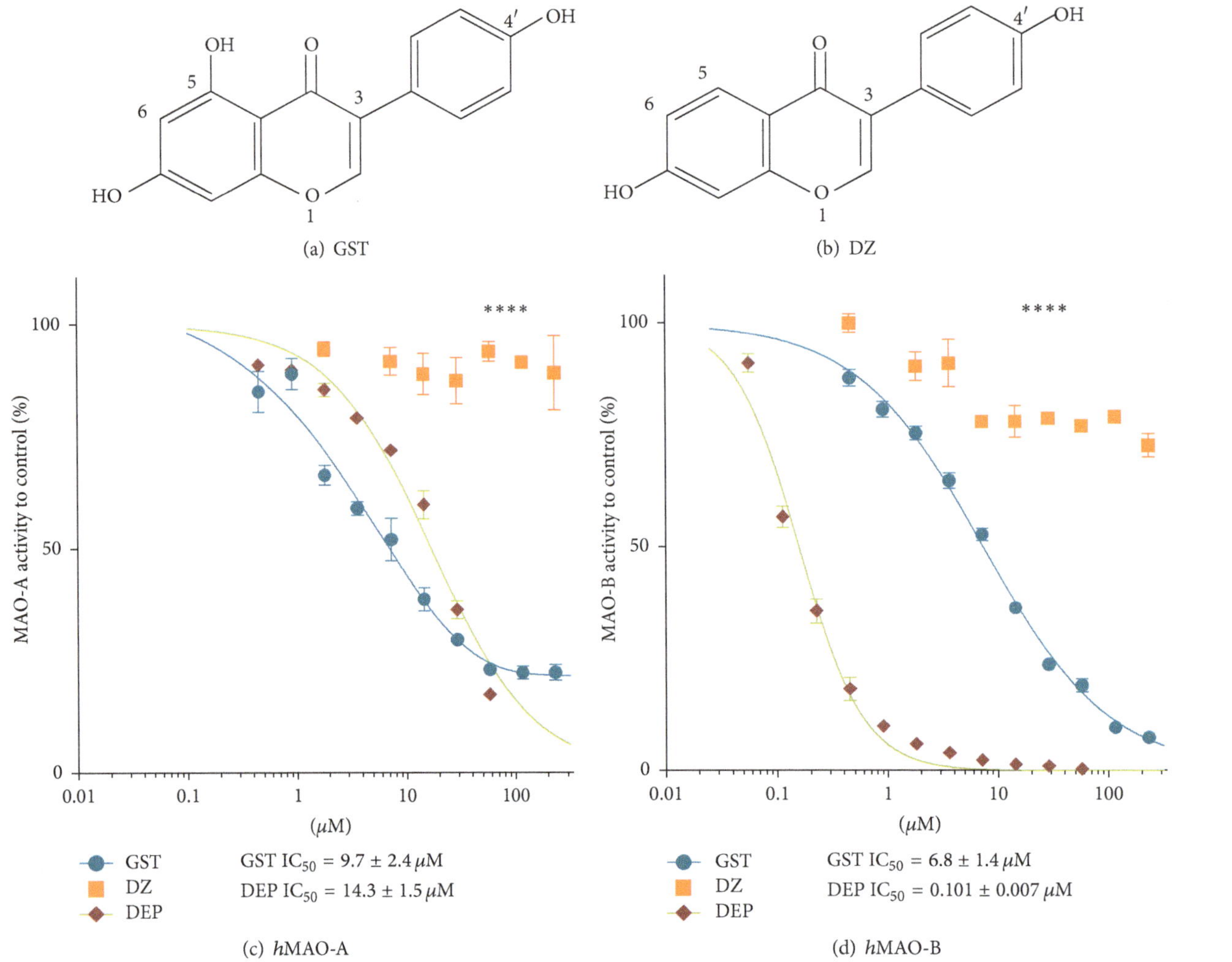

FIGURE 1: Comparison between (a) genistein (GST) and (b) daidzein (DZ) analogs inhibition of *h*MAO-A (c) and *h*MAO-B (d). Arbitrary Light Units (ALU) were measured at 25°C. Data points were presented as the mean ± SEM, $n = 3$, for two separate experiments. The significance of difference between the isoforms inhibitory effects by GST and DZ was determined using two-way ANOVA followed by Sidak's multiple comparisons test. $^{****}p < 0.0001$.

*h*MAO-A and $p < 0.0001$ for *h*MAO-B). Interestingly, GST increased LDS K_m for *h*MAO-B more significantly (14.9-fold) than LDS K_m for *h*MAO-A (8.1-fold) by more than 1.8-fold at 20 μM GST concentration.

To further assess the GST competitiveness, the alpha parameter was determined. The alpha value is used in Prism software to determine the degree at which the inhibitor can change the affinity with increasing substrate concentration. In the mixed model of inhibition analysis, alpha values were "too large" in all GST concentrations and both isozymes. The large alpha value indicates that GST reduced the substrate-binding affinity to the isozyme. The above studies exclude the noncompetitive, uncompetitive, or even mixed mode of GST inhibition to favor a competitive mode of inhibition on both MAOs.

The competitive behavior model was used for the determination of GST inhibition constant (K_i) for both isozymes by Prism (Figures 3(e) and 3(f)). GST in the competitive model of inhibition of *h*MAO-A and *h*MAO-B activities had the best-fit R^2 of 99% and 97%, respectively. GST mean *h*MAO-B K_i of 1.45 μM (Figure 3(f)) was lower than *h*MAO-A K_i of 4.31 μM (Figure 3(e)) by 3.0-fold. The lower K_i indicates lower GST concentration needed to reduce *h*MAO-B activity rate to 50%.

3.2.3. Tyramine Selective Oxidation by MAOs. Tyramine oxidation MAO assay was conducted to define RS of GST for *h*MAO-A and *h*MAO-B inhibition (Figure 4). Separate continuous *h*MAO-A and *h*MAO-B tests have shown that H_2O_2 was produced time-dependently at RT and was inhibited by DEP and CLORG standards (data not shown). After 2 h incubation, GST inhibited the H_2O_2 production by *h*MAO-B more selectively (IC_{50} 2.9 ± 0.2 μM) than of *h*MAO-A (IC_{50} 28.9 ± 0.1 μM) by about 10-fold ($p < 0.0001$) when

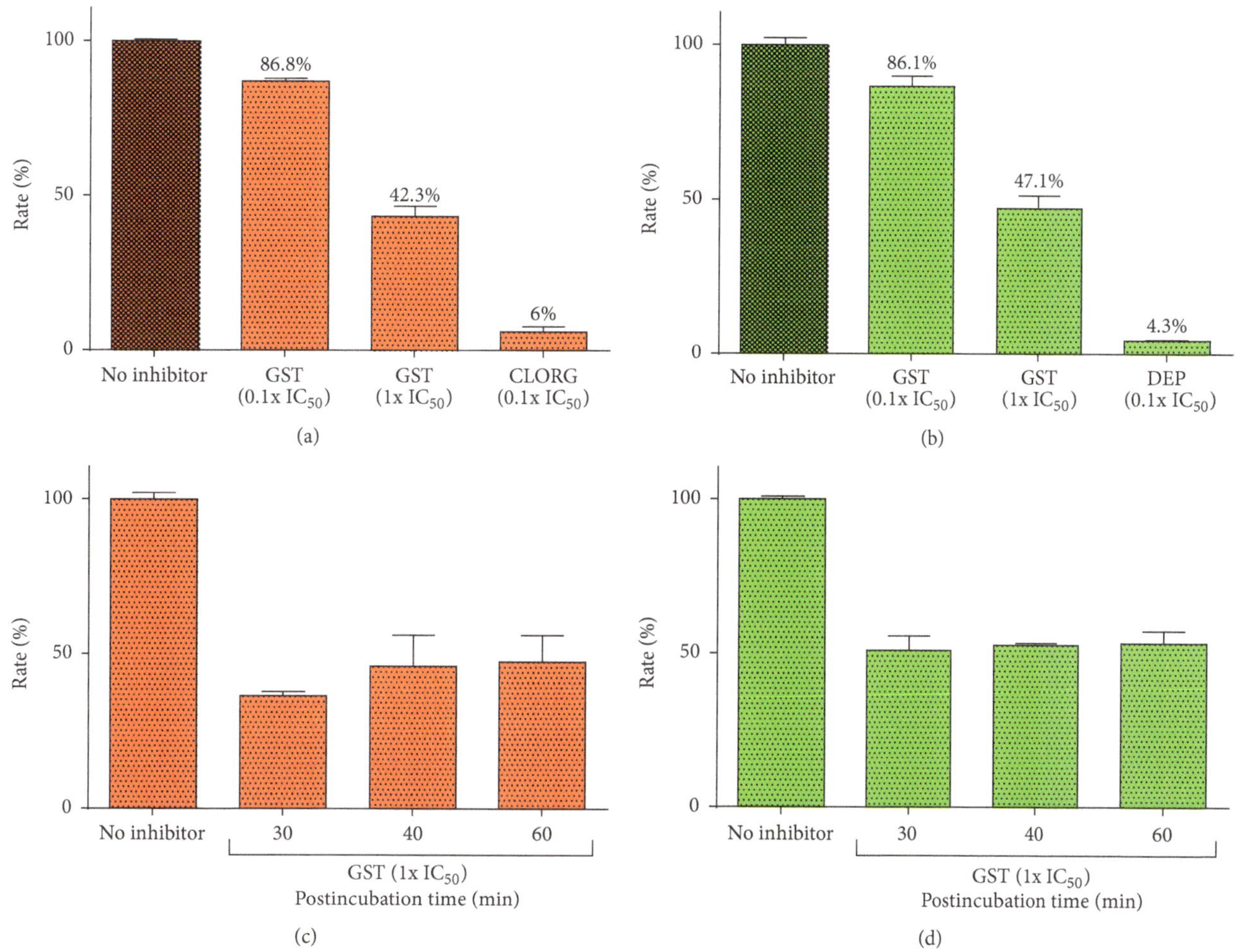

Figure 2: Recovery of the inhibition of recombinant monoamine oxidases, *h*MAO-A (a) and *h*MAO-B (b), by genistein (GST) after 40 min preincubation and GST dilution to 0.1x IC_{50} and 1x IC_{50}. The recovery of GST 1x IC_{50} is stable in *h*MAO-A (c) and *h*MAO-B (d). Clorgyline (CLORG) and deprenyl (DEP) were used as standard controls for *h*MAO-A and *h*MAO-B, respectively. The percentage of residual enzymes catalytic rates compared to their related negative control was expressed as mean ± SEM, $n = 3$. Data represent two experiments for each isozyme.

using tyramine as a substrate (Figure 4(a)). GST inhibited *h*MAO-B H_2O_2 byproduct formation more potently and time-dependently than *h*MAO-A H_2O_2 (Figures 4(b) and 4(c)).

3.3. Docking Studies. Both analogs of GST and DZ were successfully docked to the same *human* MAO-A and MAO-B crystal structure active sites at which standards of RAS, 2Z5X, and 2XCG interacted. Affinity scores and orientation predictions results are illustrated in Figure 5 and Table 1. In Figure 5, GST and DZ in MAO-A and MAO-B shared close docking poses orientations. In the *human* MAO-A model, GST and DZ within the MAO-A active site cavity in Figure 5(a)(1) and 5(a)(2) were illustrated with 2Z5X. Their chromone moieties were located in the compact entrance cavity and close to the FAD, but their hydroxy-phenyl moiety was attracted to the hydrophobic active site entrance surfaces (brown zones). Orientations of both isoflavones matched and crossed with 2Z5X standard orientation. However, a slight pull of GST toward a hydrophilic zone at its C5-OH group gave a better-matched pose to the standard without H-bonds predictions.

In the *human* MAO-B model with 2XCG (Figure 5(a)(1) and 5(a)(2)), the substrate cavity structure is illustrated with both GST and DZ isoflavones. Similarly, both analogs chromone moieties were located entirely in the hydrophobic zone of the active site cavity in the substrate-binding domain (brown zone). Both analogs were away from FAD or its surrounding tyrosine residues by having their hydroxy-phenyl moiety close to the entrance cavity. However, GST C4′-OH group moiety had more H-bonds predictions away from the hydrophobic residues than DZ. That orientation may enhance more reversibility by not affecting the FAD structure and having reversible hydrophobic and H-bond interactions.

On the other hand, the affinity of the active GST and the partially active DZ were predicted as docking scores (Table 1). The analogs were compared to RAS instead of

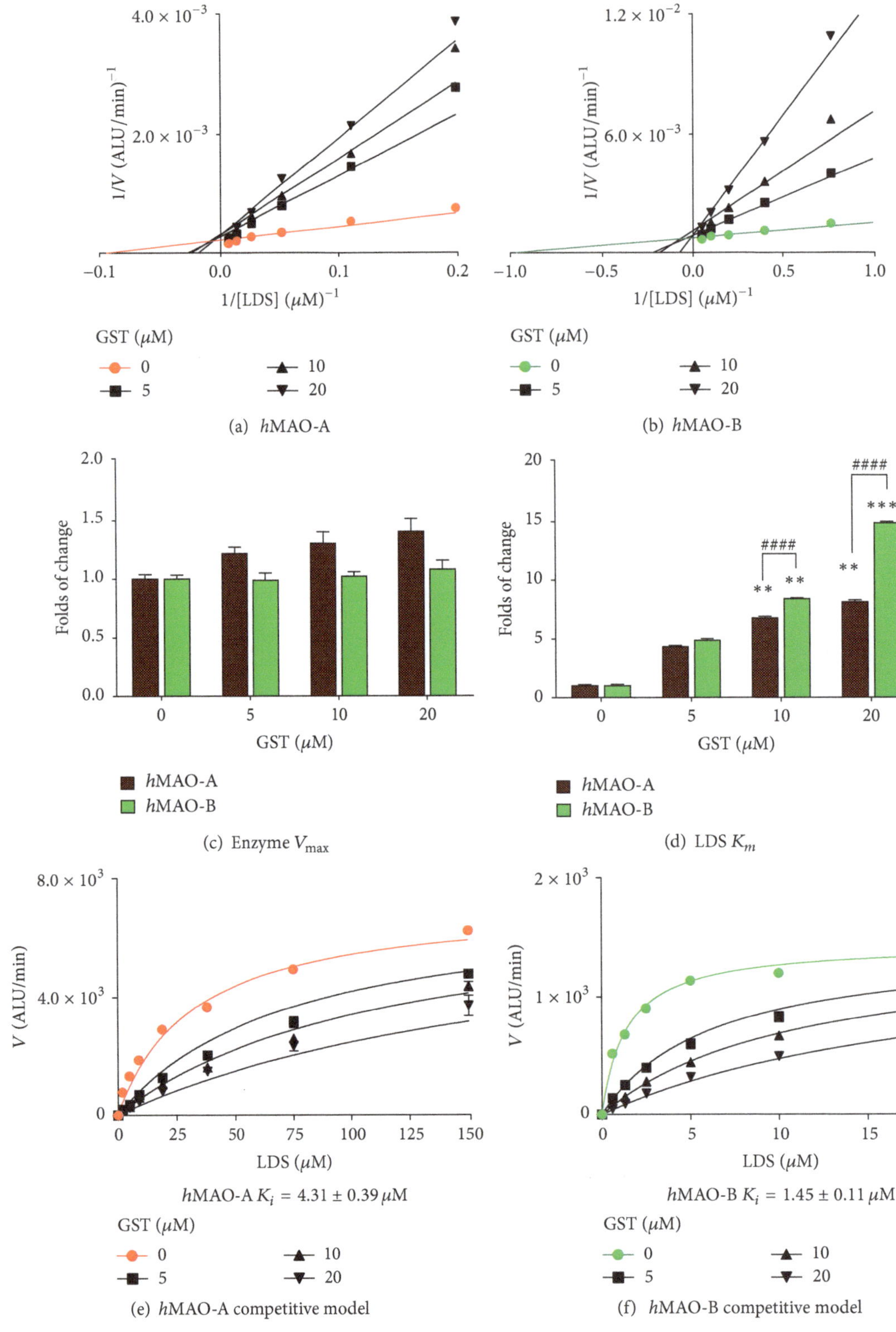

FIGURE 3: Mode of inhibition of *recombinant human* monoamine oxidases (*h*MAO-A and *h*MAO-B) by genistein (GST) compared to control the initial velocity (V). Lineweaver-Burk plots for *h*MAO-A (a) and *h*MAO-B (b) with a gradual increase of luciferin derivative substrate (LDS). Linear regression data are presented as mean ± SEM of $n = 3$. The maximum velocity (V_{max} ± SEM) (c) and Michaelis constant (K_m ± SEM) of LDS (d) parameters folds of change were measured with a gradual increase of GST concentrations in both isozymes. GST inhibitor constant (K_i) was determined using the competitive inhibition model for *h*MAO-A (e) and *h*MAO-B (f) as the best fit. Regression data are presented as the mean ± SEM of $n = 3$. The significance of difference between the controls and treatments was determined using one-way ANOVA followed by Dunnett's multiple comparisons test and between two groups of each concentration using t-test. $^{**}p < 0.01$; **** or $^{\#\#\#\#}p < 0.0001$.

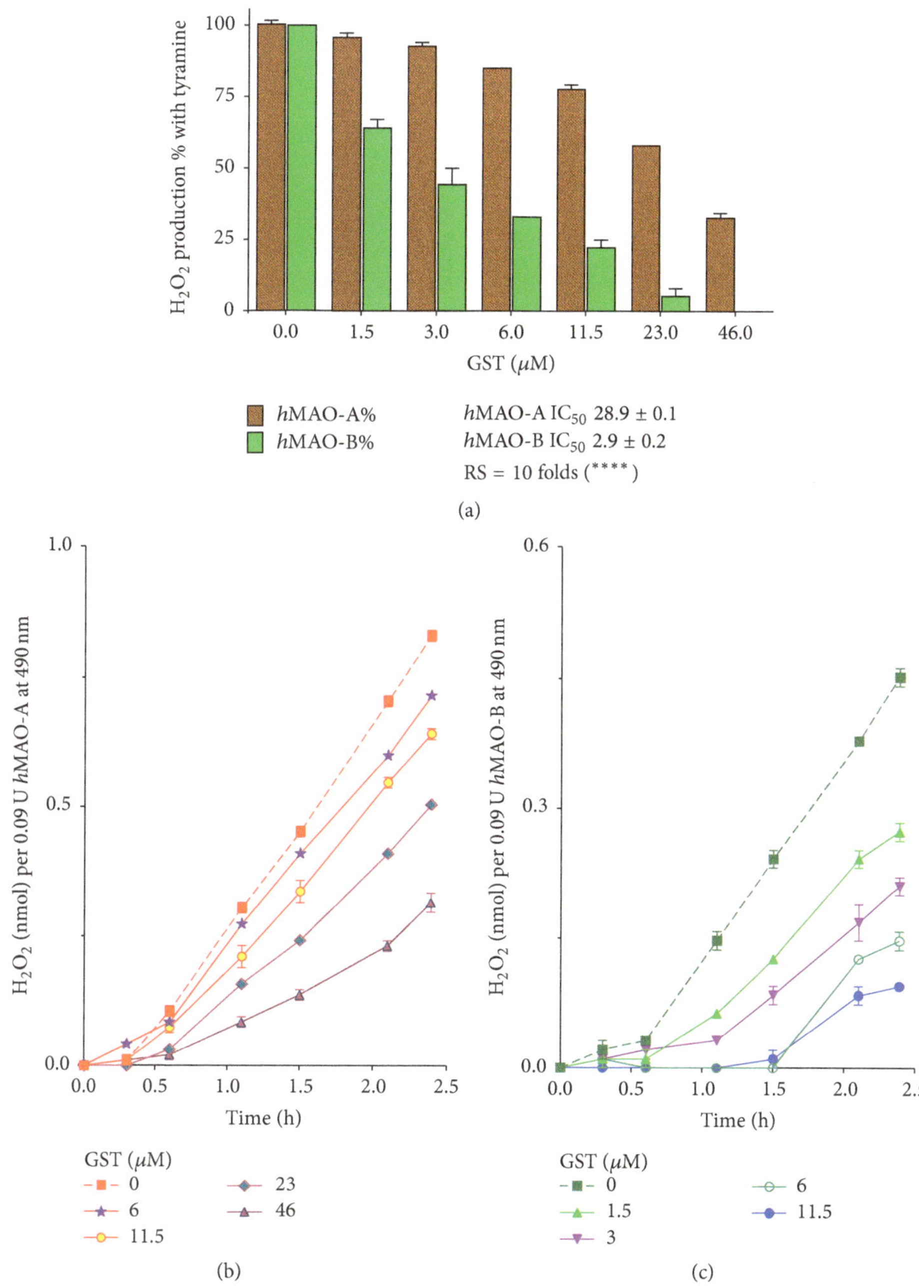

FIGURE 4: Genistein (GST) inhibited *human* monoamine oxidases (*h*MAO-A and *h*MAO-B isozymes) H_2O_2 byproduct formation differently ($^{****}p < 0.0001$) by using tyramine as a substrate (a). The enzymatic reaction was monitored in *h*MAO-A (b) and *h*MAO-B (c) without GST (dotted line) or in the presence of different GST concentrations at RT. IC_{50}s and data points were presented as the mean ± SEM, $n = 3$. RS is relative selectivity to inhibit B isozyme. The significance of difference of RS against hMAO-B was determined using unpaired t-test.

DEP because it showed H-bond interactions while DEP did not (data not shown). The affinities were similar to both isozymes including the type of H-bond interactions formed with MAO-B. The analogs' high MAO-B affinity scores (>1.8-fold MAO-A scores) were concomitants of the prediction of H-bond interactions between threonine (THR: 201: A) and analogs' oxygen donor and acceptor of C4′-OH which acted as an acceptor here. Although their interaction distances were similar (2.27 and 2.32 Å, resp.), the same oxygen in GST served as a donor and a stronger extra H-bond was predicted with threonine (1.41 Å), making the distances comparable to 2XCG. However, predicted affinities, site, and type of H-bond interactions were different with the standard ligands.

4. Discussion

The two natural isoflavone analogs GST and DZ showed a dramatic difference in their MAO inhibitory properties

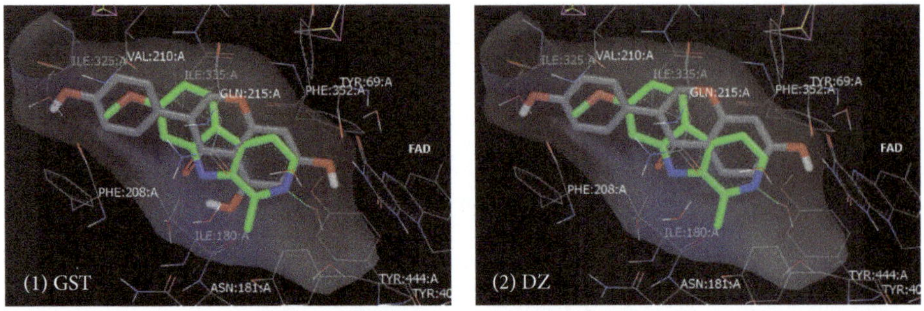

(a) *human* MOA-A (2Z5X)

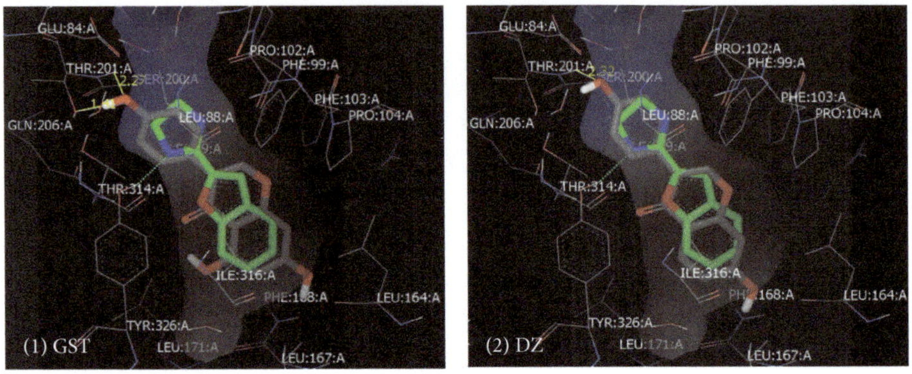

(b) *human* MOA-B (2XCG)

FIGURE 5: Predicted docking orientations of genistein (GST) and its analog daidzein (DZ) at *human* monoamine oxidase-A (MAO-A) (a) and MAO-B (b) active sites. ((a)(1)) GST and ((a)(2)) DZ with harmine (2Z5X) within MAO-A. ((b)(1)) GST and ((b)(2)) DZ with 2-(2-benzofuranyl)-2-imidazoline (2XCG) within MAO-B. Key: the hydrophobic zones are in brown color, the neutral zones are in gray, the hydrophilic zones are in blue, docked standard ligands are in green, and tested compounds are in gray.

TABLE 1: Docking scores of GST and DZ within X-ray *human* monoamine oxidase-A and -B (MAO-A and MAO-B) active sites, in comparison with MAO selective inhibitors.

Ligand[a]	MAO-A		MAO-B		Å	Type[c]	Amino acid
	Docking score[b]	H-bonds predicted	Docking score[b]	H-bonds predicted			
DZ	−6.9	0	−12.8	1	2.32	O··· HN	THR: 201: A
GST	−7.0	0	−12.8	2	2.27	OH··· N	THR: 201: A
					1.41	O··· HN	THR: 201: A
RAS	−8.8	0	−10.7	1	2.22	NH··· O	PRO: 102: A
2Z5X	−8.4	0*	−11.6	1	1.76	NH··· O	PRO: 102: A
2XCG	−12.7	0	−9.8	2	1.32	NH··· O	PRO: 102: A
					2.24	N··· HO	TYR: 326: A

[a] Ligands docked: daidzein (DZ); genistein (GST), with reported standards; rasagiline (RAS); harmine (2Z5X); 2-(2-benzofuranyl)-2-imidazoline (2XCG).
[b] HYBRID Chemgauss 4 scores.
[c] The type of H-bond between the ligand and the amino acid active site.
* H-bond formed between the ligand and the water molecule active site.

with GST being highly more potent than DZ. The chemical structure similarities of DZ to GST enabled us to explain GST MAO-A and MAO-B inhibitory actions. With using the chemical analog DZ, the structure-activity relationship between their functional groups and *h*MAO-A and *h*MAO-B inhibitions indicates that it is not the lipophilic chromone-core structure of GST and DZ causing GST MAOs inhibitory activities. Rather, the C5-OH extra group ruled the observed activity. The obtained data (Figure 1) highlights the role of C5 substitution in the isoflavones chromone-core structure on *h*MAOs inhibition. The data further suggest a crucial role of C5-OH and the threonine 201 of MAO-B in MAOs inhibitory action and selective inhibition. GST was also compared with DEP, the standard therapy for PD recently used in MDD

[6, 16]. The obtained results indicated GST higher potency than DEP to inhibit *h*MAO-A with much less *h*MAO-B selectivity. However, GST had a reversible and competitive MAO inhibition with higher affinity to MAO-B than MAO-A. That encouraged us to propose the use of GST for PD with depression.

In contrast to the irreversible inhibitors DEP and CLORG, GST allowed the recovery of both *h*MAO-A and *h*MAO-B isozymes time-independently (Figure 2). Furthermore, the Lineweaver-Burk linear regression and the severalfold increase of LDS K_m clearly indicated GST competitive mode of inhibition for both *h*MAO isoforms (Figure 3). A similar MAO mode of inhibition by other flavonoids was previously reported [29, 30]. The GST competitiveness with the substrate confirms its reversible mode of inhibition [31]. Therefore, GST *in vivo* withdrawal may easily recover both isozymes activities. Likewise, recovery of isozymes may occur with an occasional sharp increase of tyramine, DA, NE, and 5-HT, which is crucial in reducing undesirable associated adverse effects [32].

Although LDS binding affinity to *h*MAO-B is higher than *h*MAO-A [25], with GST, LDS K_m was increasing more sensitively in *h*MAO-B than *h*MAO-A (Figure 3(d)). The obtained results of *h*MAO-A GST K_i values are found to be close to our previously reported DEP K_i of 3.1 μM reported using similar conditions [30]. However, the GST K_i value in *h*MAO-A is still higher than *h*MAO-B. Those results indicate GST higher competitiveness and binding affinity to *h*MAO-B more than *h*MAO-A. In the presence of tyramine substrate (Figure 4), GST needed 10-fold of *h*MAO-B inhibitory concentrations to inhibit *h*MAO-A activity equivalently. GST *h*MAO-B inhibition selectivity is consistent with Figure 3 results and may have increased by tyramine's better affinity to *h*MAO-A than *h*MAO-B [25]. Thus, GST may allow tyramine metabolism by uninhibited *h*MAO-A without losing the capability to diminish MAO-B H_2O_2 and aldehydes cytotoxic byproducts.

To understand the molecular interactions involved in GST affinity and the C5-OH role of inhibition, we conducted a molecular docking study for both analogs. Both analogs matched the standards orientations at the isozymes entrance cavities with identical high affinity-binding predictions (Figure 5 and Table 1). The attractiveness of C5-OH to MAO-A hydrophilic zone may have contributed to GST reversible inhibition. However, the analogs' isoflavone structure may form more stable lipophilic interactions with MAO-B highly lipophilic zones than MAO-A. In addition, unlike MAO-A, MAO-B constitutes high H-bonding forming polar residues that surround the entrance cavity outer part [33]. The MAO-B acceptor and donor H-bonds may improve flavonoids affinity scores or/and inhibition [34] which may also depend on the site and strength of interaction. The formation of two acceptor and donor H-bonds between threonine and GST may have led to the complete MAO-B inhibition. Consistently in our previous report, flavonoid bavachinin was predicted to bind to threonine 201 and showed close *h*MAO-B inhibitory activity [30]. That may underline the importance of threonine contribution in flavonoid inhibitory activity. The obtained results emphasize C5-OH role in stronger H-bonds formation with threonine but eliminate its effects on increasing affinity. Thus, with the assumption that the C5-OH (the absent group in DZ) is required for GST inhibitory role, GST can bind to MAO-B better than MAO-A with the strength to impede LDS and tyramine from binding and theoretically reduce its H_2O_2 byproduct in the brain.

On the other hand, overly active and/or highly expressed MAOs contribute significantly to oxidative stress, mitochondrial toxicity, DNA damage, lipid peroxidation, and cancer [35, 36] in addition to the catalysis of neurotoxic production from MPTP [37]. Meanwhile, GST has been reported to have anti-inflammatory, antioxidant, anticancer effects [38–40] and induced the different antioxidant enzymes [41]. *In vitro*, GST had been protected against H_2O_2-induced cellular DNA damage in an aging-related prostate cancer [42] and reduced Amyloid β- and H_2O_2-induced neurotoxicity in human neuroblastoma cells [43]. Moreover, GST protected the dopaminergic neurons and enhanced Bcl-2 gene expression in the MPTP-induced PD mice model [44], which may indicate its ability to cross the blood-brain barrier and inhibit MAO-B, since its bioavailability is reasonable in human [45]. Clinically, GST oral administration improved cognitive functions and memory in males and females [46, 47].

The determination of the proper dosage in patients to achieve MAOs inhibitory concentrations of GST based on the current *in vitro* study needs more research at the basic and the clinical levels. Considerations of GST metabolism and pharmacokinetics should be taken. In a clinical investigation using oral GST to manage postmenopausal osteoporosis in women, a dose of 54 mg/day was needed to achieve a steady-state level up to 1.00 μM [48]. We believe that the required dose of GST to achieve adequate therapeutic MOA inhibition might be less than the extrapolated dose available in the literature for three reasons. Firstly, GST was reported to be metabolized to its precursor biochanin A by intracellular enzymes [49, 50]. In our laboratory, we have found that biochanin A is more potent and selective *h*MAO-BI with an IC_{50} of 0.09 μM and an *h*MAO-A IC_{50} of 3.4 μM (Zarmouh et al., data to be published). Secondly, the dose of GST can be more than 54 mg/day as reported in a clinical trial in elderly [51]. Thus, both GST and metabolites may reach their target in the brain. Thirdly, we compared the MAOI of GST to DEP that needs higher doses for MAO inhibition. DEP was first investigated as an antidepressant but was not used because of its low bioavailability and the need for high oral doses as an MAO-AI [52] (greater than GST). DEP low bioavailability is mainly due to its high first-pass metabolism to amphetamine metabolites [6]. Nonetheless, DEP was formulated for skin delivery as DEP (Emsam) and, consequently, became a well-established effective MAOI used for depression in the elderly as a transdermal patch. This route of administration allowed higher bioavailability and also fewer restrictions on diet [53]. Similarly, GST bioavailability could be improved using the transdermal patch. Therefore, clinical and pharmacokinetic parameters investigations are needed to search for the best GST preparations or route of administration to achieve effective therapeutic concentrations in the brain for MAOs inhibition.

5. Conclusions

The obtained results indicate that the isoflavone GST has potent *h*MAO-A and *h*MAO-B inhibitory activities compared to its analog DZ negligible inhibitory effects. GST MAO-A inhibition potency was more than the standard DEP. However, its affinity and potency to inhibit *h*MAO-B were higher than *h*MAO-A. GST valuable MAO inhibitory capacity over DZ and selectivity to inhibit MAO-B may be due to the presence of C5-OH substitution that may have worked as an inhibitory group. The data obtained clearly show that GST is a reversible and competitive MAO-A and MAO-B inhibitor and, consequently, can safely decrease *h*MAOs toxic H_2O_2 byproduct, with the least chance to have the cheese effect incidence. Based on the data obtained in this study we recommend further investigations to examine the use of GST as a possible agent for the therapeutic management of PD patients with depression.

Abbreviations

2-BFI:	2-(2-Benzofuranyl)-2-imidazoline
5-HT:	Serotonin
2XCG:	2-(2-Benzofuranyl)-2-imidazoline-MAO-B complex
2Z5X:	Harmine-MAO-A complex
AD:	Alzheimer's disease
ALU:	Arbitrary Light Units
CLORG:	Clorgyline
DA:	Dopamine
DEP:	(R)-(−)-Deprenyl HCl
DZ:	Daidzein
FAD:	Flavin adenine dinucleotide
GST:	Genistein
H_2O_2:	Hydrogen peroxide
HBSS:	Hank's Balanced Salt Solution
*h*MAO:	*Recombinant human* MAO
*h*MAO-AIs:	*Recombinant human* MAO-A inhibitors
*h*MAO-BIs:	*Recombinant human* MAO-B inhibitors
K_i:	Inhibitor constant
K_m:	Michaelis constant
LDS:	Luciferin derivative substrate
MDD:	Major depressive disorder
MAO:	Monoamine oxidase
MAOIs:	MAO inhibitors
MPTP:	1-Methyl-4-phenyl-1,2,3,6-tetrahydropyridine
NE:	Norepinephrine
PD:	Parkinson's disease
PDB:	Protein Data Bank pdf
RAS:	Rasagiline
RLDR:	Reporter luciferin detection reagent
RS:	Relative selectivity
V_{max}:	Maximum velocity.

Competing Interests

The authors declare that there are no competing interests regarding the publication of this paper.

Acknowledgments

This work was supported by NIH grants from NIMHD [G12 MD007582] and P20 [MD006738]. The authors acknowledge the financial support provided to the first author Najla O. Zarmouh by the National Board for Technical and Vocational Education, Misrata, Libya. The authors are also thankful to Open Eye Scientific Software, Inc. (Santa Fe, NM), for the free academic licensing of the software tools. Also, the authors recognize Dr. Suresh V. K. Eyunni for assisting in performing the molecular docking studies and Dr. David M. Bauer for proofreading the paper.

References

[1] A. Storch, G. Ebersbach, G. Fuchs et al., "Depression in Parkinson's disease—part 1: epidemiology, signs and symptoms, pathophysiology and diagnosis," *Fortschritte der Neurologie Psychiatrie*, vol. 76, no. 12, pp. 715–724, 2008.

[2] L. Chiuccariello, S. Houle, L. Miler et al., "Elevated monoamine oxidase A binding during major depressive episodes is associated with greater severity and reversed neurovegetative symptoms," *Neuropsychopharmacology*, vol. 39, no. 4, pp. 973–980, 2014.

[3] J.-P. Azulay, F. Durif, R. Rogez, C. Tranchant, I. Bourdeix, and K. Rerat, "Precoce survey: a new self-assessment patient card for early detection and management of Parkinson disease fluctuations," *Revue Neurologique*, vol. 164, no. 4, pp. 354–362, 2008.

[4] J. K. Mallajosyula, D. Kaur, S. J. Chinta et al., "MAO-B elevation in mouse brain astrocytes results in Parkinson's pathology," *PLoS ONE*, vol. 3, no. 2, Article ID e1616, 2008.

[5] S. Johnson, C. A. Stockmeier, J. H. Meyer et al., "The reduction of R1, a novel repressor protein for monoamine oxidase a, in major depressive disorder," *Neuropsychopharmacology*, vol. 36, no. 10, pp. 2139–2148, 2011.

[6] G. M. Asnis and M. A. Henderson, "EMSAM (deprenyl patch): how a promising antidepressant was underutilized," *Neuropsychiatric Disease and Treatment*, vol. 10, pp. 1911–1923, 2014.

[7] A. W. Bach, N. C. Lan, D. L. Johnson et al., "cDNA cloning of human liver monoamine oxidase A and B: molecular basis of differences in enzymatic properties," *Proceedings of the National Academy of Sciences of the United States of America*, vol. 85, no. 13, pp. 4934–4938, 1988.

[8] U. Bonnet, "Moclobemide: therapeutic use and clinical studies," *CNS Drug Reviews*, vol. 9, no. 1, pp. 97–140, 2003.

[9] T. Thomas, "Monoamine oxidase-B inhibitors in the treatment of Alzheimers disease," *Neurobiology of Aging*, vol. 21, no. 2, pp. 343–348, 2000.

[10] P. Riederer, W. Danielczyk, and E. Grünblatt, "Monoamine oxidase-B inhibition in alzheimer's disease," *NeuroToxicology*, vol. 25, no. 1-2, pp. 271–277, 2004.

[11] K. N. Westlund, R. M. Denney, R. M. Rose, and C. W. Abell, "Localization of distinct monoamine oxidase A and monoamine oxidase B cell populations in human brainstem," *Neuroscience*, vol. 25, no. 2, pp. 439–456, 1988.

[12] A. Sturza, M. S. Leisegang, A. Babelova et al., "Monoamine oxidases are mediators of endothelial dysfunction in the mouse aorta," *Hypertension*, vol. 62, no. 1, pp. 140–146, 2013.

[13] L. Barros-Miñones, B. Goñi-Allo, V. Suquia, G. Beitia, N. Aguirre, and E. Puerta, "Contribution of dopamine to mitochondrial complex I inhibition and dopaminergic deficits caused by

methylenedioxymethamphetamine in mice," *Neuropharmacology*, vol. 93, pp. 124–133, 2015.

[14] M. Gerlach, P. Riederer, and M. B. H. Youdim, "The molecular pharmacology of L-deprenyl," *European Journal of Pharmacology*, vol. 226, no. 2, pp. 97–108, 1992.

[15] P. Vezina, E. Mohr, and D. Grimes, "Deprenyl in Parkinson's disease: mechanisms, neuroprotective effect, indications and adverse effects," *Canadian Journal of Neurological Sciences*, vol. 19, no. 1, supplement, pp. 142–146, 1992.

[16] M. B. H. Youdim and Y. S. Bakhle, "Monoamine oxidase: isoforms and inhibitors in Parkinson's disease and depressive illness," *British Journal of Pharmacology*, vol. 147, supplement 1, pp. S287–S296, 2006.

[17] S. Kumar and A. K. Pandey, "Chemistry and biological activities of flavonoids: an overview," *The Scientific World Journal*, vol. 2013, Article ID 162750, 16 pages, 2013.

[18] N. Yanagihara, H. Zhang, Y. Toyohira et al., "New insights into the pharmacological potential of plant flavonoids in the catecholamine system," *Journal of Pharmacological Sciences*, vol. 124, no. 2, pp. 123–128, 2014.

[19] X. H. Han, S. S. Hong, J. S. Hwang, M. K. Lee, B. Y. Hwang, and J. S. Ro, "Monoamine oxidase inhibitory components from Cayratia japonica," *Archives of Pharmacal Research*, vol. 30, no. 1, pp. 13–17, 2007.

[20] L. D. Kong, R. X. Tan, A. Y. H. Woo, and C. H. K. Cheng, "Inhibition of rat brain monoamine oxidase activities by psoralen and isopsoralen: implications for the treatment of affective disorders," *Pharmacology and Toxicology*, vol. 88, no. 2, pp. 75–80, 2001.

[21] L. Xu, B. Du, and B. Xu, "A systematic, comparative study on the beneficial health components and antioxidant activities of commercially fermented soy products marketed in China," *Food Chemistry*, vol. 174, pp. 202–213, 2015.

[22] N. L. Booth, C. R. Overk, P. Yao et al., "The chemical and biologic profile of a red clover (*Trifolium pratense* L.) phase II clinical extract," *Journal of Alternative and Complementary Medicine*, vol. 12, no. 2, pp. 133–139, 2006.

[23] W. M. Keung, "Biogenic aldehyde(s) derived from the action of monoamine oxidase may mediate the antidipsotropic effect of daidzin," *Chemico-Biological Interactions*, vol. 130-132, pp. 919–930, 2001.

[24] T. Hatano, T. Fukuda, T. Miyase, T. Noro, and T. Okuda, "Phenolic constituents of licorice. III. Structures of glicoricone and licofuranone, and inhibitory effects of licorice constituents of monoamine oxidase," *Chemical and Pharmaceutical Bulletin*, vol. 39, no. 5, pp. 1238–1243, 1991.

[25] M. P. Valley, W. Zhou, E. M. Hawkins et al., "A bioluminescent assay for monoamine oxidase activity," *Analytical Biochemistry*, vol. 359, no. 2, pp. 238–246, 2006.

[26] L. J. Legoabe, A. Petzer, and J. P. Petzer, "Selected C7-substituted chromone derivatives as monoamine oxidase inhibitors," *Bioorganic Chemistry*, vol. 45, pp. 1–11, 2012.

[27] A. Holt, D. F. Sharman, G. B. Baker, and M. M. Palcic, "A continuous spectrophotometric assay for monoamine oxidase and related enzymes in tissue homogenates," *Analytical Biochemistry*, vol. 244, no. 2, pp. 384–392, 1997.

[28] P. C. D. Hawkins, A. G. Skillman, G. L. Warren, B. A. Ellingson, and M. T. Stahl, "Conformer generation with OMEGA: algorithm and validation using high quality structures from the protein databank and cambridge structural database," *Journal of Chemical Information and Modeling*, vol. 50, no. 4, pp. 572–584, 2010.

[29] N. D. Chaurasiya, M. A. Ibrahim, I. Muhammad, L. A. Walker, and B. L. Tekwani, "Monoamine oxidase inhibitory constituents of propolis: kinetics and mechanism of inhibition of recombinant human MAO-A and MAO-B," *Molecules*, vol. 19, no. 11, pp. 18936–18952, 2014.

[30] N. O. Zarmouh, E. A. Mazzio, F. M. Elshami, S. S. Messeha, S. V. Eyunni, and K. F. Soliman, "Evaluation of the inhibitory effects of bavachinin and bavachin on human monoamine oxidases A and B," *Evidence-Based Complementary and Alternative Medicine*, vol. 2015, Article ID 852194, 14 pages, 2015.

[31] L. H. A. Prins, J. P. Petzer, and S. F. Malan, "Inhibition of monoamine oxidase by indole and benzofuran derivatives," *European Journal of Medicinal Chemistry*, vol. 45, no. 10, pp. 4458–4466, 2010.

[32] M. C. Anderson, F. Hasan, J. M. McCrodden, and K. F. Tipton, "Monoamine oxidase inhibitors and the cheese effect," *Neurochemical Research*, vol. 18, no. 11, pp. 1145–1149, 1993.

[33] L. Novaroli, A. Daina, E. Favre et al., "Impact of species-dependent differences on screening, design, and development of MAO B inhibitors," *Journal of Medicinal Chemistry*, vol. 49, no. 21, pp. 6264–6272, 2006.

[34] S. Vilar, G. Ferino, E. Quezada, L. Santana, and C. Friedman, "Predicting monoamine oxidase inhibitory activity through ligand-based models," *Current Topics in Medicinal Chemistry*, vol. 12, no. 20, pp. 2258–2274, 2012.

[35] J. B. Wu, C. Shao, X. Li et al., "Monoamine oxidase A mediates prostate tumorigenesis and cancer metastasis," *Journal of Clinical Investigation*, vol. 124, no. 7, pp. 2891–2908, 2014.

[36] N. Kaludercic, J. Mialet-Perez, N. Paolocci, A. Parini, and F. Di Lisa, "Monoamine oxidases as sources of oxidants in the heart," *Journal of Molecular and Cellular Cardiology*, vol. 73, pp. 34–42, 2014.

[37] V. Perez and M. Unzeta, "PF 9601N [N-(2-propynyl)-2-(5-benzyloxy-indolyl) methylamine], a new MAO-B inhibitor, attenuates MPTP-induced depletion of striatal dopamine levels in C57/BL6 mice," *Neurochemistry International*, vol. 42, no. 3, pp. 221–229, 2003.

[38] Y. Li, D. Kong, A. Ahmad, B. Bao, and F. H. Sarkar, "Antioxidant function of isoflavone and 3,3/-diindolylmethane: are they important for cancer prevention and therapy?" *Antioxidants and Redox Signaling*, vol. 19, no. 2, pp. 139–150, 2013.

[39] H. Wei, R. Bowen, X. Zhang, and M. Lebwohl, "Isoflavone genistein inhibits the initiation and promotion of two-stage skin carcinogenesis in mice," *Carcinogenesis*, vol. 19, no. 8, pp. 1509–1514, 1998.

[40] D. Giles and H. Wei, "Effect of structurally related flavones/isoflavones on hydrogen peroxide production and oxidative DNA damage in phorbol ester-stimulated HL-60 cells," *Nutrition and Cancer*, vol. 29, no. 1, pp. 77–82, 1997.

[41] Q. Cai and H. Wei, "Effect of dietary genistein on antioxidant enzyme activities in SENCAR mice," *Nutrition and Cancer*, vol. 25, no. 1, pp. 1–7, 1996.

[42] M. Raschke, I. R. Rowland, P. J. Magee, and B. L. Pool-Zobel, "Genistein protects prostate cells against hydrogen peroxide-induced DNA damage and induces expression of genes involved in the defence against oxidative stress," *Carcinogenesis*, vol. 27, no. 11, pp. 2322–2330, 2006.

[43] O. Y. Bang, H. S. Hong, D. H. Kim et al., "Neuroprotective effect of genistein against beta amyloid-induced neurotoxicity," *Neurobiology of Disease*, vol. 16, no. 1, pp. 21–28, 2004.

[44] L.-X. Liu, W.-F. Chen, J.-X. Xie, and M.-S. Wong, "Neuroprotective effects of genistein on dopaminergic neurons in the mice

model of Parkinson's disease," *Neuroscience Research*, vol. 60, no. 2, pp. 156–161, 2008.

[45] Y. Chang and R. Choue, "Plasma pharmacokinetics and urinary excretion of isoflavones after ingestion of soy products with different aglycone/glucoside ratios in South Korean women," *Nutrition Research and Practice*, vol. 7, no. 5, pp. 393–399, 2013.

[46] L. R. Fournier, T. A. Ryan-Borchers, L. M. Robison et al., "The effects of soy milk and isoflavone supplements on cognitive performance in healthy, postmenopausal women," *Journal of Nutrition, Health and Aging*, vol. 11, no. 2, pp. 155–164, 2007.

[47] A. A. Thorp, N. Sinn, J. D. Buckley, A. M. Coates, and P. R. C. Howe, "Soya isoflavone supplementation enhances spatial working memory in men," *British Journal of Nutrition*, vol. 102, no. 9, pp. 1348–1354, 2009.

[48] H. Marini, A. Bitto, D. Altavilla et al., "Breast safety and efficacy of genistein aglycone for postmenopausal bone loss: a follow-up study," *Journal of Clinical Endocrinology and Metabolism*, vol. 93, no. 12, pp. 4787–4796, 2008.

[49] M. Hu, K. Krausz, J. Chen et al., "Identification of CYP1A2 as the main isoform for the phase I hydroxylated metabolism of genistein and a prodrug converting enzyme of methylated isoflavones," *Drug Metabolism and Disposition*, vol. 31, no. 7, pp. 924–931, 2003.

[50] S. Yoshihara, "A memoir of my researches on xenobiotic metabolism for 48 years—researches on Kanemi Yusho and endocrine disrupting chemicals," *Yakugaku Zasshi*, vol. 133, no. 7, pp. 747–772, 2013.

[51] E. Messing, J. R. Gee, D. R. Saltzstein et al., "A phase 2 cancer chemoprevention biomarker trial of isoflavone G-2535 (genistein) in presurgical bladder cancer patients," *Cancer Prevention Research*, vol. 5, no. 4, pp. 621–630, 2012.

[52] M.-S. Song, D. Matveychuk, E. M. MacKenzie, M. Duchcherer, D. D. Mousseau, and G. B. Baker, "An update on amine oxidase inhibitors: multifaceted drugs," *Progress in Neuro-Psychopharmacology and Biological Psychiatry*, vol. 44, pp. 118–124, 2013.

[53] A. A. Patkar, C.-U. Pae, and M. Zarzar, "Transdermal selegiline," *Drugs of Today*, vol. 43, no. 6, pp. 361–377, 2007.

12

Acute and Subchronic Oral Toxicity Evaluation of Aqueous Root Extract of *Dicoma anomala* Sond. in Wistar Rats

Fatai Oladunni Balogun and Anofi Omotayo Tom Ashafa

Phytomedicine and Phytopharmacology Research Group, Department of Plant Sciences, University of the Free State, Qwaqwa Campus, Private Bag X13, Phuthaditjhaba, Free State 9866, South Africa

Correspondence should be addressed to Anofi Omotayo Tom Ashafa; ashafaaot@ufs.ac.za

Academic Editor: Jose M. Prieto

The present study evaluated the safety of aqueous root extract of *Dicoma anomala* (AQRED) through acute and subchronic toxicity studies. Single oral dose of AQRED at the concentration of 0, 5, 300, and 2000 mg/kg as well as 125, 250, and 500 mg/kg/day was administered to rats for 14-day acute and 90-day subchronic oral toxicity studies. The results revealed no mortalities or observed clinical signs of toxicity in all the rats during both investigation periods. In subchronic toxicity testing, administration of AQRED also did not cause any changes in body weight as well as food and water consumption patterns. The haematological parameters and blood chemistry revealed no significant difference ($p > 0.05$) between the treatment and the control except in platelet count, alkaline phosphatase, and sodium levels where there was a significant increase ($p < 0.05$), although there was also a significant reduction ($p < 0.05$) in alanine transaminase, aspartate transaminase, and creatinine when compared to control. However, these changes were not reflecting the results from histology. Conclusively, the obtained results suggested that the LD_{50} of AQRED is in excess of 2000 mg/kg and its oral administration for 90 days revealed that it is unlikely to be toxic, hence, safe.

1. Introduction

Dicoma anomala belongs to the family of Asteraceae and is locally called Hloenya (South Sotho) or fever or stomach bush (Afr.). This herbaceous plant which grows in grasslands or stony places has erected stems, thinly covered with hairs, and originates from a woody rootstock. The leaves are simple, alternate, stalkless, linear, or narrowly lanceolate. The flower heads are terminal, solitary or in small pairs, narrow, with sharply pointed bracts and slender, with white, mauve, purple, or pink tubular florets [1]. *D. anomala* is widely distributed in sub-Saharan Africa including most provinces such as Limpopo, North West, Gauteng, Mpumalanga, Free State, Northern Cape, and KwaZulu-Natal within South Africa [1]. The plant is traditionally used for the treatment of cold and coughs, fever, ulcers, and dermatosis mostly among the Basotho tribe of eastern Free State. A number of documented pharmacological potentials such as antiplasmodial, antibacterial, anthelmintic, antiviral, and anti-inflammatory have been reported [2]. However, despite the various pharmacological efficacies in relation to numerous health-related benefit of the plant, it is noteworthy not to rule out issues of safety. Moreover, based on documented reports, continuous intake of high dose of medicinal plants and/or associated chemical compounds could alter hepatic and thyroid function adversely [3–6] and to date the potential toxicities of *Dicoma anomala* have not gotten enough attentions when taken in increased concentration despite the recently reported antioxidant activity of this plant by our research group. In this study, we evaluated the toxicity of the aqueous root extract with the dietary administration to male and female Wistar rats for acute 14 days and subchronic 90 days as parts of a safety assessment according to the internationally acceptable guidelines. We also subjected the extract to gas chromatography/mass spectrophotometric (GC/MS) analysis for possible identification of the phytoconstituents present in the plant.

2. Materials and Methods

2.1. Plant Collection and Extraction. Fresh root stocks of *D. anomala* were procured in April 2014 from Setsing market, Phuthaditjhaba, Qwaqwa, Free State province, South Africa. The sample was confirmed by Dr. AOT Ashafa of Plant Sciences Department, University of the Free State, Qwaqwa Campus, Free State, and a voucher specimen with (BalMed/01/2015/QHB) was thereafter prepared and deposited at the Department of Plant Sciences herbarium. A total of 5.2 kg of the root sample was cut into smaller pieces, oven-dried (40°C) for 96 hr, and pulverized using a Waring Commercial blender (USA) to yield 3.063 kg fine powder. Approximately, 600 g of the powdered root material was extracted with 5 L of distilled water on a platform shaker for 5 days. The resulting mixture was centrifuged at 1285 g for 5 min using a BHG Roto-Uni II centrifuge and afterwards filtered using Whatman number 1 filter paper. The filtrates obtained were pooled together and concentrated to dryness on a water bath (Memmert W600, Schwabach, Germany) at 40°C. The extraction yielded 137.27 g of brown gum (22.88% w/w of dry plant material) crude extract. The crude extract was reconstituted in water to afford various concentrations used in this study.

2.2. Experimental Animals. A total of one hundred (both sexes) 5-week-old Wistar rats were purchased from animal facility of University of the Free State, Bloemfontein, and were used after a week of acclimatization. Individual body weights were recorded and detailed physical examinations were performed twice during the acclimation period to ensure the use of healthy animals. Animals were housed in clean metabolic cages placed in a ventilated house and allowed free access to commercial laboratory feed (Epol rat cubes, South Africa) and tap water *ad libitum*. Animals were subjected to housing condition of the controlled system of the light-dark cycle (12-12 h), ventilation (air-exchange rate of 18 times per hour), temperature (23 ± 2°C), and relative humidity (55 ± 5%) during the study. The cages and the chip bedding were exchanged twice weekly and feed intake and water consumption, on a daily basis (by measuring the left-over feed/water and subtracting it from the initial weight or volume) and body weight measurement was taken on a weekly basis. Ethical approval for use of animals was obtained from Interfaculty Ethics Committee of the University of the Free State (NR/02/13) prior to the commencement of the study and the study was performed in accordance with the stipulation for the care and use of laboratory animals, prepared by National Institute of Health, USA (Guide for the Care and Use of Laboratory Animals, 1996).

2.3. Acute Oral Toxicity Study of Aqueous Root Extract of D. anomala (AQRED). The single dose acute oral toxicity study was evaluated following the recommendations by The Organisation for Economic Co-operation and Development (OECD, 2001) [7]. Animals (female rats) were randomly divided into four groups of 5 animals. After overnight fasting (i.e., withdrawal of feeds only and not water for about 12–15 h), they were administered a single oral dose of 0, 5, 300, and 2000 mg/kg body weight AQRED by oral gavage. Distilled water was administered to the control group. Feeding was commenced 4 h after the administration and all animals were observed for clinical signs including mortality and moribundity immediately at 1, 2, 4, 8, and 12 h and then twice daily until day 14. Body weights, food consumption, and water intake were measured on days 0, 1, 5, 10, and 14. On the 14th day, all animals were sacrificed and all organs and tissues were observed macroscopically. The organs were fixed in 10% neutral buffered formalin and observed for histopathological examination.

2.4. Subchronic 90-Day Oral Toxicity Study of AQRED

2.4.1. Experimental Design. The subchronic 90-day oral toxicity study was evaluated following the recommendations by OECD (1998) [8]. Four groups of ten (10) male and female Wistar rats received doses of 0, 125, 250, and 500 mg/kg body weight (BW) of AQRED at daily gavage of 1 mL/100 g (BW) for 90 consecutive days. Observations were made twice daily for mortality and changes in general appearance or behaviour. The body weights were recorded every week and the individual dose administered to the animals was adjusted weekly for the body weight to maintain the target dose level for all rats. Additionally, detailed clinical examination and measurement of food and water consumption were made daily.

2.4.2. Blood Preparation and Organ Isolation. The animals were anaesthetized with halothane at the end of the experimental period (i.e., day 90 of treatment) and blood was collected by clearing the neck region of fur to locate the jugular vein. An aliquot (2 mL) of the blood was collected into ethylene diamine tetra-acetic acid (EDTA) bottle and was used for the analysis of haematological parameters, while another 5 mL of the blood collected in nonheparinized bottle was centrifuged at 1285 g for 10 minutes; the resulting serum was aspirated and used for other serum bioassays. The animals were quickly dissected and the liver, kidney, heart, lungs, spleen, stomach, testes, ovary, brain, and pancreas were excised, freed of fat, blotted with clean tissue paper, and weighed for evaluation of organ-to-body weight ratios. Defined samples of the liver, brain, pancreas, kidney, and testes were placed in 10% neutral buffered formalin for histopathological examination. All organs were visually inspected and weighed directly after dissection to reduce mechanical damage.

2.4.3. Hematology and Blood Chemistry. One blood sample (approximately 20 μL) was treated with EDTA-2K for white blood cells (WBC), red blood cells (RBC), haemoglobin (Hb), platelets (PLT), percent of lymphocytes (LY), percent of monocytes (MO), haematocrit (HCT), mean corpuscular haemoglobin (MCH), mean corpuscular haemoglobin concentration (MCHC), mean corpuscular volume (MCV), mean platelet volume (MPV), platelet haematocrit (PCT), platelet distribution width (PDW), and red blood cell distribution width (RDW) using a hematology analyzer MEK-6318K (Nihon Kohden Co., Ltd.). Serum from blood samples

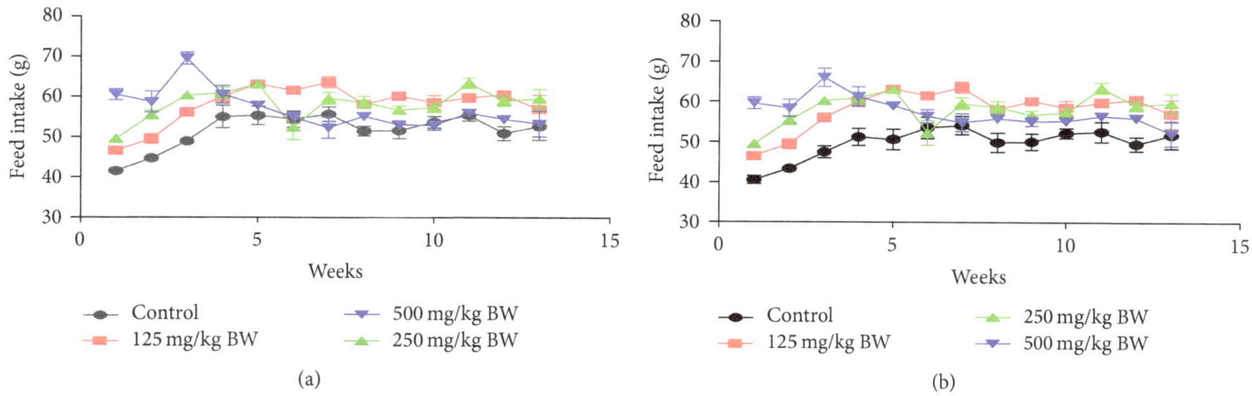

FIGURE 1: Effect of aqueous root extract of *Dicoma anomala* on food consumption for male and female Wistar rats during a 90-day subchronic toxicity study. Values were calculated and data expressed as mean ± (standard error of mean) SEM [BW: body weight].

collected in separator tubes were measured using a BS-200 automatic biochemistry analyzer (Mindray Co., Ltd.) including aspartate aminotransferase (AST), alanine aminotransferase (ALT), urea, nitrogen, creatinine (Cr), total cholesterol (TC), triglyceride (TG), total protein (TP), albumin (Alb), and glucose (Glu). Total calcium (TCa) was measured using the 7020 automatic biochemistry analyzer (Hitachi Co., Ltd.) as well as sodium (Na), potassium (K), and chloride (Cl).

2.4.4. Histopathological Studies. Pieces of vital organs from each group were fixed immediately in 10% neutral formalin for a period of at least 24 h, dehydrated in graded (50–100%) alcohol, cleaned with xylene, embedded in paraffin, cut into 4-5 μm thick sections, and stained with hematoxylin-eosin. The microscopic features of the organs of male and female rats were compared with that of the control group.

2.4.5. Statistical Analysis. Statistical analysis was performed using GraphPad Prism 5 statistical package (GraphPad Software, San Diego, CA, USA). Data were expressed as means of ten replicates ± standard error of mean (SEM) for all assays and were subjected to one-way analysis of variance (ANOVA) followed by Dunnett's multiple comparison test. Statistical significance was considered at $p < 0.05$.

2.5. Gas Chromatography/Mass Spectrophotometric Analysis. The GC/MS analysis of the extract was performed on a QP-2010 system (Shimadzu, Japan) via electron ionization (EI) at 70 eV. GC separation was achieved on a capillary column (0.25 mm i.d × 30 m, film 0.5 mm) of HP-5MS (Hewlett Packard, USA). The injection of the extract (1 mL) was done using the splitless injection method. The initial column temperature was 50°C, then went up to 250°C at a rate of 10°C/min, and finally held at 250°C for 5 min. The injection port was set at 120°C. Helium gas was used as the carrier at a flow rate of 0.6 mL/min [9]. The mass spectra of the constituents were compared with known spectra stored in Wiley library.

3. Results

3.1. Single Dose Subacute Oral Toxicity Study of AQRED in Wistar Rats. No deaths occurred during the 14-day study. There were no significant differences in body weights and food consumption of rats between the AQRED administrated group and the controls (data not shown). A short time of sluggish movement appeared in some AQRED treated rats immediately after oral gavage at 2000 mg/kg body weight concentration in the first hour, but the rats continued to live afterwards. Aside from this observation, there were no abnormal findings of other clinical signs and autopsy performed in all the experimental and control animals. It was based on these findings that the LD_{50} value of AQRED was assumed to be greater than 2000 mg/kg since no mortality or signs of toxicity were observed in all experimental animals.

3.2. Subchronic 90-Day Oral Toxicity Study of AQRED in Wistar Rats

3.2.1. Clinical Signs and Mortality. There was no mortality attributed to any effect of AQRED during the 90-day administration. Similarly, there was no treatment-related change at the autopsy in the AQRED groups or control group.

3.2.2. Feed and Water Intake. The effect of aqueous root extract of *Dicoma anomala* on feed intake is shown in Figures 1(a) and 1(b). From the results, it was observed that, during the 90-day study, there were no significant differences ($p > 0.05$) in mean food consumption among all the experimental animals. There seems to be an increase in feed intake as the experimental days increased.

The result of the effect of aqueous extract of *Dicoma anomala* on water intake (Figures 2(a) and 2(b)) revealed no significant difference ($p > 0.05$) in water intake during the 13-week study for both sexes of the animals.

3.2.3. Organ Weights. The results of relative organ weight of the animals are shown in Tables 1 and 2. It was observed that

TABLE 1: Effect of oral administration of aqueous extract of *Dicoma anomala* for 90 days on relative organ-to-body weight ratio of male Wistar rats.

Organ	Dose (mg/kg/day)			
	Control	125	250	500
Initial weight[a]	122.60 ± 2.55	123.00 ± 2.94	117.60 ± 4.09	106.60 ± 5.17
Body weight[a]	234.50 ± 6.92	394.20 ± 17.77*	371.10 ± 15.08*	342.60 ± 4.70*
% weight change	91.27	220.48	215.56	221.39
Liver[a]	5.27 ± 0.19	9.63 ± 0.95	10.22 ± 0.23	8.22 ± 0.39
Brain[a]	1.23 ± 0.05	1.35 ± 0.05	1.28 ± 0.22	3.17 ± 0.16
Heart[a]	0.82 ± 0.03	1.42 ± 0.03	1.42 ± 0.06	1.22 ± 0.12
Lungs[a]	2.02 ± 0.36	3.26 ± 0.62	3.39 ± 0.32	1.95 ± 0.20
Kidney[a]	1.69 ± 0.18	2.45 ± 0.28	2.45 ± 0.10	2.22 ± 0.16
Spleen[a]	0.46 ± 0.03	0.62 ± 0.08	0.69 ± 0.02	0.60 ± 0.07
Stomach[a]	2.65 ± 0.12	2.94 ± 0.44	3.02 ± 0.52	3.17 ± 0.05
Testes[a]	3.16 ± 0.12	4.58 ± 1.16	3.41 ± 0.21	3.33 ± 0.25
Pancreas[a]	0.96 ± 0.03	1.52 ± 0.01	1.64 ± 0.26	1.36 ± 0.18
Liver[b]	2.25	2.44	2.75	2.4
Brain[b]	0.52	0.34	0.34	0.93
Heart[b]	0.35	0.36	0.38	0.36
Lungs[b]	0.86	0.83	0.91	0.57
Kidney[b]	0.72	0.62	0.66	0.65
Spleen[b]	0.20	0.16	0.19	0.18
Stomach[b]	1.13	0.75	0.81	0.93
Testes[b]	1.35	1.16	0.92	0.97
Pancreas[b]	0.41	0.39	0.44	0.40

Mean organ-to-body weight ratio was calculated and expressed as mean ± SEM ($n = 10$).
[a]Unit: g.
[b]Unit: % body weight.
*Statistically significant compared to control ($p < 0.05$).

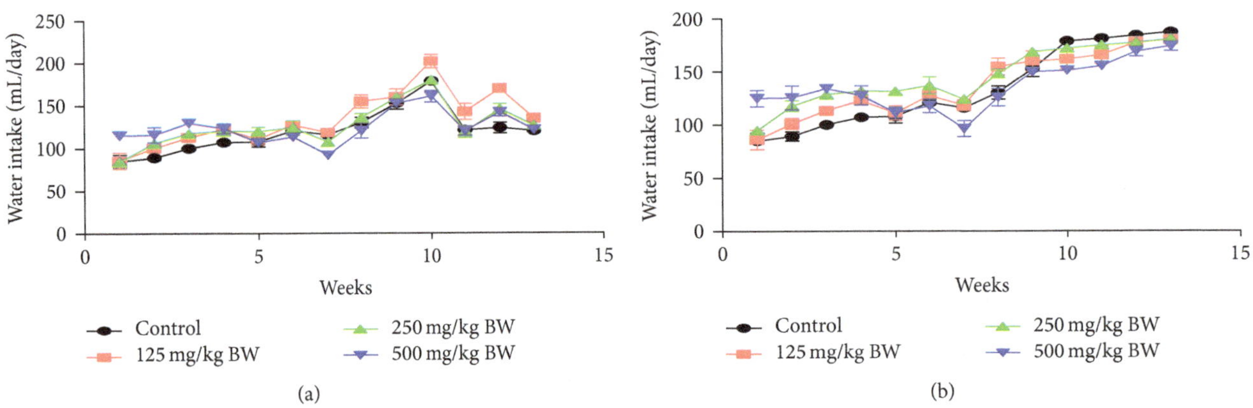

FIGURE 2: Effect of aqueous root extract of *Dicoma anomala* on water intake of male and female Wistar rats during a 90-day subchronic toxicity study. Values were calculated and data expressed as mean ± SEM.

there was no statistical difference ($p > 0.05$) in all the excised organs as compared with the control group.

3.2.4. Body Weights. The mean body weights of the animals at all concentrations were compared to the values of control (Figures 3(a) and 3(b)). The rats in all AQRED groups had statistically ($p < 0.05$) higher mean body weights (394.20 g, 371.10 g, and 342.60 g in 125, 250, and 500 mg/kg/day group, resp.) of males as compared to the control group (234.50 g). Moreover, there was a significant difference ($p < 0.05$) in body weight of female rats at all the three concentrations 125, 250, and 500 mg/kg body weight (269 g, 299 g, and 306 g, resp.) compared to control (244 g).

3.2.5. Haematology and Blood Chemistry. The results from haematological parameters only revealed statistically

TABLE 2: Effect of oral administration of aqueous extract of *Dicoma anomala* for 90 days on relative organ-to-body weight ratio of female Wistar rats.

Organ	Dose (mg/kg/day)			
	Control	125	250	500
Initial weight[a]	120.60 ± 2.55	121.00 ± 2.94	119.60 ± 4.09	116.60 ± 5.17
Body weight[a]	244.50 ± 6.94	269.20 ± 0.76	299.40 ± 3.22	306.00 ± 4.91*
% weight change	102.74	122.48	150.33	162.44
Liver[a]	6.87 ± 0.19	5.99 ± 0.95	6.29 ± 0.23	6.22 ± 0.32
Brain[a]	1.01 ± 0.05	1.15 ± 0.05	1.23 ± 0.21	1.17 ± 0.16
Heart[a]	0.52 ± 0.03	0.62 ± 0.03	0.58 ± 0.06	0.60 ± 0.12
Lungs[a]	1.52 ± 0.36	1.36 ± 0.62	1.39 ± 0.12	1.45 ± 0.20
Kidney[a]	1.39 ± 0.18	1.40 ± 0.28	1.45 ± 0.10	1.35 ± 0.06
Spleen[a]	0.32 ± 0.03	0.40 ± 0.08	0.39 ± 0.02	0.41 ± 0.07
Stomach[a]	2.05 ± 0.12	2.44 ± 0.44	2.12 ± 0.52	2.17 ± 0.05
Ovary[a]	3.16 ± 0.12	4.58 ± 1.16	3.41 ± 0.21	3.33 ± 0.25
Pancreas[a]	0.76 ± 0.03	0.78 ± 0.01	1.64 ± 0.26	1.36 ± 0.18
Liver[b]	2.81	2.23	2.10	2.03
Brain[b]	0.41	0.43	0.41	0.38
Heart[b]	0.21	0.23	0.19	0.20
Lungs[b]	0.62	0.51	0.46	0.47
Kidney[b]	0.57	0.52	0.48	0.44
Spleen[b]	0.13	0.15	0.13	0.13
Stomach[b]	1.84	0.91	0.71	0.71
Ovary[b]	1.29	1.70	0.14	1.09
Pancreas[b]	0.31	0.29	0.55	0.44

Mean organ-to-body weight ratio was calculated and expressed as mean ± SEM ($n = 10$).
[a]Unit: g.
[b]Unit: % body weight.
*Statistically significant compared to control ($p < 0.05$).

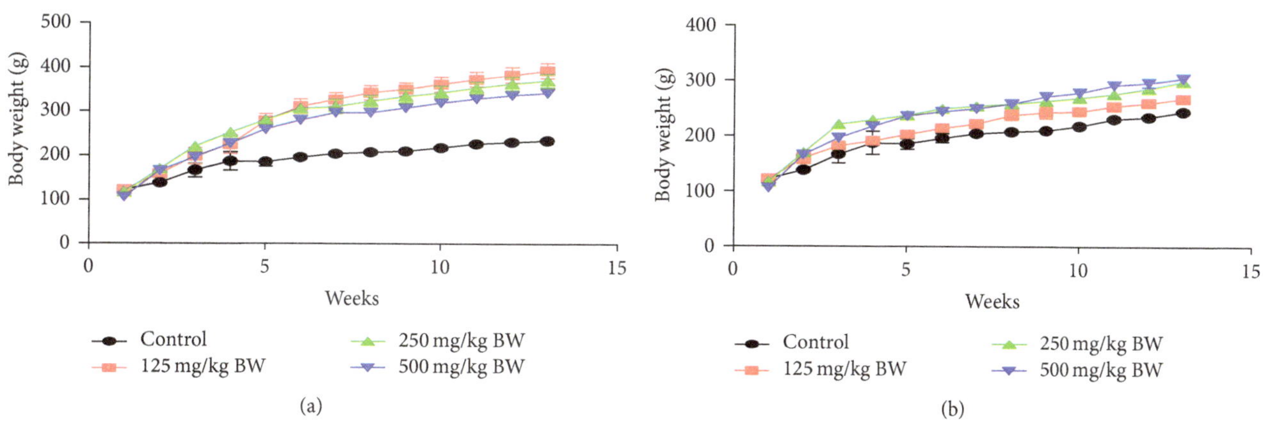

FIGURE 3: Effects of oral administration of aqueous root extracts of *Dicoma anomala* on mean body weights of male and female Wistar rats. Body weight was calculated and data expressed as mean ± SEM.

significant decrease ($p < 0.05$) in platelet count compared with control groups for both sexes, while there was no significant difference in other parameters compared to the control groups (Tables 3 and 4). Moreover, the result obtained from the blood chemistry showed a dose-dependent decrease ($p < 0.05$) in creatinine level and alanine transaminase activity, while it recorded a dose-dependent increase ($p < 0.05$) in sodium level. Serum activity of alkaline phosphatase also showed a statistical increase ($p < 0.05$) in the entire dose regimen, while the reverse is the case for aspartate transaminase when compared with control groups. Beyond all the reported results, there was no treatment-related or statistically significant ($p < 0.05$) effects observed in all the other tested blood chemistry parameters (Tables 5 and 6).

TABLE 3: Haematological data for male rats given aqueous root extracts of *Dicoma anomala* for 90 days.

Parameters	Unit	Dose (mg/kg/day)			
		Control	125	250	500
RBC	millions/μL	8.42 ± 0.10	9.44 ± 0.01	9.3 ± 0.05	9.18 ± 0.02
Haemoglobin	g/dL	16.4 ± 0.01	17.6 ± 0.02	16.9 ± 0.01	16.9 ± 0.01
Haematocrit	L/L	0.55 ± 0.05	0.61 ± 0.01	0.58 ± 0.02	0.59 ± 0.00
MCV	fL	65.00 ± 0.00	64.00 ± 0.00	62.00 ±0.00	64.00 ± 0.00
MCH	pg	19.00 ± 0.01	19.00 ± 0.01	18.00 ± 0.01	19.00 ± 0.01
MCHC	g/dL	30.00 ± 0.10	29.00 ± 0.10	29.00 ± 0.10	29.00 ± 0.10
RDW	fL	12.60 ± 0.01	13.40 ± 0.10	14.00 ± 0.00	14.10 ± 0.2
WBC	thous/μL	5.80 ± 0.02	6.50 ± 0.01	6.40 ± 0.02	6.90 ± 0.02
Neutrophils	$\times 10^9$/L	0.22 ± 0.00	0.46 ± 0.01	0.51 ± 0.02	0.62 ± 0.01
Lymphocytes	%	4.58 ± 0.10	4.45 ± 0.20	4.37 ± 0.20	4.89 ± 0.10
Monocytes	%	0.92 ± 0.00	1.43 ± 0.01	1.38 ± 0.01	1.28 ± 0.02
Eosinophils	$\times 10^9$/L	0.07 ± 0.00	0.16 ± 0.02	0.09 ± 0.00	0.08 ± 0.00
Basophils	$\times 10^9$/L	0.01 ± 0.00	0.02 ± 0.00	0.03 ± 0.01	0.02 ± 0.01
Platelet	thous/L	979.00 ± 0.50	803.00 ± 0.03*	701.00 ± 0.10*	754.00 ± 0.49*

Values are presented as mean ± SEM ($n = 10$).
*Significantly different compared to control at $p < 0.05$.

TABLE 4: Haematological data for female rats given aqueous root extracts of *Dicoma anomala* for 90 days.

Parameters	Unit	Dose (mg/kg/day)			
		Control	125	250	500
RBC	millions/μL	7.45 ± 0.10	7.44 ± 0.01	7.53 ± 0.05	7.88 ± 0.02
Haemoglobin	g/dL	14.41 ± 0.01	13.96 ± 0.02	15.09 ± 0.01	15.19 ± 0.01
Haematocrit	L/L	0.50 ± 0.05	0.49 ± 0.01	0.56 ± 0.02	0.59 ± 0.00
MCV	fL	61.00 ± 0.00	60.00 ± 0.00	62.00 ±0.00	63.00 ± 0.00
MCH	pg	16.00 ± 0.01	17.00 ± 0.01	17.00 ± 0.01	18.00 ± 0.01
MCHC	g/dL	27.00 ± 0.10	27.00 ± 0.10	28.00 ± 0.10	28.00 ± 0.10
RDW	fL	10.60 ± 0.01	11.40 ± 0.10	11.09 ± 0.00	11.91 ± 0.2
WBC	thous/μL	5.80 ± 0.02	6.30 ± 0.01	6.70 ± 0.02	6.91 ± 0.02
Neutrophils	$\times 10^9$/L	0.12 ± 0.00	0.16 ± 0.01	0.15 ± 0.02	0.16 ± 0.01
Lymphocytes	%	4.08 ± 0.10	4.05 ± 0.20	4.07 ± 0.20	4.80 ± 0.10
Monocytes	%	0.73 ± 0.00	0.93 ± 0.01	1.08 ± 0.01	1.12 ± 0.02
Eosinophils	$\times 10^9$/L	0.09 ± 0.00	0.12 ± 0.02	0.08 ± 0.00	0.08 ± 0.00
Basophils	$\times 10^9$/L	0.01 ± 0.00	0.02 ± 0.00	0.03 ± 0.01	0.02 ± 0.01
Platelet	thous/L	1007.00 ± 0.50	893.00 ± 0.03*	871.00 ± 0.10*	944.00 ± 0.49*

Values are presented as mean ± SEM ($n = 10$).
*Significantly different compared to control at $p < 0.05$.

3.2.6. Histopathological Examination. The result from histological analysis revealed no macroscopic observations considered to be treatment-related. No gross deformities could be considered to be related to the test article for any of the euthanized animals necropsied at the expiration of the 90-day experimental study. Histopathological observation including presence of hyperplasia and lymph nodes was only noticeable in one of the sections of the stomach for the 125 mg/kg body weight male rats as well as presence of renal calculi in the collecting tubes of the kidney for untreated control animals; as such, these changes could not be treatment-related.

3.3. GC/MS Analysis. The GC/MS chromatogram of *Dicoma anomala* extract revealed the presence of rich amounts of eighty phytochemical compounds. The major identifiable constituents are 5-(Hydroxymethyl)-2-furancarboxyaldehyde, 2-(1-methyl-2,5-dioxoimidazolidin-4-yl) acetic acid, n-tridecane, 9-octadecenoic acid, hexadecanoic acid, phosphine, 1,6-anhydro-β-D-glucopyranoside, 3-(Bromophenyl) triphenyl phosphonium bromide, Guanosine, and Xanthosine. The compound name, molecular formula, and peak area (%) of the majority of the constituents are presented in Table 7.

TABLE 5: Effect of aqueous root extracts of *Dicoma anomala* for 90 days on biochemical parameters of male Wistar rats.

Parameters	Unit	Dose (mg/kg/day)			
		Control	125	250	500
Total cholesterol	mmol/L	2.50 ± 0.23	2.10 ± 0.15	2.20 ± 0.13	2.00 ± 0.20
Triglycerides	mmol/L	0.65 ± 0.00	1.21 ± 0.11	0.87 ± 0.20	0.86 ± 0.01
HDL-c	mmol/L	1.60 ± 0.23	1.30 ± 0.17	1.40 ± 0.25	1.30 ± 0.19
LDL-c	mmol/L	0.90 ± 0.00	0.80 ± 0.11	0.80 ± 0.14	0.70 ± 0.50
ALT	U/L	51.00 ± 0.85	48.00 ± 0.55*	47.00 ± 0.77*	47.00 ± 0.74*
AST	U/L	215.00 ± 0.85	188.00 ± 0.90*	145.00 ± 0.87*	192.00 ± 0.88*
ALP	U/L	185.00 ± 0.87	200.00 ± 0.90*	264.00 ± 0.47*	220.00 ± 0.75*
Glucose	mg/dL	4.23 ± 0.10	3.70 ± 0.11	4.27 ± 0.05	4.47 ± 0.23
Sodium	mmol/L	137.00 ± 0.67	141.00 ± 0.85*	142.00 ± 0.44*	142.00 ± 0.53*
Potassium	mmol/L	5.40 ± 0.01	5.20 ± 0.01	4.80 ± 0.02	5.60 ± 0.00
Chloride	mmol/L	104.00 ± 0.11	103.00 ± 0.21	104.00 ± 0.12	104.00 ± 0.01
Calcium	mmol/L	2.38 ± 0.01	2.31 ± 0.10	2.32 ± 0.14	2.34 ± 0.20
Magnesium	mmol/L	0.99 ± 0.40	0.87 ± 0.02	0.95 ± 0.14	0.88 ± 0.01
Urea	mmol/L	8.10 ± 0.01	7.50 ± 0.00	7.90 ± 0.12	7.50 ± 0.24
Creatinine	μmol/L	44.00 ± 0.23	41.00 ± 0.21*	40.00 ± 0.17*	35.00 ± 0.20*
Albumin	g/L	34.00 ± 0.15	32.00 ± 0.20	31.00 ± 0.10*	32.00 ± 0.05
Total protein	g/L	65.00 ± 0.3	65.00 ± 0.25	63.00 ± 0.33	64.00 ± 2.0
Total bilirubin	μmol/L	3.00 ± 0.11	3.00 ± 0.12	2.00 ± 0.00	2.00 ± 0.15
Conj. bilirubin	μmol/L	1.00 ± 0.1	1.00 ± 0.01	1.00 ± 0.10	1.00 ± 0.01
Unconj. bilirubin	μmol/L	2.00 ± 0.01	2.00 ± 0.01	1.00 ± 0.00	1.00 ± 0.00

Values are presented as mean ± SEM ($n = 10$).
*Significantly different compared to control at $p < 0.05$.

TABLE 6: Effect of aqueous root extracts of *Dicoma anomala* for 90 days on biochemical parameters of female Wistar rats.

Parameters	Unit	Dose (mg/kg/day)			
		Control	125	250	500
Total cholesterol	mmol/L	2.30 ± 0.23	2.00 ± 0.15	2.20 ± 0.13	2.10 ± 0.20
Triglycerides	mmol/L	0.56 ± 0.00	0.67 ± 0.11	0.85 ± 0.20	0.89 ± 0.01
HDL-c	mmol/L	1.65 ± 0.23	1.15 ± 0.17	1.30 ± 0.25	1.30 ± 0.19
LDL-c	mmol/L	0.80 ± 0.00	0.70 ± 0.11	0.70 ± 0.14	0.60 ± 0.50
ALT	U/L	49.00 ± 0.85	46.00 ± 0.55*	45.00 ± 0.77*	45.00 ± 0.74*
AST	U/L	210.00 ± 0.85	178.00 ± 0.90*	150.00 ± 0.87*	182.00 ± 0.88*
ALP	U/L	165.00 ± 0.87	170.00 ± 0.90*	235.00 ± 0.47*	210.00 ± 0.75*
Glucose	mg/dL	3.23 ± 0.10	3.10 ± 0.11	4.29 ± 0.05	4.74 ± 0.23
Sodium	mmol/L	107.00 ± 0.67	115.00 ± 0.85*	123.00 ± 0.44*	144.00 ± 0.53*
Potassium	mmol/L	5.49 ± 0.01	5.29 ± 0.01	4.99 ± 0.02	5.61 ± 0.00
Chloride	mmol/L	107.00 ± 0.11	106.00 ± 0.21	107.00 ± 0.12	107.00 ± 0.01
Calcium	mmol/L	2.32 ± 0.67	2.30 ± 0.10	2.31 ± 0.14	2.33 ± 0.20
Magnesium	mmol/L	0.80 ± 0.40	0.82 ± 0.02	0.85 ± 0.14	0.88 ± 0.01
Urea	mmol/L	7.99 ± 0.01	7.65 ± 0.00	7.89 ± 0.12	8.05 ± 0.24
Creatinine	μmol/L	43.00 ± 0.23	40.00 ± 0.21*	40.00 ± 0.17*	37.00 ± 0.20*
Albumin	g/L	35.00 ± 0.15	33.00 ± 0.20	32.00 ± 0.10*	34.00 ± 0.05
Total protein	g/L	65.00 ± 0.3	65.00 ± 0.25	65.00 ± 0.33	64.00 ± 2.0
Total bilirubin	μmol/L	2.00 ± 0.11	2.00 ± 0.12	3.00 ± 0.00	3.00 ± 0.15
Conj. bilirubin	μmol/L	1.00 ± 0.1	1.00 ± 0.01	1.00 ± 0.10	1.00 ± 0.01
Unconj. bilirubin	μmol/L	2.00 ± 0.01	2.00 ± 0.01	1.00 ± 0.00	1.00 ± 0.00

Values are presented as mean ± SEM ($n = 10$).
*Significantly different compared to control at $p < 0.05$.

TABLE 7: Reported biological activities of the identified bioactive compounds from *D. anomala*.

Compound	% Composition	Biological activity
5-(Hydroxymethyl)-2-furancarboxyaldehyde [$C_6H_6O_3$]	40.64	Antimicrobial preservative, antifungal [10], anti-inflammatory [11–13], antihepatotoxic [14] activity
2,3-Dihydro-3,5-dihydroxyl-6-methyl-4H-pyran-4-one [$C_{11}H_8O_4$]	1.52	Antimicrobial, anti-inflammatory activity [15]
n-Tridecane [$C_{13}H_{28}$]	5.56	Antimicrobial activity [16]
1,6-Anhydro-β-D-glucopyranoside [$C_6H_{10}O_5$]	3.48	Nontoxic on cell-cell communication systems [17]
2-(1-methyl-2,5-dioxoimidazolidin-4-yl) acetic acid [$C_6H_8N_2O_4$]	10.90	Nontoxic, antihepatotoxic activity [18]
Acetamide [$C_4H_9NO_2$]	1.85	Anticonvulsant activity [19]
Hexadecanoic acid [$C_{16}H_{32}O_2$]	4.36	Antioxidant, hypocholesteroemic, nematicide, pesticide, lubricant, antiandrogenic, flavour, haemolytic 5-α-reductase inhibitor [15]
9-Octadecenoic acid [$C_{57}H_{104}O_6$]	4.46	Antioxidant, anticancer [20, 21]
Globulol [$C_{15}H_{26}O$]	1.68	Antimicrobial [22, 23], antibacterial, antiglutamatergic, sedative activity [24]
Phosphine [$C_{18}H_{15}P$]	4.69	Antihypertensive, diuretic, uric acid excretion stimulant, saluretic activity [25]

4. Discussion

The recognition of herbal treatment or phytomedicine as the most common form of alternative medicine has been around since time immemorial [26]. This is because a larger percentage of the world's population (about 80% according to World Health Organization's estimation) depends on these plant-based remedies as a viable option to diseased conditions most especially in developing and/or developed countries where conventional or modern drugs are majorly used [27]. Similarly, it is worth mentioning that the popularity, as well as the usage of these traditional medicines, has continued to increase all over the world [28]. Despite this popularity and wide usage, the safety of these herbal therapies has, in recent times, raised a lot of questions as a result of revelations due to illnesses and fatalities [29, 30] such as hepatotoxicity [31] and nephrotoxicity [32, 33] and only a few of them have been evaluated through various phases of clinical trials [34].

Toxicity studies encompass acute, subacute, chronic, or subchronic toxicity. In the present study, acute and subchronic toxicities studies were evaluated on *Dicoma anomala* aqueous root extract that paved the way for the meaningful interpretation of its toxic effect. The single oral dose administration of AQRED to Wistar albino rats at the highest concentration of 2000 mg/kg body weight did not cause any mortality and revealed no clinical signs, like changes in fur and skin, eyes, mucus membrane, respiratory rate, circulatory signs, autonomic effects, and central nervous system. In general, exposure of the animals to a single oral dose of AQRED did not produce any mortality or any treatment-related effect [35]; as such, the lethal dose (LD_{50}) was assumed to be greater than 2000 mg/kg suggesting that the extract could be generally regarded as nontoxic. This report corroborates the work of M. L. Clarke and E. G. C. Clarke [36] who maintained that any drug with oral LD_{50} greater than 1000 mg/kg BW could be regarded as safe and of low toxicity.

The administration of AQRED for 90 days revealed no clinical signs of toxicity or mortality in both sexes of the animals used in this study. There was no significant reduction in feed and water intake of the treated rats in either sex through the 90-day study; this is a pointer to the fact that the diet and water were well accepted by the rats, suggesting that the extracts did not in any way alter the metabolism of carbohydrate, protein, and fats in the rats. It may also signify the fact that the nutritional status (weight gain and appetite stability) which was expected to be seen in prolonged-fed animals was not adversely affected by the extracts. This corroborates the traditional usage of the plant by the oral route.

The body weight changes may reflect the general health status of animals [37]. However, the body weight gain witnessed in all the animals treated with AQRED suggests that the extracts did not interfere with normal body metabolism of the animals as the increment in food and water intake is synonymous to an increase in body weight. The essence of weighing organs in studies relating to toxicity provides facts on their sensitivity to toxicity, physiologic perturbations, induction of enzymes, and acute organ damage [38]. An insignificant difference in the weight of the excised vital organs compared to that of the control obtained for this study was an indication that AQRED on prolonged use or intake might not have an effect on normal growth; and since there was no reduction in body and/or relative organ weight in all the tested doses of the treated rats, it is assumed that the extract is not toxic to the excised and evaluated organs.

The assessment of blood hematology and clinical biochemistry provides an insight to possible damage brought about by the extract in the hepatic and renal functions. In toxicity studies, assessment of liver and kidney functions is germane because both organs are essential for the survival of an organism [39]. Alanine aminotransferase (ALT), aspartate transaminase (AST), and alkaline phosphatase (ALP) are sensitive enzymes used in assessing the severity of liver damage [40]. Elevated activities of these enzymes are associated with liver or heart damage [41–43]. The significant reduction in ALT and AST of the treated animals in both sexes compared with normal control could suggest that AQRED may not have hepatotoxic effect [44] and, equally, might not have deleterious effect on the heart [45], while the increase in ALP might suggest obstruction of the biliary tract which may be present in the liver. Evaluation of total protein gives an estimation of the nutritional status and diagnostic measurement of liver and kidney diseases [46]. A reduction in total protein, albumin, and globulin is an indication of impaired hepatocellular function [47]; however, an insignificant difference in serum level of these parameters upon prolonged administration of *D. anomala* when compared with the control further corroborates the fact that the extracts do not destroy the secretory functions of the liver. Measurement of serum urea, creatinine, and uric acid concentration reflects the likelihood of renal problems or dysfunction [48]. The insignificant changes in urea and the significant reduction in creatinine levels obtained in this study as compared to the normal control could suggest an indication of the potentials of AQRED in maintaining a normal renal function [45]. The result was in consonance with the report of Patrick-Iwuanyanwu et al. [49] for Baker cleansers bitters.

Abnormalities in the concentration of major lipids like cholesterol (TC), high-density lipoprotein cholesterol (HDL-c), and triglycerides (TG) can give useful information on the lipid metabolism as well as the predisposition of the animals to atherosclerosis and its complications. The insignificant changes in the value of TC, LDL-c, HDL-c, and triglycerides recorded in this study might signify the intact position of the myocardial membrane [50] and could also suggest the hypolipidemic potentials of the plant [51].

A prominent role in the exchange of gas and the intercompartmental water balance is played by electrolytes. Increase or decrease in the levels of these electrolytes within the serum may be a consequence of the hypo- or hyperfunctioning of the concerned organ or tissue. Sodium, potassium, and chlorides are examples of these clinical electrolytes used in assessing the functioning of the kidney. In the present study, there was no significant change in the treated rats in these parameters when compared with the control; this could be attributed to a normal functioning status of the kidney.

Haematological evaluation is used to determine the extent of the deleterious effect on the blood. It can also explain the blood relating functions of a plant extract or its products [52]. The result from the present study revealed no significant effects on red blood cells (RBC), MCV, and haemoglobin values of the treated rats when compared to the control, suggesting that the erythropoiesis, morphology, or osmotic fragility of RBC are not affected [53]. Similarly, the insignificant changes in neutrophils, lymphocytes, and monocytes witnessed in all the tested concentrations similarly suggested the intact state of the immune system and lack of injury to the tissues, while the significant increase in platelets concentration for all the treated groups compared to control may be attributed to the elevated secretion and production of thrombopoietin, the primary regulator of platelet production [54], by AQRED suggesting its homeostatic property [55]. This result was in line with the report of Patrick-Iwuanyanwu et al. [49]. Generally, the result obtained from the hematology examinations further justified the safety potential of AQRED.

The histological examination of all the analysed (vital) organs revealed that none of the organs from the extract treated rats revealed alteration and there were no abnormalities in the cell structure of these vital organs.

Besides being antioxidative [15, 20, 21], most of the identified compounds from the GC/MS chromatogram of the plant have been implicated in other biological and pharmacological activities. 5-(Hydroxymethyl)-2-furancarboxyaldehyde, 2,3-dihydro-3,5-dihydroxyl-6-methyl-4H-pyran-4-one, n-tridecane, and globulol are reported to possess antimicrobial activity [10, 15, 16, 22, 23]. The presence of 5-(Hydroxymethyl)-2-furancarboxyaldehyde and 2,3-dihydro-3,5-dihydroxyl-6-methyl-4H-pyran-4-one in the phytonutrients is attributed to their anti-inflammatory potentials [11–13, 15]. 2-(1-methyl-2,5-dioxoimidazolidin-4-yl) acetic acid and 5-(Hydroxymethyl)-2-furancarboxyaldehyde have been reported to have antihepatotoxic effect [14, 18]. Some of the other pharmacological activities such as anticancer [20, 21] and antihypertensive [25] exhibited by the phytonutrients are shown in Table 7.

5. Conclusions

In conclusion, the administration of aqueous root extract of *Dicoma anomala* to Wistar rats was not toxic in all the tested doses and did not reveal any toxic signs in the two studied toxicities. The extract did not have a direct impact on the liver and kidney functions as evidenced from the haematological and blood chemistry results and did not cause any change in food intake, water consumption, and body weight and produces no evident histopathological damage in the rats. The presented results might give an insight to exploring the pharmaceutical and therapeutic benefit of AQRED as a viable candidate to conventional drugs with lots of side effects. Moreover, the presence of various bioactive compounds as revealed by the GC/MS result and the confirmation of some of the therapeutic properties justify the usage of the plants for various ailments by traditional healers. Further studies to ascertain the effects of the herb on pregnant animals, animal foetus, and their reproductive capability are however encouraged to fully explore the safety profile of the plant.

Competing Interests

The authors both read the paper and declared that there are no competing interests.

Acknowledgments

The authors acknowledge research committee of the University of the Free State, Qwaqwa campus, for financing the study. The authors also acknowledge Dr. OT Ojuromi, Mr. S Sabiu, and Ms. G Mahanke for their assistance during the blood sample collection, paper proofreading, and daily data recording, respectively.

References

[1] J. Mnegwane and M. Koekemoer, "*Dicoma anomala* Sond.," South African National Biodiversity Institute, 2007, http://www.plantzafrica.com/plantcd/dicomanom.htm.

[2] J. V. Becker, M. M. Van der Merwe, A. C. Van Brummelen et al., "*In Vitro* anti-plasmodial activity of *Dicoma anomala* subsp. *gerrardii* (Asteraceae): identification of its main active constituent, structure-activity relationship studies and gene expression profiling," *Malaria Journal*, vol. 10, pp. 295–304, 2011.

[3] M. Schmidt, H.-J. Schmitz, A. Baumgart et al., "Toxicity of green tea extracts and their constituents in rat hepatocytes in primary culture," *Food and Chemical Toxicology*, vol. 43, no. 2, pp. 307–314, 2005.

[4] H. L. Bonkovsky, "Hepatotoxicity associated with supplements containing Chinese green tea (*Camelia inensis*)," *Annals of Internal Medicine*, vol. 144, no. 1, pp. 68–71, 2006.

[5] S. S. Bun, H. Bun, D. Guédon, C. Rosier, and E. Ollivier, "Effect of green tea extracts on liver functions in Wistar rats," *Food and Chemical Toxicology*, vol. 44, no. 7, pp. 1108–1113, 2006.

[6] A. K. Chandra and N. De, "Goitrogenic/antithyroidal potential of green tea extract in relation to catechin in rats," *Food and Chemical Toxicology*, vol. 48, no. 8-9, pp. 2304–2311, 2010.

[7] Organization of Economic Co-operation and Development (OECD), *The OECD Guideline for Testing of Chemicals: 423 Acute Oral Toxicity—Acute Toxic Class Method*, OECD, Paris, France, 2001.

[8] Organization of Economic Co-operation and Development (OECD), *The OECD Guideline for Testing of Chemicals: 408 Subchronic Oral Toxicity—Rodent: 90 Day Study*, OECD, Paris, France, 1998.

[9] M. Nitta, H. Kobayashi, M. Ohnishi-Kameyama, T. Nagamine, and M. Yoshida, "Essential oil variation of cultivated and wild Perilla analyzed by GC/MS," *Biochemical Systematics and Ecology*, vol. 34, no. 1, pp. 25–37, 2006.

[10] H. J. Zeringue Jr., "Identification and effects of maize silk volatiles on cultures of *Aspergillus flavus*," *Journal of Agricultural and Food Chemistry*, vol. 48, no. 3, pp. 921–925, 2000.

[11] J. Brustugun, H. H. Tønnesen, R. Edge, and S. Navaratnam, "Formation and reactivity of free radicals in 5-hydroxymethyl-2-furaldehyde—the effect on isoprenaline photostability," *Journal of Photochemistry and Photobiology B: Biology*, vol. 79, no. 2, pp. 109–119, 2005.

[12] Y.-H. Li and X.-Y. Lu, "Investigation on the origin of 5-HMF in Shengmaiyin decoction by RP-HPLC method," *Journal of Zhejiang University: Science*, vol. 6, no. 10, pp. 1015–1021, 2005.

[13] Q. Xu, Y.-H. Li, and X.-Y. Lü, "Investigation on influencing factors of 5-HMF content in Schisandra," *Journal of Zhejiang University of Science B*, vol. 8, no. 6, pp. 439–445, 2007.

[14] C. L. Graff and G. M. Pollack, "Nasal drug administration: potential for targeted central nervous system delivery," *Journal of Pharmaceutical Sciences*, vol. 94, no. 6, pp. 1187–1195, 2005.

[15] S. Gopalakrishnan and T. Kalaiarasi, "Determination of biologically active constituents of the fruits of *Cucumis sativum* Linn. using GC-MS analysis," *International Journal of Biological and Pharmaceutical Research*, vol. 4, no. 7, pp. 523–527, 2013.

[16] N. Rahbar, A. Shafaghat, and F. Salimi, "Antimicrobial activity and constituents of the hexane extracts from leaf and stem of *Origanum vulgare* L. ssp. Viride (Boiss.) Hayek. growing wild in Northwest Iran," *Journal of Medicinal Plants Research*, vol. 6, no. 13, pp. 2681–2685, 2012.

[17] D. Deryabin and A. Tolmacheva, "Antibacterial and anti-quorum sensing molecular composition derived from *Quercus cortex* (Oak bark) extract," *Molecules*, vol. 20, no. 9, pp. 17093–17108, 2015.

[18] S. Q. Tang, Y. Y. I. Lee, D. S. Packiaraj, H. K. Ho, and C. L. L. Chai, "Systematic evaluation of the metabolism and toxicity of thiazolidinone and imidazolidinone heterocycles," *Chemical Research in Toxicology*, vol. 28, no. 10, pp. 2019–2033, 2015.

[19] K. Kamiński, J. Obniska, B. Wiklik, and D. Atamanyuk, "Synthesis and anticonvulsant properties of new acetamide derivatives of phthalimide, and its saturated cyclohexane and norbornene analogs," *European Journal of Medicinal Chemistry*, vol. 46, no. 9, pp. 4634–4641, 2011.

[20] F. A. Syeda, A. M. Habib-ur-Rahman, F. A. Syeda, and M. I. Khan Choudahry, "Gas Chromatography-Mass Spectrometry (GC-MS) analysis of petroleum ether extract (oil) and bioassays of crude extract of *Iris germanica*," *International Journal of Genetics and Molecular Biology*, vol. 3, no. 7, pp. 95–100, 2011.

[21] R. Hema, S. Kumaravel, and J. Alagusundaram, "GC/MS determination of bioactive components of *Murraya koenigii*," *Journal of American Science*, vol. 7, pp. 80–83, 2011.

[22] M. Tan, L. Zhou, Y. Huang, Y. Wang, X. Hao, and J. Wang, "Antimicrobial activity of globulol isolated from the fruits of *Eucalyptus globulus* Labill," *Natural Product Research*, vol. 22, no. 7, pp. 569–575, 2008.

[23] S. Mulyaningsih, F. Sporer, S. Zimmermann, J. Reichling, and M. Wink, "Synergistic properties of the terpenoids aromadendrene and 1,8-cineole from the essential oil of *Eucalyptus globulus* against antibiotic-susceptible and antibiotic-resistant pathogens," *Phytomedicine*, vol. 17, no. 13, pp. 1061–1066, 2010.

[24] L. L. Silva, Q. I. Garlet, S. C. Benovit et al., "Sedative and anesthetic activities of the essential oils of *Hyptis mutabilis* (Rich.) Briq. and their isolated components in silver catfish (*Rhamdia quelen*)," *Brazilian Journal of Medical and Biological Research*, vol. 46, no. 9, pp. 771–779, 2013.

[25] T. Mallikadevi, S. Paulsamy, S. Jamuna, and K. Karthika, "Analysis for phytoceuticals and bioinformatics approach for the evaluation of therapetic properties of whole plant methanolic extract of *Mukia maderaspatana* (L.) M.Roem. (Cucurbitaceae)-a traditional medicinal plant in Western districts of Tamil Nadu, India," *Asian Journal of Pharmaceutical and Clinical Research*, vol. 5, no. 4, pp. 163–168, 2012.

[26] S. O. Ogbonnia, G. O. Mbaka, E. N. Anyika, J. E. Emordi, and N. Nwakakwa, "An evaluation of acute and subchronic toxicities of a Nigerian polyherbal tea remedy," *Pakistan Journal of Nutrition*, vol. 10, no. 11, pp. 1022–1028, 2011.

[27] S. Ogbonnia, A. A. Adekunle, M. K. Bosa, and V. N. Enwuru, "Evaluation of acute and subacute toxicity of *Alstonia congensis* Engler (Apocynaceae) bark and *Xylopia aethiopica* (Dunal) A. Rich (Annonaceae) fruits mixtures used in the treatment of diabetes," *African Journal of Biotechnology*, vol. 7, no. 6, pp. 701–705, 2008.

[28] G. P. Daswani, S. Brijesh, and J. T. Birdi, "Preclinical testing of medicinal plants: advantages and approaches," in *Workshop Proceedings on Approaches Towards Evaluation of Medicinal Plants Prior to Clinical Trial*, pp. 60–77, The Foundation for Medical Research at Yashwantrao Chavan Academy of Development Administration (YASHADA), Pune, India, 2006.

[29] V. F. Veiga Jr., A. C. Pinto, and M. A. M. Maciel, "Medicinal plants: safe cure?" *Quimica Nova*, vol. 28, no. 3, pp. 519–528, 2005.

[30] M.-Y. Park, H.-Y. Choi, J.-D. Kim, H.-S. Lee, and S.-K. Ku, "28 Days repeated oral dose toxicity test of aqueous extracts of mahwangyounpae-tang, a polyherbal formula," *Food and Chemical Toxicology*, vol. 48, no. 8-9, pp. 2477–2482, 2010.

[31] B. Saad, H. Azaizeh, G. Abu-Hijleh, and O. Said, "Safety of traditional Arab herbal medicine," *Evidence-Based Complementary and Alternative Medicine*, vol. 3, no. 4, pp. 433–439, 2006.

[32] C. R. D. Colson and M. E. De Broe, "Kidney injury from alternative medicines," *Advances in Chronic Kidney Disease*, vol. 12, no. 3, pp. 261–275, 2005.

[33] F. D. Debelle, J.-L. Vanherweghem, and J. L. Nortier, "Aristolochic acid nephropathy: a worldwide problem," *Kidney International*, vol. 74, no. 2, pp. 158–169, 2008.

[34] C.-W. Cheng, Z.-X. Bian, and T.-X. Wu, "Systematic review of Chinese herbal medicine for functional constipation," *World Journal of Gastroenterology*, vol. 15, no. 39, pp. 4886–4895, 2009.

[35] A. Wallace Hayes, *Principles and Methods of Toxicology*, CRC Press, Boca Raton, Fla, USA, 4th edition, 2001.

[36] M. L. Clarke and E. G. C. Clarke, *Veterinary Toxicology*, Bailliere Tindall, London, UK, 1967.

[37] J. El Hilaly, Z. H. Israili, and B. Lyoussi, "Acute and chronic toxicological studies of *Ajuga iva* in experimental animals," *Journal of Ethnopharmacology*, vol. 91, no. 1, pp. 43–50, 2004.

[38] B. Michael, B. Yano, R. S. Sellers et al., "Evaluation of organ weights for rodent and non-rodent toxicity studies: a review of regulatory guidelines and a survey of current practices," *Toxicologic Pathology*, vol. 35, no. 5, pp. 742–750, 2007.

[39] O. S. Olorunnisola, G. Bradley, and A. J. Afolayan, "Acute and sub-chronic toxicity studies of methanolic extract of *Tulbaghia violacea* rhizomes in Wistar rats," *African Journal of Biotechnolology*, vol. 11, pp. 14934–14940, 2012.

[40] S. K. Ramaiah, "Preclinical safety assessment: current gaps, challenges, and approaches in identifying translatable biomarkers of drug-induced liver injury," *Clinics in Laboratory Medicine*, vol. 31, no. 1, pp. 161–172, 2011.

[41] K. M. Wasan, S. Najafi, J. Wong et al., "Assessing plasma lipid levels, body weight and hepatic and renal toxicity following chronic oral administration of a water soluble phytostanol compound FM-VP4 to gerbils," *Journal of Pharmaceutical Sciences*, vol. 4, pp. 228–234, 2001.

[42] N. Brautbar and J. Williams II, "Industrial solvents and liver toxicity: risk assessment, risk factors and mechanisms," *International Journal of Hygiene and Environmental Health*, vol. 205, no. 6, pp. 479–491, 2002.

[43] R. Mythilypriya, P. Shanthi, and P. Sachdanandam, "Oral acute and subacute toxicity studies with *Kalpaamruthaa*, a modified indigenous preparation, on rats," *Journal of Health Science*, vol. 53, no. 4, pp. 351–358, 2007.

[44] F. O. Balogun and A. O. T. Ashafa, "Comparative study on the antioxidant activity of *Dicoma anomala* and *G. krebsiana* used in Basotho traditional medicine," *South African Journal of Botany*, vol. 98, p. 170, 2015.

[45] M. A. Crook, *Clinical Chemistry and Metabolic Medicine*, Hodder Arnold, Dacie, London, UK, 2006.

[46] J. Ozer, M. Ratner, M. Shaw, W. Bailey, and S. Schomaker, "The current state of serum biomarkers of hepatotoxicity," *Toxicology*, vol. 245, no. 3, pp. 194–205, 2008.

[47] M. T. Yakubu, L. S. Bilbis, M. Lawal et al., "Effect of repeated administration of sildenafil citrate on selected enzyme activities of liver and kidney of male albino rate," *Nigerian Journal of Pure and Applied Sciences*, vol. 18, pp. 1395–1400, 2003.

[48] M. E. Davis and N. D. Bredt, "Renal methods for toxicity," in *Principles and Methods of Toxicology*, Raven Press, New York, NY, USA, 1994.

[49] K. C. Patrick-Iwuanyanwu, C. C. Onyemaenu, M. O. Wegwu, and E. O. Ayalogu, "Hepatotoxic and nephrotoxic effects of kerosene and petrol-contaminated diets in Wistar albino rats," *Research Journal of Environmental Toxicology*, vol. 5, no. 1, pp. 49–57, 2011.

[50] H. B. Brewer Jr., "Hypertriglyceridemia: changes in the plasma lipoproteins associated with an increased risk of cardiovascular disease," *American Journal of Cardiology B*, vol. 83, no. 9, pp. 3F–12F, 1999.

[51] T. O. Sunmonu and A. J. Afolayan, "Protective effect of *Artemisia afra* Jacq. on isoproterenol-induced myocardial injury in Wistar rats," *Food and Chemical Toxicology*, vol. 48, no. 7, pp. 1969–1972, 2010.

[52] M. T. Yakubu, M. A. Akanji, and A. T. Oladiji, "Haematological evaluation in male albino rats following chronic administration of aqueous extract of *Fadogia agrestis* stem," *Pharmacognosy Magazine*, vol. 3, pp. 34–38, 2007.

[53] A. C. Guyton and J. E. Hall, *Textbook of Medical Physiology*, W. B. Saunders, Philadelphia, Pa, USA, 2000.

[54] K. Kaushansky, "Thrombopoietin: the primary regulator of megakaryocyte and platelet production," *Thrombosis and Haemostasis*, vol. 74, no. 1, pp. 521–525, 1995.

[55] S. B. Olaleye, J. A. Akinniyi, H. A. Salami et al., "Preliminary study on the toxicity and antimicrobial effects of extracts of *Securidaca longipedunculata*," *African Journal of Biomedical Research*, vol. 1, no. 1, pp. 39–44, 1998.

13

Rannasangpei Is a Therapeutic Agent in the Treatment of Vascular Dementia

Peng Wu,[1,2] Yuandai Luo,[2] Lifang Zhen,[2] Xianda Hu,[2] Ying Shang,[3] Yinuo Liao,[1] Huiyuan Xue,[1] Fukai Huang,[2] and Wei Xiao[1]

[1]*Southern Medical University, Guangzhou 510515, China*
[2]*Beijing Tibetan Hospital, China Tibetology Research Center, Beijing 100029, China*
[3]*Beijing Mentougou Hospital of Traditional Chinese Medicine, Beijing 102300, China*

Correspondence should be addressed to Fukai Huang; zgzxyjzxbjzyy@126.com and Wei Xiao; xw76888@126.com

Academic Editor: Ching-Liang Hsieh

Rannasangpei (RSNP) is used as a therapeutic agent in the treatment of cardiovascular diseases, neurological disorders, and neurodegeneration in China; however, its potential use in the treatment of vascular dementia (VD) was unclear. In this study, our aim was to examine the neuroprotective effect of RSNP in a VD rat model, which was induced by permanent bilateral common carotid artery occlusion (2VO). Four-week administration with two doses of RSNP was investigated in our study. Severe cognitive deficit in the VD model, which was confirmed in Morris water maze (MWM) test, was significantly restored by the administration of RSNP. ELISA revealed that the treatments with both doses of RSNP could reinstate the cholinergic activity in the VD animals by elevating the production of choline acetyltransferase (ChAT) and reducing the acetylcholinesterase (AChE); the treatment of RSNP could also reboot the level of superoxide dismutase (SOD) and decrease malondialdehyde (MDA). Moreover, Western blot and quantitative PCR (Q-PCR) results indicated that the RSNP could suppress the apoptosis in the hippocampus of the VD animals by increasing the expression ratio of B-cell lymphoma-2 (Bcl-2) to Bcl-2-associated X protein (Bax). These results suggested that RSNP might be a therapeutic agent in the treatment of vascular dementia in the future.

1. Introduction

Vascular dementia (VD), which is caused by chronic cerebral hypoperfusion (CCH), hampers the intelligence of an individual, leading to the development of cognitive dysfunction syndrome [1, 2]. Epidemiological studies have shown that the prevalence of VD is remarkably high—VD is diagnosed in 20–30% of the total number of cases with dementia—in the elderly population of China and other countries of the world. Patients with VD are serious economic burdens to their families and the society [3, 4]. Several evidences have indicated that CCH aggravates cerebrovascular pathological changes [5, 6], such as central cholinergic dysfunction, oxidative injury, and apoptosis in hippocampus [7]. It is a well-known fact that central cholinergic neurotransmission is closely associated with learning and memory in humans [8]; reactive oxygen species cause oxidative stress that activates various signal transduction pathways involved in apoptosis. As a result, many cognitive deficits are caused in individuals [9]. All the above situations can eventually exacerbate the process of VD. However, the pathogenesis of VD is not fully understood till date. Owing to the complicated etiology and pathology of VD, it is difficult to develop a single-target therapy for patients with VD.

Rannasangpei (RSNP) (it is also known as *Ratna Samphel* or *70 Flavors Pearl Pill*), a traditional Tibetan medicine [10], acts as a multitarget therapeutic agent in the treatment of cerebrovascular diseases. It has enormous therapeutic efficacy as it contains many ingredients, which are obtained from herbal, nonherbal, and mineral sources [11, 12]. RSNP originated from the classical prescription of *Ershiwuwei Zhenzhu*

(*25 Flavors Pearl Pill*), which was recorded in the Tibetan medical masterpiece "Four Medical Tantra" in the 8th century. Thereafter, the classical prescription was improved and perfected by many generations of Tibetan physicians. The prescription used today was developed by Surkhar Nyamnyi Dorjé, a representative of the Southern School of Tibetan Medicine, in the mid-15th century. This Tibetan prescription mentions 70 different ingredients, including six superlative medicines [13], three myrobalan fruits [14], bellflower (*Codonopsis pilosula*), sandalwood (*lignum santali albi*), heartwood of rosewood (*lignun dalbergiae odoriferae*), bezoar (*calculus bovis*), and musk (*moschus*). RSNP also contains *Tsothel*—the king of essence [15]. *Tsothel* is a form of detoxified mercury, which is carefully prepared through a series of standard detoxifying processes. Calcinated powder, which is prepared from precious stones and metals, such as pearl, turquoise, coral, nine-eye stone, gold, silver, copper, and iron, is also included in RSNP [16]. Because RSNP is a confidential Tibetan prescription, its precise composition and preparation method have still been kept as a secret (see Pharmacopoeia of the People's Republic of China for details [17]).

For hundreds of years, RSNP has been widely used in the treatment of various acute or chronic cerebrovascular and neuropsychological diseases, such as hypertension, stroke, cerebral hemorrhage, cerebral embolism, sequelae of traumatic brain injury, cerebral concussion, epilepsy, and cognitive impairment [18]. In particular, there was significant improvement in cognitive symptoms and daily living of patients with Alzheimer's disease when they were treated with RSNP at a high altitude [12]. To understand its therapeutic mechanisms, various preclinical studies have been conducted. Previous studies showed that RSNP can suppress the occlusion of middle cerebral artery, which induces neurologic deficits; it exerts neuroprotective effects by increasing superoxide dismutase (SOD), reducing lipid peroxidation, and regulating neuron-specific enolase and S-100β protein levels [19, 20]. Furthermore, animal experiments have proved that RSNP improves Alzheimer's disease by either preventing or degrading the aggregation of beta-amyloid, which reduces the formation of senile plaque [21, 22]. However, no previous research study has reported about its therapeutic effect on patients with VD. Therefore, the therapeutic mechanism through which RSNP improves the condition of patients with VD is unclear.

To determine the therapeutic effect of RSNP on patients with VD, we used a VD model in rat, which was induced by permanent, bilateral common carotid artery occlusion (2VO) [23]. We also included the ginkgo biloba extract (EGB) as a positive control; it contains ginkgo flavone glycosides, ginkgolides, and bilobalide. EGB is a well-known free radical scavenger and antioxidant drug. It can increase cerebral blood flow, prevent thrombosis, improve brain functions, and enhance memory [24, 25]. We evaluated whether RSNP improved the cognitive functions of VD in the animal model. Thereafter, we further investigated its therapeutic mechanisms by determining factors, such as the alteration of central cholinergic system, oxidative stress, cell apoptosis, and the related molecular regulations.

2. Materials and Methods

2.1. Drugs and Preparation. RSNP was purchased from a medicine pharmaceutical company named JinHei Tibetan (Qinghai, China). In this study, RSNP solution was freshly prepared for oral administration. Pills of RSNP were first crushed into a fine powder using mortar and pestle and then dissolved in distilled water at final concentrations of 14.09 and 56.35 mg/mL in separate patches. To dissolve the powder in distilled water, we stirred the suspensions at 300 rpm on a magnetic stirrer (Tianjin Wei Yi Technology Development Company, Tianjin, China) at room temperature till uniform suspensions were produced. The injection volume was 5 mL/kg. EGB was provided by Dr. Willmar Schwabe Gmbh & Co. Kg (Karlsruhe, Germany), which was also dissolved in distilled water (3.41 mg/mL) for further use. The preparation of EGB was the same as that of RSNP. All the other chemicals and materials were obtained from Beijing Tibetan Hospital, which is affiliated to the China Tibetology Research Center, Beijing, China.

2.2. Animal Models and Experimental Study Design. We obtained healthy male Sprague-Dawley rats (aged 3 months, weighing 220 ± 20 grams) from Si Beifu Laboratory Animal Science and Technology Co., Ltd. (Beijing, China). The rats were placed in cages; each cage contained a group of five rats. The cages were maintained at room temperature (23 ± 2°C); a relative humidity of 55 ± 5% was maintained in these cages; these rats were subjected to a light-dark cycle of 12 h (light from 7 a.m.–7 p.m.). These rats were provided *ad libitum* access to food and water throughout the study. The experimental protocols were approved by the Ethics Committee of Beijing Tibetan Hospital, China Tibetology Research Center. The animal experiments were performed according to the regulations of laboratory animal management, which were promulgated by the Ministry of Science and Technology of the People's Republic of China [1988] number 134. These regulations are in accordance with the internationally recognized guidelines of National Institute of Health (NIH), New York City, NY, USA.

In this study, 50 rats were randomly divided into five groups: (1) sham-operated group; (2) 2VO-induced VD model group; (3) RSNP-L (low dose) + 2VO group; (4) RSNP-M (medium dose) + 2VO group; (5) EGB + 2VO group. The rats were kept in cages for a week before the 2VO or sham surgeries. Five days after the surgery, the animals were orally given a definite volume of indicated drugs (5 mL/kg) or distilled water (5 mL/kg) once every day for four weeks; the sham-operated group and the VD model group were given same volume of distilled water (5 mL/kg). The administered doses of RSNP were 70.44 mg/kg (low dose) and 281.76 mg/kg (medium dose); EGB was administered at a dosage of 17.03 mg/kg.

2.3. Preparation of VD Model. The VD model of rats was produced by the bilateral common carotid arteries occlusion (2VO) method [26]. In brief, rats were anesthetized with choral hydrate at a dosage of 350 mg/kg. Throughout the surgery, the rectal temperature was maintained at 37 ± 0.5°C by placing a heating pad underneath the rat. The bilateral common carotid arteries were exposed by incising the ventral midline neck. Then, these carotid arteries were gently separated from the attached muscles, adjacent blood vessels, and nerves using glass dissecting tools. The bilateral common carotid arteries were double ligated with silk suture; a cut was made between the ligations to ensure a permanent ligature. At the end of the surgery, both the muscle layer and the skin layer were closed. After the surgery, the wound was disinfected with iodophil for seven days. In the sham-operated animals, none of the arteries were ligated.

2.4. Learning and Memory Assessment. For determining the spatial learning and memory capability, we carried out Morris water maze (MWM) test on the animals, after completing the four-week drug administration [26]. The experiment was performed in a circular water pool (150 cm in diameter), which was filled with opaque water (water was mixed with black ink) at 23 ± 1°C till a depth of 30 cm. The pool was equally divided into 4 quadrants, and an escape platform (10 cm × 10 cm) was placed at the center of one quadrant; the escape platform was submerged 2 cm under the surface of water. A video camera, which was connected to a computer, was placed above the pool to record and track the swimming paths of rats for subsequent analysis. During the entire experiment, same spatial signs and decorations were maintained around the maze.

During the first five consecutive days, each animal was trained four times per day to find the hidden platform. Every time, they were placed in the maze at the different starting points of different quadrants. All the animals followed the same sequence of starting positions. During each trial, each animal was given 90 s to find and mount on the hidden platform; they were allowed to rest on the platform for 30 s. If the animal did not find the platform within 90 s, it was gently guided onto the platform by the observer. Then, the animal was allowed to rest on the platform for 30 s. In each trial, the escape latency, which was defined as the amount of time spent by the animal in locating and mounting on the platform, was recorded and analyzed using the video analysis system, EthoVision (Noldus Information Technology, Wageningen, The Netherlands). These trials were called navigation tests. On the sixth day, a probe test was performed. In this test, the platform was removed to assess the spatial learning and memory capability of these animals. The percentage of the swimming time and the distance covered in the target quadrant, where the platform was originally placed, were recorded and analyzed.

2.5. Determination of Central Cholinergic Neurotransmission and Oxidative Stress Using Biochemical Analysis. The cholinergic neurotransmission was determined by detecting the activities of choline acetyltransferase (ChAT) and acetylcholinesterase (AChE); the oxidative stress in the brain was assessed by measuring the activity of superoxide dismutase (SOD) and the level of malondialdehyde (MDA). After the MWM experiment, the animals were sacrificed by overdosed choral hydrate (0.35 g/kg). The brain was immediately removed and placed on an ice-cold sterilized surface. Then, the hippocampi from both sides of the brain were dissected and weighed. The hippocampus of one side was stored at −80°C, and it was later used for performing quantitative polymerase chain reaction (Q-PCR). The tissues of the hippocampus from the other side were homogenized at 4°C with nine times its volume of 0.1 M phosphate buffer (pH = 7.4). About half of the homogenate was centrifuged at 4000 ×g for 15 min; the supernatant was collected for determining the amount of ChAT, AChE, SOD, and MDA, which was using ELISA kits according to the manufacturer's instructions (Beijing Cheng Lin Biological Technology Co., Beijing, China). The remaining homogenate of hippocampus was stored at −80°C for performing Western blot analysis subsequently.

2.6. Detection of Apoptotic Protein Expression Using Western Blotting. The expression of apoptotic regulatory protein, B-cell lymphoma-2 (Bcl-2), as well as a decrease in the level of Bcl-2-associated X protein (Bax), was assessed by both Western blotting and Q-PCR. The remaining homogenate was centrifuged at 1600 ×g for 10 min at 4°C; the supernatant was collected and the total supernatant protein was determined by Bradford assay. Samples containing 40 μg of protein were denaturalized and separated on 10% sodium dodecyl sulfate polyacrylamide gel electrophoresis (SDS-PAGE) gels by electrophoresis. Then, the separated proteins were transferred onto nitrocellulose filter membranes. In Western blotting, the membranes were blocked for one hour with tris-buffered saline (TBS) containing 10% skimmed milk powder and 0.05% of Tween-20. Then, they were incubated for 2 h at 4°C with a primary antibody, which was diluted to 1 : 1000 in the blocking solution. In this experiment, the following primary antibodies were used: Bcl-2 antibody (mouse anti-rat, Novus Biologicals, USA), Bax antibody (mouse anti-rat, Abcam, Cambridge, UK), or β-actin antibody (rabbit anti-rat, Shanghai Kang Bioengineering Limited Company, Shanghai, China). The membranes were washed thrice with TBS containing 0.05% Tween-20 before they were incubated for 1.5 h at room temperature with a secondary antibody diluted to 1 : 5000 in the blocking solution. In this experiment, we used goat anti-rabbit IgG (Southern Biotech Associates, Birmingham, USA) as the secondary antibody. The relative intensity of the detected protein was quantified by gel image analysis system (Shanghai Day Technology Co., Shanghai, China).

2.7. Detection of Apoptotic mRNA Expression Using Real-Time Q-PCR. To determine the mRNA levels of Bcl-2, Bax, and β-actin n the hippocampus, real-time Q-PCR was performed. Total RNA was extracted from the hippocampus tissue using TRIzol reagent (Invitrogen, Carlsbad, USA). The purity as well as quantity of total RNA was detected by performing UV spectrophotometry using Biophotometer (Eppendorf, Hamburg, Germany). The integrity of the RNA was examined by performing agarose gels electrophoresis and visualized by an imaging system (Shanghai Day Technology Co., Shanghai,

TABLE 1: Primer sequences used for Q-PCR.

Gene name	Primer sequences	Product length
Bcl-2-F	5′-GGGACGCGAAGTGCTATTGGT-3′	208 bp
Bcl-2-R	5′-CTCAGGCTGGAAGGAGAAGAT-3′	208 bp
Bax-F	5′-GTTTCATCCAGGATCGAGCAGA-3′	265 bp
Bax-R	5′-GCAAAGTAGAAGAGGGCAACCAC-3′	265 bp
β-actin-F	5′ AGGGAAATCGTGCGTGACAT	150 p
β-actin-R	5′ GAACCGCTCATTGCCGATAG	150 p

China). The qualified total RNA samples were treated with DNase I, and they were reverse transcribed into cDNA using Oligo(dT)15 primer (Promega, Madison, USA) and M-MLV Reverse Transcriptase (Promega, Madison, USA) according to the manufacturer's instruction. Quantitative Q-PCR was performed using synthesized cDNA, specific primers of interested genes (Table 1), and 2x SYBR Green PCR Master Mix (TOYOBO, Osaka, Japan) under the following reaction conditions: 1 cycle of 95°C for 10 min, 40 cycles of 95°C for 15 s, 60°C for 15 s, and 72°C for 30 s (ABI PRISM® 7500 Sequence Detection System, Applied Biosystems, Foster City, USA). Each amplification was performed in triplet. After amplification, the melting curve was used to verify the specificity of PCR products. β-actin was considered as an internal reference for normalization. Thus, we analyzed the relative mRNA level of Bcl-2 or Bax using the comparative cycle threshold method [27].

2.8. Statistical Analysis. Data were presented as mean ± SD. A two-way repeat measures analysis of variance (ANOVA) was applied to analyze the escape latencies of different groups in MWM test over a period of five days. Other data were analyzed using one-way ANOVA followed by the least significant difference (LSD) test. All the statistical analyses were performed using SPSS version 20.0 (IBM, Armonk, NY, USA). The results were assumed to be statistically significant when $P < 0.05$.

3. Results

3.1. RSNP Improved the Spatial Learning and Memory Deficits Induced by 2VO. The MWM test was used to observe the effect of RSNP on the spatial learning and memory capability of VD rat model, which was induced by 2VO.

As shown in Figure 1(b), the result of escape latency in the navigation test indicated a significant decrease in the escape latency with the passage of time ($F = 924.053$, $P < 0.05$). This indicates that the animals were indeed learning to memorize the position of the platform. There was statistically significant difference among the groups ($F = 6.467$, $P < 0.05$); the statistically significant difference among the groups depended on the day on which the trial was carried out during the five days of navigation test ($F = 75.489$, $P < 0.05$). Post hoc analysis showed that there was no significant difference in the escape latency of different groups in the first two days ($P > 0.05$); however, significant difference was detected from day 3 till day 5 of the navigation test ($P < 0.05$). Compared with the sham-operated group, the model group demonstrated significantly higher escape latency in the last 3 days ($P < 0.05$). This indicates that a clear learning disability was developed in the VD model group. Compared with the VD model group, both the RSNP-M treatment group, which received RSNP at a medium dose (281.76 mg/kg), and the EGB treatment group had a significantly lower escape latency of VD animals on day 3 to day 5 ($P < 0.05$), while the group that received RSNP at a low dose (70.44 mg/kg) (RSNP-L) also showed lower escape latency of VD animals on day 3 and day 5 ($P < 0.05$). Owing to the difference between the two doses of RSNP, the RSNP-M group spent significantly less time in finding the platform than the RSNP-L group on day 3 to day 5 ($P < 0.05$); there was no significant difference between RSNP-M and EGB groups ($P > 0.05$). These results indicated that both doses of RSNP improved the learning disability of VD animals, which was induced by 2VO; the medium dose of RSNP probably showed a better effect than the low dosage, and there was no significant difference in the recovery of learning ability of VD animals in RSNP-M group and EGB group.

The probe test was performed one day after the navigation test. The platform was removed before conducting the probe test. The percentage of swimming time and the distance of the target quadrant were used as indicators of memory capacity (Figures 1(c) and 1(d)). Compared to the sham-operated group, the VD model group spent considerably lesser time and covered lesser distance in the target quadrant ($P < 0.05$). This indicates that a memory deficit was induced by 2VO. In the RSNP-M and EGB groups, the VD animals' focus on the target quadrant was significantly better than those of the model group ($P < 0.05$); however, the memory capacity of RSNP-L group was not better than that of model group. Compared with the RSNP-L group, RSNP-M and EGB groups covered a significantly greater distance in the target quadrant ($P < 0.05$). Moreover, there was no significant difference between RSNP-M and EGB groups ($P > 0.05$). The results indicate that only a medium dose of RSNP alleviated the spatial memory deficit, which was previously induced in the experimental animals by 2VO.

In summary, RSNP treatment significantly improved the impaired learning and memory in the VD animal model. Furthermore, medium doses of RSNP definitely brought about a better improvement.

3.2. Effect of RSNP on the Cholinergic Activity of the Hippocampus of VD Animals. Since cholinergic neurotransmission was closely associated with the ability of learning and memory, we wanted to determine whether RSNP improved the learning and memory deficits in the VD animals by altering the cholinergic activities in the hippocampus. Therefore, we measured the levels of ChAT and AChE in the hippocampus of VD animals. The results (Figure 2) indicate that, in the model group, the level of ChAT was significantly lower than that in the sham-operated control group ($P < 0.05$). After being treated with either RSNP (70.44 or 281.76 mg/kg) or EGB, the level of ChAT in the treatment groups was

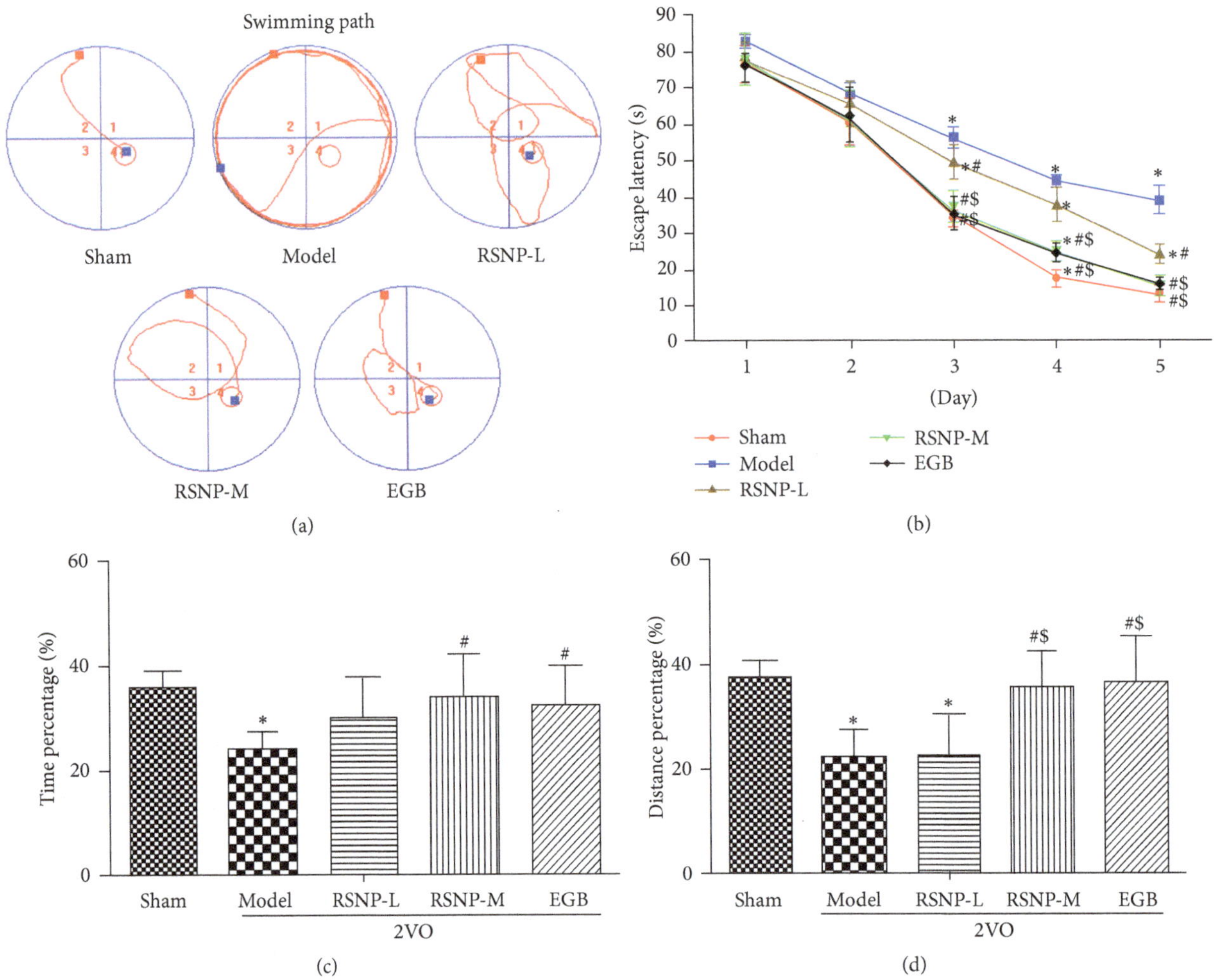

FIGURE 1: RSNP improves the impaired spatial learning and memory capability in VD animal model, which is proved by MWM test. (a) Representative pathways on the fifth day of navigation test, red block: start position, blue block: platform position; (b) escape latencies of rats in each group; (c) percentage of the time spent in the target quadrant in the probe test; (d) percentage of distance in the target quadrant in the probe test. Values were expressed as mean ± SD. Sham or sham-operated: sham-operated group; model: 2VO induced VD model group; RSNP-L: the group of VD model, which was administered with 70.44 mg/kg of RSNP for four weeks after the surgery; RSNP-M: the group of VD model, which was administered with 281.76 mg/kg of RSNP for four weeks after the surgery; EGB: the group of VD model, which was administered with 17.03 mg/kg of EGB for four weeks after the surgery; $n = 10$ per group; ∗: compared to the sham-operated group, $P < 0.05$; #: compared to the model group, $P < 0.05$; $: compared to the RSNP-L group, $P < 0.05$.

significantly higher than that in the nontreated model group ($P < 0.05$). However, the level of ChAT was not completely restored to normal levels in the control group ($P < 0.05$).

Inversely, the content of AChE in the VD model group was significantly higher than that in the control group ($P < 0.05$); however, the AChE activity clearly decreased to normal levels in VD animals when they were treated with either RSNP or EGB ($P < 0.05$). Compared with the RSNP-L group, the RSNP-M treatment group showed a better recovery ($P < 0.05$). Furthermore, there was no significant difference between RSNP-M and EGB groups ($P > 0.05$).

These results indicate that there is a correlation between learning and memory capacity and cholinergic activity in the hippocampus. Both low and medium doses of RSNP could restore the altered cholinergic activity to normal levels in VD animals; however, the VD animals treated with the medium dose of RSNP showed better improvement in cholinergic activity.

3.3. Effect of RSNP on the Oxidative Stress Induced by 2VO in the Hippocampus. We also wanted to determine the effect of RSNP on oxidative stress, which plays a crucial role in damaging the brain of VD animals. For this purpose, we measured the levels of total SOD and MDA in the hippocampus (Figure 3). The results indicate that, in the VD model group, the total SOD was significantly lower than that in the sham-operated control group ($P < 0.05$). After being treated with either RSNP (70.44 or 281.76 mg/kg) or EGB, the activity of total SOD in VD animals increased sharply to become significantly higher than that in the model group

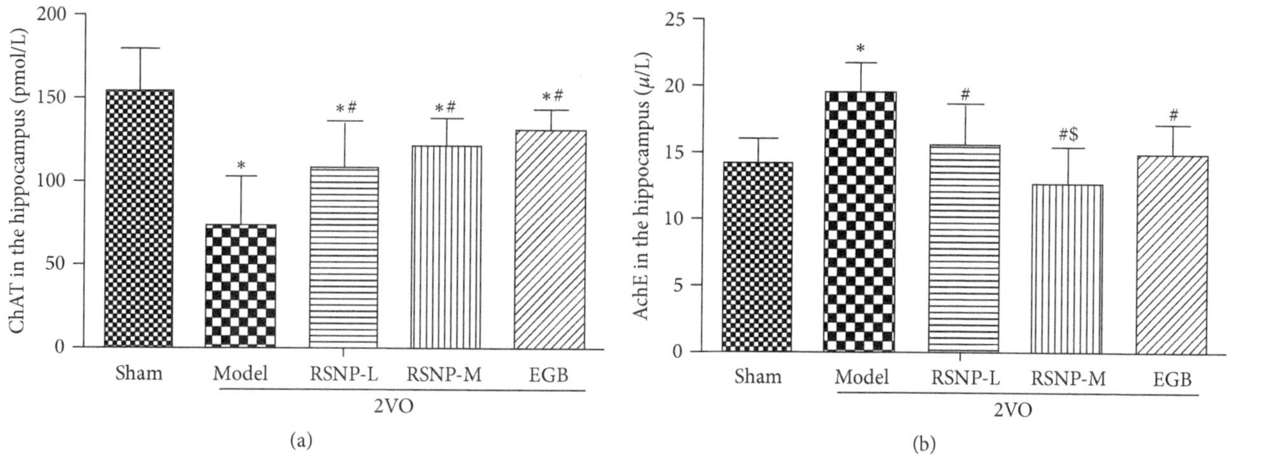

FIGURE 2: Effect of RSNP on the levels of ChAT (a), AChE (b) in the hippocampus of 2VO-induced VD rats. All the data were shown as mean ± SD, $n = 10$ per group. $^{*}P < 0.05$, compared with the sham-operated group; $^{\#}P < 0.05$, compared with the model group; $^{\$}P < 0.05$, compared with the RSNP-L group.

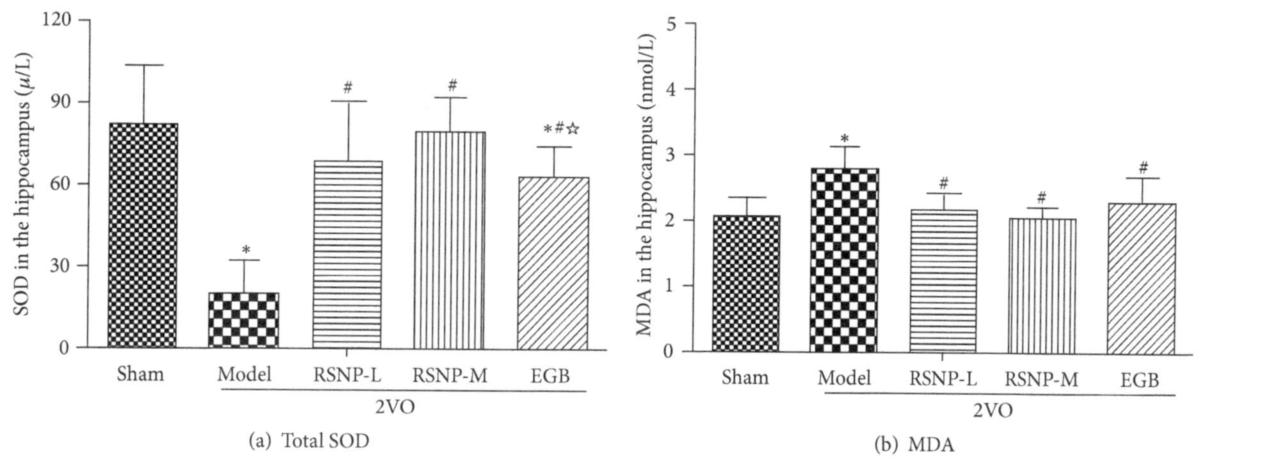

FIGURE 3: Effect of RSNP on the abnormal activity of SOD (a) and MDA (b) in the hippocampus of 2VO-induced VD rats. All data were shown as mean ± SD, $n = 10$ per group. $^{*}P < 0.05$, compared to the sham-operated group; $^{\#}P < 0.05$, compared with the VD model group; $^{☆}P < 0.05$, compared with the RSNP-M group.

($P < 0.05$). Furthermore, in RSNP-M treatment group, the activity of SOD was even higher than that in EGB group ($P < 0.05$).

The content of MDA in the hippocampus of VD model group was significantly higher than that in the sham-operated control group ($P < 0.05$). Both doses of RSNP could effectively reduce the abnormally higher levels of MDA. Moreover, the abnormally higher MDA levels were also restored to normal levels in EGB group ($P < 0.05$). No significant difference was observed between RSNP and EGB groups ($P > 0.05$).

These results indicated that, in the VD animal model, RSNP could significantly decrease the oxidative stress induced by 2VO. Therefore, this Tibetan prescription has numerous beneficial effects on the brain.

3.4. Effects of RSNP on Apoptosis Regulatory Factors, Bcl-2 and Bax, and the Ratio of Bcl-2/Bax in the Hippocampus of VD Rat Model. To determine the effect of RSNP on the apoptosis regulatory factors, Bcl-2 and Bax, in this VD animal model, we used Western blotting analysis to detect the protein expression of Bcl-2 and Bax (Figure 4(a)). Then, a semiquantitative measurement was used to determine the ratio of Bcl-2/Bax (Figure 4(b)). The Western blotting results indicate that there was a decrease in the protein expression of Bcl-2, while the protein expression of Bax increased in the VD animal model. Furthermore, both RSNP (70.44 or 281.76 mg/kg) and EGB restored the protein expression of Bcl-2 and Bax to normal levels (the sham-operated control group showed normal levels of Bcl-2 and Bax) at different degrees. The result of semiquantitative analysis confirmed

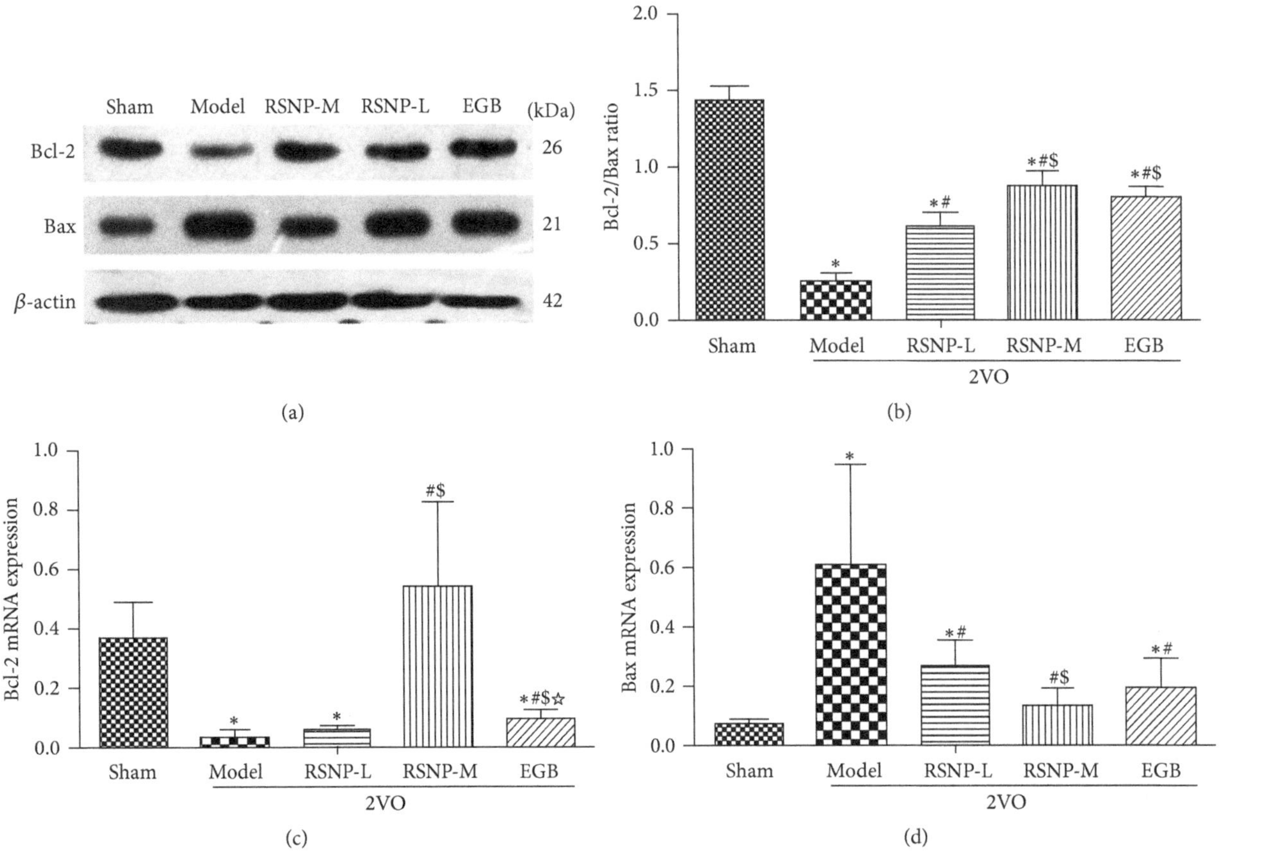

FIGURE 4: Effects of RSNP on the Bax and Bcl-2 levels in the hippocampus of VD model induced by 2VO. After completing the behavior test, the hippocampus was segregated and used to assess the expression of Bax and Bcl-2 by Western blot analysis (a). The intensities of Bcl-2 and Bax protein bands were used to determine the Bax/Bcl-2 ratio (b). The transcript levels of Bcl-2 (c) and Bax (d) genes in the hippocampus were also measured to verify the profile of protein expression. All the data were shown as mean ± SD, $n = 10$ per group. $^*P < 0.05$, compared with the sham-operated group; $^\#P < 0.05$, compared with the VD model group; $^\$P < 0.05$, compared with the RSNP-L group. $^☆P < 0.05$, compared with the RSNP-M group.

this observation: it showed a significant reduction in the Bcl-2/Bax ratio in VD model group ($P < 0.05$). Both RSNP and EGB could effectively prevent the 2VO-induced upregulation of Bax and the downregulation of Bcl-2. Therefore, the Bcl-2/Bax ratio was significantly increased ($P < 0.05$) in VD animals when they were treated with either RSNP or EGB. Compared with RSNP-L group, the RSNP-M and EGB groups had a higher Bcl-2/Bax ratio ($P < 0.05$). There was no significant difference between RSNP-M and EGB groups ($P > 0.05$).

To verify the protein expression data obtained by Western blotting, we performed real-time Q-PCR to examine the transcript levels of Bcl-2 and Bax (Figures 4(c) and 4(d)). The Q-PCR results indeed confirmed the protein expression of Bcl-2 and Bax. This indicates that when the VD animals were treated with RSNP (70.44 and 281.76 mg/kg) for four weeks, the abnormal transcript levels of Bcl-2 and Bax were improved in the hippocampus of VD rats; moreover, the medium dose of RSNP was more effective than the low dose of RSNP on both transcripts ($P < 0.05$). Interestingly, the RSNP-M group demonstrated a more protective effect than the EGB group, as indicated by the transcript level of Bcl-2 in the VD animals after the treatments ($P < 0.05$).

4. Discussion

In this study, we used the 2VO method to induce VD in experimental animals. This method was also used to prepare the model of chronic cerebral ischemia [28, 29] in which a persistent ischemia was developed in the animal's brain, causing cognitive dysfunction. Our current VD model showed serious impairment of learning and memory, which was caused by cerebral hypoperfusion [7, 30]. Therefore, this VD model was suitable for investigating the pharmacological mechanisms of RSNP, which has therapeutic effects on VD. After a 4-week oral administration of RSNP, the ability of learning and memory was improved greatly in the VD animal model. Further investigations proved that RSNP improved the cognitive dysfunction in VD animals by regulating cholinergic neurotransmission, reducing oxidative stress, and managing apoptotic regulators, such as Bax and Bcl-2, in the hippocampal area.

Although China is a multiethnic country, most people are of the Han Chinese race. In China, there are two major alternative systems of medicine: traditional Chinese medicine and ethnic medicine. Ethnic medicine has been quite effective in treating certain diseases. Traditional Tibetan medicine is one of the representative branches of ethnic medicine, and it has been practiced for many centuries [31]. RSNP, one of the most famous formulations of Tibetan medicine, is used to treat a wide range of diseases, such as hypertension, stroke, cerebral infarction, cerebral hemorrhage, and cardiomyopathy [18]. Previous research studies have reported that RSNP can be used to greatly reduce amnesia in patients with Alzheimer's disease [12, 32]. In this study, after administering RSNP orally for four weeks, the animals of VD model showed significantly lower escape latency in the navigation test. Moreover, in the probe test, their swimming time and distance in the target quadrant were also significantly lower. These results indicate that RSNP is efficient in improving the dysfunction of spatial learning and memory.

Central cholinergic system plays an important role in the spatial learning and memory. Acetylcholine (ACh), the actual neurotransmitter, is synthesized from a reaction between choline and acetyl coenzyme A; this reaction is catalyzed by ChAT in cholinergic synapses. After ACh is released into synaptic cleft, AChE rapidly degrades it to avoid excessive cholinergic neurotransmission. Therefore, ChAT and AChE actively control the homeostasis of cholinergic system [33]. In patients with cerebral ischemia, the lesions are located in the hippocampus and cortex where the activity of ChAT increases, while the activity of AChE decreases. As a result, the synthesis of ACh is reduced, resulting in the dysfunction of cholinergic system. All these events cause the disability of learning and memory, which eventually leads to dementia in these patients [34]. In this study, both doses of RSNP were effective in reducing AChE and enhancing ChAT activity. This indicates that RSNP improves impaired learning and memory in VD animal model by increasing cholinergic neurotransmission.

Free radicals are found extensively in organisms. They cause damage to proteins and DNAs, triggering serious diseases [35–37]. There were many endogenous antioxidants in the human body, including SOD, catalase, and cytochrome. These antioxidants scavenge free radicals and maintain a dynamic equilibrium. However, oxidative stress is significant in patients with cerebral ischemia. Since the brain is rich in lipids, free radicals can easily stimulate lipid peroxidation [38], leading to the generation of many toxic free radicals; these free radicals cannot be scavenged by the endogenous antioxidants in a timely manner. Therefore, these excessive free radicals cause damage to proteins and DNAs, triggering an intense damage to the brain [39]. SOD, which was an important antioxidant enzyme in the body, can remove superoxide anion radicals and inhibit lipid peroxidation. Thus, it can protect cells from further damage [40]. On the other hand, MDA is a product of lipid peroxidation; its content in the brain indicates not only the level of lipid peroxidation but also the severity with which body cells are attacked by free radicals [28, 41]. In this study, we have measured the activity of SOD and the level of MDA in the hippocampus to estimate the antioxidant activity and the level of oxidative stress, respectively. RSNP efficiently recovered the pathologically reduced SOD and the increased MDA in VD animals induced with 2VO surgery. This indicates that RSNP is beneficial to the animals of VD model as it eliminates the excessive accumulation of free radicals, which are produced due to chronic cerebral ischemia.

Hippocampus, a crucial structure that governs learning ability and memory, is found to be closely associated with spatial cognitive function. Therefore, it is very vulnerable to apoptosis in patients inflicted with brain ischemia and hypoperfusion. Previous studies have reported that the Bcl-2 protein family plays a vital role in the regulation of apoptosis [42]. Bcl-2 and Bax are the two major factors influencing the regulation of apoptosis; Bcl-2 prevents the release of cytochrome C from mitochondria, and it also activates caspases to inhibit apoptosis. In contrast, Bax protein directly induces the release of cytochrome C from mitochondria into the cytoplasm, thereby promoting apoptosis [43]. To further explore the function of RSNP in inhibiting cell apoptosis, we performed Western blot and real-time Q-PCR. With these methods, we detected the expression levels of Bcl-2 and Bax both as protein and as mRNA. In the VD model group, the level of Bax increased significantly, while the level of Bcl-2 decreased significantly. After the administration of RSNP for four weeks, the level of Bcl-2 increased significantly, while the level of Bax decreased. Thus, the Bcl-2/Bax ratio increased in VD animals. This result indicated that RSNP reduces apoptosis in the brain by regulating the levels of Bcl-2 and Bax.

For many centuries, RSNP has been widely used in the treatment of chronic cerebrovascular diseases and neural system diseases, but the therapeutic mechanisms of RSNP have not yet been deciphered. Ours was the first study to elucidate the neuroprotective effects of RSNP in the animal model of VD. The protective mechanisms of RSNP probably involve the reduction of oxidative stress, which ultimately leads to a decrease in proapoptotic Bax/Bcl-2 ratio and the restoration of cholinergic neurotransmission. A medium dose of RSNP (281.76 mg/kg) provided neuroprotective effects, which were the same as those offered by EGB. This study proves that RSNP can be considered as a potential therapeutic agent in the treatment of VD.

Competing Interests

The authors declare that they have no conflict of interests.

Authors' Contributions

Yuandai Luo and Peng Wu collaborated equally to this work.

Acknowledgments

This work was supported by the National Special Financial Foundation in China (1981420400011).

References

[1] T. L. Sudduth, D. K. Powell, C. D. Smith, A. Greenstein, and D. M. Wilcock, "Induction of hyperhomocysteinemia models vascular dementia by induction of cerebral microhemorrhages and neuroinflammation," *Journal of Cerebral Blood Flow and Metabolism*, vol. 33, no. 5, pp. 708–715, 2013.

[2] A. R. Ramos, S. I. Dib, and C. B. Wright, "Vascular dementia," *Current Translational Geriatrics and Experimental Gerontology Reports*, vol. 2, no. 3, pp. 188–195, 2013.

[3] J. Yuan, Z. Zhang, H. Wen et al., "Incidence of dementia and subtypes: a cohort study in four regions in China," *Alzheimer's and Dementia*, vol. 12, no. 3, pp. 262–271, 2016.

[4] R. N. Kalaria, G. E. Maestre, R. Arizaga et al., "Alzheimer's disease and vascular dementia in developing countries: prevalence, management, and risk factors," *The Lancet Neurology*, vol. 7, no. 9, pp. 812–826, 2008.

[5] G. C. Román, T. Erkinjuntti, A. Wallin, L. Pantoni, and H. C. Chui, "Subcortical ischaemic vascular dementia," *Lancet Neurology*, vol. 1, no. 7, pp. 426–436, 2002.

[6] H. Liu and J. Zhang, "Cerebral hypoperfusion and cognitive impairment: the pathogenic role of vascular oxidative stress," *International Journal of Neuroscience*, vol. 122, no. 9, pp. 494–499, 2012.

[7] Y. Xi, M. Wang, W. Zhang et al., "Neuronal damage, central cholinergic dysfunction and oxidative damage correlate with cognitive deficits in rats with chronic cerebral hypoperfusion," *Neurobiology of Learning and Memory*, vol. 109, pp. 7–19, 2014.

[8] S. Deiana, B. Platt, and G. Riedel, "The cholinergic system and spatial learning," *Behavioural Brain Research*, vol. 221, no. 2, pp. 389–411, 2011.

[9] K. Toyama, N. Koibuchi, K. Uekawa et al., "Apoptosis signal-regulating kinase 1 is a novel target molecule for cognitive impairment induced by chronic cerebral hypoperfusion," *Arteriosclerosis, Thrombosis, and Vascular Biology*, vol. 34, no. 3, pp. 616–625, 2014.

[10] K. P. Reuter, T. E. Weißhuhn, and C. M. Witt, "Tibetan medicine: a systematic review of the clinical research available in the west," *Evidence-Based Complementary and Alternative Medicine*, vol. 2013, Article ID 213407, 16 pages, 2013.

[11] M.-C. Wan, J.-S. Lou, and Y.-W. Qin, "Application of Rannasangpei in the treatment of cardiovascular and cerebrovascular diseases," *Pharmaceutical Care and Research*, vol. 9, no. 4, pp. 283–285, 2009.

[12] A. Zhu, "P2-376: effect of tibet medicine in patients with Alzheimer's disease at high altitude," *Alzheimer's & Dementia*, vol. 4, no. 4, p. T483, 2008.

[13] B. Clark, *The Quintessence Tantras of Tibetan Medicine*, Shambhala Publications, 2014.

[14] T. Dakpa, "Unique aspect of tibetan medicine," *Acupuncture and Electro-Therapeutics Research*, vol. 39, no. 1, pp. 27–43, 2014.

[15] X. Y. Zhao, M. Sun, J. X. Wang et al., "Characterization of tibetan medicine zuota by multiple techniques," *Bioinorganic Chemistry and Applications*, vol. 2013, Article ID 198545, 11 pages, 2013.

[16] Men-Tsee-Khang (Tibetan Medical & Astro. Institute). Precious Pill: Rinchen Ratna Samphel, http://www.men-tsee-khang.org/medicine/rinchen-pills/ratna.htm.

[17] C. Commission, *Pharmacopoeia of the People's Republic of China*, China Medical Science Press, Beijing, China, 2015.

[18] W. B. Du, F. K. Huang, Y. D. Shaouo, L. F. Zhen, Y. L. Liu, and Y. Shang, "Progress in pharmacological and clinical research of Qishiwei Zhenzhu Wan," *Chinese Journal of Experimental Traditional Medical Formulae*, vol. 6, article 107, 2013.

[19] L. Zhen, Y. Luo, F. Huang et al., "Neural protective effect of Rannasangpei on local cerebral ischemia in rats," *Pharmacology and Clinics of Chinese Materia Medica*, vol. 30, no. 1, pp. 90–92, 2014.

[20] L. Zhen, Y. Luo, and F. Huang, "Effect of rannasangpei on the SOD, CAT and MDA in brain tissues of rats with local cerebral ischemia," *World Journal of Traditional Chinese Medicine*, vol. 9, no. 3, pp. 347–354, 2014.

[21] Z. Bai, E. Jin, and X. Lu, "Effects of Tibetan Medicine Panansongpei on learning memory functions and superoxide dismutase and maleic dialdehyde in Alzheimer's disease model rats," *Journal of Qinghai Medical College*, vol. 32, no. 1, pp. 29–31, 2011.

[22] Q. Zhu, D. Zhu, and G. Li, "Effect of Tibet-medicine Ratanasampil on serum β-amyloid protein and inflamatory cytokine levels in patients with Alzheimer's disease," *Chinese Journal of Geriatrics*, vol. 30, no. 2, pp. 133–137, 2011.

[23] N. S. Jiwa, P. Garrard, and A. H. Hainsworth, "Experimental models of vascular dementia and vascular cognitive impairment: a systematic review," *Journal of Neurochemistry*, vol. 115, no. 4, pp. 814–828, 2010.

[24] N. Bachinskaya, R. Hoerr, and R. Ihl, "Alleviating neuropsychiatric symptoms in dementia: the effects of Ginkgo biloba extract EGb 761®. Findings from a randomized controlled trial," *Neuropsychiatric Disease and Treatment*, vol. 7, no. 1, pp. 209–215, 2011.

[25] S. Gauthier and S. Schlaefke, "Efficacy and tolerability of Ginkgo biloba extract EGb 761(R) in dementia: a systematic review and meta-analysis of randomized placebo-controlled trials," *Clinical Interventions in Aging*, vol. 9, pp. 2065–2077, 2014.

[26] C. Liu, J. Wu, J. Gu et al., "Baicalein improves cognitive deficits induced by chronic cerebral hypoperfusion in rats," *Pharmacology Biochemistry and Behavior*, vol. 86, no. 3, pp. 423–430, 2007.

[27] K. J. Livak and T. D. Schmittgen, "Analysis of relative gene expression data using real-time quantitative PCR and the $2^{-\Delta\Delta CT}$ method," *Methods*, vol. 25, no. 4, pp. 402–408, 2001.

[28] R.-R. Zhao, F. Xu, X.-C. Xu et al., "Effects of alpha-lipoic acid on spatial learning and memory, oxidative stress, and central cholinergic system in a rat model of vascular dementia," *Neuroscience Letters*, vol. 587, pp. 113–119, 2015.

[29] H.-J. Ji, J.-F. Hu, Y.-H. Wang, X.-Y. Chen, R. Zhou, and N.-H. Chen, "Osthole improves chronic cerebral hypoperfusion induced cognitive deficits and neuronal damage in hippocampus," *European Journal of Pharmacology*, vol. 636, no. 1–3, pp. 96–101, 2010.

[30] Y. Peng, S. Xu, G. Chen, L. Wang, Y. Feng, and X. Wang, "l-3-n-Butylphthalide improves cognitive impairment induced by chronic cerebral hypoperfusion in rats," *Journal of Pharmacology and Experimental Therapeutics*, vol. 321, no. 3, pp. 902–910, 2007.

[31] J. V. Alphen and A. Aris, *Oriental Medicine: An Illustrated Guide to the Asian Arts of Healing*, Serindia, 1995.

[32] B. X. Liao, A. Q. Zhu, and A. Q. Xi, "Effect of Ratnasampil on Alzheimer's disease patient's cognitive function and oxidative stress," *Chinese Journal of Gerontology*, vol. 19, p. 11, 2009.

[33] A. Blokland, "Acetylcholine: a neurotransmitter for learning and memory?" *Brain Research Reviews*, vol. 21, no. 3, pp. 285–300, 1995.

[34] H. Ishimaru, A. Takahashi, Y. Ikarashi, and Y. Maruyama, "Effect of transient cerebral ischaemia on acetylcholine release in the gerbil hippocampus," *NeuroReport*, vol. 5, no. 5, pp. 601–604, 1994.

[35] R. A. Floyd and J. M. Carney, "Free radical damage to protein and DNA: mechanisms involved and relevant observations on brain undergoing oxidative stress," *Annals of Neurology*, vol. 32, pp. S22–S27, 1992.

[36] B. A. Freeman and J. D. Crapo, "Biology of disease: free radicals and tissue injury," *Laboratory Investigation*, vol. 47, no. 5, pp. 412–426, 1982.

[37] B. K. Siesjö, C. D. Agardh, and F. Bengtsson, "Free radicals and brain damage," *Cerebrovascular and Brain Metabolism Reviews*, vol. 1, no. 3, pp. 165–211, 1989.

[38] S. Yoshida, S. Inoh, T. Asano et al., "Effect of transient ischemia on free fatty acids and phospholipids in the gerbil brain. Lipid peroxidation as a possible cause of postischemic injury," *Journal of Neurosurgery*, vol. 53, no. 3, pp. 323–331, 1980.

[39] S. Love, "Oxidative stress in brain ischemia," *Brain Pathology*, vol. 9, no. 1, pp. 119–131, 1999.

[40] P. H. Chan, "Role of oxidants in ischemic brain damage," *Stroke*, vol. 27, no. 6, pp. 1124–1129, 1996.

[41] H. Liu, M. Zhao, S. Yang, D.-R. Gong, D.-Z. Chen, and D.-Y. Du, "(2*R*,3*S*)-Pinobanksin-3-cinnamate improves cognition and reduces oxidative stress in rats with vascular dementia," *Journal of Natural Medicines*, vol. 69, no. 3, pp. 358–365, 2015.

[42] J. C. Reed, "Proapoptotic multidomain Bcl-2/Bax-family proteins: mechanisms, physiological roles, and therapeutic opportunities," *Cell Death and Differentiation*, vol. 13, no. 8, pp. 1378–1386, 2006.

[43] L. Wu, Q.-S. Zhao, T.-W. Li et al., "Yifei Xuanfei Jiangzhuo formula, a Chinese herbal decoction, improves memory impairment through inhibiting apoptosis and enhancing PKA/CREB signal transduction in rats with cerebral ischemia/reperfusion," *Molecular Medicine Reports*, vol. 12, no. 3, pp. 4273–4283, 2015.

14

The *In Vitro* and *In Vivo* Wound Healing Properties of the Chinese Herbal Medicine "Jinchuang Ointment"

Tsung-Jung Ho,[1,2,3] Shinn-Jong Jiang,[4] Guang-Huey Lin,[5] Tzong Shiun Li,[6,7,8] Lih-Ming Yiin,[9] Jai-Sing Yang,[10] Ming-Chuan Hsieh,[5] Chun-Chang Wu,[1] Jaung-Geng Lin,[11] and Hao-Ping Chen[4]

[1] *Division of Chinese Medicine, China Medical University Beigang Hospital, Yulin 65152, Taiwan*
[2] *Division of Chinese Medicine, An Nan Hospital, China Medical University, Tainan 70965, Taiwan*
[3] *College of Chinese Medicine, China Medical University, Taichung 40421, Taiwan*
[4] *Department of Biochemistry, School of Medicine, Tzu Chi University, Hualien 97004, Taiwan*
[5] *Department of Microbiology, School of Medicine, Tzu Chi University, Hualien 97004, Taiwan*
[6] *Department of Plastic Surgery, China Medical University Beigang Hospital, Yulin 65152, Taiwan*
[7] *School of Medicine, China Medical University, Taichung 40421, Taiwan*
[8] *Department of Plastic Surgery, China Medical University Hospital, Taichung 40447, Taiwan*
[9] *Department of Public Health, School of Medicine, Tzu Chi University, Hualien 97004, Taiwan*
[10] *Department of Medical Research, China Medical University Hospital, China Medical University, Taichung 40447, Taiwan*
[11] *Graduate Institute of Chinese Medicine, China Medical University, Taichung 40421, Taiwan*

Correspondence should be addressed to Shinn-Jong Jiang; sjjiang@mail.tcu.edu.tw and Hao-Ping Chen; hpchen@mail.tcu.edu.tw

Academic Editor: Yoshiji Ohta

"Jinchuang ointment" is a traditional Chinese herbal medicine complex for treatment of incised wounds. For more than ten years, it has been used at China Medical University Hospital (Taichung, Taiwan) for the treatment of diabetic foot infections and decubitus ulcers. Three different cases are presented in this study. "Jinchuang" ointment is a mixture of natural product complexes from nine different components, making it difficult to analyze its exact chemical compositions. To further characterize the herbal ingredients used in this study, the contents of reference standards present in a subset of the ointment ingredients (dragon's blood, catechu, frankincense, and myrrh) were determined by HPLC. Two *in vitro* cell based assay platforms, wound healing and tube formation, were used to examine the biological activity of this medicine. Our results show that this herbal medicine possesses strong activities including stimulation of angiogenesis, cell proliferation, and cell migration, which provide the scientific basis for its clinically observed curative effects on nonhealing diabetic wounds.

1. Introduction

It is well-known that diabetic foot ulcers are extremely difficult to be treated and are the dominant complication leading to amputations [1]. "Jinchuang ointment" is a traditional Chinese herbal medicine complex for treatment of incised wounds. Its recipe was first described in one ancient Chinese book of medicine, *Medicine Comprehended*, published in 1732. Clinical applications of this herbal medicine for diabetic foot infections and decubitus ulcers have been a successful course of treatment in the Division of Chinese Medicine, China Medical University Hospital, Taichung, Taiwan, for more than ten years. Despite its track record of curative effects, there is no literature published in the English language describing the clinical efficacy of "Jinchuang ointment" [2]. Moreover, neither a biological mechanism nor the compositions of effective components have yet to be systematically investigated. Like many Chinese herbal medicines, "Jinchuang ointment" is also a mixture of natural product complexes. The combination of compounds results in complications when it determines the chemical composition and bioactivity of each component [3].

"Jinchuang ointment" is composed of lard, wax, starch, synthetic borneol, camphor, frankincense, dragon's blood, myrrh, and catechu. To further characterize the chemical content of each component in this complex, the ratio of stereoisomers in chemically synthesized borneol used in this study was analyzed by chiral gas chromatography (GC). Meanwhile, the content of reference standards in the herbal components, like frankincense, myrrh, dragon's blood, and catechin, was determined by high performance liquid chromatography (HPLC). Lard is the major component in this complex, and its weight percentage is as high as 67%. It is of great interest to determine the role of lard in this complex. Lard was therefore substituted for synthetic triacylglycerol, coconut oil, Vaseline®, and sesame oil. The activity of these reconstituted complexes was examined in this study.

"Jinchuang ointment" is directly applied to the wound surface during treatment. The components in this complex are neither digested nor absorbed in the gastrointestinal tract. It is therefore reasonable to evaluate its bioactivity by direct addition of this complex into media containing cultured human skin or endothelial cells. Wound healing is a very complicated process. In this study, an *in vitro* tube formation assay, a wound healing assay, and a cell proliferation test were carried out to examine the activity of "Jinchuang ointment." Here, we report the outcomes of treating patients with "Jinchuang ointment," the results of cell based activity assays, and characterization of herbal components by HPLC.

2. Materials and Methods

2.1. Materials. The reference standards of dracorhodin perchlorate, acetyl-11-keto-β-boswellic acid, catechin, and epicatechin were purchased from the National Institute for the Control of Pharmaceutical and Biological Products (Beijing, China). (E)-Guggulsterone and (+)-borneol were obtained from Sigma-Aldrich (St. Louis, MO, USA). (−)-Borneol and (±)-isoborneol were purchased from Alfa Assar (Lancashire, UK). DMEM high glucose with sodium pyruvate media, Catalog number: I-26F55-I, was bought from Amimed® BioConcept (Allschwil, Switzerland). Chemically synthesized borneol and camphor were bought from Cheng Yi Chemical Co., Ltd. (Taipei, Taiwan). Herbal medicine, dragon's blood, catechu, frankincense, and myrrh were bought from Healthy Beautiful Biotech. Co. Ltd. (Taichung, Taiwan). Vascular endothelial growth factor (VEGF) was bought from B&D Systems (Minneapolis, MN, USA). Antibodies for western blot analysis were bought from Santa Cruz Biotechnology, Inc. (Dallas, Texas, USA). Food-grade lard was obtained from I-Mei Food Company (Taipei, Taiwan). Synthetic triacylglycerol (glyceryl tricaprylate-caprate, $C_8 : C_{10}$, 60 : 40) was obtained from InterMed Manufacturing Sdn. Bhd. (Kuala Lumpur, Malaysia). Food-grade sesame oil was from Fwusow Industry Co. Ltd. (Taichung, Taiwan). Coconut oil was bought from First Chemical Co., Ltd. (Taipei, Taiwan). Vaseline was bought from Unilever (Trumbull, Connecticut, USA).

The composition of "Jinchuang ointment" (100 g) is as follows: lard 67.3 g, dragon's blood 2.1 g, catechu 2.1 g, frankincense 2.1 g, myrrh 2.1 g, camphor 6.3 g, borneol 0.1 g, corn starch 8.4 g, and wax 9.5 g. For wound healing and tube formation assays, the DMSO stock solution of "Jinchuang ointment" is prepared as follows: two grams of "Jinchuang ointment" is dissolved in 10 mL DMSO and homogenized by ultrasonication just before use.

2.2. Determination of Reference Standard Content in Dragon's Blood, Catechu, Frankincense, and Myrrh by HPLC. All experiments were carried out on a Hitachi L-7000 HPLC system, equipped with L-7100 quaternary gradient pump and a L-7450 photo diode array detector. Hitachi HSM software was used for machine controlling, data collecting, and processing. A Mightysil, RP-18, 5 μm, 250 × 4.6 mm, analytic column (Kanto Chemical Co., Inc., Tokyo, Japan) was used for analysis.

For samples of dragon's blood, catechu, and frankincense, 0.1 g grounded solids were weighed and dissolved in 10 mL of methanol. After ultrasonicating for 30 minutes at room temperature, methanol extracts were transferred to a new glass vial by using disposable glass Pasteur pipettes. 4 mL of methanol was then added and ultrasonicated for another 30 minutes at room temperature. The final volume of the extract was adjusted to 25 mL by adding methanol. Undissolved particles were removed by centrifugation at 2500 ×g for 10 minutes at room temperature and filtrated through a 0.22 μm syringe filter. For myrrh, 95% ethanol was used for extraction rather than methanol. Other preparation steps were identical to those of dragon's blood, catechu, frankincense, and myrrh.

The methanol extract of dragon's blood was separated using a gradient elution of solvent A (10% CH_3CN containing 0.1% formic acid) and solvent B (90% CH_3CN containing 0.1% formic acid) with a flow rate of 1 mL/min [4]. The elution program is given in Table 1. The UV detection wavelength was 254 nm.

The catechu methanol extract was separated using a gradient elution of A (H_2O containing 0.1% formic acid), B (10% CH_3CN containing 0.1% formic acid), and C (90% CH_3CN containing 0.1% formic acid) with a flow rate of 1 mL/min [5]. The elution program is given in Table 1. The UV detection wavelength was 270 nm.

The frankincense methanol extract was separated using a gradient elution of solvent A (9.5% methanol containing 0.5% H_3PO_4, 85%) and solvent B (45% methanol, 55% CH_3CN containing 0.5% H_3PO_4, 85%) with a flow rate of 1 mL/min [6]. The elution program is given in Table 1. The UV detection wavelength was 250 nm.

To determine the content of (E)-guggulsterones in myrrh, an ethanol extract was separated using an isocratic elution of 0.1% $H_3PO_4 : CH_3CN$ (45 : 55, v/v) with a flow rate of 1 mL/min for 25 minutes [7]. The UV detection wavelength was 240 nm.

2.3. Determination of the Ratio of Stereoisomers in Synthetic Borneol. Chiral GC was used to determine the ratio of stereoisomers in synthetic borneol. Analysis was performed

Table 1: HPLC elution program for dragon's blood, catechu, and frankincense.

Dragon's blood		Catechu		Frankincense	
Time (min)	Eluent (B%)	Time (min)	Eluent (B, C%)	Time (min)	Eluent (B%)
0–2	19	0–5	0,0	0–5	90
2–20	19–100	5–7	0,0–100,0	5–11	90–100
20-21	100	7–12	100,0–20,80	11–23	100
		12–26	20,80–0,100		

using an Agilent GC system model HP 6890N (Santa Clara, CA, USA) equipped with a split/splitless injector, liner of silanized quartz with a 4 mm i.d. (effective volume 0.49 mL), and an Agilent 6890 autosampler for 100 vials. A Cydex-B chiral GC column (25 m × 0.22 mm ID; 0.25 μm) was obtained from SGE Analytical Science (Austin, TX, USA). Chromatographic conditions were as follows: helium used as a gas carrier; a constant flow of 1.0 mL/min; 2 μL injection volume (splitless model), and a 280°C injector temperature. The GC temperature program was as follows: 90°C (1 min), 90°C to 130°C (41 min), 130°C (10 min), and 200°C (3 min). An Agilent 5973N quadrupole mass spectrometer was operated in selective ion monitoring (SIM) mode, with ionization source by electron impact at 70 eV, transfer line at 280°C, ion source at 280°C, and quadrupole at 150°C.

2.4. In Vitro Wound Healing Assay. Confluent HaCaT cells in 12-well plates were starved overnight in DMEM medium. The surface of the plate was scraped with a 200 μL pipette tip to generate a cell-free zone. Free cells were then removed by two HBSS washes, and cells were incubated in DMEM medium containing 200 μg/mL, 20 μg/mL, or 2 μg/mL "Jinchuang ointment." After 24 hours of incubation, cells were imaged using microscopy. The area of wound closure was quantitatively determined using Image J software (National Institutes of Health, Bethesda, MD).

Stimulation effects on *in vitro* wound healing assay by "Jinchuang ointment" were also examined using human microvascular endothelial cells (HMEC-1). Ibidi Culture-Inserts (Ibidi Gmbh, Martinsried, Germany) were placed on the chamber of 24-well cell culture plates. About 70 μL of HMEC-1 (5×10^5 cells/mL) was seeded per well and plates were incubated at 37°C and 5% CO_2. After 24-hour incubation, Ibidi Culture-Inserts were removed, and 1 mL of MCDB131 media containing 1 μL DMSO solution of "Jinchuang ointment" was then added into individual wells. The migration of cells was observed by microscopy over a period of 6–24 hours. The gap size was measured by using software Image J.

2.5. Cell Proliferation Assay. HaCaT cells (5×10^4/well) were seeded in 96-well plates. The medium containing "Jinchuang ointment" at various concentrations was then added after cell adhesion. Cells were incubated in DMEM medium for the indicated time. The proliferation of HaCaT cells was subsequently determined by using Cell Proliferation Reagent WST-1 (Roche, Indianapolis, IN, USA). The statistical method used is Student's t-test.

2.6. Western Blotting. Confluent monolayers of HaCaT cells were treated with various concentrations of Jinchuang ointment for the indicated time. Equal quantities of cell lysate proteins were separated by 10% SDS-PAGE and electroblotted onto PVDF membranes (Millipore, Billerica, MA). Membranes were blocked for 1 h with 5% low-fat milk powder solubilized in phosphate-buffered saline (PBS) containing 0.05% Tween 20. Levels of Cdc25b, Cdc25c, CDK2, CDC D2, Cyclin B, Cyclin D3, and α-tubulin were determined by western blotting using specific antibodies and enhanced chemiluminescence detection methods. The intensity of the resulting bands was measured by densitometric analysis using Image J software and presented as the ratio relative to the internal control.

2.7. In Vitro Tube Formation Assay. Human umbilical vein endothelial cells (HUVEC) were bought from Bioresource Collection and Research Center (Hsinchu, Taiwan). 1 mL of HUVEC (1×10^5 cells/well) was placed into the wells of a 24-well flat bottomed plates precoated with 200 μL Matrigel (BD Biosciences, Bedford, MA, USA). Cells were then mixed with 1 mL medium containing "Jinchuang ointment" (final concentration of 200 μg/mL). Cells were incubated at 37°C for a 24 h exposure [8]. After incubation, cell tube or network formation was observed using a phase-contrast microscope.

2.8. Statistical Analysis. Results are expressed as the means ± SD from at least three independent experiments. Differences between groups were assessed by one-way analysis of variance (ANOVA). A P value less than 0.05 was considered statistically significant.

3. Results and Discussion

3.1. Clinical Treatment Observations on a Nonhealing Diabetic Wound by Treating with "Jinchuang Ointment". To the best of our knowledge, there are no English language case reports describing "Jinchuang ointment" treatment for nonhealing diabetic wounds. Three different cases are presented in this study. The first subject, Mrs. Wu, is a 75-year-old female patient with type II insulin-dependent diabetes accompanied by peripheral arterial occlusion disease (PAOD) which led to left lateral leg and ankle necrotizing fasciitis. She was treated with percutaneous transluminal angiography (PTA) to improve lower limb circulation on Feb 6, 2013. As a result of reperfusion injury, the ulcer had enlarged with erythema. After examination, a below-knee amputation was immediately scheduled two weeks later at the Surgery Division,

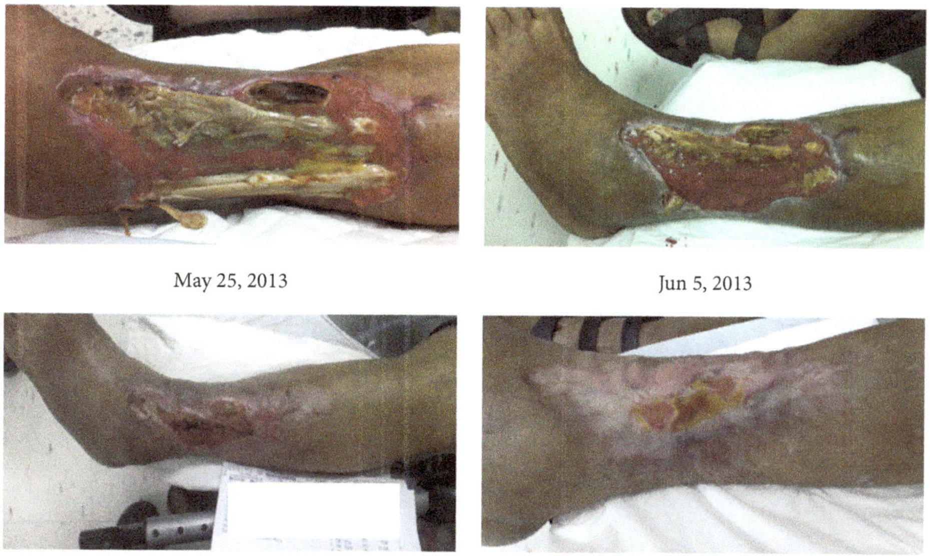

May 25, 2013 Jun 5, 2013 Sep 4, 2013 Aug 27, 2014

FIGURE 1: The wound area of the patient Mrs. Wu during "Jinchuang ointment" treatment. Wound dimensions measured on the date specified are as follows: May 25, 2013, 26 × 9 cm; Jun 5, 2013, 26 × 9 cm; Sep 4, 2013, 8 × 4 cm; Aug 27, 2014, 2.5 × 3 cm.

the China Medical University Beigang Hospital. As suggested by a doctor from the Division of Chinese Medicine, she decided to use traditional Chinese medicine to treat her wound. She was referred to the Division of Chinese Medicine for wound management. Normal saline was first used to clean the wound. About 2-3 g "Jinchuang ointment" was applied directly to the wound once daily. Pictures depicting wound healing under treatment with "Jinchuang ointment" are shown in Figure 1.

Mr. Tsai, a 71-year-old male, with past history of type II diabetes was diagnosed on September 8, 2013. He had a 3 × 0.8 cm and a 4 × 1.5 cm grade 3 pressure sore in the sacral region. 1 g of "Jinchuang ointment" was applied topically to the wound area once per day. Pictures documenting wound healing under treatment of "Jinchuang ointment" are shown in Figure 2. It is well-known that all treatments for bedsores are to prevent wounds from worsening. Complete wound closure was observed on October 27, 2013.

Mr. Wang, a 64-year-old male with a past history of hypertension, had a chronic wound measuring 6.2 × 5.3 cm which had not healed for more than six months. He received the topical application of "Jinchuang ointment" once per day beginning November 26, 2014. A great improvement was observed after two months of treatment as shown in Figure 3.

3.2. Content of Reference Standards Present in Dragon's Blood, Catechu, Frankincense, and Myrrh. One of the main problems associated with herbal medicine is the high level of batch to batch variation in the amounts of active components. The content of pure chemical reference standards in herbal products is therefore used as an indicator for the purposes of quality control and standardization. Accordingly, the content of reference standards in dragon's blood, catechu, frankincense, and myrrh used was measured by HPLC in this study. All the calibration curves of reference compounds were linear over the concentration range studied (Table 2). A linear interpolation method was used to calculate the percentage by mass of each reference standard in the herbal extract that we examined.

Dracorhodin is a red anthocyanin pigment that is a major component in "dragon's blood" resin of the plant *Daemonorops draco*. It possesses antimicrobial, anticancer, and cytotoxic activity [9, 10]. Figure 4(a) shows the separation of dracorhodin in dragon's blood. The mass percentage of dracorhodin in the "dragon's blood" used in this study is 0.15%.

Both catechin and epicatechin are phenol-type antioxidants in catechu, an extract of acacia trees. Catechu is a common component of herbal medicine. In addition to their ability to scavenge free radicals in plasma, the health benefits of catechin and epicatechin also include stimulation of fat oxidation, expansion of the brachial artery, and resistance of LDLs to oxidation [11]. At the cellular and molecular level, catechin can enhance the expression of human PTGS2 (a dioxygenase gene), 1L1B (cyclooxygenase-2 gene), SOD (superoxide dismutase gene), MAPK1 (Mitogen-activated protein kinase 1), and MAPK3 [12–14]. Figure 4(b) shows the separation of catechin and epicatechin in catechu. The mass percentage of catechin and epicatechin in the catechu used in this study is 24.2% and 1.7%, respectively.

Frankincense is a resin from plants in the genus *Boswellia*. In Africa and Asia, it is widely used in incense, perfume, and traditional medicine. Boswellic acids, a series of pentacyclic triterpene molecules, are one of the major components of frankincense. Theiranti-inflammatory properties and ability to induce cancer cell apoptosis have been reported *in vitro* [15–17]. The expression of TOP1 (DNA topoisomerase I) and TOP2A (DNA topoisomerase II) genes can be altered in the presence of 11-keto-β-boswellic acid derivatives and

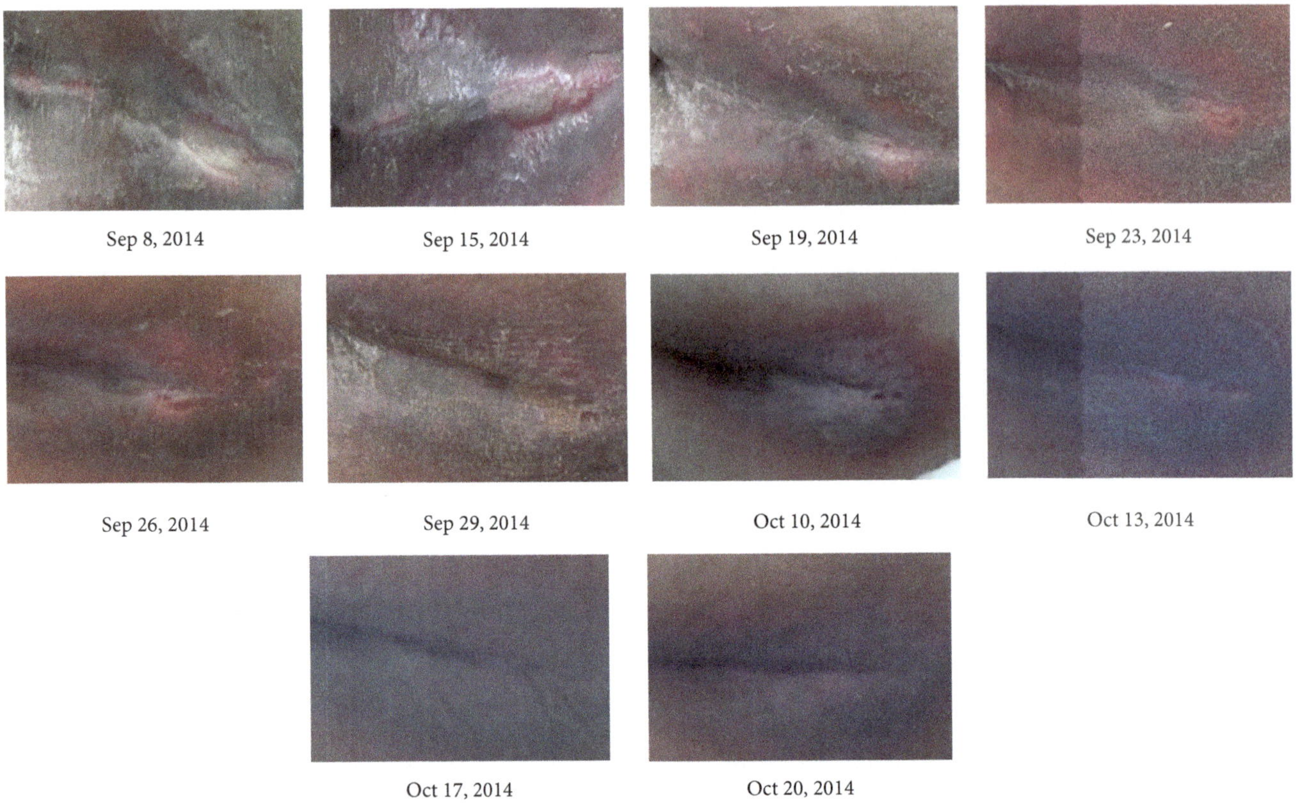

FIGURE 2: The pressure sore of the patient Mr. Tsai during "Jinchuang ointment" treatment. This wound was located at the sacral region and was completely closed after a 50-day treatment.

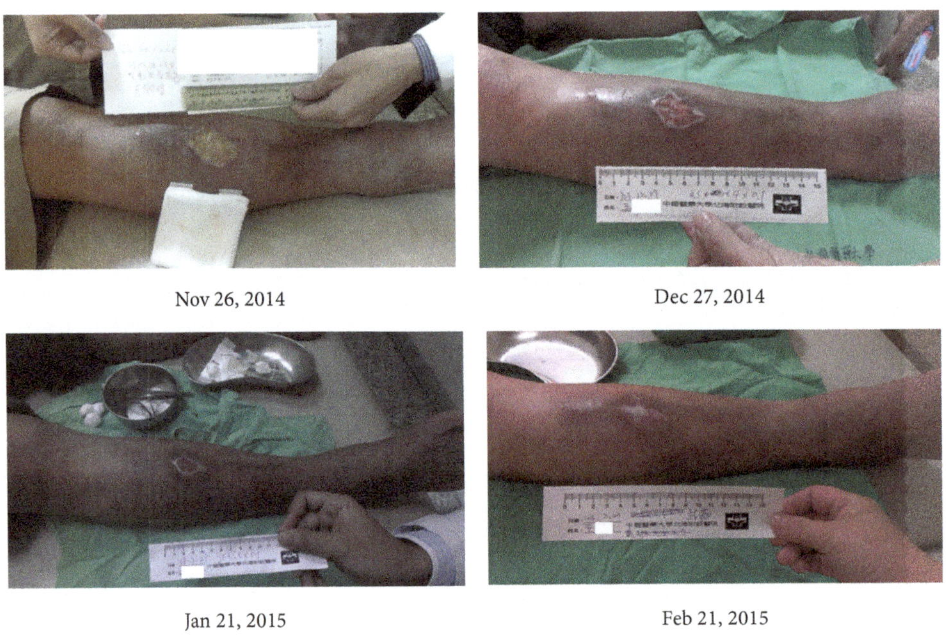

FIGURE 3: The previously nonhealing wound of patient Mr. Wang during "Jinchuang ointment" treatment. Wound dimensions were measured on the following dates: Nov 26, 2014, 6.2 × 5.3 × 0.3 cm; Dec 27, 2014, 4.5 × 4 × 0.1 cm; Jan 21, 2015, 2.5 × 1.5 × 0.1 cm; Feb 21, 2015, wound complete closure.

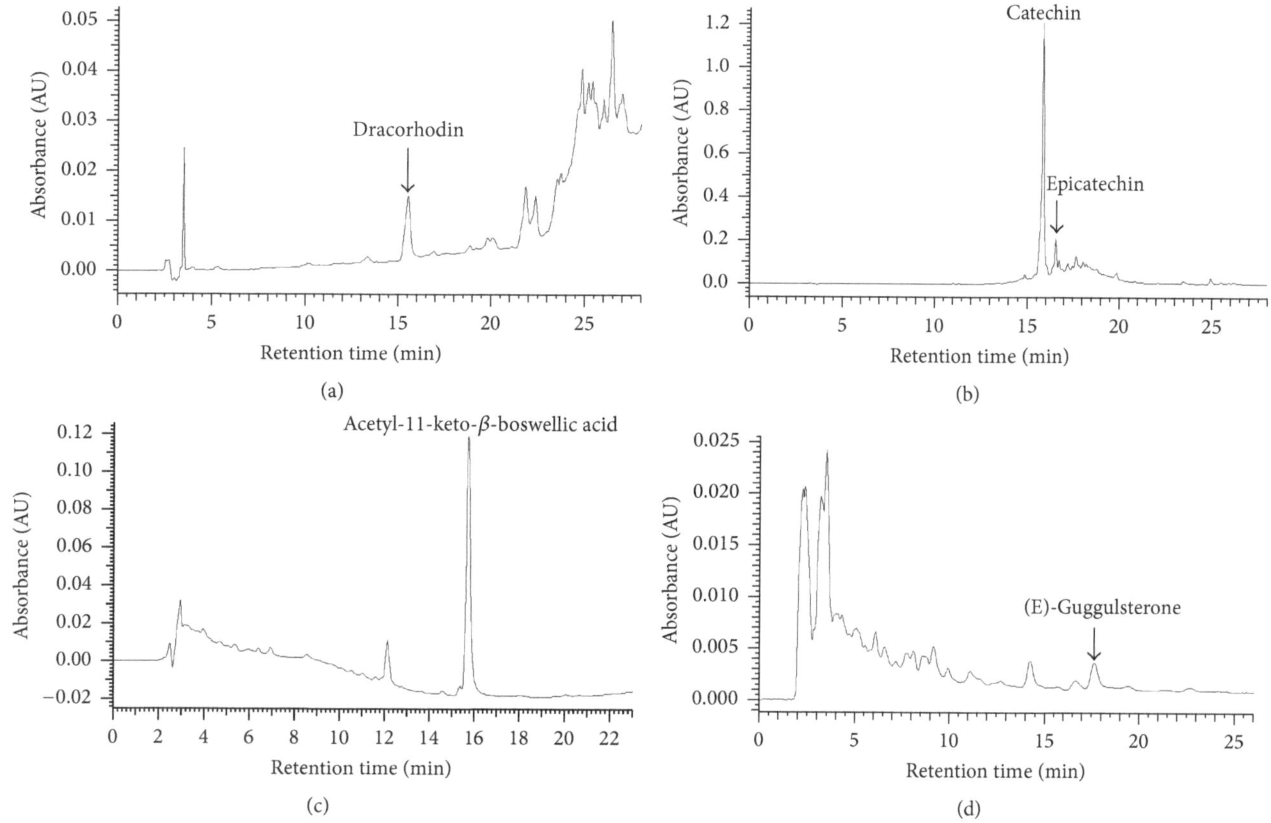

FIGURE 4: HPLC separation of reference compounds present in extracts of herbal components. HPLC traces of (a) dracorhodin in "dragon's blood," (b) catechin and epicatechin in catechu, (c) acetyl-11-keto-β-boswellic acid in frankincense, and (d) (E)-guggulsterone in myrrh.

acetyl-boswellic acid [16, 18]. Figure 4(c) shows the separation of acetyl-11-keto-β-boswellic acid in frankincense. The mass percentage of acetyl-11-keto-β-boswellic acid in the frankincense used in this study is 1.62%.

Myrrh is also a resin from plants in the genus *Commiphora*. The usage of myrrh is similar to that of frankincense. In fact, both myrrh and frankincense are frequently used in concert in many traditional Chinese medicine recipes. In western medicine, myrrh is also used in liniment and healing salves for minor skin ailments. The chemical composition of myrrh is rather complicated [19]. Notably, both (Z)- and (E)-isomers of guggulsterone possess high affinity toward a variety of steroid receptors [20]. Both isomers seem equipotent as inhibitors of HUVEC tube formation [21]. The mass percentage of (E)-guggulsterone in the myrrh used in this study is 0.02%. Figure 4(d) shows the separation of (E)-guggulsterone in myrrh.

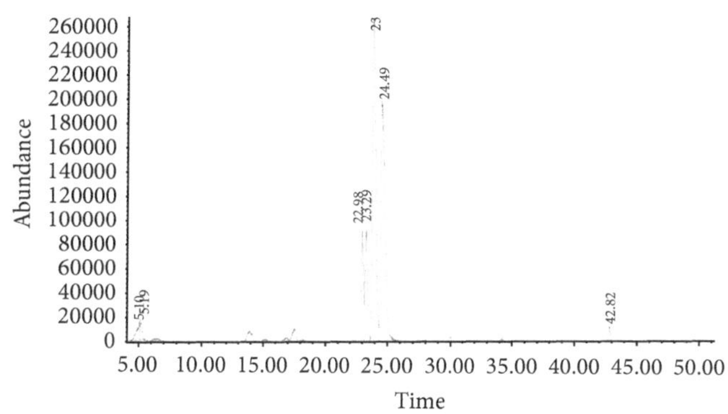

FIGURE 5: Chiral GC separations of synthetic borneol. The four major peaks from 22.0 to 26.0 min are (+)-isoborneol, (−)-isoborneol, (−)-borneol, and (+)-borneol, respectively.

3.3. The Ratio of Stereoisomers in Chemically Synthesized Borneol. Borneol is a bicyclic monoterpene plant secondary metabolite. (+)-Borneol, mainly isolated from the plant family of Dipterocarpaceae, is the major form used for analgesia and anesthesia in traditional Chinese medicine. More recently, chemically synthesized borneol and (−)-borneol isolated from the plant species *Blumea balsamifera* have enjoyed more widespread use. The price of synthetic borneol is the lowest among the sources discussed above. Previous results show that borneol stereoisomers can interact with GABA receptors [22, 23] and possess antimicrobial activity [24]. Chiral GC was used to analyze the composition of borneol stereoisomers in synthetic borneol used in this study. Our results show that (+)-isoborneol : (−)-isoborneol : (−)-borneol : (+)-borneol is in the ratio of 8.9 : 10.9 : 41.6 : 38.6 (Figure 5).

TABLE 2: HPLC calibration curves of reference compounds including regression equations, the coefficients of determination (R^2), and calibration ranges.

Reference compound	Regression equation	R^2	Calibration range	Mass percentage
Dracorhodin perchlorate	$y = 2000000x - 19368$	0.999	0.0125–0.2 μg	0.15%
Catechin	$y = 26508x - 35003$	0.997	0.25–4 μg	24.2%
Epicatechin	$y = 33500x - 65614$	0.999	0.5–4 μg	1.7%
Acetyl-11-keto-β-boswellic acid	$y = 79427x - 54832$	0.999	0.125–2 μg	1.62%
(E)-Guggulsterone	$y = 2466634x + 12554$	0.999	0.0625–1 μg	0.02%

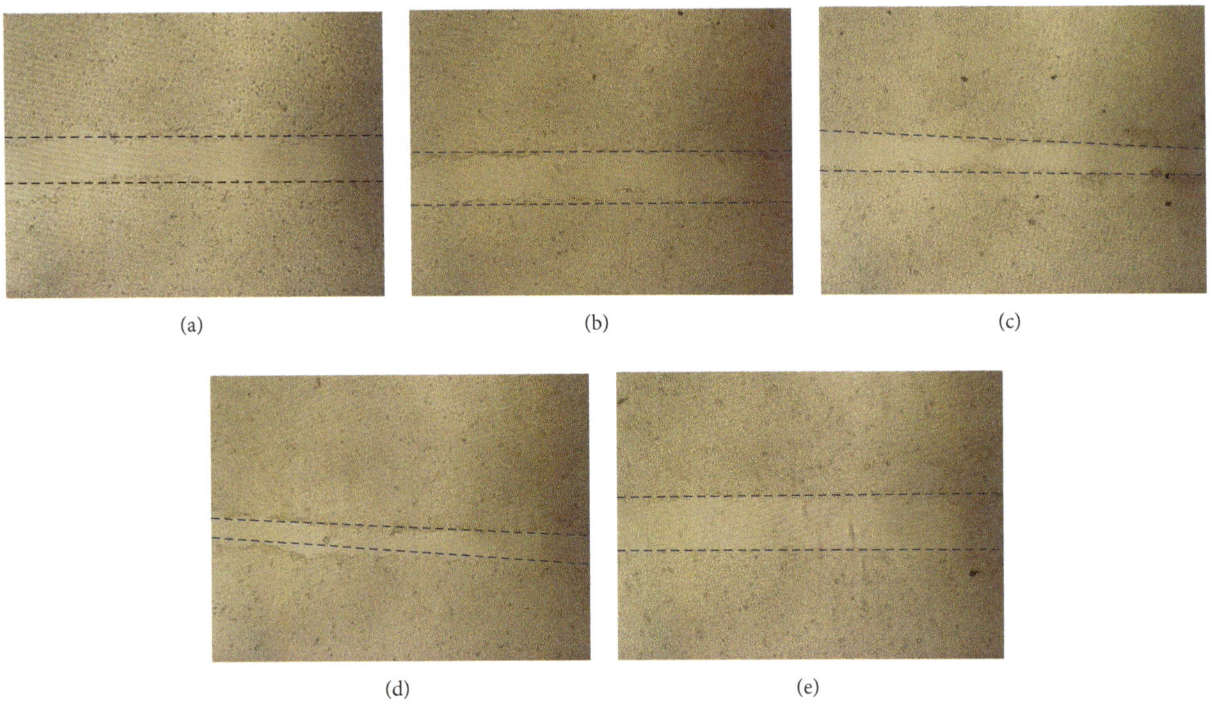

FIGURE 6: Wound healing assay with HaCaT cells displaying the increased cell migration induced by "Jinchuang ointment." Cells were treated with (a) DMSO alone (control), (b) 100 ng/mL EGF (positive control), (c) 200 μg/mL "Jinchuang ointment," (d) 20 μg/mL "Jinchuang ointment," and (e) 2 μg/mL "Jinchuang ointment." Cell migration was documented by phase contrast microscopy over a 24-hour time course where time 0 is the time of wound scratching.

3.4. In Vitro Wound Healing Assay. Confluent HaCaT cells were scratched and treated with "Jinchuang ointment." The wound area was measured after 24 hours of treatment. All experiments were performed in triplicate. The percentage of wound closure was calculated as follows: (initial wound area − 24 h posttreatment wound area)/initial wound area × 100%. The wound closure percentage with 200 μg/mL, 20 μg/mL, and 2 μg/mL "Jinchuang ointment" treatment was 78.2±5.3%, 78.2 ± 4.3%, and 63.8 ± 1.7%, respectively. In contrast, the negative control HaCaT cells without "Jinchuang ointment" treatment only showed 64.4 ± 4.0% wound closure. The positive control treated with 100 ng/mL EGF treatment showed 71.8 ± 1.0% wound closure. It is obvious that application of 200 μg/mL or 20 μg/mL "Jinchuang ointment" is more potent than 100 ng/mL EGF in promoting *in vitro* wound closure, showing statistically significant differences when compared to both positive and negative controls (Figure 6).

The wound-healing assay was also used to assess the stimulatory effect of "Jinchuang ointment" on the migration of HMEC-1 cells. The wound closure percentage with 200 μg/mL "Jinchuang ointment" 24 hours after treatment was 85.0 ± 12.3%, whereas the wound closure percentage observed with the DMSO control was only 43.3 ± 8.2% (Figures 7(a) and 7(b)). The weight percentage of lard is as high as 67% in "Jinchuang ointment," and sesame oil is used to prepare another famous traditional Chinese herbal ointment, Shiunko. The contribution of lard to the total cell migratory activity was therefore evaluated by reconstituting "Jinchuang ointment" with various fats. It is apparent that the significant cell migration into the wound region is seen with Jinchuang ointment-treated cells when compared to the control group (Figure 8). When sesame oil, synthetic triacylglycerol, coconut oil, and Vaseline were used as lard substituents, 85%, 91%, 74%, and 105% migration activity

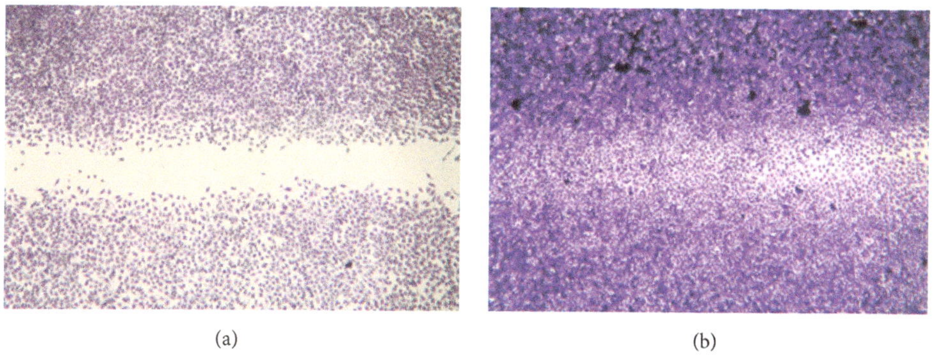

FIGURE 7: Wound healing assay with HMEC-1 cells displaying the increased cell migration induced by "Jinchuang ointment." Cells were treated with (a) DMSO alone (control) or (b) 200 μg/mL "Jinchuang ointment." Cell migration was recorded and cells were stained by microscopy over a 24-hour time course.

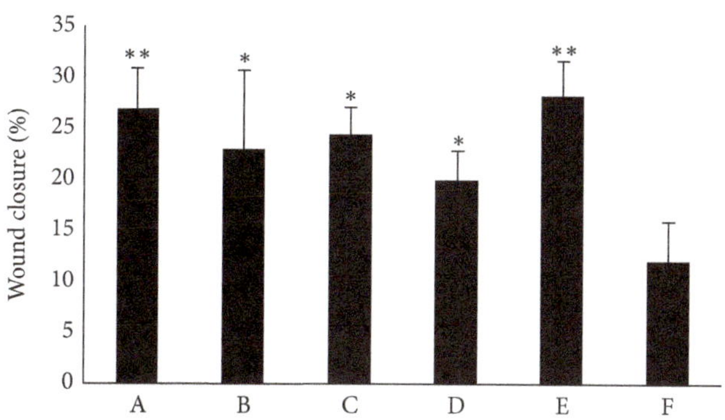

FIGURE 8: The percentage of wound closure with HMEC-1 cells after six hours of treatment in response to reconstituted variants "Jinchuang ointments." Lard is replaced by sesame oil (group B), synthetic triacylglycerol (group C), coconut oil (group D), and Vaseline (group E). Group A is the original recipe of Jinchuang ointment, and group F is DMSO only (control). Values are the mean ± SD. $^*P < 0.05$ and $^{**}P < 0.01$ compared with control.

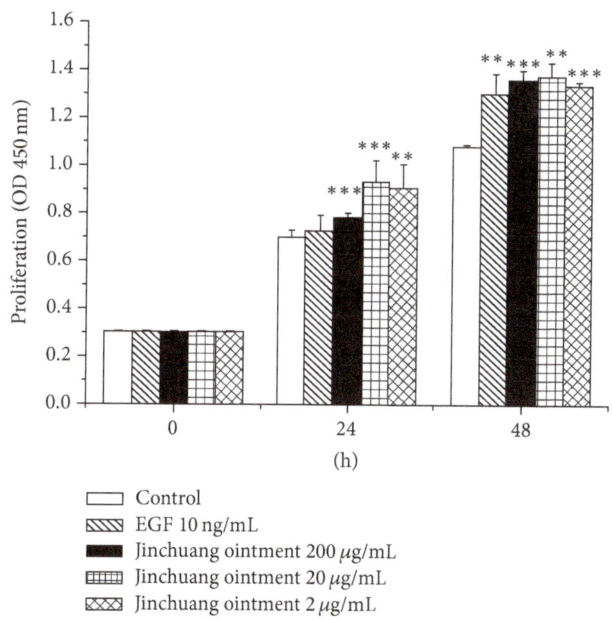

FIGURE 9: Proliferation of HaCaT cells measured by a WST-1 assay. Increased cell proliferation of HaCaT cells was observed in the presence of 200 μg/mL, 20 μg/mL, and 2 μg/mL "Jinchuang ointment." Negative and positive controls are in the presence of DMSO and 10 ng/mL EGF, respectively. Values are the mean ± SD. $^{**}P < 0.01$ and $^{***}P < 0.001$ compared with control.

can be observed (Figure 8). Unlike natural fat, Vaseline is mainly made from petroleum jelly, a semisolid mixture of hydrocarbons with carbon numbers greater than 25. The chain length of carbon atoms in the synthetic triacylglycerols used in this study is C_8 and C_{10} . These results suggest that the carbon chain length of the fat used in the ointment plays a minor role in stimulating cell migration.

3.5. The Effect of "Jinchuang Ointment" on HaCaT Cell Proliferation. The stimulatory effect of "Jinchuang ointment" on HaCaT cell proliferation was evaluated in the presence of 10% fetal bovine serum (FBS) by WST-1 assay. The increased percentages of cell proliferation by 200 μg/mL, 20 μg/mL, and 2 μg/mL "Jinchuang ointment" at 24 and 48 hours were 117±2.66%, 133±12.7%, and 129.7±14.1% and 126.4±3.5%, 127.3 ± 5.8%, and 124.1 ± 1.3%, respectively (Figure 9). These results indicate that treatment with "Jinchuang ointment" leads to an increase in HaCaT cell growth.

3.6. The Effect of "Jinchuang Ointment" on the Expression of G1/S Transition-Related Regulators. To further investigate the underlying mechanisms involved in "Jinchuang ointment"-induced effects on cell proliferation in HaCaT cells, the expression of several key cellular proteins involved in cell cycle progression was investigated by western blot analysis. As shown in Figure 10, a six-hour treatment with "Jinchuang ointment" leads to a dose-dependent increase in Cdc25b, Cdc25c, and Cyclin D3 levels. After treatment for 12 hours, significant changes in the expression pattern of those proteins between experiment and control groups were observed,

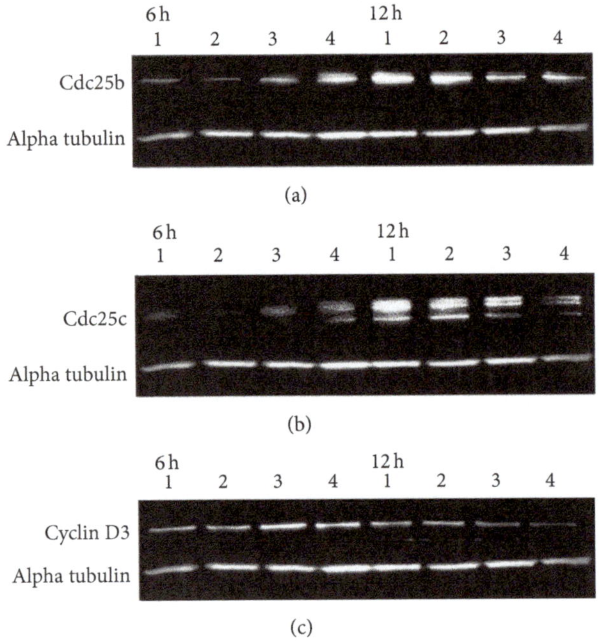

FIGURE 10: Treatment of HaCaT cells with "Jinchuang ointment" leads to altered expression of cell cycle-related proteins.Western blot analysis of (a) Cdc25b, (b) Cdc25c, and (c) cyclic D3 protein expression in HaCaT cell extracts after six and 12 hours of treatment. Lanes one to four are as follows: control, 100 ng/mL EGF, 200 μg/mL "Jinchuang ointment," and 20 μg/mL "Jinchuang ointment," respectively.

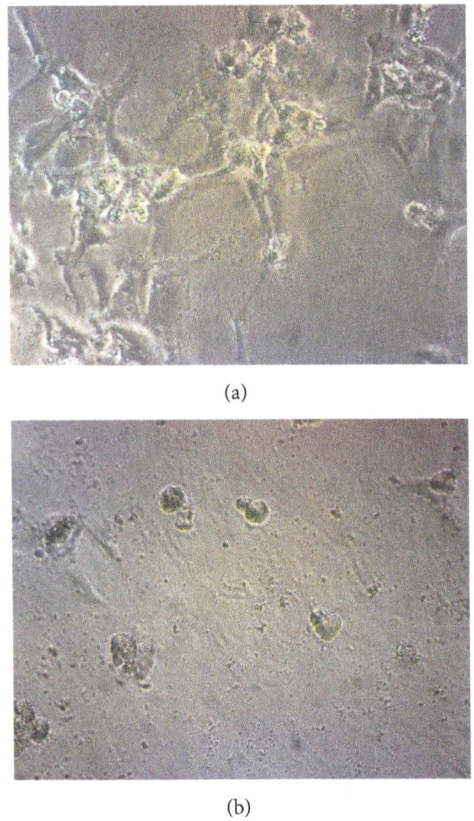

FIGURE 11: *In vitro* tube formation assay displaying the stimulation of angiogenesis by "Jinchuang ointment" in HUVEC cells. Cells were treated with (a) 200 μg/mL "Jinchuang ointment" and (b) DMSO only (negative control).

suggesting that "Jinchuang ointment" alters HaCaT cell cycle progression.

3.7. Tube Formation Assay. The process of wound healing has been divided into three different stages, inflammatory, proliferative, and remodeling phases [25]. Angiogenesis is responsible for new blood vessel formation and oxygen and nutrient supply and plays an important role in the proliferative phase of wound healing [26]. The tube formation assay was used to evaluate the *in vitro* angiogenic effect of "Jinchuang ointment" on HUVEC cells. As shown in Figure 11, treatment of HUVEC cell with 200 μg/mL "Jinchuang ointment" for 24 hours can efficiently induce endothelial cell capillary tubes and network formation.

3.8. Conclusions. "Jinchuang ointment" is a Chinese herbal medicine complex. It has been clinically used in the treatment of diabetic foot infection and decubitus ulcers in China Medical University Hospital for more than ten years. Because of its complicated composition, its biological activities have never been investigated. To further characterize its herb ingredients, the content of reference standards present in dragon's blood, catechu, frankincense, and myrrh was determined by HPLC. Two cell based assay platforms, *in vitro* wound healing and tube formation, were used to examine activity. Our results show that this herbal medicine possesses potent activities stimulating cell proliferation, migration, and angiogenesis. This provides a scientific rationale to account for the observed clinical curative effects on wound healing by "Jinchuang ointment."

According to current pharmaceutical regulations in Taiwan, only traditional Chinese herbal medicine manufactured from cGMP pharmaceutical factories can be sold in drug stores or by hospital marketing channels. However, for homemade traditional Chinese herbal medicine, they can only be administered to patients by the doctors who made the respective medicine. For this reason, "Jinchuang ointment" cannot be widely used in the Taiwan area since many clinicians are not able or unwilling to prepare this remedy. To facilitate the manufacturing process of "Jinchuang ointment" by cGMP factories, it will be very important to find out the activity indicator markers for components, such as dragon's blood, catechu, frankincense, and myrrh.

Competing Interests

The authors declare no conflict of interests.

Authors' Contributions

Tsung-Jung Ho, Tzong Shiun Li, Chun-Chang Wu, and Jaung-Geng Lin are responsible for "Jinchuang ointment" preparations, clinical treatment, and observations; Shinn-Jong Jiang helped in western blot analysis, cell proliferation, and wound healing assay of HaCaT cells; Guang-Huey Lin and Ming-Chuan Hsieh helped in wound healing assay of HMEC-1 cells; Jai-Sing Yang helped in tube formation assay; Lih-Ming Yiin helped in GC analysis; Hao-Ping Chen helped in HPLC analysis, experiment design, "Jinchuang ointment" preparation, and paper preparation.

Acknowledgments

This work was supported by Grant CMUBH R104-007 from China Medical University Beigang Hospital, Grant TCMRC-P-101014 from Tzu Chi University, and, in part, Grant MOST 104-2320-B-039-023 from the Ministry of Science and Technology, Taiwan.

References

[1] L. R. Braun, W. A. Fisk, H. Lev-Tov, R. S. Kirsner, and R. R. Isseroff, "Diabetic foot ulcer: an evidence-based treatment update," *American Journal of Clinical Dermatology*, vol. 15, no. 3, pp. 267–281, 2014.

[2] C. Y. Tu, H. C. Hsu, and J. J. Lu, "To examine the quality, safety, and efficacy of Jin Chuang Gao without moshus," *The Journal of Taiwan Pharmacy*, vol. 27, 2011.

[3] M. Yang, J. Sun, Z. Lu et al., "Phytochemical analysis of traditional Chinese medicine using liquid chromatography coupled with mass spectrometry," *Journal of Chromatography A*, vol. 1216, no. 11, pp. 2045–2062, 2009.

[4] T. Yi, Y. Tang, J. Zhang, Z. Zhao, Z. Yang, and H. Chen, "Characterization and determination of six flavonoids in the ethnomedicine 'Dragon's Blood' by UPLC-PAD-MS," *Chemistry Central Journal*, vol. 6, article 116, 2012.

[5] D. Shen, Q. Wu, M. Wang, Y. Yang, E. J. Lavoie, and J. E. Simon, "Determination of the predominant catechins in *Acacia catechu* by liquid chromatography/electrospray ionization-mass spectrometry," *Journal of Agricultural and Food Chemistry*, vol. 54, no. 9, pp. 3219–3224, 2006.

[6] M. A. Tawab, A. Kaunzinger, U. Bahr, M. Karas, M. Wurglics, and M. Schubert-Zsilavecz, "Development of a high-performance liquid chromatographic method for the determination of 11-keto-β-boswellic acid in human plasma," *Journal of Chromatography B: Biomedical Sciences and Applications*, vol. 761, no. 2, pp. 221–227, 2001.

[7] A. L. Gottumukkala, T. Ramakrishna, S. K. Babu, and G. V. Subbaraju, "Determination of (E) & (Z)-Guggulsterones in Guggul formulations by high performance liquid chromatography," *Asian Journal of Chemistry*, vol. 17, no. 3, pp. 1789–1793, 2005.

[8] J.-H. Chiang, J.-S. Yang, C.-C. Lu et al., "Newly synthesized quinazolinone HMJ-38 suppresses angiogenetic responses and triggers human umbilical vein endothelial cell apoptosis through p53-modulated Fas/death receptor signaling," *Toxicology and Applied Pharmacology*, vol. 269, no. 2, pp. 150–162, 2013.

[9] M. Xia, D. Wang, M. Wang et al., "Dracorhodin perchlorate induces apoptosis via activation of caspases and generation of reactive oxygen species," *Journal of Pharmacological Sciences*, vol. 95, no. 2, pp. 273–283, 2004.

[10] J. Shi, R. Hu, Y. Lu, C. Sun, and T. Wu, "Single-step purification of dracorhodin from dragon's blood resin of Daemonorops draco using high-speed counter-current chromatography combined with pH modulation," *Journal of Separation Science*, vol. 32, no. 23-24, pp. 4040–4047, 2009.

[11] G. Williamson and C. Manach, "Bioavailability and bioefficacy of polyphenols in humans. II. Review of 93 intervention studies," *The American Journal of Clinical Nutrition*, vol. 81, no. 1, pp. 243S–255S, 2005.

[12] C.-H. Wu, C.-F. Wu, H.-W. Huang, Y.-C. Jao, and G.-C. Yen, "Naturally occurring flavonoids attenuate high glucose-induced expression of proinflammatory cytokines in human monocytic THP-1 cells," *Molecular Nutrition and Food Research*, vol. 53, no. 8, pp. 984–995, 2009.

[13] S. Y. H. Lee, B. Munerol, S. Pollard et al., "The reaction of flavanols with nitrous acid protects against N-nitrosamine formation and leads to the formation of nitroso derivatives which inhibit cancer cell growth," *Free Radical Biology and Medicine*, vol. 40, no. 2, pp. 323–334, 2006.

[14] Y. M. Li, H. Y. E. Chan, Y. Huang, and Z. Y. Chen, "Green tea catechins upregulate superoxide dismutase and catalase in fruit flies," *Molecular Nutrition and Food Research*, vol. 51, no. 5, pp. 546–554, 2007.

[15] H. P. T. Ammon, N. Safayhi, T. Mack, and J. Sabieraj, "Mechanism of antiinflammatory actions of curcumine and boswellic acids," *Journal of Ethnopharmacology*, vol. 38, no. 2-3, pp. 113–119, 1993.

[16] G. Chashoo, S. K. Singh, P. R. Sharma et al., "A propionyloxy derivative of 11-keto-β-boswellic acid induces apoptosis in HL-60 cells mediated through topoisomerase I & II inhibition," *Chemico-Biological Interactions*, vol. 189, no. 1-2, pp. 60–71, 2011.

[17] J.-J. Liu, Å. Nilsson, S. Oredsson, V. Badmaev, W.-Z. Zhao, and R.-D. Duan, "Boswellic acids trigger apoptosis via a pathway dependent on caspase-8 activation but independent on Fas/Fas ligand interaction in colon cancer HT-29 cells," *Carcinogenesis*, vol. 23, no. 12, pp. 2087–2093, 2002.

[18] T. Syrovets, B. Büchele, E. Gedig, J. R. Slupsky, and T. Simmet, "Acetyl-boswellic acids are novel catalytic inhibitors of human topoisomerases I and IIα," *Molecular Pharmacology*, vol. 58, no. 1, pp. 71–81, 2000.

[19] Y. Chen, C. Zhou, Z. Ge et al., "Composition and potential anticancer activities of essential oils obtained from myrrh and frankincense," *Oncology Letters*, vol. 6, no. 4, pp. 1140–1146, 2013.

[20] T. P. Burris, C. Montrose, K. A. Houck et al., "The hypolipidemic natural product guggulsterone is a promiscuous steroid receptor ligand," *Molecular Pharmacology*, vol. 67, no. 3, pp. 948–954, 2005.

[21] D. Xiao and S. V. Singh, "z-Guggulsterone, a constituent of Ayurvedic medicinal plant *Commiphora mukul*, inhibits angiogenesis *in vitro* and *in vivo*," *Molecular Cancer Therapeutics*, vol. 7, no. 1, pp. 171–180, 2008.

[22] R. E. Granger, E. L. Campbell, and G. A. R. Johnston, "(+)- And (−)-borneol: efficacious positive modulators of GABA action at human recombinant $\alpha 1\beta 2\gamma 2L$ GABAA receptors," *Biochemical Pharmacology*, vol. 69, no. 7, pp. 1101–1111, 2005.

[23] A. C. Hall, C. M. Turcotte, B. A. Betts, W.-Y. Yeung, A. S. Agyeman, and L. A. Burk, "Modulation of human GABAA and glycine receptor currents by menthol and related monoterpenoids," *European Journal of Pharmacology*, vol. 506, no. 1, pp. 9–16, 2004.

[24] K. A. Al-Farhan, I. Warad, S. I. Al-Resayes, M. M. Fouda, and M. Ghazzali, "Synthesis, structural chemistry and antimicrobial activity of −(−) borneol derivative," *Central European Journal of Chemistry*, vol. 8, no. 5, pp. 1127–1133, 2010.

[25] R. J. Mendonça and J. Coutinho-Netto, "Cellular aspects of wound healing," *Anais Brasileiros de Dermatologia*, vol. 84, no. 3, pp. 257–262, 2009.

[26] M. Schäfer and S. Werner, "Cancer as an overhealing wound: an old hypothesis revisited," *Nature Reviews Molecular Cell Biology*, vol. 9, no. 8, pp. 628–638, 2008.

15

Effects of Guchang Capsule on Dextran Sulphate Sodium-Induced Experimental Ulcerative Colitis in Mice

Baoshan Liu,[1] Tong Liu,[2] Xiaohong Wang,[1] Xin Zheng,[2] Hong Wang,[1] and Lin Ma[1]

[1]*Department of Traditional Chinese Medicine, Tianjin Medical University General Hospital, Tianjin 300052, China*
[2]*Tianjin Zhongxin Pharmaceutical Group Corporation LTD., Tianjin 300457, China*

Correspondence should be addressed to Baoshan Liu; baoshanliu621@163.com

Academic Editor: Ho Lin

Guchang capsule (GC) is a Chinese materia medica standardized product extracted from 15 Chinese traditional medical herbs and it has been clinically used in the treatment of intestinal disease. In this study, in order to extend the research of GC in intestinal disease, we were aiming to evaluate potential effects of GC on dextran sulphate sodium- (DSS-) induced murine experimental colitis and to elucidate the underlying mechanisms. GC treatment attenuated DSS-induced body weight loss and reduced the mortality. Moreover, GC treatment prevented DSS-induced colonic pathological damage; meanwhile it inhibited proinflammatory cytokines production in colon tissues. *In vitro*, GC significantly reduced LPS-induced proinflammatory cytokines production via inhibiting the activation of NF-κB in macrophage cells, and the expressions of several long noncoding RNAs (lncRNAs) which were reported in regulating NF-κB signaling pathway were obviously affected by adding GC into culture medium. In conclusion, our data suggested that administration of GC exhibits therapeutic effects on DSS-induced colitis partially through regulating the expression of NF-κB related lncRNAs in infiltrating immune cells.

1. Introduction

Ulcerative colitis (UC) and Crohn's disease (CD), which are considered inflammatory bowel diseases (IBDs), are chronic gastrointestinal disorders characterized by inflammation in the intestine and colon, as well as mucosal tissue damage [1]. Although many studies suggest that genetic and environmental factors, infection, and immune system disorders are involved in the development of UC, its cause and underlying mechanisms remain unclear [2]. Several animal models of experimental colitis have been developed to help investigate the molecular and cellular mechanisms of the disease. Among these, the dextran sodium sulfate- (DSS-) induced experimental colitis model is one of the best studied. It is initiated by DSS-induced damage to the intestinal epithelial cells but is dependent on the presence of both commensal microflora [3, 4]. Similar to human IBD, DSS-induced colitis is limited to the colonic mucosa and is characterized by diarrhea, bloody feces, weight loss, colonic ulceration, and a histopathological picture of inflammation, consisting mainly of infiltrating macrophages and granulocytes [3, 4].

NF-κB has represented a paradigm for signal transduction and gene regulation implicated in numerous diseases including malignancies and chronic inflammatory disorders [5, 6]. NF-κB is normally sequestered in the cytoplasm by a family of inhibitory proteins known as inhibitors of NF-κB (IκBs). Upon activation, IκB is phosphorylated by the IκB kinase (IKK) complex, and the phosphorylation of IκB results in its degradation [7]. Subsequently, NF-κB is translocated to the nucleus and initiates downstream target genes transcription related to inflammation and immunity [6]. It has been reported that NF-κB plays a critical role at IBD onset in Crohn's disease (CD) and UC patients as well as experimental colitis models [8, 9].

Recently, pathogenic mechanism of UC is considered to be dysregulation of the intestinal immune response to intestinal environmental antigens, such as gut microbiota [10, 11]. Lipopolysaccharide (LPS), major constituent of outer membranes of Gram-negative bacteria, is a pivotal risk factor and prominent stimulus for inflammatory mediators releasing [12]. LPS would trigger the innate immune systems by activating Toll-like receptors (TLRs) superfamily in innate immune cells such as dendritic cells and macrophages [13, 14]. Among TLRs, TLR4 is a major LPS receptor and mediates the most of inflammation responses to LPS by activating NF-κB protein, via myeloid differentiation factor 88- (MyD88-) dependent and MyD88-independent pathway [13–15]. Then, the activated NF-κB induces the productions of proinflammatory cytokines such as tumor necrosis factor-α (TNFα), interleukin-1β (IL-1β), and IL-6 [14–16], resulting in severe intestinal injury and formation of UC. Alteration in cytokines production by macrophages is one major component of the pathology of UC. Therefore, strategies for targeting inflammatory macrophages and focusing on downregulating the TLR4/NF-κB signaling pathways inflammatory responses would provide potential therapeutic effects for UC.

Recent advances in large-scale RNA sequencing (RNA-seq) have led to the identification of novel RNA species encoded in the genome, many of which are long noncoding RNAs (lncRNAs) [17, 18]. lncRNAs are arbitrarily defined as having ≥200 nt, which discriminates them from small noncoding RNAs. lncRNAs have emerged as important regulators of gene expression, with an accumulating body of evidence linking lncRNAs to a plethora of human pathologies, including inflammatory diseases [19]. Meanwhile, the role of lncRNAs in intestinal diseases remains poorly understood.

Irritable bowel syndrome (IBS) is characterized by abdominal pain or discomfort associated with altered bowel function, such as constipation or diarrhea, without significant structural changes or inflammation [20]. IBD is characterized by abundant inflammation in the bowel which can result in symptoms such as abdominal pain, cramping, diarrhea, and bloody stools. Approximately 60–80% of patients with IBD suffer from irritable IBS-like symptoms such as increased abdominal pain, bloating, distention, and stool alteration [21, 22].

Traditional Chinese medicine has been widely used in many kinds of diseases and has shown excellent curative effect [23, 24]. Guchang capsule (GC) is a Chinese materia medica standardized product extracted from 15 Chinese traditional medical herbs and is widely used for treatment of patients with irritable bowel syndrome (IBS) in clinical setting. However, the function of GC in IBD and the molecular mechanisms still remain unclear. Because of the overlapping symptom of IBS and IBD, we hypothesized if GC could have beneficial effect on IBD. In this paper, we described the effect of GC in DSS-induced experimental colitis which extended the research of GC in intestinal disease and explored the underlying mechanisms which may be associated with the production of inflammation related lncRNAs.

2. Materials and Methods

2.1. Vegetal Materia and Reagents. Guchang capsule (GC) consists of Halloysite, *Coptis*, *Phellodendron amurense*, Myrobalan, Nutmeg, *Cortex Magnoliae officinalis*, Fructus Evodiae, Qu Jian, Cinnamon, Rhizoma Zingiberis, Chinese Prickly Ash, *Ligusticum wallichii*, Concha Ostreae, Gallnut, and Dark Plum Fruit (Zhongxin Pharmaceutical Corporation, Tianjin, China). We dissolved the drug powder in sterile water at 0.1 g/mL GC for the further study: *in vivo*, GC were given intragastrically (2 g/kg); *in vitro*, GC were added into culture medium at a final concentration of 1 mg/mL. LPS (*E. coli*: Serotype O55:B5) and phorbol 12-myristate 13-acetate (PMA) were purchased from Sigma-Aldrich (St. Louis, MO, USA) and used at a final concentration of 100 ng/mL. Dextran sulfate sodium (DSS, molecular weight 36–50 kDa) was obtained from MP Biomedicals Inc. (Irvine, CA, USA).

2.2. Mice and Cells. Male C57BL/6J mice weighing 20–25 g (aged 8–10 weeks) were used in this study; all mice were obtained from Beijing Vital River Laboratory Animal Technology Co., Ltd. (Beijing, China). The animals were fed a standard diet and water was provided ad libitum. The mice were kept at room temperature (controlled at 25°C) with a light-dark cycle of 12 h each day. The experiments were carried out according to the National Institutes of Health Guide for the Care and Use of Laboratory Animals approved by the Animal Ethics Committee of the Scientific Investigation Board of Tianjin Medical University. Mouse macrophage cell line RAW264.7 and human monocytic leukemia cell line THP-1 were obtained from American Type Culture Collection (Manassas, VA). The cells were cultured at 37°C under 5% CO_2 in DMEM supplemented with 10% FBS (Invitrogen, Life Technologies), 100 U/mL penicillin, and 100 mg/mL streptomycin. Differentiation of THP-1 monocytes to human macrophages was induced by 0.5 mM phorbol 12-myristate 13-acetate (PMA) for 3 h; the differentiated cells were washed three times with PBS, followed by the further experiments.

2.3. Induction and Evaluation of DSS-Induced Colitis. The mice were randomly assigned to control, GC, control + DSS-treated, and GC + DSS-treated groups. Experimental colitis was induced by adding DSS to the drinking water to a final concentration of 4% (w/v) for 6 days; subsequently, mice were sacrificed at day 6 to separate the colons for tissue experiments or switched to regular drinking water until 15 days for survival data monitoring. The animals were given free access to water containing DSS for 6 days. Control animals received water without DSS. GC were given intragastrically once per day for 6 days from the first day, respectively. Mice were examined daily to determine their clinical disease activity index (DAI), which was based on the degree of body weight loss, stool consistency, and fecal blood (ranging from 0 to 12). Briefly, DAI was scored as follows: weight loss (no change = 0; <5% = 1; 6–10% = 2; 11–20% = 3; >20% = 4), stool (normal = 0; soft, well-formed = 1; soft without pellets = 2; diarrhea = 4), and blood (no blood = 0; visible blood in rectum = 1; gross bleeding in rectum = 2; visible blood on fur = 4). For histological analysis, the distal colonic specimens were fixed in 10% buffered formalin and embedded in paraffin. Sections were stained with H&E, and pathological scores, ranging from 0 to 6 (combining inflammatory cell infiltration score and tissue damage score), were determined as follows: inflammatory cell infiltration in the lamina propria (occasional inflammatory cells = 0; increased inflammatory cells = 1; confluence of inflammatory

TABLE 1: List of primers used in the study.

Number	Gene	Primer sequence	Primer length
1	TNFα	Forward 5′-GCCACCACGCTCTTCTGTCT-3′ Reverse 5′-TGAGGGTCTGGGCCATAGAAC-3′	20 bp 21 bp
2	IL-6	Forward 5′-ACAACCACGGCCTTCCCTAC-3′ Reverse 5′-CATTTCCACGATTTCCCAGA-3′	20 bp 20 bp
3	IL-1β	Forward 5′-ACCTTCCAGGATGAGGACATGA-3′ Reverse 5′-AACGTCACACACCAGCAGGTTA-3′	22 bp 22 bp
4	GAPDH	Forward 5′-ACCACAGTCCATGCCATCAC-3′ Reverse 5′-TCCACCACCCTGTTGCTGTA-3′	20 bp 20 bp
5	lncRNA Lethe	Forward 5′-CAGGACTGAGGAGGACATCA-3′ Reverse 5′-GCCTCTCTTCTCAGCGTTGT-3′	20 bp 20 bp
6	lncRNA-Cox2	Forward 5′-AAGGAAGCTTGGCGTTGTGA-3′ Reverse 5′-GAGAGGTGAGGAGTCTTATG-3′	20 bp 20 bp
7	lncRNA AS-IL1α	Forward 5′-AGCTCCCATGGATGCCTTTAG-3′ Reverse 5′-GCCCTAAGAACAGGGCTAGG-3′	21 bp 20 bp
8	lncRNA NKILA	Forward 5′-GAAACAGGTGCACGTTTCAGG-3′ Reverse 5′-ACAGATGTACCCTGGCAACC-3′	21 bp 20 bp
9	lncRNA THRIL	Forward 5′-AACTCCTGACCTCAGGTGATCCAT-3′ Reverse 5′-AAGGGAGTTTCAGAAGGTGTGGCT-3′	24 bp 24 bp
10	lncRNA-IL7R	Forward 5′-CCAGCCTTTGCCTCTTCCTTCAAT-3′ Reverse 5′-CCGTACCAAGTCTCTTAGCCCCTC-3′	24 bp 23 bp

cells extending to the submucosa = 2; transmural extension = 3) and tissue damage (no mucosal damage = 0; lymphoepithelial lesions = 1; surface mucosal erosion = 2; extensive mucosal damage and extension into deeper structures of the bowel wall = 3).

2.4. ELISA. Distal parts of colons were homogenized in CelLytic buffer (Sigma-Aldrich, St. Louis, MO) supplemented with complete protease inhibitor mixture (Roche, Indianapolis, IN). Protein concentration was measured by BCA assay (Pierce, Rockford, USA). Cytokine content was determined as pg/mg of total colon protein. Antibodies, which include purified and biotinylated rat anti-mouse TNFα, IL-6, and IL-1β, were purchased from eBioscience and BD Biosciences Pharmingen. Quantitative ELISA was performed according to the manufacturer's instructions.

2.5. RNA Isolation and Quantitative PCR Analysis. The tissue samples were frozen and mechanically dissociated in TRIzol reagent (Invitrogen, Carlsbad, CA). Total RNA was extracted with TRIzol reagent according to the manufacturer's instructions. A LightCycler (ABI PRISM 7000; Applied Biosciences) and a SYBR RT-PCR kit (Takara Biotechnology, Dalian, China) were used for real time PCR analysis. GAPDH was used as the internal control, and $2^{-\Delta\Delta CT}$ method was used to evaluate the relative quantities of each amplified product in the samples. For each qPCR analysis, three technical replicates were performed. Primer sequences used in quantitative PCR were shown in Table 1.

2.6. Western Blot Analysis. The cells were harvested after stimulation and washed three times by ice-cold PBS (MDL biotech, Beijing, China) on ice, and the cells were lysed with RIPA buffer (MDL biotech, Beijing, China) with proteasome inhibitor cocktail (Roche, Indianapolis, IN), followed by sonication. After centrifugation for 15 min at 13,000 g, supernatants were collected and the protein concentration of lysates was measured using Bio-Rad quantification assay (Bio-Rad Laboratories, Hercules, CA). Twenty micrograms of protein sample was incubated with loading buffer (Beyotime, Beijing, China) at 95°C for 10 minutes. Proteins were separated using 10% SDS-PAGE and transferred to a PVDF membrane (Millipore, Billerica, USA). The membrane was then blocked with 2.5% nonfat dry milk for 1 h. The antibodies specific for p65, phospho-p65, IκBα, phospho-IκBα, IKKβ, phospho-IKKβ (Cell Signaling Technology Inc., Beverly, USA), and β-Actin (Santa Cruz Biotechnology, Santa Cruz, USA) were added and incubated overnight at 4°C. After incubation with the corresponding horseradish peroxidase-conjugated secondary antibody (Santa Cruz Biotechnology, Santa Cruz, USA), the target protein was visualized by enhanced chemiluminescence (Thermo Fisher Scientific, Bremen, Germany).

2.7. Assay of Luciferase Reporter Gene Expression. RAW264.7 macrophages were cotransfected with NF-κB luciferase reporter plasmid and pRL-TK-Renilla-luciferase plasmid using Jet-PEI transfection reagent (Polyplus, Illkirch, France) as previously reported [25]. 24 hours after transfection, the cells were left untreated or treated with LPS, with 1 mg/mL GC or sterile water coapplied into culture medium for 4 hours. The cells were harvested and washed by ice-cold PBS for three times and luciferase activities were measured with Dual-Luciferase Reporter Assay System (Promega, Madison, USA), according to the manufacturer's instructions. Data are normalized for transfection efficiency by dividing Firefly luciferase activity with that of Renilla luciferase. NF-κB luciferase reporter plasmid and pRL-TK-Renilla-luciferase plasmid were gifts of X. Cao (Second Military Medical University, Shanghai, China).

2.8. Statistical Analysis. All data are presented as mean ± SD of three independent experiments. Statistical significance was determined with the two-tailed Student's t-test to compare two groups. One-way ANOVA was performed to compare three or more groups. If the ANOVA analysis was significant, the Newman-Keuls test was applied for comparison between each two groups. The survival curves were plotted according to the Kaplan-Meier method and compared using the log-rank test. A p value of less than 0.05 was considered statistically significant.

3. Results

3.1. Effect of GC on Body Weight, DAI, and Survival Rate in DSS-Treated Mice. To determine the potential role of Guchang capsule (GC) in experimental ulcerative colitis, mice were given 4% DSS for 6 days to induce acute colitis. The consumption of food and water was measured throughout the experiment, and there were no significant differences between the groups (data not shown). As shown in Figure 1(a), DSS-treated colitis mice exhibited profound body weight loss, whereas GC administration could significantly attenuate the loss of body weight. The clinical manifestation of the disease, as reflected by disease activity index (DAI), was markedly higher in the DSS-treated group compared with nontreated control group, but the treatment with GC significantly reduced the clinical scores of the DSS-induced colitis in mice (Figure 1(b)). Furthermore, the mortality of DSS-treated mice was improved by about 50% after GC administration (Figure 1(c)).

3.2. Effect of GC on Histology of Colon in DSS-Treated Mice. Histological examination was also performed to validate the clinical data. DSS treatment induced significant histopathological changes in the colons of control mice that were characterized by massive inflammatory infiltrates and disruption of mucosal structures (Figure 2(a)). However, GC treated mice displayed less severe injury compared with control mice after DSS feeding (Figure 2(a)). The histopathological score of GC treated mice was significantly lower than that of control mice after DSS treatment (Figure 2(b)). After DSS-induced injury, the colon weight of GC treated mice was heavier than that of control mice (Figure 2(d)), and GC treated mice had longer colon length compared to control group after DSS feeding.

3.3. GC Administration Decreased Proinflammatory Cytokines Production in DSS-Treated Mice. To evaluate whether the protection from colitis induced by DSS in mice with GC treatment was associated with a reduction in the production of proinflammatory cytokines, after DSS challenge, expression levels of TNFα, IL-1β, and IL-6 in colons of control or GC treated mice were detected using ELISA (Figure 3(a)) and qPCR (Figure 3(b)). Significantly, both the mRNA and protein levels of proinflammatory cytokine were decreased in GC treated group.

3.4. GC Treatment Decreased Proinflammatory Cytokines Production in LPS Stimulated RAW264.7 Cells. During intestinal mucosa damage, LPS secreted by the intestinal flora will stimulate infiltration of macrophages to activate the production of inflammatory factors, so we examined the effect of GC on LPS stimulated proinflammatory cytokines production in RAW264.7 cells. The same as the above results, the anti-inflammatory activity of GC was also confirmed in LPS stimulated RAW264.7 cells *in vitro*. Both the mRNA and protein levels of proinflammatory cytokines were decreased in GC treated group compared with control group after LPS stimulation (Figures 4(a) and 4(b)).

3.5. GC Suppressed NF-κB Activation after LPS Stimulation in RAW264.7 Cells. Production of proinflammatory cytokines upon LPS depends mainly on the NF-κB activation, so we hypothesized if GC would affect NF-κB activation. To determine the function of GC on NF-κB activation, first we transfected NF-κB luciferase reporter plasmid into RAW264.7 cells; 24 hours later we stimulated cells with LPS together with GC or PBS treatment for 4 hours and measured luciferase activity. LPS-induced NF-κB activation was greatly decreased by GC treatment compared with control group (Figure 5(a)). Western blotting showed that LPS-induced phosphorylation of NF-κB/p65 and IKKβ and IκBα phosphorylation were all suppressed by GC treatment (Figure 5(b)).

3.6. GC Regulated NF-κB Related lncRNAs Expression. In recent years, lots of long noncoding RNAs (lncRNAs) have been identified in the mammalian genomes, many of which have been implicated in a range of developmental processes and diseases [18, 26–28]. Though most of lncRNAs have been primarily studied in the context of genomic imprinting, developmental process, and cancer, lncRNAs are now emerging as important regulators of both innate and adaptive immune responses [29]. We hypothesized that GC could regulate lncRNAs expression in DSS-induced colitis; then we examined the expression of lncRNAs which were reported in regulating activation of NF-κB pathway. Interestingly, lncRNA Lethe, reported as a negative regulator of NF-κB, was significantly upregulated in GC group after LPS stimulation (Figure 6(a)) or DSS treatment (Figure 6(b)), but lncRNA-Cox2 and lncRNA AS-IL1α expressions were not affected (Figures 6(a) and 6(b)). We also examined the effect of GC on expression of lncRNAs which were reported in human THP-1-derived macrophages after LPS stimulation; we found that expressions of the negative regulatory lncRNA NKILA and lncRNA-IL7R were both upregulated, and the expression of lncRNA THRIL which was reported to downregulate TNFα production was suppressed (Figure 6(c)). These results indicated GC could regulate multiple NF-κB related lncRNAs expressions in murine and human macrophage.

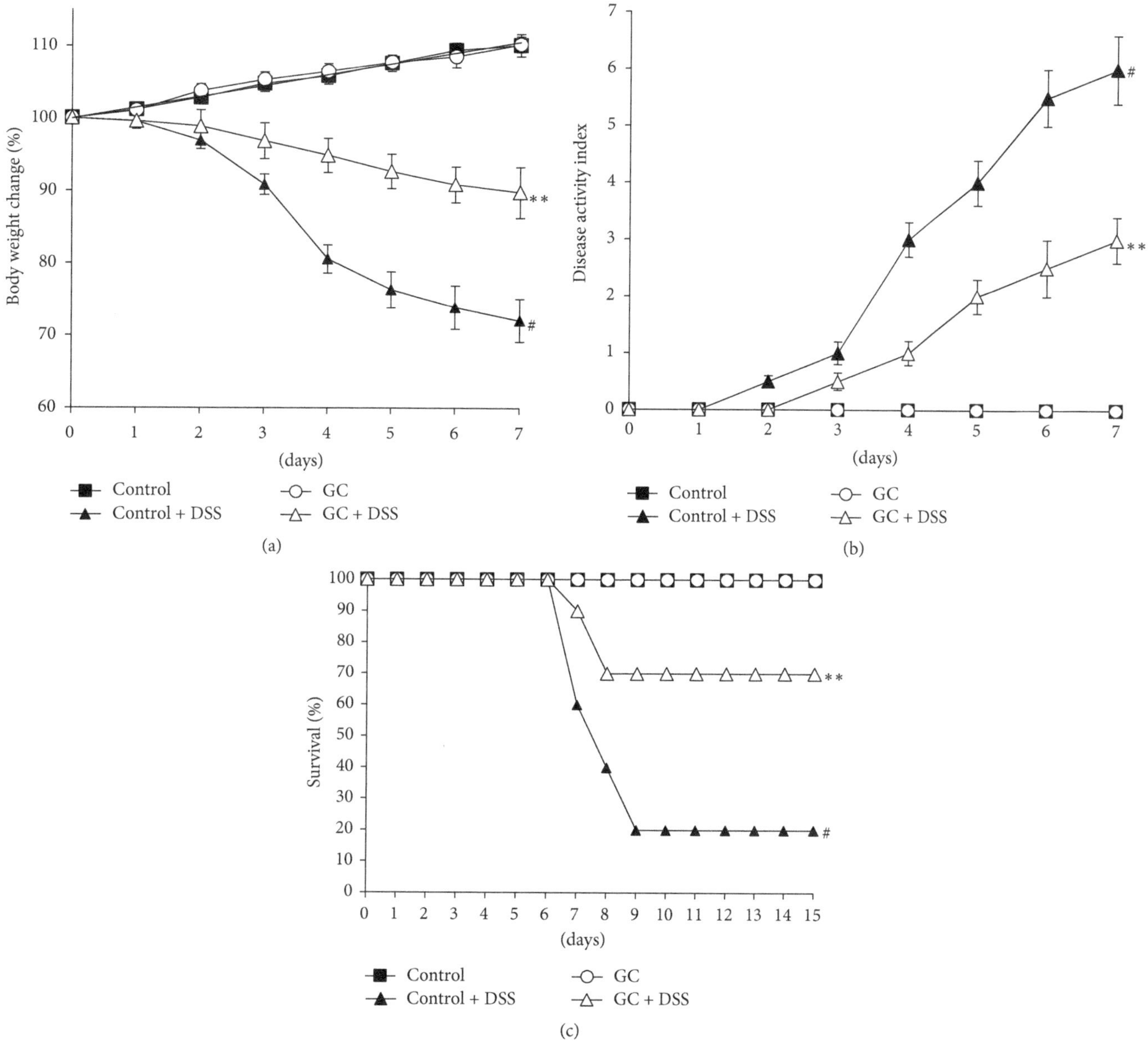

FIGURE 1: Effect of GC on body weight, DAI, and survival rate in DSS-treated mice. (a) Body weight change; (b) disease activity index; and (c) survival rate. Experimental model of ulcerative colitis was induced by administration of 4% dextran sulfate sodium (DSS) for 6 days and then switched to regular drinking water for data monitoring. GC were given intragastrically once per day for 6 days from the first day, respectively. Body weight change (a) and disease progression (b) were monitored daily from day 1 to day 7. Survival rate (c) was monitored until day 15 after the initiation of DSS. The data are representative of three independent experiments ($n = 5$ per group in (a-b) and $n = 10$ per group in (c), mean ± SD). $^{**}p < 0.01$ versus control + DSS group; $^{\#}p < 0.05$ versus control group.

4. Discussion

Guchang capsule has been widely used for treatment of patients with IBS in clinical setting in China; because of the overlapping symptom between IBS and IBD, we wonder if GC could affect IBD progressing and we investigated the effect of GC in murine experimental colitis and revealed the potential molecular mechanisms in current study. To the best of our knowledge, this study is the first to systematically demonstrate the function of GC in DSS-induced murine experimental colitis and reveal the special effect of GC on regulating inflammation associated lncRNA expression. Our results suggested that GC treatment could attenuate DSS-induced injury and suppressed proinflammatory cytokines production in DSS-treated mice or LPS stimulated RAW264.7 cells. Furthermore, we found that GC treatment would inhibit the activation of NF-κB and GC had different regulating effect on several kinds of NF-κB/inflammation associated lncRNA.

Ulcerative colitis (UC) is one of the two major forms of inflammatory bowel diseases (IBDs), which are chronic, relapsing, idiopathic, and inflammatory conditions that are

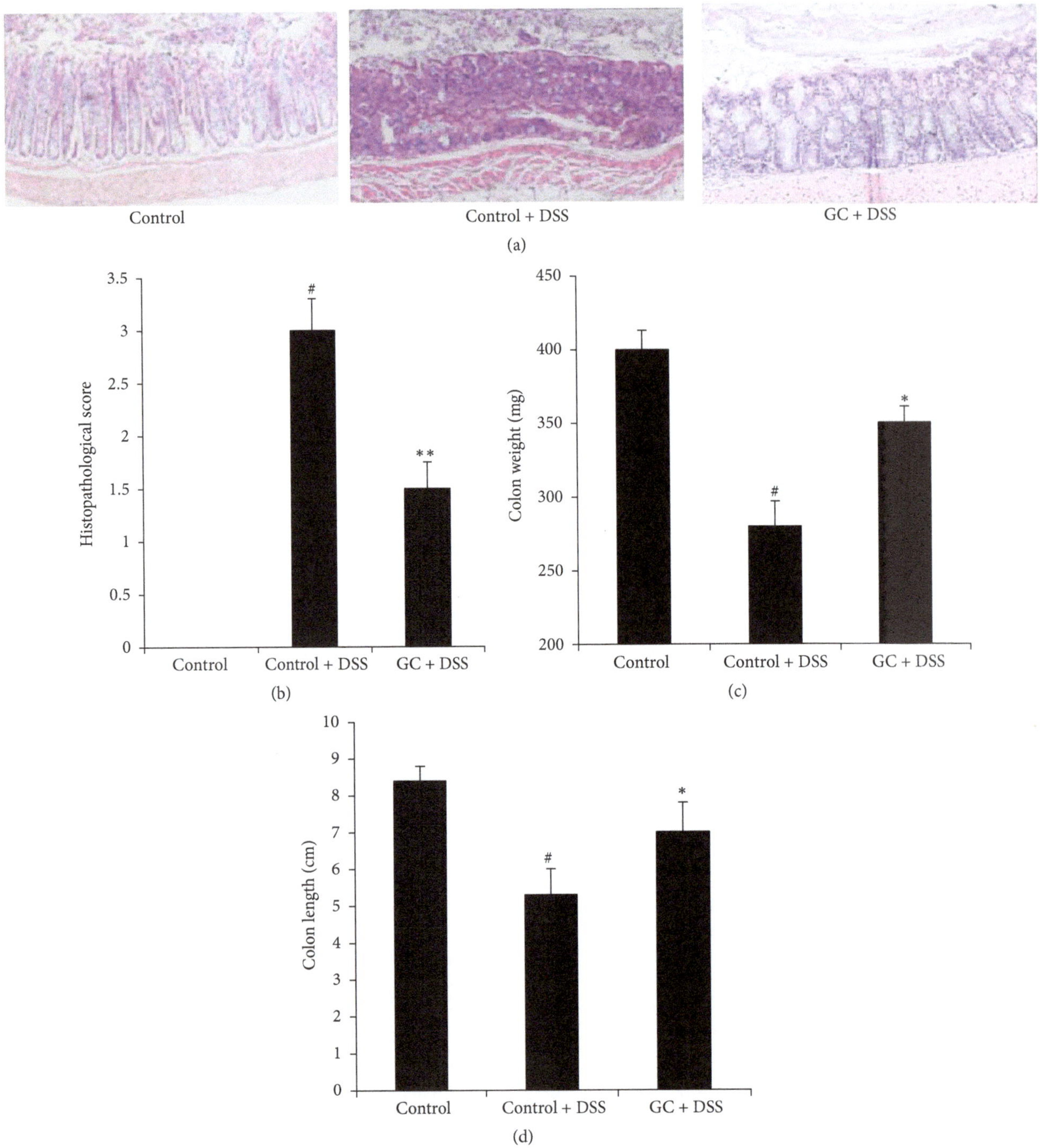

FIGURE 2: Effect of GC on histology of colon in DSS-treated mice. (a) Hematoxylin and eosin- (H&E-) stained sections of colons (original magnification ×100); (b) histopathological score; (c) colon weight; (d) colon length. Colitis was induced by administration of 4% DSS for 6 days. GC were given intragastrically once per day for 6 days from the first day, respectively. The mice were sacrificed at day 6 and colons were excised for indicated experiments. The data are representative of three independent experiments ($n = 5$ per group, mean ± SD). $^{*}p < 0.05$ versus control + DSS group, $^{**}p < 0.01$ versus control + DSS group, and $^{\#}p < 0.05$ versus control group.

immunologically mediated. Diarrhea, abdominal pain, and bloody mucopurulent stool are the main clinical symptoms for UC [1, 2]. Currently, there are various evolving therapeutic options for UC. Immunosuppressive drugs such as TNFα antibody [30], azathioprine (AZA), and methotrexate (MTX) [31] have been adopted to control the symptoms. However, these immunosuppressants have their limitations in efficacy and safety [32, 33]. Therefore, novel strategies with high efficacy and safety are urgently required.

Establishment of UC by oral administration of DSS in the mouse is a widely used model for studies on this disease because this model resembles human UC and the resulting

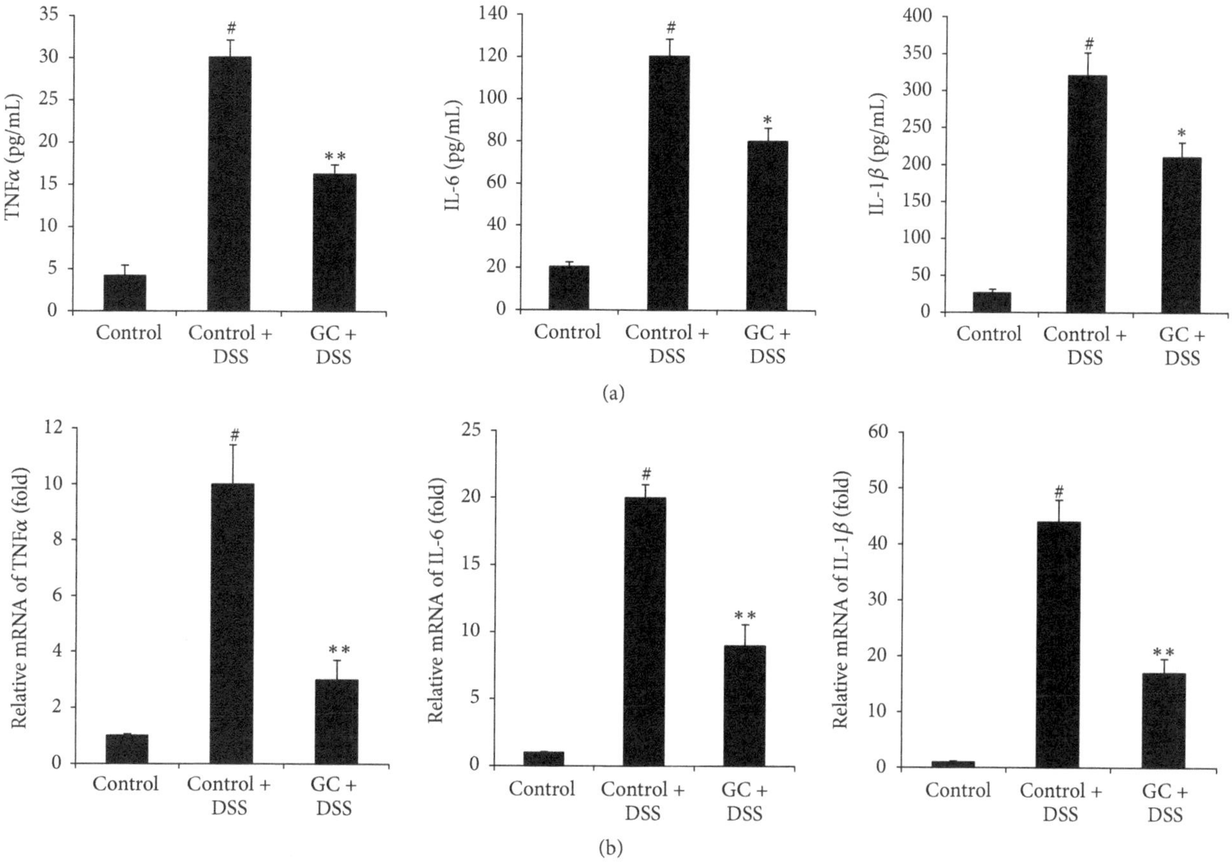

FIGURE 3: GC administration decreased proinflammatory cytokines production in DSS-treated mice. (a) ELISA analysis of secreted proinflammatory cytokines; (b) qPCR analysis of mRNA level of proinflammatory cytokines. Colitis was induced by administration of 4% DSS for 6 d. GC were given intragastrically once per day for 6 days from the first day, respectively. The mice were sacrificed at day 6. The protein level (a) or mRNA level (b) of TNFα, IL-6, and IL-1β in distal part of colons was analyzed. The data are representative of three independent experiments ($n = 5$ per group, mean ± SD). $^*p < 0.05$ versus control + DSS group, $^{**}p < 0.01$ versus control + DSS group, and $^{\#}p < 0.05$ versus control group.

pathological conditions correspond very well to human. Acute ulcerative colitis induced by DSS showed intestinal bacterial infection and was characterized by massive infiltration of proinflammatory cells, such as macrophages, neutrophils, and CD4+ T cells, within the colonic walls, which destroy epithelium and shorten the colon length [34]. These infiltrated inflammatory cells are major producers of inflammatory mediators, such as TNFα, IL-6, and IL-1β, which contribute to pathogenesis [4]. Activation of NF-κB is thought of as a strong inducer of these proinflammatory cytokine expressions [35, 36] and has been proposed as a major culprit and therapeutic target for IBD. Recent studies showed that many traditional Chinese medicines showed protective effect on DSS-induced colitis in mice. Song et al. reported that black tea extract could prevent LPS-induced NF-κB signaling and attenuates DSS-induced experimental colitis [37]; Li et al. showed that Calculus Bovis Sativus (CBS) had protective effect on DSS-induced colitis and CBS significantly downregulated the mRNA expression of TNFα, IL-1β, and IL-6 in the colon tissue [38]. Dave et al. found that mulberry fruit prevents LPS-induced NF-κB/pERK/MAPK signals in macrophages and suppresses acute colitis and colorectal tumorigenesis in mice [39]. Similar to their data, we found that GC showed beneficial effect on DSS-induced colitis in mice, such as less body weight loss, improved survival rate, weaker pathological damage, and decreased production of proinflammatory cytokines compared to the control group exposed to DSS, and GC treatment also attenuated cytokines production and suppressed NF-κB activation in RAW264.7 cells after LPS stimulation.

In recent years, tens of thousands of long noncoding RNAs (lncRNAs) have been identified in the mammalian genomes, many of which have been implicated in TLRs/NF-κB pathways. lncRNA Lethe was found to interact with NF-κB subunit RelA to inhibit RelA DNA binding and target gene activation; furthermore, Lethe level decreases with organismal age, a physiological state associated with increased NF-κB activity [19]. TLR signaling could induce lncRNA-Cox2, which serves as both repressor and activator of genes through interactions with various regulatory complexes [40].

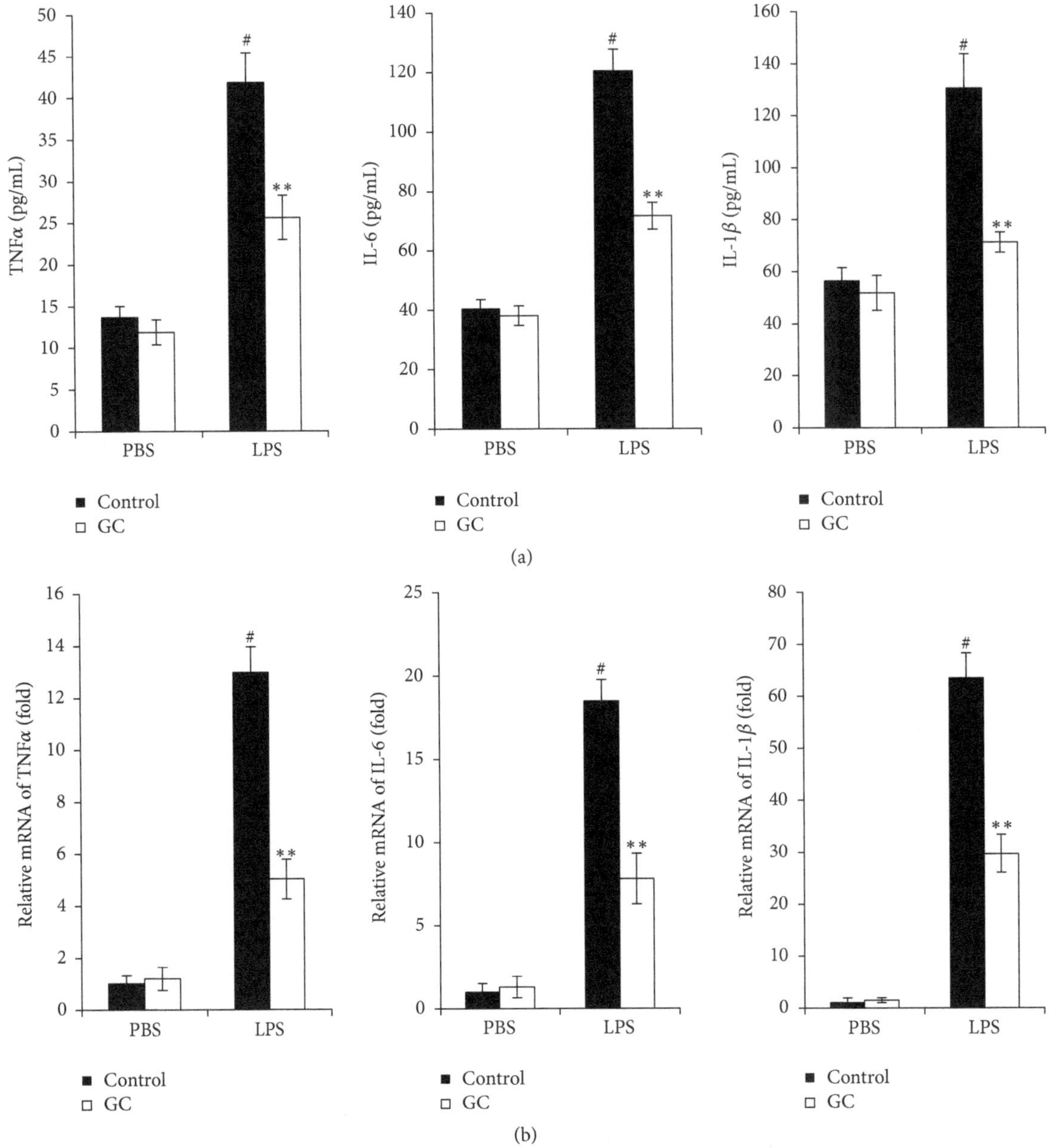

Figure 4: GC treatment decreased proinflammatory cytokines production in LPS stimulated RAW264.7 cells. (a) ELISA analysis of secreted proinflammatory cytokines; (b) qPCR analysis of mRNA level of proinflammatory cytokines. RAW264.7 cells were stimulated with LPS (100 ng/mL) together with GC (1 mg/mL) for 4 hours and the protein level (a) or mRNA level (b) of TNFα, IL-6, and IL-1β was analyzed. The data are representative of three independent experiments (mean ± SD). $^{**}p < 0.01$ versus control + DSS group; $^{\#}p < 0.05$ versus PBS + control group.

A natural antisense transcript, AS-IL1α, was found to control inducible transcription of the proinflammatory cytokine IL-1α upon TLRs stimulations [41]. Liu et al. report that NKILA is an essential lncRNA that regulates NF-κB signaling and represses inflammation; NKILA can bind to NF-κB/IκB complex and inhibits NF-κB signaling by blocking the phosphorylation sites of IκB and stabilizing the complex [42]. Li et al. identified that lncRNA THRIL was essential for induction of TNFα expression through its interaction with hnRNPL during innate activation of THP-1 macrophages [43]. Cui et al. identified lncRNA-IL7R which inhibited LPS-induced proinflammatory response through regulating trimethylation of histone H3 at K27 at the proximal promoters of inflammatory mediators [44]. We then examined the effect of GC on the expression of these lncRNAs in DSS-treated mice and LPS stimulated macrophages. Interestingly, we found that, in mouse macrophage cell line RAW264.7, lncRNA Lethe was decreased after DSS challenge or LPS stimulation in control group, while GC treatment significantly increased Lethe expression in these conditions. The expressions of

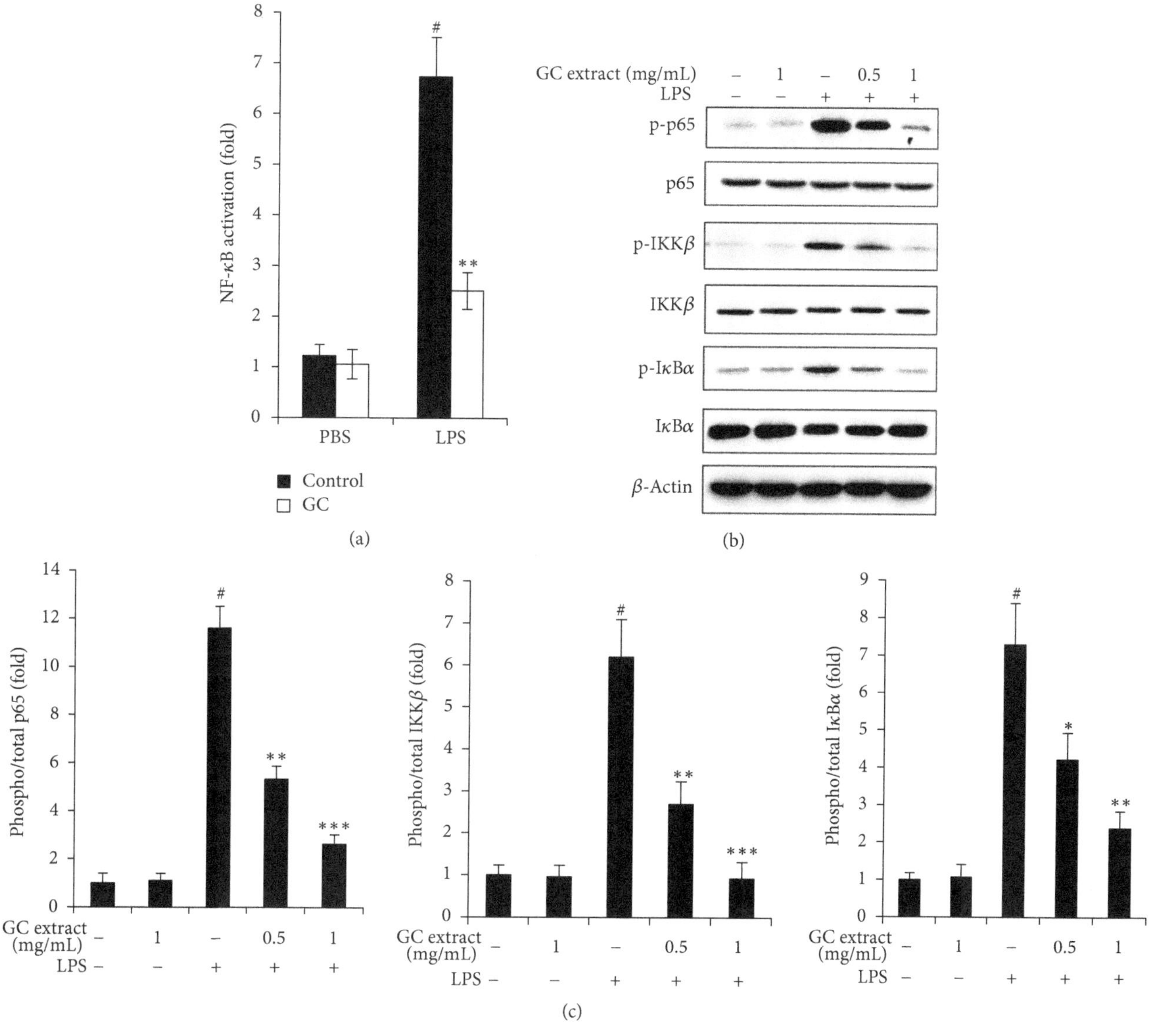

FIGURE 5: GC suppressed NF-κB activation after LPS stimulation in RAW264.7 cells. (a) Luciferase reporter assay; (b) Western blot analysis; (c) quantification of protein level. RAW264.7 cells were transfected with NF-κB luciferase reporter plasmid together with pRL-TK-Renilla-luciferase plasmid (internal control); 24 hours later the cells were stimulated with LPS (100 ng/mL) together with GC (1 mg/mL) for 4 hours; the luciferase reporter assay was performed to examine the activation of NF-κB promoter (a); $^{**}p < 0.01$ versus control + DSS group; $^{\#}p < 0.05$ versus PBS + control group. The expressions of p-p65, p65, p-IKKβ, IKKβ, p-IκBα, and IκBα were examined by WB in RAW264.7 cells after stimulation with LPS and treatment with different quality of GC (b). Quantification of protein level of p-p65, p-IKKβ, p-IκBα in (b) and (c); $^{*}p < 0.05$ versus control + LPS group, $^{**}p < 0.01$ versus control + LPS group, $^{***}p < 0.001$ versus control + LPS group, and $^{\#}p < 0.05$ versus untreated control group. The data are representative of three independent experiments (mean ± SD in (a, c)).

lncRNA-Cox2 and AS-IL1α were not changed between GC group and control group after DSS treatment or LPS stimulation. We also detected the expression of inflammation associated lncRNAs such as NKILA, lncRNA THRIL, and lncRNA-IL7R which were discovered in human immune cells. In THP-1-derived macrophages, the expressions of NKILA and lncRNA-IL7R were significantly upregulated, and mRNA level of lncRNA THRIL which could inhibit TNFα expression was decreased. These findings suggested that GC could regulate diverse lncRNAs expressions; for example, in NF-κB pathway and during proinflammatory cytokines production, GC could upregulate the negative regulatory lncRNAs expression; meanwhile it suppressed the expression of positive regulatory lncRNAs related to NF-κB pathway, which resulted in ameliorate effect on ulcerative colitis.

5. Conclusions

In conclusion, our current study provided the evidence that Guchang capsule could ameliorate DSS-induced colitis and illustrated its potential mechanism by inhibiting NF-κB

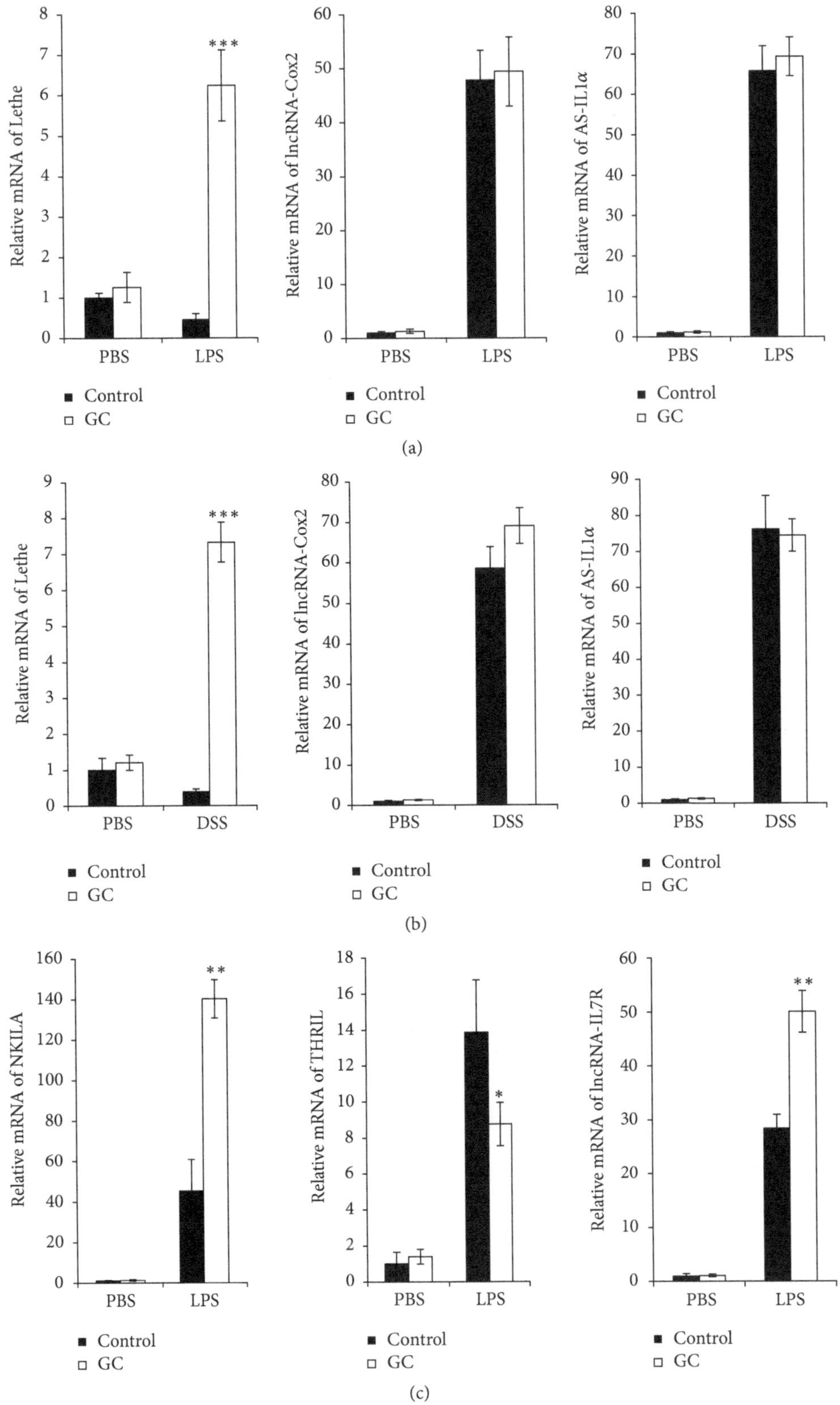

FIGURE 6: GC regulated NF-κB related lncRNAs expression. (a) QPCR analysis of lncRNA Lethe, lncRNA-Cox2, and lncRNA AS-IL1α expression in RAW264.7 cells after LPS (100 ng/mL) and GC (1 mg/mL) treatment for 4 hours; (b) qPCR analysis of lncRNA Lethe, lncRNA-Cox2, and lncRNA AS-IL1α mRNA level in mice after DSS (4%) and GC (2 g/kg) treatment for 6 days; (c) qPCR analysis of expression of lncRNA NKILA, lncRNA THRIL, and lncRNA-IL7R in THP-1-derived macrophages after LPS (100 ng/mL) and GC (1 mg/mL) treatment for 4 hours. The data are representative of three independent experiments ($n = 5$ per group in (b), mean ± SD). $^{*}p < 0.05$; $^{**}p < 0.01$; $^{***}p < 0.001$ versus control + LPS (DSS) group.

activation through regulating expression of NF-κB related lncRNAs. This study enriched the function of Guchang capsule in the treatment of ulcerative colitis and expanded our understanding of the mechanism of traditional Chinese medicine.

Competing Interests

The authors declare that there are no competing interests.

Authors' Contributions

Baoshan Liu and Tong Liu contributed equally to this work.

Acknowledgments

The authors thank Dr. Xuetao Cao for providing NF-κB luciferase reporter plasmid and pRL-TK-Renilla-luciferase plasmid.

References

[1] D. K. Podolsky, "Inflammatory bowel disease," *New England Journal of Medicine*, vol. 347, no. 6, pp. 417–429, 2002.

[2] D. C. Baumgart and S. R. Carding, "Inflammatory bowel disease: cause and immunobiology," *Lancet*, vol. 369, no. 9573, pp. 1627–1640, 2007.

[3] I. Okayasu, S. Hatakeyama, M. Yamada, T. Ohkusa, Y. Inagaki, and R. Nakaya, "A novel method in the induction of reliable experimental acute and chronic ulcerative colitis in mice," *Gastroenterology*, vol. 98, no. 3, pp. 694–702, 1990.

[4] I. Ordás, L. Eckmann, M. Talamini, D. C. Baumgart, and W. J. Sandborn, "Ulcerative colitis," *The Lancet*, vol. 380, no. 9853, pp. 1606–1619, 2012.

[5] M. Karin and A. Lin, "NF-κB at the crossroads of life and death," *Nature Immunology*, vol. 3, no. 3, pp. 221–227, 2002.

[6] S. S. Makarov, "NF-κB as a therapeutic target in chronic inflammation: recent advances," *Molecular Medicine Today*, vol. 6, no. 11, pp. 441–448, 2000.

[7] M. S. Hayden and S. Ghosh, "Signaling to NF-κB," *Genes and Development*, vol. 18, no. 18, pp. 2195–2224, 2004.

[8] G. Rogler, K. Brand, D. Vogl et al., "Nuclear factor κB is activated in macrophages and epithelial cells of inflamed intestinal mucosa," *Gastroenterology*, vol. 115, no. 2, pp. 357–369, 1998.

[9] S. Schreiber, S. Nikolaus, and J. Hampe, "Activation of nuclear factor κB inflammatory bowel disease," *Gut*, vol. 42, no. 4, pp. 477–484, 1998.

[10] F. Rafii, J. G. H. Ruseler-Van Embden, and L. M. C. van Lieshout, "Changes in bacterial enzymes and PCR profiles of fecal bacteria from a patient with ulcerative colitis before and after antimicrobial treatments," *Digestive Diseases and Sciences*, vol. 44, no. 3, pp. 637–642, 1999.

[11] F. Peris-Bondia, A. Latorre, A. Artacho, A. Moya, and G. D'Auria, "The active human gut microbiota differs from the total microbiota," *PLoS ONE*, vol. 6, no. 7, Article ID e22448, 2011.

[12] M. Rojas, C. R. Woods, A. L. Mora, J. Xu, and K. L. Brigham, "Endotoxin-induced lung injury in mice: structural, functional, and biochemical responses," *American Journal of Physiology-Lung Cellular and Molecular Physiology*, vol. 288, no. 2, pp. L333–L341, 2005.

[13] Y. Imai, K. Kuba, G. G. Neely et al., "Identification of oxidative stress and toll-like receptor 4 signaling as a key pathway of acute lung injury," *Cell*, vol. 133, no. 2, pp. 235–249, 2008.

[14] H.-Z. Yang, J.-P. Wang, S. Mi et al., "TLR4 activity is required in the resolution of pulmonary inflammation and fibrosis after acute and chronic lung injury," *The American Journal of Pathology*, vol. 180, no. 1, pp. 275–292, 2012.

[15] G. Bonizzi and M. Karin, "The two NF-κB activation pathways and their role in innate and adaptive immunity," *Trends in Immunology*, vol. 25, no. 6, pp. 280–288, 2004.

[16] M. T. Ganter, J. Roux, B. Miyazawa et al., "Interleukin-1beta causes acute lung injury via alphavbeta5 and alphavbeta6 integrin-dependent mechanisms," *Circulation Research*, vol. 102, no. 7, pp. 804–812, 2008.

[17] S. Katayama, Y. Tomaru, T. Kasukawa et al., "Antisense transcription in the mammalian transcriptome," *Science*, vol. 309, no. 5740, pp. 1564–1566, 2005.

[18] T. Derrien, R. Johnson, G. Bussotti et al., "The GENCODE v7 catalog of human long noncoding RNAs: analysis of their gene structure, evolution, and expression," *Genome Research*, vol. 22, no. 9, pp. 1775–1789, 2012.

[19] N. A. Rapicavoli, K. Qu, J. Zhang, M. Mikhail, R.-M. Laberge, and H. Y. Chang, "A mammalian pseudogene lncRNA at the interface of inflammation and anti-inflammatory therapeutics," *eLife*, vol. 2, Article ID e00762, 2013.

[20] D. A. Drossman, "The functional gastrointestinal disorders and the rome III process," *Gastroenterology*, vol. 130, no. 5, pp. 1377–1390, 2006.

[21] S. J. Halpin and A. C. Ford, "Prevalence of symptoms meeting criteria for irritable bowel syndrome in inflammatory bowel disease: systematic review and meta-analysis," *American Journal of Gastroenterology*, vol. 107, no. 10, pp. 1474–1482, 2012.

[22] J. Keohane, C. O'Mahony, L. O'Mahony, S. O'Mahony, E. M. Quigley, and F. Shanahan, "Irritable bowel syndrome-type symptoms in patients with inflammatory bowel disease: a real association or reflection of occult inflammation?" *The American Journal of Gastroenterology*, vol. 105, no. 8, pp. 1788–1795, 2010.

[23] J.-L. Tang, B.-Y. Liu, and K.-W. Ma, "Traditional Chinese medicine," *The Lancet*, vol. 372, no. 9654, pp. 1938–1940, 2008.

[24] D. Normile, "The new face of traditional Chinese medicine," *Science*, vol. 299, no. 5604, pp. 188–190, 2003.

[25] H. An, H. Xu, M. Zhang et al., "Src homology 2 domain-containing inositol-5-phosphatase 1 (SHIP1) negatively regulates TLR4-mediated LPS response primarily through a phosphatase activity- and PI-3K-independent mechanism," *Blood*, vol. 105, no. 12, pp. 4685–4692, 2005.

[26] J. T. Y. Kung, D. Colognori, and J. T. Lee, "Long noncoding RNAs: past, present, and future," *Genetics*, vol. 193, no. 3, pp. 651–669, 2013.

[27] M. Cabili, C. Trapnell, L. Goff et al., "Integrative annotation of human large intergenic noncoding RNAs reveals global properties and specific subclasses," *Genes and Development*, vol. 25, no. 18, pp. 1915–1927, 2011.

[28] J. L. Rinn and H. Y. Chang, "Genome regulation by long noncoding RNAs," *Annual Review of Biochemistry*, vol. 81, pp. 145–166, 2012.

[29] K. A. Fitzgerald and D. R. Caffrey, "Long noncoding RNAs in innate and adaptive immunity," *Current Opinion in Immunology*, vol. 26, no. 1, pp. 140–146, 2014.

[30] M. Noti, N. Corazza, C. Mueller, B. Berger, and T. Brunner, "TNF suppresses acute intestinal inflammation by inducing local glucocorticoid synthesis," *Journal of Experimental Medicine*, vol. 207, no. 5, pp. 1057–1066, 2010.

[31] O. H. Nielsen, J. T. Bjerrum, H. Herfarth, and G. Rogler, "Recent advances using immunomodulators for inflammatory bowel disease," *Journal of Clinical Pharmacology*, vol. 53, no. 6, pp. 575–588, 2013.

[32] S. Danese, "New therapies for inflammatory bowel disease: from the bench to the bedside," *Gut*, vol. 61, no. 6, pp. 918–932, 2012.

[33] J. Meier and A. Sturm, "Current treatment of ulcerative colitis," *World Journal of Gastroenterology*, vol. 17, no. 27, pp. 3204–3212, 2011.

[34] H. Y. Won, E. J. Jang, K. Lee et al., "Ablation of peroxiredoxin II attenuates experimental colitis by increasing FoxO1-induced Foxp3^{+} regulatory T cells," *The Journal of Immunology*, vol. 191, no. 8, pp. 4029–4037, 2013.

[35] L. Andresen, V. L. Jørgensen, A. Perner, A. Hansen, J. Eugen-Olsen, and J. Rask-Madsen, "Activation of nuclear factor κB in colonic mucosa from patients with collagenous and ulcerative colitis," *Gut*, vol. 54, no. 4, pp. 503–509, 2005.

[36] S. Schreiber, "The complicated path to true causes of disease: role of nuclear factor κB in inflammatory bowel disease," *Gut*, vol. 54, no. 4, pp. 444–445, 2005.

[37] Y.-A. Song, Y.-L. Park, K.-Y. Kim et al., "Black tea extract prevents lipopolysaccharide-induced NF-κB signaling and attenuates dextran sulfate sodium-induced experimental colitis," *BMC Complementary and Alternative Medicine*, vol. 11, article 91, 2011.

[38] X. Li, Y. Xu, C. Zhang et al., "Protective effect of calculus bovis sativus on dextran sulphate sodium-induced ulcerative colitis in mice," *Evidence-Based Complementary and Alternative Medicine*, vol. 2015, Article ID 469506, 8 pages, 2015.

[39] R. K. Dave, M. E. Dinger, M. Andrew, M. Askarian-Amiri, D. A. Hume, and S. Kellie, "Regulated expression of *PTPRJ*/CD148 and an antisense long noncoding RNA in macrophages by proinflammatory stimuli," *PLoS ONE*, vol. 8, no. 6, Article ID e68306, 2013.

[40] N. E. Iiott, J. A. Heward, B. Roux et al., "Long non-coding RNAs and enhancer RNAs regulate the lipopolysaccharide-induced inflammatory response in human monocytes," *Nature Communications*, vol. 5, article 3979, 2014.

[41] J. Chan, M. Atianand, Z. Jiang et al., "Cutting edge: a natural antisense transcript, AS-IL1α, controls inducible transcription of the proinflammatory cytokine IL-1α," *The Journal of Immunology*, vol. 195, no. 4, pp. 1359–1363, 2015.

[42] B. Liu, L. Sun, Q. Liu et al., "A cytoplasmic NF-κB interacting long noncoding RNA blocks IκB phosphorylation and suppresses breast cancer metastasis," *Cancer Cell*, vol. 27, no. 3, pp. 370–381, 2015.

[43] Z. Li, T.-C. Chao, K.-Y. Chang et al., "The long noncoding RNA THRIL regulates TNFα expression through its interaction with hnRNPL," *Proceedings of the National Academy of Sciences of the United States of America*, vol. 111, no. 3, pp. 1002–1007, 2014.

[44] H. Cui, N. Xie, Z. Tan et al., "The human long noncoding RNA lnc-IL7R regulates the inflammatory response," *European Journal of Immunology*, vol. 44, no. 7, pp. 2085–2095, 2014.

16

Hataedock Treatment Has Preventive Therapeutic Effects in Atopic Dermatitis-Induced NC/Nga Mice under High-Fat Diet Conditions

Ho-Yeol Cha,[1] Sang-hyun Ahn,[2] Jin-Hong Cheon,[1] In-Sik Park,[3] Jin-Tack Kim,[3] and Kibong Kim[1,4]

[1] *Department of Korean Pediatrics, Hospital of Korean Medicine, Pusan National University, 20 Geumo-ro, Mulgeum-eup, Yangsan-si, Gyeongsangnam-do 50612, Republic of Korea*
[2] *Research Institute for Korean Medicine, Pusan National University, 49 Pusandaehak-ro, Mulgeum-eup, Yangsan-si, Gyeongsangnam-do 50612, Republic of Korea*
[3] *Department of Anatomy, College of Korean Medicine, Dongguk University, Seokjang-dong, Gyeongju-si, Gyeongsangbuk-do 38066, Republic of Korea*
[4] *Department of Korean Pediatrics, School of Korean Medicine, Pusan National University, 49 Pusandaehak-ro, Mulgeum-eup, Yangsan-si, Gyeongsangnam-do 50612, Republic of Korea*

Correspondence should be addressed to Kibong Kim; kkb2630@gmail.com

Academic Editor: Arpita Basu

This study investigated the preventive therapeutic effects of Hataedock (HTD) treatment on inflammatory regulation and skin protection in AD-induced NC/Nga mice under high-fat diet conditions. Before inducing AD, the extract of *Coptidis Rhizoma* and *Glycyrrhiza uralensis* was administered orally to the 3-week-old mice. After that, AD-like skin lesions were induced by applying DNFB. All groups except the control group were fed a high-fat diet freely. We identified the effects of HTD on morphological changes, cytokine release and the induction of apoptosis through histochemistry, immunohistochemistry, and TUNEL assay. HTD downregulated the levels of IL-4 and PKC but increased the levels of LXR. HTD also suppressed the mast cell degranulation and release of MMP-9, Substance P. The levels of TNF-α, p-IκB, iNOS, and COX-2 were also decreased. The upregulation of inflammatory cell's apoptosis is confirmed by our results as increase of apoptotic body and cleaved caspase-3 and decrease of Bcl-2. HTD also reduced edema, angiogenesis, and skin lesion inflammation. Our results indicate HTD suppresses various inflammatory response on AD-induced mice with obesity through the regulation of Th2 differentiation and the protection of lipid barrier. Therefore, HTD could be used as an alternative and preventive therapeutic approach in the management of AD.

1. Introduction

Atopic dermatitis (AD) is a chronic and relapsing inflammatory skin disease with a typical distribution of pruritic skin lesions. As with any other inflammatory skin disease, it greatly affects the quality of life of patients [1, 2]. Many studies have supported the definition of AD as a complex trait, in that interactions between genes and environmental factors and the interplay between multiple genes contribute to disease manifestation [3].

Traditionally, it was thought that the primary pathogenic mechanism of AD was initiated largely due to immune dysfunction, with the key roles played by Th1/Th2 cell dysregulation, IgE production, dendritic cell signaling, and mast cell hyperactivity, leading to pruritic, inflammatory dermatosis, and the secondary disruption of the epidermal barrier [4–6].

Recently, the importance of environmental factors during infancy and early childhood in the expression of AD has become well-recognized. It was suggested that the immune and respiratory systems are relatively immature during infancy and that they continue to develop during early childhood [7]. In addition, it was suggested that allergic diseases have their origins in early life and that the priming of the immune system starts in utero [8]. Previous studies have found that obesity is associated with defective skin barrier function [9, 10]. In addition, obesity results in a chronic low-grade inflammatory condition that may directly contribute to inflammatory pathways in AD [11]. Although the precise link between obesity and AD has not been well established, adiposity is believed to induce systemic inflammation, which may negatively influence the immature immune system and atopic disorders [12]. Based on these studies, we can conclude that early life is a crucial period of development for the immune system and that excess fat may influence the pathogenesis or expression of allergic diseases among susceptible infants and children.

Within traditional Korean Medicine, AD is thought to be caused by children being influenced by "heat" during fetal development, which is referred to as "fetal heat" [13]. This "fetal heat" is influenced by maternal diet or mentality during pregnancy. Therefore, traditional Korean Medicine treats AD with "heat-clearing" medicines to reduce accumulated heat in the skin [14]. Hataedock (HTD) treatment is a "heat-clearing" treatment that dispels "fetal heat" and the meconium collected by the fetus via orally administering herbal extracts to a newborn baby. In our previous study, HTD treatment alleviated inflammatory skin damages in NC/Nga mice through regulating of inflammation and downregulation of protein kinase C (PKC) and Th2 cytokines, which are involved in the initial steps of AD development [15, 16].

An extract of *Coptidis Rhizoma* and *Glycyrrhiza uralensis* is traditionally used in HTD treatment. Recent studies have indicated that *Coptidis Rhizoma*, a kind of classical heat-clearing and detoxifying herb according to traditional Korean pharmacology, has antihyperglycemia, antihyperlipidemia, antihypertension, anti-inflammatory, and antioxidant effects [17]. It is also known that *Coptidis Rhizoma* and its main active compound, berberine, improve glucose and lipid metabolism disorders and have antiobesity activities [18, 19]. *Glycyrrhiza uralensis* is used to treat several inflammatory disorders, enhance the activity of other ingredients, reduce toxicity, and improve flavor [20]. The antioxidant and anti-inflammatory activities of flavonoids separated from *Glycyrrhiza uralensis* have been reported in recent years [21, 22]. The combination of these effects may lead to enhanced lipid metabolism and reduced skin inflammation in AD.

Based on this background, we evaluated the preventive therapeutic effects of HTD treatment on inflammatory regulation and skin protection in AD-induced NC/Nga mice fed a high-fat diet.

2. Materials and Methods

2.1. Preparation of HTD Herb Extract. The procedure used to manufacture the herb extract for HTD treatment was as follows: 100 g of *Coptidis Rhizoma* and 100 g of *Glycyrrhiza uralensis* were decocted in 1,000 mL of distilled water for 3 hours and then filtered; after concentrating this mixture to 50 mL under reduced pressure using a rotary evaporator, the filtrate was freeze-dried. We obtained 31 g of the extract (yield: 15.5%) for use.

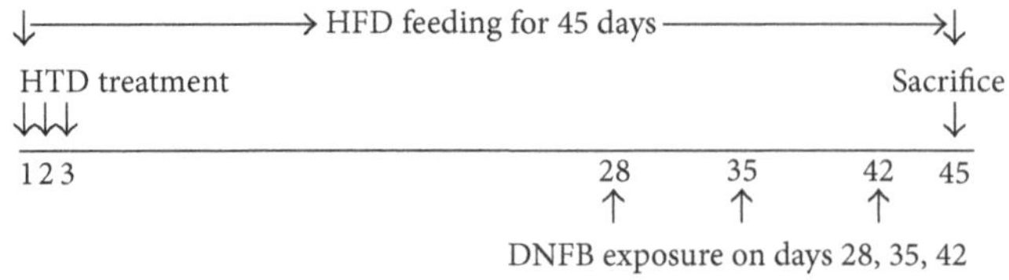

Group	HFD feeding	HTD treatment	Dermatitis elicitation
Ctrl	−	−	PBS
HF	+	−	PBS
HDE	+	−	DNFB
HTT	+	+	DNFB

Figure 1: Experimental design. Before inducing AD, the extract of *Coptidis Rhizoma* and *Glycyrrhiza uralensis*, which is traditionally used in HTD treatment, was administered orally to the HTT group on days 1, 2, and 3. Mice were challenged by DNFB on days 28, 35, and 42. During the experimental period, all groups except the Ctrl group were fed a high-fat diet freely. Ctrl: normal feeding, HF: high-fat diet, HDE: high-fat diet and untreated AD-induced, HTT: high fat diet and Hataedock treated AD-induced, HFD: high-fat diet, HTD: Hataedock, PBS: phosphate-buffered saline, and DNFB: dinitrofluorobenzene.

2.2. Animal and AD Induction. Male 3-week-old NC/Nga mice (13–15 g each) were obtained from Central Lab Animal Inc. (Seoul, Korea). The mice were divided into four groups ($n = 10$ per group) as follows: the normal feeding group (Ctrl group), high-fat diet group (HF group), high-fat diet and AD-induced with no treatment group (HDE group), and high-fat diet and AD-induced with HTD treatment group (HTT group). In the HTT group, 3-week-old mice were given HTD treatment; they were given the extract of *Coptidis Rhizoma* and *Glycyrrhiza uralensis* orally (20 mg/kg) on days 1, 2, and 3. To induce AD-like skin lesions, the back regions of the mice were stripped, and 1 mL of 5% sodium dodecyl sulfate (SDS) (Sigma-Aldrich, St. Louis, MO, USA) was rubbed on the back of each mouse 20 times using a cotton swab to remove the lipid lamella of the stratum corneum. On day 28, the mice were sensitized via exposure to 100 μL of 1% dinitrofluorobenzene (DNFB) in acetone/olive oil (4 : 1). On days 35 and 42, the mice were challenged with 2% DNFB 100 μL. On day 45, the mice were deeply anesthetized with sodium pentobarbital and killed. Mice in the HF, HDE, and HTT groups except the control group were fed a high-fat diet (fat, 60%; carbohydrate, 20%; protein, 20%; DIO DIET, USA) freely for the experimental period.

All animal experiments were approved by the Institutional Animal Care and Use Committee of Pusan National University (IACUC number: PNU-2014-0732). We followed the NIH Guide for the Care and Use of Laboratory Animals throughout this study. The experimental design is summarized in Figure 1.

2.3. Fingerprinting Analysis. High-performance liquid chromatography- (HPLC-) based fingerprinting was performed with an Agilent 1200 Series HPLC System (Agilent Technologies, Santa Clara, CA, USA), binary solvent delivery pump (G1312A), autosampler (G1329A), column oven

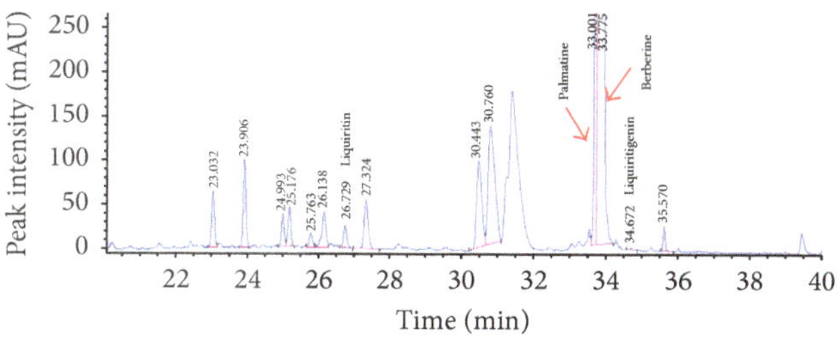

FIGURE 2: The HPLC analysis of the extract of *Coptidis Rhizoma* and *Glycyrrhiza uralensis*. Palmatine was detected at approximately 33.001 minutes, Berberine was detected at approximately 33.775 minutes, Liquritin was detected at approximately 26.729 minutes, and Liquiritigenin was detected at approximately 34.672 minutes. HPLC: High-performance liquid chromatography.

(G1316A), diode array detector (DAD; G1315D), vacuum degasser (G1322A), and Capcell PAKMGII C18 column (3.0 × 150 mm, 3.0 μm; Shiseido, Tokyo, Japan). The flow rate of the column was set at 0.6 mL/min, the temperature was maintained at 35°C, and the injection volume was set at 15 μL. The mobile phase consisted of 0.5% formic acid in water (v/v; A) and acetonitrile (B) with the following linear gradient profile: initiation 5 min, 2% B, 12 min, 10% B, 20 min, 25% B, 27 min, 25% B, 25 min, 80% B, 37 min, 80% B, 40 min, 30% B, and 45 min, 2% B. A standard solution containing Palmatine, Berberine (ChemFaces, Wuhan, China), Liquritin, and Liquiritigenin (Sigma-Aldrich, USA) was prepared by dissolving these compounds in distilled water (10 mg/100 mL). The solution was filtered through a 0.45 μm syringe filter, after which HPLC was performed.

To identify the constituents of the herb extract used for HTD treatment (the extract of *Coptidis Rhizoma* and *Glycyrrhiza uralensis*) in the study, we conducted HPLC fingerprinting. The standard constituents of our component analysis of the extract were Palmatine, Berberine, Liquritin, and Liquritigenin. The HPLC analysis is shown in Figure 2.

2.4. Tissue Process and Histochemistry. After the mice were sacrificed, dorsal skins were obtained and fixed in 10% NBF at room temperature for 24 h and embedded in paraffin for serial sectioning (5 μm).

To investigate histological changes such as epithelial hyperplasia, capillary distribution, and collagen fiber distribution, we performed Masson's trichrome staining, which is used to detect collagen fibers and collagen deposition. The samples were fixed using Bouin's fluid (50–60°C) for 1 hr. The picric acid was then removed with 70% ethanol. The samples were incubated in Weigert's iron hematoxylin working solution for 10 min to stain the nuclei, and then, the collagen fibers were stained blue with Biebrich scarlet-acid fuchsin solution and phosphomolybdic-phosphotungstic acid for 15 min each and aniline blue solution for 5 min.

To investigate the distribution and morphological changes of the mast cells that were activated by neuropeptide, we performed histochemical staining with Luna's stain. We stained the mast cell granules using an aldehyde fuchsin solution for 30 minutes and Weigert's iron hematoxylin working solution for 10 minutes and then counterstained in methyl orange solution for 5 minutes.

To investigate changes in the lipid lamella in the stratum corneum, we used the oil red O staining method. To create frozen sections for lipid staining, the samples were fixed with 10% NBF and 10% formol-calcium. We immersed the sample in a cryoprotection solution of 30% sucrose and made the frozen sections 10 mm in width by freezing microtome (Microm, Germany). After that, we placed the slices in oil red O for 10 minutes to drain off the water, counterstained with Harris hematoxylin for 2 minutes, rinsed in distilled water, then mounted the sample with glycerin jelly, and observed the slices.

2.5. Immunohistochemistry. The skin slices were steeped in proteinase K solution (20 μg/mL) to undergo proteolysis for 5 minutes. The proteolysed slices were incubated in blocking serum (10% normal goat serum) for 4 hours. Then, the slices were incubated with goat anti-LXR (1:200, Santa Cruz Biotec, USA), goat anti-PKC (1:100, Santa Cruz Biotec, USA), goat anti-IL-4 (1:100, Santa Cruz Biotec, USA), goat anti-Substance P (1:100, Santa Cruz Biotec, USA), goat anti-MMP-9 (1:200, Santa Cruz Biotec, USA), goat anti-TNF-α (1:100, Santa Cruz Biotec, USA), goat anti-p-IκB (1:500, Santa Cruz Biotec, USA), goat anti-iNOS (1:200, Santa Cruz Biotec, USA), goat anti-COX-2 (1:200, Santa Cruz Biotec, USA), goat anti-Bcl-2 (1:100, Santa Cruz Biotec, USA), and goat anti-cleaved caspase-3 (1:100, Santa Cruz Biotec, USA), all of which are primary antibodies, for 72 hours in a 4°C humidified chamber. Next, the slices were linked with biotinylated rabbit anti-goat IgG (1:100, Santa Cruz Biotec), which is a secondary antibody, for 24 hours at room temperature. After the slices were exposed to the secondary antibody, an avidin biotin complex kit (Vector Lab, USA) was applied for 1 hour at room temperature. Finally, the slices were developed with 0.05 M tris-HCl buffer solution (pH 7.4), which consisted of 0.05% 3, 3′-diaminobenzidine and 0.01% HCl, and then counterstained with hematoxylin.

2.6. TUNEL Assay. To investigate apoptosis, a TUNEL assay was performed using an *in situ* apoptosis detection kit (Apoptag, Intergen, USA). We carried out proteolysis using proteinase K for 5 minutes and then applied equilibration buffer for 5 seconds. The proteolysed slices were added strength TdT enzyme (36 μL TdT enzyme: 72 μL reaction buffer). Then, the slices were incubated in a humidified chamber at 37°C for 1 hour and then agitated for 10 minutes in strength stop/wash buffer. Next, the slices were treated with anti-digoxigenin peroxidase and DAB for 1 hour. Finally, we observed the sections counterstained with eosin using an optical microscope.

2.7. Image Analysis and Statistical Analysis. To produce numerical data from our immunohistochemistry, an image analysis was performed using image Pro Plus (Media cybernetics, USA). In image analysis of our 400x magnification exposure photography, the positive reacted particle as pixel cells (80–100 intensity range) was counted in 10 randomly

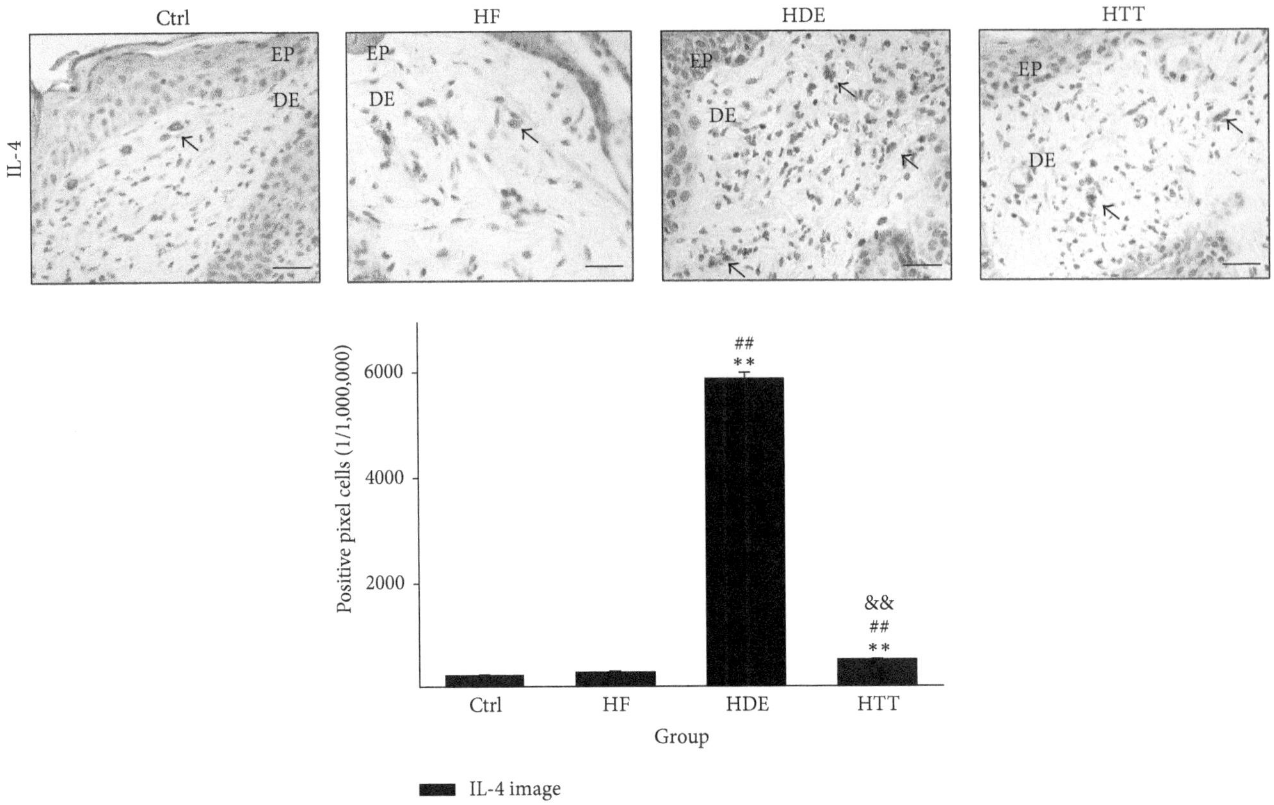

Figure 3: The regulation of Th2 differentiation. IL-4-positive reaction (arrow indicates dark brown) decreased in the HTT group compared with the HDE group (IL-4 immunohistochemistry; bar size, 50 μm). Data of IL-4 image analysis was also showing the same result ($p < 0.01$). Ctrl: normal feeding, HF: high-fat diet, HDE: high-fat diet and untreated AD-induced, HTT: high fat diet and Hataedock treated AD-induced, EP: epidermis, and DE: dermis. $^{**}p < 0.01$, compared with the Ctrl group; $^{\#\#}p < 0.01$, compared with the HF group; $^{\&\&}p < 0.01$, compared with the HDE group.

selected fields of each group (total pixel cells 100,000,000 or 1,000,000 by various results of immunohistochemistry condition such as nonspecific structure and artificiality). The data were presented as the means ± standard error. The statistical significances of the differences were analyzed with SPSS software (SPSS 23, SPSS Inc., USA), using a one-way ANOVA and Levene's (LSD) test with a significance level of $p < 0.01$.

3. Results

3.1. The Regulation of Th2 Differentiation. The regulation of Th2 differentiation was estimated by measuring the IL-4-positive reaction. The IL-4-positive reaction was seen in the cytoplasm of dermal papilla cells. The levels of IL-4 in the HTT group were shown to be decreased by 54% ($p < 0.01$) as compared with the HDE group (Figure 3).

3.2. The Maintenance of Lipid Barrier in Epidermis. The protective effects of the lipid barrier were estimated by measuring the liver X receptor- (LXR-) and PKC-positive reactions. The levels of LXR-positive reaction that were seen diffusely in the cytoplasm of cells in the stratum corneum and the stratum granulosum were remarkably decreased in the HDE group, but the levels of the HTT group were increased by 148% ($p < 0.01$) as compared with the HDE group (Figure 4).

An increase in the levels of PKC-positive reaction appearing in damaged keratinocytes and in the intercellular space was observed in the HDE group as compared with the Ctrl and HF group. This elevation was significantly decreased by HTD treatment. The levels of PKC in the HTT group were shown to be decreased by 54% ($p < 0.01$) as compared with the HDE group (Figure 4).

Moreover, we observed that skin damage, such as the elimination of the intercellular lipid lamellae in the stratum corneum, was remarkably reduced in the HTT group as compared with HDE group (Figure 4).

3.3. The Regulation of Mast Cells Activation. The regulation of mast cells activation was estimated by measuring the Substance P and matrix metallopeptidase 9- (MMP-9-) positive reaction in dermal papilla. Marked increases of Substance P and MMP-9-positive reactions, which were seen in the cytoplasm, were observed in the HDE group. Treatment with Hataedock suppressed the production of Substance P and MMP-9 significantly. The levels of Substance P in the HTT

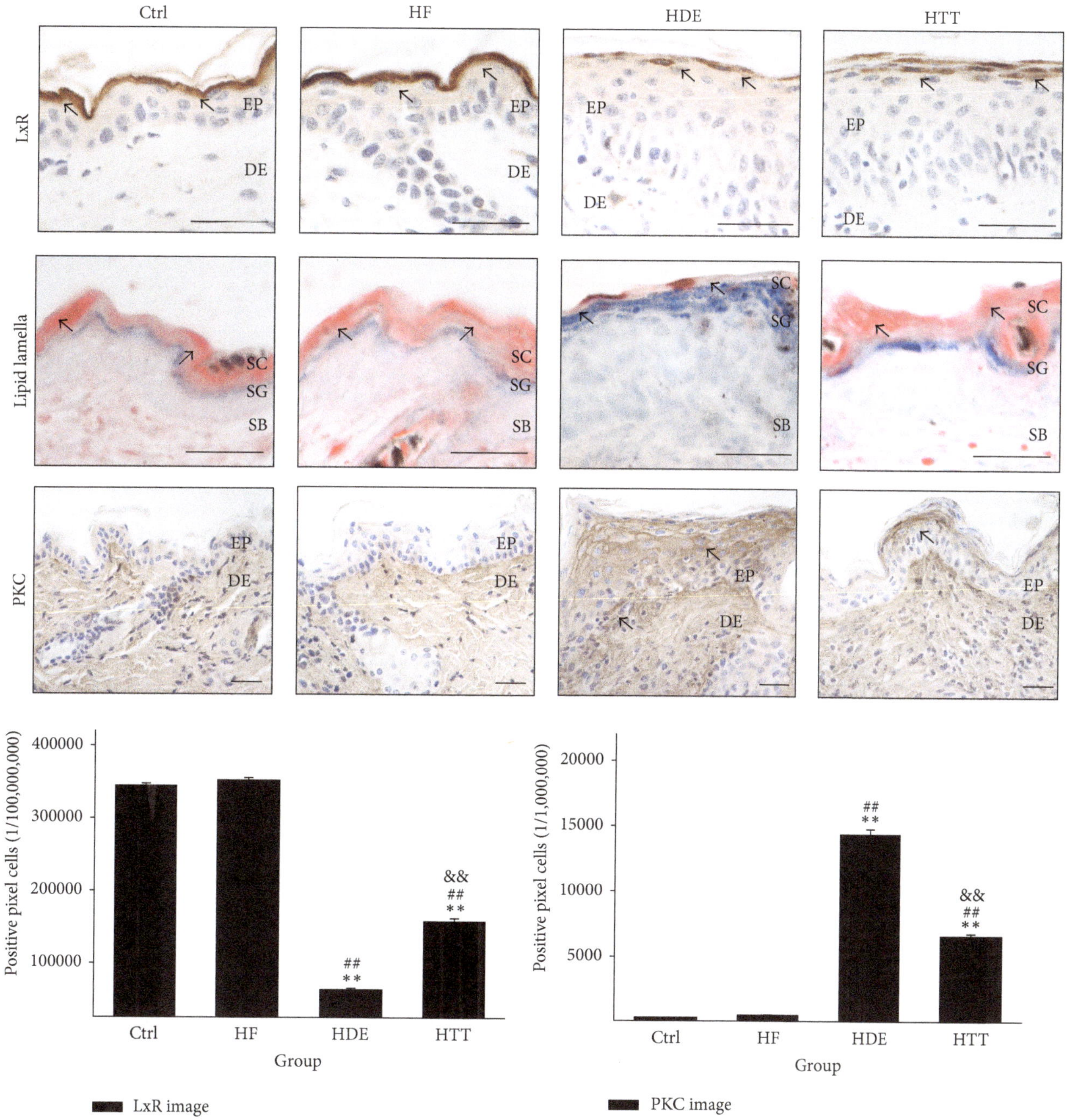

Figure 4: The maintenance of lipid barrier in epidermis. The LXR-positive reaction (arrow indicates dark brown) in HDE remarkably decreased but was maintained in HTT (LXR immunohistochemistry; bar size, 50 μm). The intercellular lipid lamellae (arrow indicates reddish line) of the stratum corneum disappeared in HDE but appeared in HTT (oil red O; bar size, 50 μm). The PKC-positive reaction (arrow indicates dark brown) in HTT remarkably decreased (PKC immunohistochemistry; bar size, 50 μm). Data of LXR and PKC image analysis was also showing the same result ($p < 0.01$). Ctrl: normal feeding, HF: high-fat diet, HDE: high-fat diet and untreated AD-induced, HTT: high fat diet and Hataedock treated AD-induced, EP: epidermis, DE: dermis, SC: stratum corneum, SG: stratum granulosum, SB: stratum basale, LXR: liver X receptor, and PKC: protein kinase C. $^{**}p < 0.01$, compared with the Ctrl group; $^{\#\#}p < 0.01$, compared with the HF group; $^{\&\&}p < 0.01$, compared with the HDE group.

group were shown to be decreased by 54% ($p < 0.01$) as compared with the HDE group. The levels of MMP-9 in the HTT group were also shown to be decreased by 48% ($p < 0.01$) as compared with the HDE group (Figure 5).

Furthermore, the results of Luna's staining showed that many degranulated mast cells from the dermal papilla to the area around the subcutaneous layer were observed in the HDE group. On the other hand, decreases in degranulated

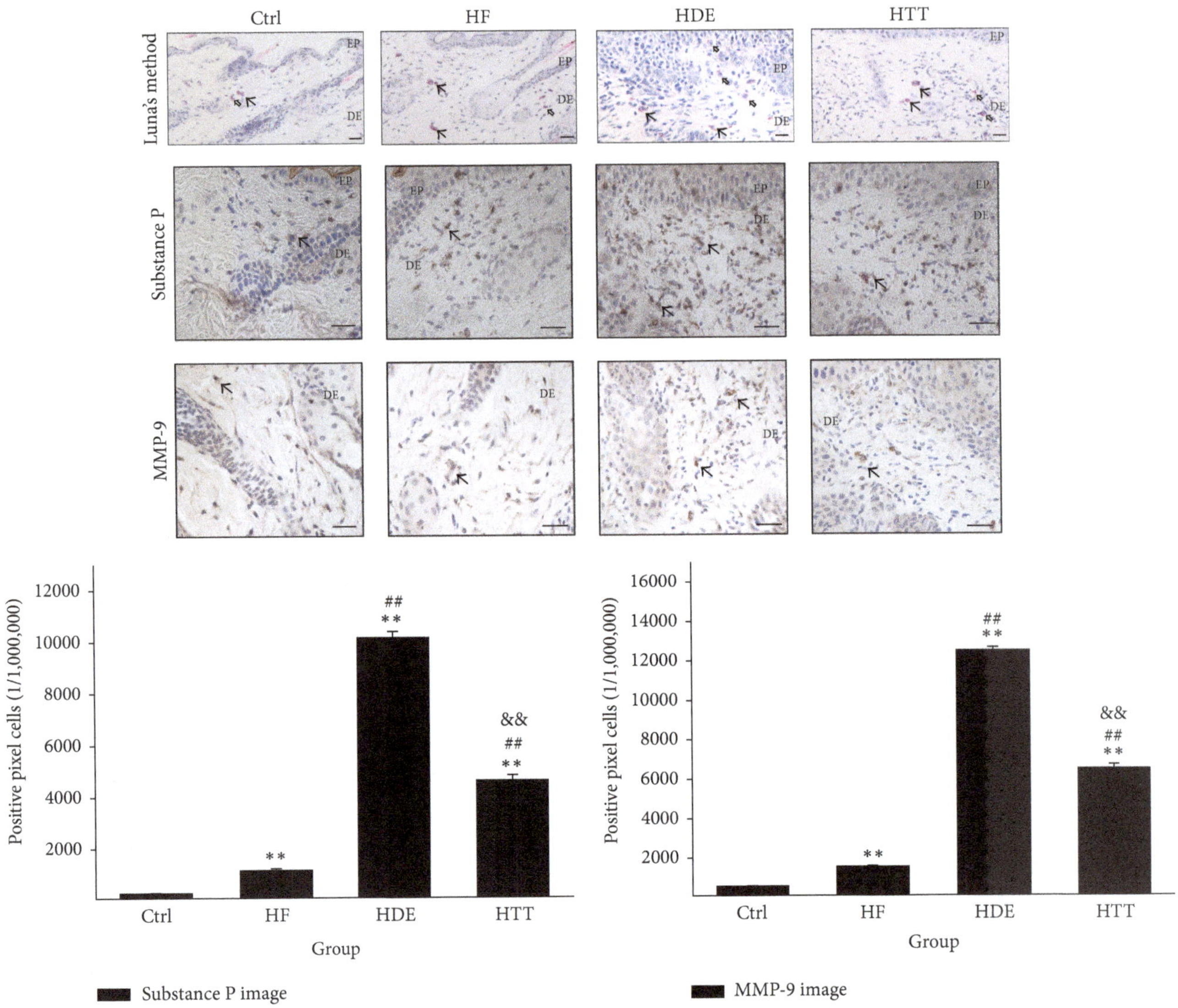

FIGURE 5: The regulation of mast cells activation. The distribution of degranulated mast cell (vacant arrow) in dermal papillae was increased in the HDE group but decreased in the HTT group (Luna's method; bar size, 50 μm). The Substance P positive reaction (arrow indicates dark brown) in HTT significantly decreased (Substance P immunohistochemistry; bar size, 50 μm). The MMP-9 positive reaction (arrow indicates dark brown) in HTT remarkably decreased (MMP-9 immunohistochemistry; bar size, 50 μm). Data of Substance P and MMP-9 image analysis was also showing the same result ($p < 0.01$). Ctrl: normal feeding, HF: high-fat diet, HDE: high-fat diet and untreated AD-induced, HTT: high fat diet and Hataedock treated AD-induced, EP: epidermis, DE: dermis, and MMP-9: matrix metalloproteinases-9. $^{**}p < 0.01$, compared with the Ctrl group; $^{\#\#}p < 0.01$, compared with the HF group; $^{\&\&}p < 0.01$, compared with the HDE group.

mast cells were observed in the HTT group as compared with the HDE group (Figure 5).

3.4. Downregulation of Inflammation. To estimate the anti-inflammatory effects of HTD, we measured the levels of TNF-α-, p-IκB-, iNOS-, and COX-2-positive reactions in stratum basale and dermal papilla. The results of the immunohistochemical staining showed the appearance of TNF-α-, p-IκB-, iNOS-, and COX-2-positive reactions in the cytoplasm. Compared with the HDE group, HTD treatment significantly decreased the levels of TNF-α-, p-IκB-, iNOS-, and COX-2-positive reactions. The HTT group showed a 32% ($p < 0.01$) decrease in TNF-α as compared with the HDE group. The HTT group showed a 61% ($p < 0.01$) decrease in p-IκB as compared with the HDE group. The levels of iNOS in the HTT group were also shown to be decreased by 63% ($p < 0.01$) as compared with the HDE group. In addition, COX-2-positive reaction levels were decreased by 51% ($p < 0.01$) in the HTT group (Figure 6).

3.5. Upregulation of Apoptosis. The results of the TUNEL assay indicated the upregulation of apoptosis in the dermal papilla cells via the HTD treatment. In the HTT group, the apoptotic body as synonymous with gathering of DNA fragmentation on nucleus was remarkably increased by 373% ($p < 0.01$) as compared to the HDE group (Figure 7).

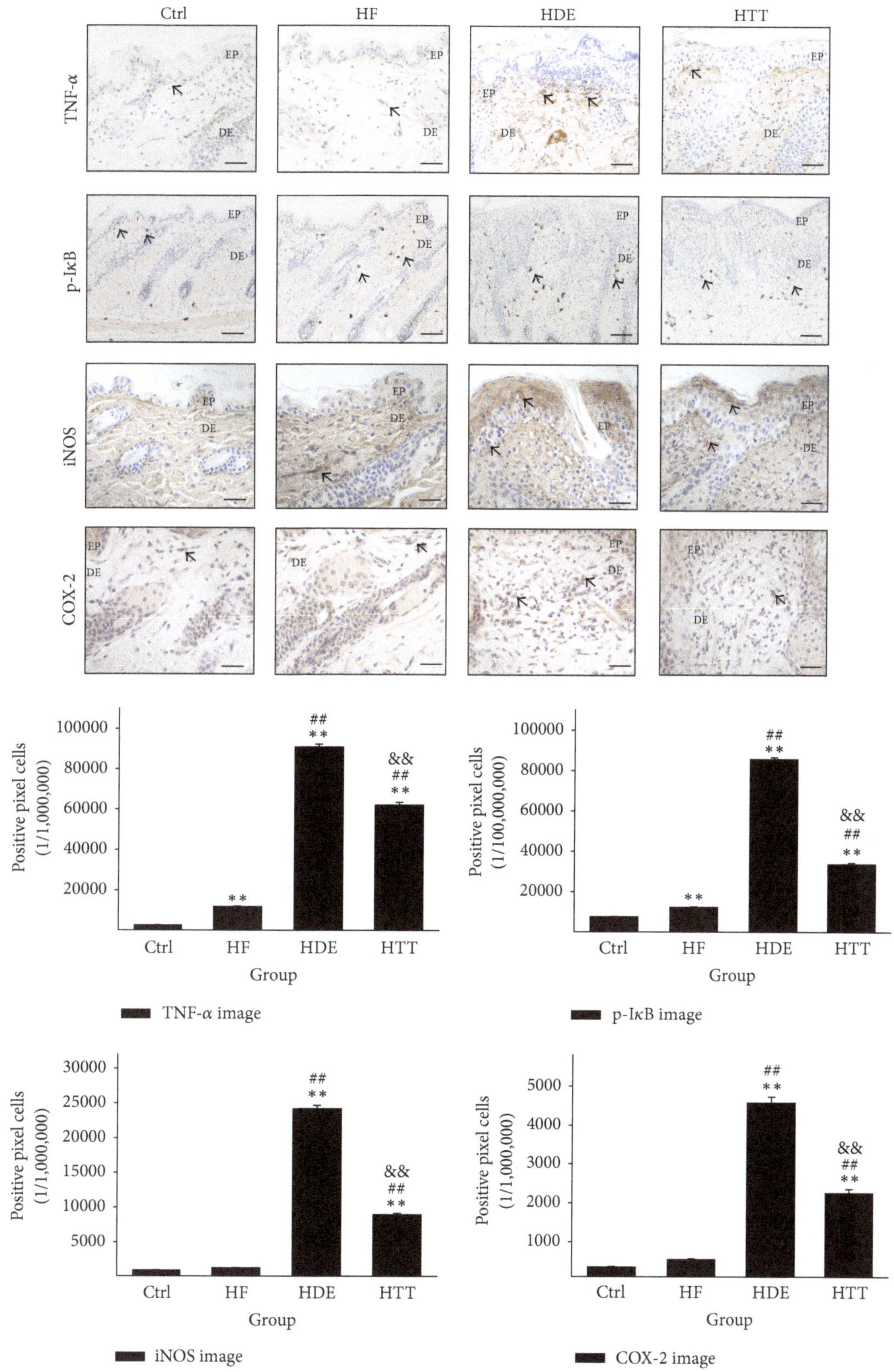

FIGURE 6: Downregulation of inflammation. In HTT group, the excessive inflammation condition such as increase of TNF-α, p-IκB, iNOS, and COX-2 was ameliorated by HTD treatment. These positive reactions (arrow indicates dark brown) were remarkably decreased compared with those of the HDE group (immunohistochemistry; bar size, 50 μm, only p-IκB bar size 100 μm). Data of TNF-α, p-IκB, iNOS, and COX-2 image analysis was also showing the same result ($p < 0.01$). Ctrl: normal feeding, HF: high-fat diet, HDE: high-fat diet and untreated AD-induced, HTT: high fat diet and Hataedock treated AD-induced, EP: epidermis, DE: dermis. $^{**}p < 0.01$, compared with the Ctrl group; $^{\#\#}p < 0.01$, compared with the HF group; $^{\&\&}p < 0.01$, compared with the HDE group.

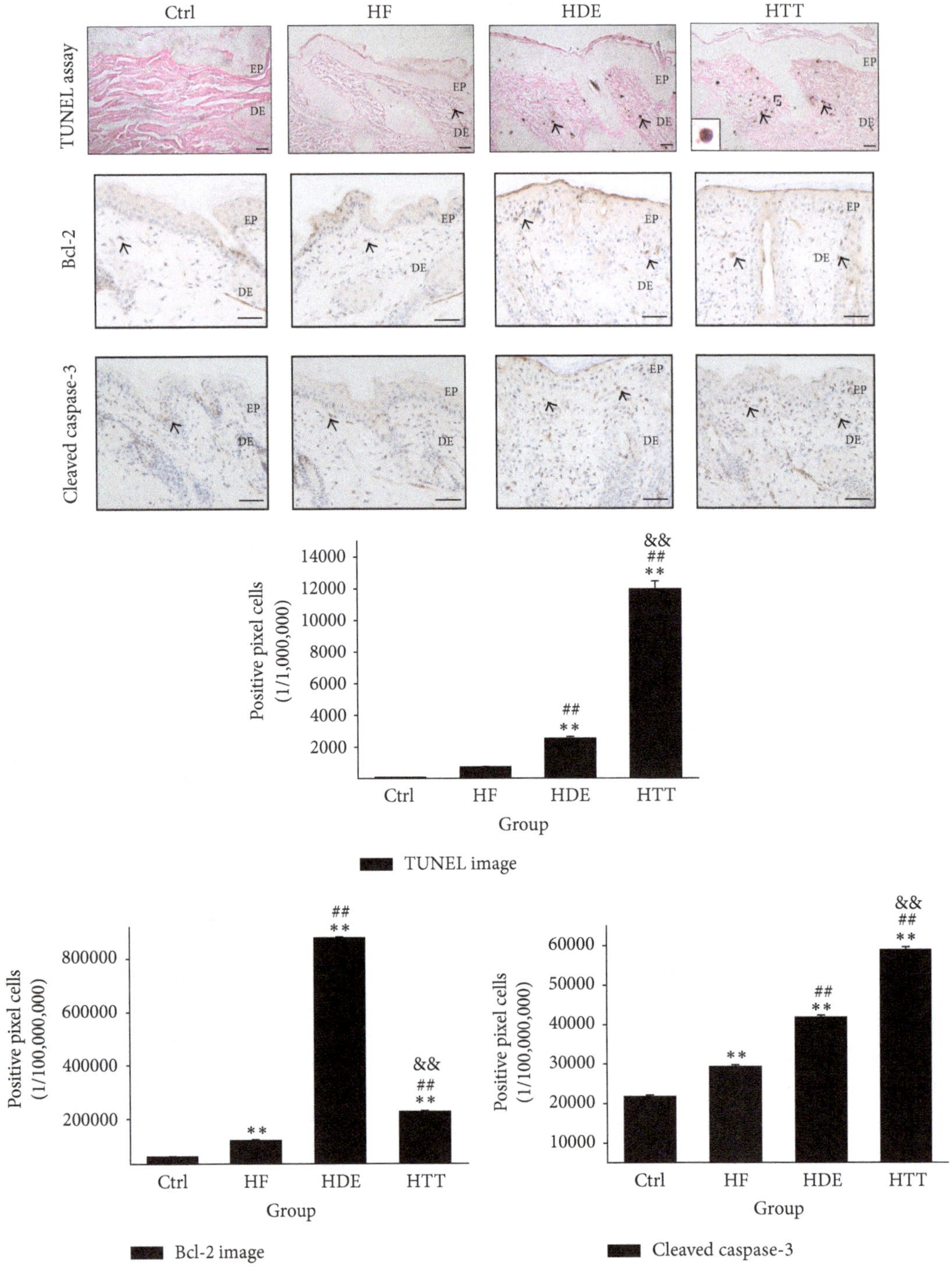

FIGURE 7: Upregulation of apoptosis. Upregulation of apoptosis in dermatitis induced by HTD treatment. The apoptotic body (arrow indicates dark brown) in the HTT group was remarkably increased compared to the HDE group (TUNEL assay; square box, enlarged DNA fragmentation of nucleus with TUNEL positive reaction; bar size, 50 μm). The Bcl-2 positive reaction (arrow indicates dark brown) in HTT group was remarkably decreased compared with those of the HDE group (immunohistochemistry; bar size, 50 μm). The cleaved caspase-3 positive reaction (arrow indicates dark brown) in HTT group was increased compared with those of the HDE group (immunohistochemistry; bar size, 50 μm). Data of TUNEL, Bcl-2, and cleaved caspase-3 image analysis was also showing the same result ($p < 0.01$). Ctrl: normal feeding, HF: high-fat diet, HDE: high-fat diet and untreated AD-induced, HTT: high fat diet and Hataedock treated AD-induced, EP: epidermis, and DE: dermis. $^{**}p < 0.01$, compared with the Ctrl group; $^{\#\#}p < 0.01$, compared with the HF group; $^{\&\&}p < 0.01$, compared with the HDE group.

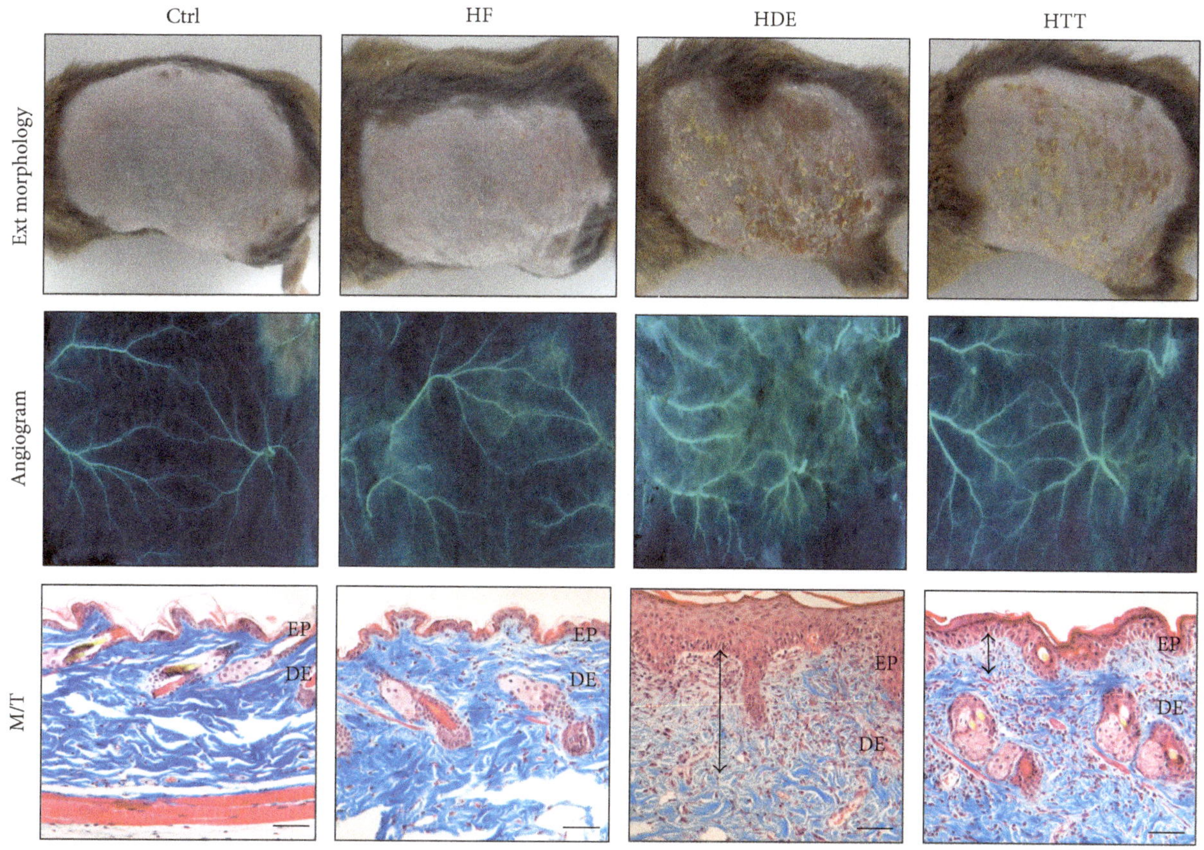

FIGURE 8: The mitigative effect of HTD treatment for dermatitis. The skin damage as eczema was mitigated in HTT group. The angiogenesis was increased in HDE group but decreased in HTT group (×4). The histological features of AD such as vacuolation of keratinocytes, hyperplasia, edema (up-down arrow), infiltration of inflammatory cells, and increase of capillary were increased in HDE group but decreased in HTT group (bar size, 100 μm). Ctrl: normal feeding, HF: high-fat diet, HDE: high-fat diet and untreated AD-induced, HTT: high fat diet and Hataedock treated AD-induced, EP: epidermis, DE: dermis, and M/T: Masson trichrome method.

Compared with the HDE group, HTD treatment significantly changes the apoptosis signal. The HTT group showed a 74% ($p < 0.01$) decrease in Bcl-2, an antiapoptotic protein, as compared with the HDE group. The HTT group showed a 41% ($p < 0.01$) increase in cleaved caspase-3, proapoptotic protein, as compared with the HDE group (Figure 7).

3.6. The Mitigative Effect of HTD Treatment on Dermatosis. The therapeutic effectiveness of HTD (administering the extract of *Coptidis Rhizoma* and *Glycyrrhiza uralensis*) was explored by examining its effect on dermatosis severity. AD-induced mice that were fed a high-fat diet and did not receive any treatment (the HDE group) showed the highest level of dermatosis severity. The obtained image of the HDE group showed various pathological features, such as severe erythema, blood clot, edema, superficial erosion, deep excoriation, and dry skin. In contrast, the high-fat-diet-fed, AD-induced mice treated with HTD (the HTT group) exhibited better control of AD symptoms (Figure 8).

A comparison of angiogenesis was conducted between the HDE and HTT groups. Our angiogram reveals that the HTT group experienced much better angiogenesis reduction than the HDE group (Figure 8).

For the results obtained from Masson's trichrome stains, the atopic mice of the HDE group also exhibited significant damage such as vacuolation of keratinocytes, hyperplasia in epidermis, disappearance of collagen fibers, the infiltration of inflammatory cells, and an increase in dermal capillary density.

On the other hand, when mice were treated with HTD, the amelioration of epidermal hyperplasia, the improvement of collagen fiber density, and fewer inflammatory cell infiltrates in the dermis were remarkably observed (Figure 8).

4. Discussion

The results of the studies suggest that HTD treatment may be an effective preventive treatment for AD. HTD treatment was effective in attenuating inflammation and maintaining the skin barrier in AD-induced NC/Nga mice under high-fat-diet conditions. Much progress has been made in understanding the genetic background and pathophysiology of AD, thus allowing more specific therapeutic interventions to be introduced [23]. Among these interventions, we paid attention to those that intervene very early in the lives of infants and young children by controlling skin inflammation at the earliest time point [24]. Moreover, there is now plenty of evidence indicating close ties between the metabolic and immune systems. It is now clear that obesity is associated with a state of chronic low-level inflammation [25]. In this respect, an unbalanced maternal diet during breastfeeding may be a risk factor underlying the later development of atopic sensitization in the infant, regardless of maternal atopic disease [26]. It was also reported that neonatal adiposity is a predictor of AD [12].

We hypothesized that both immune system dysregulation and a high-fat diet may affect inflammatory responses in the infant. Further, we hypothesized that these responses may amplify the development of AD. Based on these hypotheses, we investigated the preventive therapeutic effects of HTD treatment on inflammatory regulation and skin protection in AD-induced NC/Nga mice under high-fat diet conditions. This study differs from previous studies with regard to the timing of treatment administration. Previous studies administered the herbal extracts after AD symptom onset [27–30]. On the other hand, this study administered the herbal extracts before clinical symptom onset. We also established a high-fat-diet-induced model and so attempted to identify relevant neonatal adiposity and the development of AD.

4.1. The Regulation of Th2 Differentiation. It was known that the Th2-biased immune responses that characterize neonates may influence the later onset of allergic disease [31]. Th2 cells mediate these functions by producing various cytokines. Particularly, IL-4 is a key Th2 cytokine that is critical for Th2 cell differentiation, IgE production, and eosinophil recruitment, among other functions [32]. It was reported that high levels of IL-4-producing T cells and low levels of IFN-γ at birth may enhance the risk of the subsequent development of AD [33].

To estimate the regulation of Th2 differentiation, we measured the level of IL-4-positive reaction in the dermal papilla cells. We show that the levels of IL-4 positive reaction were remarkably increased in the HDE group but that the levels of the HTT group were decreased (Figure 3). This finding suggests that HTD treatment reduced the level of IL-4. This decrease of IL-4 may contribute to the regulation of Th2 differentiation and these results may also contribute to the improvement of AD.

4.2. The Maintenance of Lipid Barrier in Epidermis. We show that the levels of LXR-positive reaction were remarkably decreased in the HDE group but that the level of the HTT group was maintained. Moreover, the lipid barrier in the intercellular space was also maintained in the HTT group. On the other hand, an increase in the levels of PKC was observed in the HDE group as compared with the Ctrl group. This elevation was significantly decreased in the HTT group (Figure 4).

It is known that dysfunctional ceramides in the SC barrier may contribute to the disruption of the epidermal barrier, resulting in mechanisms that operate in the pathophysiology of AD [34]. This condition is induced by PKC activation, which plays a role in the initiation of epidermal barrier dysfunction [35]. The PKC signaling pathway is activated by a broad spectrum of extracellular stimuli that promote lipid hydrolysis and play a fundamental role in numerous biological facets, such as differentiation, proliferation, apoptosis, and neuronal transmitter release [36]. It is known that transactivation by LXR was decreased by the activation of the PKC signaling pathway [37].

LXRs play a critical role in the control of lipid metabolism, acting as regulators of cholesterol and fatty acid metabolism [38]. Previous studies have demonstrated that LXR activators stimulate epidermal differentiation, improve permeability barrier homeostasis, and inhibit epidermal proliferation [39, 40]. Additionally, it is known that LXR activators exhibit potent antihyperplastic and anti-inflammatory activity in irritant-contact dermatitis and acute allergic-contact dermatitis [41]. LXR activation also accelerates permeability barrier recovery following acute barrier disruption [42].

Therefore, the protective effects for the lipid barrier may be caused by the activation of LXRs and the inhibition of PKC. Such effects may influence the maintenance of the lipid barrier in the HTT group.

4.3. The Regulation of Mast Cells Activation. Mast cells play a central role in both acute and chronic allergic reactions through the release of a number of mediators and cytokines [43]. Because most studies have shown increased numbers of mast cells in skin lesions in AD models, it is generally assumed that mast cells contribute to skin inflammation [2]. Upon activation, mast cells release their membrane-bound cytosolic granules, leading to the release of several molecules that are important in the pathogenesis of AD and host defense [44].

Mast cell associated nerves in the skin are predominantly Substance P-positive [45]. Substance P, an established neurotransmitter, evokes an immune inflammatory response involving the degranulation of mast cells [46]. Interestingly, it has also been pointed out that stress and anxiety worsen dermatitis via Substance P-dependent neurogenic inflammation in mice [47]. Thus, Substance P is currently considered to be one of the key pruritogenic factors [48].

Matrix metalloproteinase- (MMP-) 9 has been recognized in the process of inflammation and tissue remodeling and repair. Also, mast cells can produce MMP-9, which may contribute to extracellular matrix degradation and absorption in the process of allergic and nonallergic responses [49]. Thus, it is assumed that MMP-9 could be important in the pathogenesis of AD [50].

In the present study, many degranulated mast cells were observed in the HDE group. On the other hand, primarily granular mast cells appeared in HTT group. Moreover, the levels of Substance P and MMP-9 were significantly decreased in the HTT group (Figure 5). Therefore, these results imply that HTD reduces the infiltration of degranulated mast cells and can prevent the release of Substance P and MMP-9.

4.4. Downregulation of Inflammation. TNF-α is one inflammatory mediator that has been implicated in AD, due to its participation in lipid and protein synthesis in the epidermis and as a consequence of effect of skin barrier lipid composition and organization [51]. It is known that facilitated translocation of NF-κB may worsen the allergic inflammation including AD by enhancing the production of inflammatory cytokines and chemokines [52]. And the phosphorylated IκB (p-IκB) allow the NF-κB subunit to translocate to the nucleus [53]. For this reason, deregulation of NF-κB and p-IκB is a hallmark of chronic inflammatory diseases [54]. iNOS and COX-2 are also known to play important roles in the regulation of inflammatory reactions [55, 56]. iNOS produces high amounts of NO induced by cytokines such as interferon gamma and TNF-α [57]. NO derived from iNOS also plays important roles in the modulation of symptoms in patients with inflammatory diseases, including AD [58]. It is also known that COX products are increased in the skin of patients with AD [59].

To elucidate the role of the anti-inflammatory effects of HTD, we analyzed the levels of TNF-α-, p-IκB-, iNOS-, and COX-2-positive reactions. Marked increases in TNF-α, p-IκB, iNOS, and COX-2 production were observed in the HDE group. These increases were effectively lowered by HTD treatment in the HTT group (Figure 6). While the inflammatory response plays important roles in protecting the host and repairing tissues, it can also damage normal skin tissues. Therefore, these results of the decrease in inflammatory cytokines imply that HTD may contribute to the reduction of inflammation and improvement of AD.

4.5. Upregulation of Apoptosis. Apoptosis is highly important in the renewal of cells and formation of epidermal structure [60]. Apoptotic cells may not stimulate inflammation if they are ingested by phagocytes before they release their intracellular substances. Moreover, during this process apoptotic cells can stimulate phagocytes to induce anti-inflammatory cytokines [61]. It has also been reported that dysregulated apoptosis may contribute to the development and persistence of AD [62].

Overexpression of the Bcl-2 has been demonstrated to prevent apoptosis either by sequestering proforms of death-driving caspases or by preventing the release of cytochrome c into the cytoplasm [63, 64]. On the other hand, sequential activation of caspases plays an important role in the execution-phase of cell apoptosis. Among them, caspase-3 is a commonly activated death protease, catalyzing the specific cleavage of many key cellular proteins [65]. The caspase-3 is known to act downstream on bax/bcl-2 control [66]. The cleavage products of bcl-2 are located to the mitochondria resulting in the release of cytochrome c and leading to more caspase-3 activation as a positive feedback effect, strengthening the apoptotic effect [67].

In the present study, apoptotic cells were determined via TUNEL assay. The apoptotic bodies in the HTT group were remarkably increased in number as compared to the HDE group. The cleaved caspase-3 positive reaction was also increased in the HTT group. In contrast, the Bcl-2 positive reaction in HTT group was remarkably decreased (Figure 7). This finding suggests that HTD treatment may contribute to stimulate the apoptotic cascade activation that ultimately leads to improvement of AD.

4.6. The Mitigative Effect of HTD Treatment on Dermatosis. In this study, we demonstrated the skin barrier maintenance and anti-inflammatory effects of HTD treatment under high-fat-diet conditions in AD. In our animal model, the repeated application of DNFB caused skin damage and increased angiogenesis and spongiosis in the HDE group. However, in the HTT group, damage to the intercellular space, hyperplasia, edema, the infiltration of inflammatory cell, and increased capillaries were decreased (Figure 8).

Therefore, these findings suggest that HTD was more effective in maintaining skin integrity during the course of dermatosis and treatment under high-fat-diet conditions. These results indicate that HTD may alleviate the underlying inflammatory reactions and effectively attenuate these skin damages.

5. Conclusions

In summary, we demonstrated that HTD treatment was effective in attenuating inflammation and maintaining the skin barrier in AD-induced NC/Nga mice under high-fat-diet conditions. These results imply that HTD may alleviate the symptom of AD through the regulation of Th2 differentiation, the maintenance of lipid barrier in epidermis, the regulation of mast cells activation, downregulation of inflammation, and upregulation of apoptosis. In conclusion, HTD could be used as an alternative and preventive therapeutic approach in the management of AD. Further studies about detailed mechanism of these protective immune responses are needed.

Competing Interests

The authors declare that there are no competing interests regarding the publication of this paper.

Acknowledgments

This research was supported by the Basic Science Research Program through the National Research Foundation of Korea (NRF) funded by the Ministry of Education (NRF-2014R1A1A2055061).

References

[1] N. Behniafard, M. Gharagozlou, E. Farhadi et al., "TNF-alpha single nucleotide polymorphisms in atopic dermatitis," *European Cytokine Network*, vol. 23, no. 4, pp. 163–165, 2012.

[2] T. Kawakami, T. Ando, M. Kimura, B. S. Wilson, and Y. Kawakami, "Mast cells in atopic dermatitis," *Current Opinion in Immunology*, vol. 21, no. 6, pp. 666–678, 2009.

[3] K. C. Barnes, "An update on the genetics of atopic dermatitis: scratching the surface in 2009," *Journal of Allergy and Clinical Immunology*, vol. 125, no. 1–3, pp. 16.e11–29.e11, 2010.

[4] S. Danby and M. J. Cork, "A new understanding of atopic dermatitis: the role of epidermal barrier dysfunction and subclinical inflammation," *Journal of Clinical Dermatology*, vol. 1, pp. 33–46, 2012.

[5] P. M. Elias and M. Schmuth, "Abnormal skin barrier in the etiopathogenesis of atopic dermatitis," *Current Opinion in*

Allergy and Clinical Immunology, vol. 9, no. 5, pp. 437–446, 2009.

[6] D. Y. M. Leung, M. Boguniewicz, M. D. Howell, I. Nomura, and Q. A. Hamid, "New insights into atopic dermatitis," *The Journal of Clinical Investigation*, vol. 113, no. 5, pp. 651–657, 2004.

[7] A. Yabuhara, C. Macaubas, S. L. Prescott et al., "TH2-polarized immunological memory to inhalant allergens in atopics is established during infancy and early childhood," *Clinical and Experimental Allergy*, vol. 27, no. 11, pp. 1261–1269, 1997.

[8] F. I. Smillie, A. J. Elderfield, F. Patel et al., "Lymphoproliferative responses in cord blood and at one year: no evidence for the effect of in utero exposure to dust mite allergens," *Clinical and Experimental Allergy*, vol. 31, no. 8, pp. 1194–1204, 2001.

[9] H. Löffler, J. U. N. Aramaki, and I. Effendy, "The influence of body mass index on skin susceptibility to sodium lauryl sulphate," *Skin Research and Technology*, vol. 8, no. 1, pp. 19–22, 2002.

[10] M. Nino, A. Franzese, N. Ruggiero Perrino, and N. Balato, "The effect of obesity on skin disease and epidermal permeability barrier status in children," *Pediatric Dermatology*, vol. 29, no. 5, pp. 567–570, 2012.

[11] A. Zhang and J. I. Silverberg, "Association of atopic dermatitis with being overweight and obese: a systematic review and metaanalysis," *Journal of the American Academy of Dermatology*, vol. 72, no. 4, pp. 606–616.e4, 2015.

[12] S. M. O'Donovan, J. O'B Hourihane, D. M. Murray et al., "Neonatal adiposity increases the risk of atopic dermatitis during the first year of life," *Journal of Allergy and Clinical Immunology*, vol. 137, no. 1, pp. 108–117, 2015.

[13] H. W. Jeong and H. S. Kim, "Oriental medical approach on the allergic disease," *Korean Journal of Oriental Physiology and Pathology*, vol. 16, no. 5, pp. 831–839, 2002.

[14] A. Baroni, E. Ruocco, T. Russo et al., "The use of traditional Chinese medicine in some dermatologic diseases: part II—autoimmune bullous disorders and lichen planus," *Skinmed*, vol. 13, no. 3, pp. 195–203, 2015.

[15] H. Y. Cha, S. H. Ahn, A. R. Jeong, J. H. Cheon, S. Y. Park, and K. B. Kim, "The effects of hataedock on 2,4-dinitrofluorobenzene induced atopic dermatitis like skin lesion in NC/Nga mice," *The Journal of Korean Oriental Pediatrics*, vol. 29, no. 4, pp. 97–107, 2015.

[16] H. Y. Cha, S. H. Ahn, A. R. Jeong et al., "Anti-inflammatory effects of hataedock extracted from coptidis rhizoma and glycyrrhiza uralensis on atopic dermatitis-like skin lesions of NC/Nga mouse," *Journal of Korean Oriental Internal Medicine*, vol. 36, no. 4, pp. 486–497, 2015.

[17] B. Pang, X.-T. Yu, Q. Zhou et al., "Effect of *Rhizoma coptidis* (Huang Lian) on treating diabetes mellitus," *Evidence-Based Complementary and Alternative Medicine*, vol. 2015, Article ID 921416, 10 pages, 2015.

[18] H. Wang, W. Mu, H. Shang, J. Lin, and X. Lei, "The antihyperglycemic effects of rhizoma coptidis and mechanism of actions: a review of systematic reviews and pharmacological research," *BioMed Research International*, vol. 2014, Article ID 798093, 10 pages, 2014.

[19] W. Xie, D. Gu, J. Li, K. Cui, and Y. Zhang, "Effects and action mechanisms of berberine and *Rhizoma coptidis* on gut microbes and obesity in high-fat diet-fed C57BL/6J mice," *PLoS ONE*, vol. 6, no. 9, Article ID e24520, 2011.

[20] B. Jayaprakasam, S. Doddaga, R. Wang, D. Holmes, J. Goldfarb, and X.-M. Li, "Licorice flavonoids inhibit eotaxin-1 secretion by human fetal lung fibroblasts *in vitro*," *Journal of Agricultural and Food Chemistry*, vol. 57, no. 3, pp. 820–825, 2009.

[21] Y. Fu, J. Chen, Y.-J. Li, Y.-F. Zheng, and P. Li, "Antioxidant and anti-inflammatory activities of six flavonoids separated from licorice," *Food Chemistry*, vol. 141, no. 2, pp. 1063–1071, 2013.

[22] H. J. Kim, J.-Y. Seo, H.-J. Suh, S. S. Lim, and J.-S. Kim, "Antioxidant activities of licorice-derived prenylflavonoids," *Nutrition Research and Practice*, vol. 6, no. 6, pp. 491–498, 2012.

[23] D. E. Cohen and N. Heidary, "Treatment of irritant and allergic contact dermatitis," *Dermatologic Therapy*, vol. 17, no. 4, pp. 334–340, 2004.

[24] T. Bieber, "Atopic dermatitis," *Annals of Dermatology*, vol. 22, no. 2, pp. 125–137, 2010.

[25] K. E. Wellen and G. S. Hotamisligil, "Inflammation, stress, and diabetes," *Journal of Clinical Investigation*, vol. 115, no. 5, pp. 1111–1119, 2005.

[26] U. Hoppu, M. Kalliomaki, and E. Isolauri, "Maternal diet rich in saturated fat during breastfeeding is associated with atopic sensitization of the infant," *European Journal of Clinical Nutrition*, vol. 54, no. 9, pp. 702–705, 2000.

[27] K.-H. Kim and S.-Y. Choung, "Oral administration of vaccinium uliginosum L. extract alleviates dncb-induced atopic dermatitis in NC/Nga mice," *Journal of Medicinal Food*, vol. 17, no. 12, pp. 1350–1360, 2014.

[28] H. Ha, H. Lee, C. S. Seo et al., "Artemisia *capillaris* inhibits atopic dermatitis-like skin lesions in *Dermatophagoides farinae*-sensitized Nc/Nga mice," *BMC Complementary and Alternative Medicine*, vol. 14, article 100, 2014.

[29] M.-C. Kim, C.-H. Lee, and T.-H. Yook, "Effects of anti-inflammatory and rehmanniae radix pharmacopuncture on atopic dermatitis in NC/Nga mice," *Journal of Acupuncture and Meridian Studies*, vol. 6, no. 2, pp. 98–109, 2013.

[30] H.-S. Lim, C.-S. Seo, H. Ha et al., "Effect of Alpinia katsumadai Hayata on house dust mite-induced atopic dermatitis in NC/Nga mice," *Evidence-Based Complementary and Alternative Medicine*, vol. 2012, Article ID 705167, 9 pages, 2012.

[31] A. Dubois, N. Deruytter, B. Adams et al., "Regulation of Th2 responses and allergic inflammation through bystander activation of $CD8^+$ T lymphocytes in early life," *The Journal of Immunology*, vol. 185, no. 2, pp. 884–891, 2010.

[32] E. B. Brandt and U. Sivaprasad, "Th2 cytokines and atopic dermatitis," *Journal of Clinical & Cellular Immunology*, vol. 2, no. 3, p. 110, 2011.

[33] G. Herberth, J. Heinrich, S. Röder et al., "Reduced IFN-γ- and enhanced IL-4-producing $CD4^+$ cord blood T cells are associated with a higher risk for atopic dermatitis during the first 2 yr of life," *Pediatric Allergy and Immunology*, vol. 21, no. 1, part I, pp. 5–13, 2010.

[34] J. Levin, S. F. Friedlander, and J. Q. Del Rosso, "Atopic dermatitis and the stratum corneum: part 1: the role of filaggrin in the stratum corneum barrier and atopic skin," *Journal of Clinical and Aesthetic Dermatology*, vol. 6, no. 10, pp. 16–22, 2013.

[35] H. Kim, R. Zamel, X.-H. Bai, and M. Liu, "PKC activation induces inflammatory response and cell death in human bronchial epithelial cells," *PLoS ONE*, vol. 8, no. 5, Article ID e64182, 2013.

[36] A. C. Newton, "Regulation of the ABC kinases by phosphorylation: protein kinase C as a paradigm," *Biochemical Journal*, vol. 370, no. 2, pp. 361–371, 2003.

[37] C. J. Delvecchio and J. P. Capone, "Protein kinase C α modulates liver X receptor α transactivation," *Journal of Endocrinology*, vol. 197, no. 1, pp. 121–130, 2008.

[38] T. Nomiyama and D. Bruemmer, "Liver X receptors as therapeutic targets in metabolism and atherosclerosis," *Current Atherosclerosis Reports*, vol. 10, no. 1, pp. 88–95, 2008.

[39] L. G. Kömüves, K. Hanley, Y. Jiang, P. M. Elias, M. L. Williams, and K. R. Feingold, "Ligands and activators of nuclear hormone receptors regulate epidermal differentiation during fetal rat skin development," *Journal of Investigative Dermatology*, vol. 111, no. 3, pp. 429–433, 1998.

[40] K. Hanley, D. C. Ng, S. S. He et al., "Oxysterols induce differentiation in human keratinocytes and increase AP-1-dependent involucrin transcription," *Journal of Investigative Dermatology*, vol. 114, no. 3, pp. 545–553, 2000.

[41] Y. Hatano, M.-Q. Man, Y. Uchida et al., "Murine atopic dermatitis responds to peroxisome proliferator-activated receptors α and β/δ (but not γ) and liver X receptor activators," *Journal of Allergy and Clinical Immunology*, vol. 125, no. 1, pp. 160–169.e5, 2010.

[42] L. G. Kömüves, M. Schmuth, A. J. Fowler et al., "Oxysterol stimulation of epidermal differentiation is mediated by liver X receptor-β in murine epidermis," *Journal of Investigative Dermatology*, vol. 118, no. 1, pp. 25–34, 2002.

[43] H. J. Gould, B. J. Sutton, A. J. Beavil et al., "The biology of IgE and the basis of allergic disease," *Annual Review of Immunology*, vol. 21, pp. 579–628, 2003.

[44] S. J. Galli and M. Tsai, "IgE and mast cells in allergic disease," *Nature Medicine*, vol. 18, no. 5, pp. 693–704, 2012.

[45] A. Naukkarinen, I. Harvima, K. Paukkonen, M.-L. Aalto, and M. Horsmanheimo, "Immunohistochemical analysis of sensory nerves and neuropeptides, and their contacts with mast cells in developing and mature psoriatic lesions," *Archives of Dermatological Research*, vol. 285, no. 6, pp. 341–346, 1993.

[46] H. Suzuki, S. Miura, Y. Y. Liu, M. Tsuchiya, and H. Ishii, "Substance P induces degranulation of mast cells and leukocyte adhesion to venular endothelium," *Peptides*, vol. 16, no. 8, pp. 1447–1452, 1995.

[47] S. Pavlovic, M. Daniltchenko, D. J. Tobin et al., "Further exploring the brain-skin connection: stress worsens dermatitis via substance P-dependent neurogenic inflammation in mice," *Journal of Investigative Dermatology*, vol. 128, no. 2, pp. 434–446, 2008.

[48] C.-F. Wahlgren, "Itch and atopic dermatitis: an overview," *Journal of Dermatology*, vol. 26, no. 11, pp. 770–779, 1999.

[49] N. Kanbe, A. Tanaka, M. Kanbe, A. Itakura, M. Kurosawa, and H. Matsuda, "Human mast cells produce matrix metalloproteinase 9," *European Journal of Immunology*, vol. 29, no. 8, pp. 2645–2649, 1999.

[50] A. C. A. Devillers, A. W. Van Toorenenbergen, G. J. Klein Heerenbrink, P. G. H. Mulder, and A. P. Oranje, "Elevated levels of plasma matrix metalloproteinase-9 in patients with atopic dermatitis: a pilot study," *Clinical and Experimental Dermatology*, vol. 32, no. 3, pp. 311–313, 2007.

[51] M. O. Danso, V. van Drongelen, A. Mulder et al., "TNF-α and Th2 cytokines induce atopic dermatitis-like features on epidermal differentiation proteins and stratum corneum lipids in human skin equivalents," *Journal of Investigative Dermatology*, vol. 134, no. 7, pp. 1941–1950, 2014.

[52] A. Tanaka, S. Muto, K. Jung, A. Itai, and H. Matsuda, "Topical application with a new NF-κB inhibitor improves atopic dermatitis in NC/NgaTnd mice," *Journal of Investigative Dermatology*, vol. 127, no. 4, pp. 855–863, 2007.

[53] A. Blaecke, Y. Delneste, N. Herbault et al., "Measurement of nuclear factor-kappa B translocation on lipopolysaccharide-activated human dendritic cells by confocal microscopy and flow cytometry," *Cytometry*, vol. 48, no. 2, pp. 71–79, 2002.

[54] P. Viatour, M.-P. Merville, V. Bours, and A. Chariot, "Phosphorylation of NF-κB and IκB proteins: implications in cancer and inflammation," *Trends in Biochemical Sciences*, vol. 30, no. 1, pp. 43–52, 2005.

[55] K. Orita, K. Hiramoto, H. Kobayashi, M. Ishii, A. Sekiyama, and M. Inoue, "Inducible nitric oxide synthase (iNOS) and α-melanocyte-stimulating hormones of iNOS origin play important roles in the allergic reactions of atopic dermatitis in mice," *Experimental Dermatology*, vol. 20, no. 11, pp. 911–914, 2011.

[56] D. Laouini, A. Elkhal, A. Yalcindag, S. Kawamoto, H. Oettgen, and R. S. Geha, "COX-2 inhibition enhances the TH2 immune response to epicutaneous sensitization," *Journal of Allergy and Clinical Immunology*, vol. 116, no. 2, pp. 390–396, 2005.

[57] L. Leifeld, M. Fielenbach, F.-L. Dumoulin, N. Speidel, T. Sauerbruch, and U. Spengler, "Inducible nitric oxide synthase (iNOS) and endothelial nitric oxide synthase (eNOS) expression in fulminant hepatic failure," *Journal of Hepatology*, vol. 37, no. 5, pp. 613–619, 2002.

[58] S. Taniuchi, T. Kojima, K. Hara Mt et al., "Increased serum nitrate levels in infants with atopic dermatitis," *Allergy*, vol. 56, no. 7, pp. 693–695, 2001.

[59] K. Fogh, T. Herlin, and K. Kragballe, "Eicosanoids in skin of patients with atopic dermatitis: prostaglandin E2 and leukotriene B4 are present in biologically active concentrations," *The Journal of Allergy and Clinical Immunology*, vol. 83, no. 2, pp. 450–455, 1989.

[60] J. Grigaitiene, I. Marciukaitiene, A. Blaziene, and A. Chomiciene, "Study of apoptosis in normal skin tissues," *Medicina (Kaunas, Lithuania)*, vol. 43, no. 4, pp. 301–305, 2007.

[61] K. L. Rock and H. Kono, "The inflammatory response to cell death," *Annual Review of Pathology: Mechanisms of Disease*, vol. 3, pp. 99–126, 2008.

[62] A. Trautmann, M. Akdis, K. Blaser, and C. A. Akdis, "Role of dysregulated apoptosis in atopic dermatitis," *Apoptosis*, vol. 5, no. 5, pp. 425–429, 2000.

[63] K. W. Yip and J. C. Reed, "Bcl-2 family proteins and cancer," *Oncogene*, vol. 27, no. 50, pp. 6398–6406, 2008.

[64] Y. Tsujimoto, "Role of Bcl-2 family proteins in apoptosis: apoptosomes or mitochondria?" *Genes to Cells*, vol. 3, no. 11, pp. 697–707, 1998.

[65] A. G. Porter and R. U. Jänicke, "Emerging roles of caspase-3 in apoptosis," *Cell Death and Differentiation*, vol. 6, no. 2, pp. 99–104, 1999.

[66] T. Rudel, "Caspase inhibitors in prevention of apoptosis," *Herz*, vol. 24, no. 3, pp. 236–241, 1999.

[67] D. G. Kirsch, A. Doseff, B. N. Chau et al., "Caspase-3-dependent cleavage of Bcl-2 promotes release of cytochrome c," *Journal of Biological Chemistry*, vol. 274, no. 30, pp. 21155–21161, 1999.

The Classification of *Sini* Decoction Pattern in Traditional Chinese Medicine by Gene Expression Profiling

Hung-Tsu Cheng,[1,2] Chaang-Ray Chen,[3] Chia-Yang Li,[4] Chao-Ying Huang,[3] Wun-Yi Shu,[5] and Ian C. Hsu[3]

[1] *Institute of Nano Engineering and Microsystems, National Tsing Hua University, No. 101, Section 2, Kuang-Fu Road, Hsinchu 300, Taiwan*
[2] *Classics Chinese Medicine Clinic, Taipei 104, Taiwan*
[3] *Department of Biomedical Engineering and Environmental Sciences, National Tsing Hua University, Hsinchu 300, Taiwan*
[4] *Department of Genome Medicine, College of Medicine and Center for Infectious Disease and Cancer Research, Kaohsiung Medical University, Kaohsiung 807, Taiwan*
[5] *Institute of Statistics, National Tsing Hua University, Hsinchu 300, Taiwan*

Correspondence should be addressed to Ian C. Hsu; ichsu@mx.nthu.edu.tw

Academic Editor: Kamal D. Moudgil

We investigated the syndromes of the *Sini* decoction pattern (SDP), a common ZHENG in traditional Chinese medicine (TCM). The syndromes of SDP were correlated with various severe *Yang deficiency* related symptoms. To obtain a common profile for SDP, we distributed questionnaires to 300 senior clinical TCM practitioners. According to the survey, we concluded 2 sets of symptoms for SDP: (1) pulse feels deep or faint and (2) reversal cold of the extremities. Twenty-four individuals from Taipei City Hospital, Linsen Chinese Medicine Branch, Taiwan, were recruited. We extracted the total mRNA of peripheral blood mononuclear cells from the 24 individuals for microarray experiments. Twelve individuals (including 6 SDP patients and 6 non-SDP individuals) were used as the training set to identify biomarkers for distinguishing the SDP and non-SDP groups. The remaining 12 individuals were used as the test set. The test results indicated that the gene expression profiles of the identified biomarkers could effectively distinguish the 2 groups by adopting a hierarchical clustering algorithm. Our results suggest the feasibility of using the identified biomarkers in facilitating the diagnosis of TCM ZHENGs. Furthermore, the gene expression profiles of biomarker genes could provide a molecular explanation corresponding to the ZHENG of TCM.

1. Introduction

Traditional Chinese medicine (TCM) has been adopted to treat the Chinese for thousands of years on the basis of some classic Chinese medicine textbooks, including *Huang Ti Nei Jing* ("The Inner Cannon of Huangti") [1], *Shénnóng Běn Cǎo Jīng* [2], and *Shang Han Za Bing Lun* ("Treatise on Cold Damage Disorders") [3]. *Shang Han Za Bing Lun* is a Chinese medical treatise written by Zhang Zhongjing before AD 220, at the end of the Han dynasty. The treatise is the oldest comprehensive clinical textbook in the world containing principles, methods, formulas, and medicine and is the clinical literature of TCM theory with practice. To obtain the appropriate decoction for a particular ZHENG requires a diagnostic system, namely, the Decoction ZHENG proposed in *Shang Han Za Bing Lun*. Through the methods of inspection, listening, smelling, inquiry, and palpation, physicians collect information on patients to identify their TCM ZHENGs according to their personal experience and then treat these patients with herbs, which is called decoction. The methods applied in TCM have been criticized as insufficiently scientific. To overcome this weakness, we conducted systems biology research to differentiate TCM ZHENGs.

Systems biology-based diagnostic principles can be used to support the relationship between TCM and current biomedicine [4, 5]. From the perspective of gene expression profile, TCM ZHENGs differentiation is closely related to gene polymorphisms and differences in gene expression profile. Therefore, applying advanced sequencing techniques and cDNA microarray studies can help to clarify the biological basis of TCM ZHENGs [4]. For example, by using microarray, real-time polymerase chain reaction, and enzyme-linked immunosorbent assay technologies, *Shen Yang Xu ZHENG* has been determined to be involved with the gene level [6] and may be primarily attributed to the insufficient activity of the mitogen-activated protein kinase (MAPK) pathway [7]. The *cold* ZHENG was discovered to be possibly caused by a physiological imbalance and disorder of metabolite processes by using microarray technology [8]. Human mRNAs in peripheral blood mononuclear cells (PBMCs) were extracted for microarray experiments to analyze differently expressed gene expressions for TCM *cold* and *hot ZHENG* differentiation [9–11].

In this study, we investigated the syndromes of *Sini* decoction pattern (SDP). *Sini* decoction was first mentioned in *Shang Han Za Bing Lun Sini* decoction consisting of three herbs: fresh *Aconitum carmichaelii*, dry *Zingiber officinale*, and *Glycyrrhiza uralensis*, which was characterized as a remedy to have essential effect of recuperating the patients from collapse. It was used to treat the syndrome of displaying coldness on the extremities, pulse feels deep or faint, continuous diarrhea with undigested cereal, profuse perspiration, abdominal fullness and distention, vomiting, and lethargy [12]. Based on the clinical applications of *Sini* decoction, SDP was then developed by Sun [13]. The syndromes of SDP were correlated with numerous symptoms, such as a slow pulse, coldness on the extremities, continuous diarrhea with undigested cereal, and severe diarrhea, but no common profile exists. According to our survey of 300 senior clinical TCM practitioners, we obtained a common profile for SDP: (1) pulse feels deep or faint and (2) reversal cold of the extremities. We collected SDP patients with these 2 symptoms. In this study, 12 patients with SDP and 12 non-SDP individuals were recruited from Taipei City Hospital, Linsen Chinese Medicine Branch, Taiwan.

We extracted the total mRNA of PBMCs from the 24 individuals for microarray experiments. Twelve individuals (including 6 SDP patients and 6 non-SDP individuals) were used as the training set to identify the biomarkers that were screened using the hypothesis test for distinguishing the SDP and non-SDP groups. The remaining 12 individuals (including 6 SDP patients and 6 non-SDP individuals) were used as the test set to examine whether the identified biomarkers can distinguish the SDP and non-SDP groups. The test results indicated that the gene expression profiling by the biomarkers could effectively distinguish the 2 groups by using a hierarchical clustering algorithm.

Our results suggested the feasibility of using biomarkers extracted from the gene expressions of PBMCs in facilitating the diagnosis of TCM ZHENGs. Furthermore, the gene expression profiles of biomarkers could provide the possible molecular mechanisms of related TCM ZHENGs.

2. Materials and Methods

2.1. Chinese Medicine Terminology. All Chinese medicine terms used in this paper were in accordance with the *International Acupuncture Nomenclature* (IAN) proposed by WHO in 1991; if not available in IAN, the standard nomenclature proposed in the *WHO International Standard Terminologies on Traditional Medicine in the Western Pacific Region* [14] was adapted. These translated Chinese medicine terms are presented in italics in this paper.

2.2. Human Participants. The syndromes of SDP were associated with a slow, deep, and faint pulse that disappeared, coldness on the extremities, severe diarrhea, continuous diarrhea with undigested cereal, generalized pain, abdominal fullness, cold-fluid retention on the diaphragm, profuse sweating, severe spasms in the feet, tight clamping of the extremities, and reversal cold in both the hands and feet; however, no common profile exists. To obtain a common profile for SDP, we distributed questionnaires to 300 senior clinical TCM practitioners. Our questionnaire listed 41 symptoms related to SDP. In the survey, each senior clinical TCM practitioner assigned a score to each symptom, indicating the correlation between the symptom and SDP from high to low (5, 4, 3, 2, 1, and 0). We identified symptoms that collectively constituted a common SDP profile according to the frequency with which participating TCM practitioners assigned a score of 5 to the symptoms; the frequency threshold was set at higher than 35% of the returned surveys. We recruited SDP patients with the aforementioned symptoms. In this study, 12 SDP patients and 12 non-SDP individuals from Taipei City Hospital, Linsen Chinese Medicine Branch, Taiwan, were recruited. All of the individuals provided informed consent. The definition of healthy subject was diagnosed by western medicine rather different from TCM. It is difficult to diagnose healthy subject. Therefore, we consider substituting non-SDP patients for healthy subject. We try our best to collect non-SDP patients who are alike healthy subjects.

2.3. Blood Sample Collection. We phlebotomized 30 mL of human peripheral blood from each donor and then separated the blood into three 10 mL plastic whole blood tubes with spray-coated K2EDTA (Becton Dickenson, Franklin Lakes, NJ, USA). The blood was transferred to a 50 mL centrifuge tube. The PBMCs were then prepared from the 30 mL of peripheral blood through Ficoll-Hypaque density gradient centrifugation. The PBMCs were added to an RNA*later* RNA Stabilization Reagent (Qiagen, Valencia, CA, USA) and then placed into a bottle with liquid nitrogen. All of these procedures were performed immediately after the blood was collected at the laboratory of Taipei City Hospital, Linsen Chinese Medicine Branch, Taiwan. The isolated PBMCs were frozen, stored in a liquid nitrogen freezer, and transported to the microarray experimental laboratory at National Tsing Hua University, Hsinchu, Taiwan, for further microarray experiments.

2.4. RNA Extraction and Microarray Hybridization. We extracted total RNA by using the RNeasy Mini Kit according to the manufacturer's protocol (Qiagen, Valencia, CA, USA). Total RNA quantity and quality were assessed using an ultraviolet absorption spectrophotometer at 260 and 280 nm. Subsequently, α- and β-globin mRNA were reduced from a portion of the total RNA samples by using the GLOBINclear™ human kit (Ambion, Austin, TX, USA), according to the manufacturer's instructions, at the recommended start quantity of 10 μg of total RNA. The quality of total RNA was evaluated using the Agilent 2100 bioanalyzer with the RNA 6000 Nano LabChip kit (Agilent Technologies, Palo Alto, CA, USA). Before reverse transcription, each RNA sample was spiked with a mixture of Arabidopsis mRNAs, which we called doping control. Fluorescence-labeled (Cy3, Cy5-3DNA Capture Reagent) cDNA was conducted using the 3DNA Array 900 labeling kit according to the manufacturer's protocols (Genisphere, Hatfield, PA, USA). Reverse transcription was performed using SuperScript II (Invitrogen, Carlsbad, CA, USA). Hybridization was performed at 65°C in a water bath for 16 to 18 h, and arrays were washed according to the manufacturer's protocol (Corning Life Sciences, New York, NY, USA). The arrays were scanned using GenePix 4000B scanner (Axon Instruments, Foster City, CA, USA).

2.5. Microarray Fabrication. A total of 9600 human cDNA clones were purchased from Incyte Genomics (Wilmington, DE, USA). These cDNAs were randomly selected from the IMAGE library. Resequencing was performed on these clones, and 7334 cDNAs were verified to have corrected DNA sequences. These 7334 sequence-verified human cDNAs (Incyte Genomics) and 10 Arabidopsis cDNAs (SpotReport™ cDNA Array Validation System; Stratagene, La Jolla, CA, USA), serving as spike-in controls, and one housekeeping gene (β-actin), serving as a positive control, were arrayed on Corning UltraGAPS slides (Corning, Corning, NY, USA). These 7334 human cDNAs and 96 Arabidopsis cDNAs and housekeeping genes were spotted in quadruplicate on each array making a total of 32248 spots to enhance the statistical confidence in the gene expression data. Each array had 32,448 spots. The arrays were postprocessed according to the Corning UltraGAPS Coated Slides instruction manual.

2.6. Experimental Design. Loop design, a type of statistical microarray experimental design, was adopted to construct an optimal design. The basic principles of optimal design are a balance among the factors, approximately equal sampling of varieties, and minimal distance between pairs of varieties [15]. Samples from 24 individuals were hybridized on 48 arrays based on the 2 loop designs presented in Figure 1. The individuals of samples L1A1, L1A2, L1A3, L1C1, L1C2, L1C3, L2A1, L2A2, L2A3, L2C1, L2C2, and L2C3 were SDP patients, and those of samples L1B1, L1B2, L1B3, L1D1, L1D2, L1D3, L2B1, L2B2, L2B3, L2D1, L2D2, and L2D3 were non-SDP individuals. Each arrow in the figure indicates a microarray hybridization experiment. The arrow heads and tails represent samples labeled with Cy5 (3DNA Capture Reagent) and Cy3 (3DNA Capture Reagent), respectively. The black solid circles stand for the SDP samples and the open circles stand for non-SDP samples. We used 12 individuals in Loop 1 experiments as the training set and the remaining 12 individuals in Loop 2 experiments as the test set.

2.7. Microarray Data Analysis and Statistical Analysis. Microarray data preprocessing, normalization, and statistical analysis were performed using the bioinformatics software suite Tsing Hua Engine for Microarray Experiment [16].

Spot-screening rules were applied to screen invalid spots on these arrays. The spot-screening rules for the data of Loop 1 (the training set) were as follows: (1) exclude the spots defined as "flag bad" or "absent" in all GenePix Results (GPR), (2) exclude the spots with diameters less than 100 μm, (3) exclude the spots with a coefficient of variation (CV) of pixel intensity of over 100% in both channels, and (4) exclude the spots with signal to noise ratios (SNRs) in both channels were less than 2 in the training set microarray experiments. The SNR is defined as $(S - B)/B$ (S: mean of pixel intensities of the signal; B: median pixel intensity of the background). The logarithm of the ratios for all valid spots on each array was normalized using global lowess normalization [17]. After the data were preprocessed, the normalized log ratios of the fluorescence intensity of each cDNA spot were analyzed using a log linear model, which was described in our previous study [18], to obtain the least-squares estimates $\widehat{\lambda_1}$, $\widehat{\lambda_2}$, $\widehat{\lambda_3}$, $\widehat{\lambda_4}$, $\widehat{\lambda_5}$, $\widehat{\lambda_6}$, $\widehat{\lambda_7}$, $\widehat{\lambda_8}$, $\widehat{\lambda_9}$, $\widehat{\lambda_{10}}$, $\widehat{\lambda_{11}}$, and $\widehat{\lambda_{12}}$ for the relative expressions among all of the samples. The relative expressions of sample i are defined as (expression of sample i)/(geometric average of the expression of all samples), for each gene, where i runs from 1 to 12. For the training set microarray data, 4951 genes satisfied the selection criteria of the spot-screening rules and log linear model. The selection criteria for the data of Loop 2 (the test set) are described in the subsequent subsection. The microarray data is available at GEO (GSE67090).

2.8. Searching Biomarkers to Distinguish SDP. We used Loop 1 experiments as the training set and Loop 2 experiments as the test set. For the 4951 genes of Loop 1 (the training set), 192 genes were identified using an F test with null hypothesis H_0: $(\widehat{\lambda_1}+\widehat{\lambda_3}+\widehat{\lambda_5}+\widehat{\lambda_7}+\widehat{\lambda_9}+\widehat{\lambda_{11}})-(\widehat{\lambda_2}+\widehat{\lambda_4}+\widehat{\lambda_6}+\widehat{\lambda_8}+\widehat{\lambda_{10}}+\widehat{\lambda_{12}}) = 0$, at a Bonferroni-adjusted significance level of 0.05/4951, where $\widehat{\lambda_1}$, $\widehat{\lambda_3}$, $\widehat{\lambda_5}$, $\widehat{\lambda_7}$, $\widehat{\lambda_9}$, and $\widehat{\lambda_{11}}$ were the least-squares estimates for the relative expressions of the SDP samples and $\widehat{\lambda_2}$, $\widehat{\lambda_4}$, $\widehat{\lambda_6}$, $\widehat{\lambda_8}$, $\widehat{\lambda_{10}}$, and $\widehat{\lambda_{12}}$ were the least-squares estimates for the relative expressions of the non-SDP samples.

The 192 biomarker genes were then used to distinguish the SDP and non-SDP groups of the test set. We applied the selection criteria to filter bad spots to perform an effective normalization and a log linear model. In order to include additional available genes to be tested, we relaxed the selection criteria of the spot-screening rules for the data of Loop 2 (the test set) as follows: (1) exclude the spots defined as "flag bad" or "absent" in all GPR files, (2) exclude the spots with diameters less than 50 μm, (3) exclude the spots with a CV of pixel standard deviation of over 150% in both channels, and (4) exclude the spots with SNRs in either channel were less than 1 in the test microarray experiments. The logarithm of the ratios for all valid spots on each array was normalized under the same normalization conditions as those for

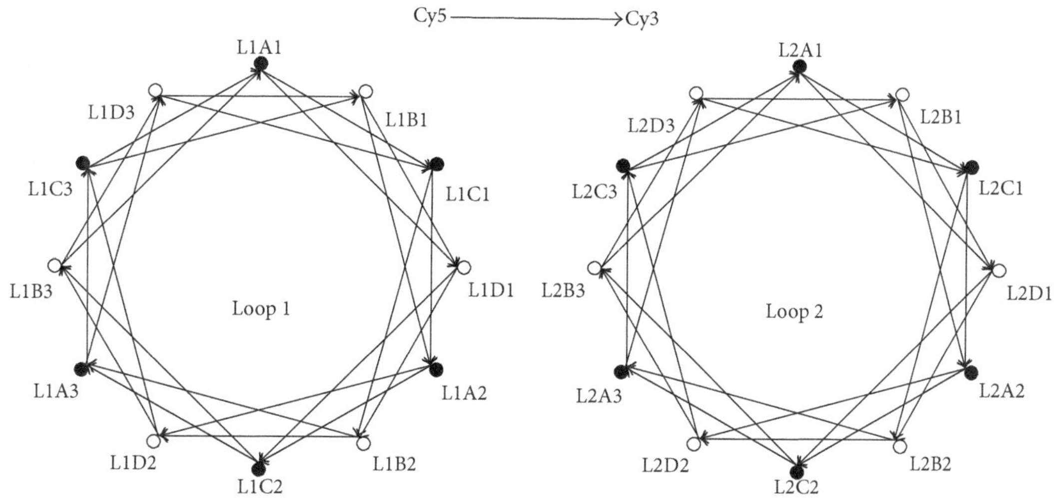

Loop 1 (for the training set)		
SDP	L1A1 L1A2 L1A3	L1C1 L1C2 L1C3
Non-SDP	L1B1 L1B2 L1B3	L1D1 L1D2 L1C3

Loop 2 (for the test set)		
SDP	L2A1 L2A2 L2A3	L2C1 L2C2 L2C3
Non-SDP	L2B1 L2B2 L2B3	L2D1 L2D2 L2C3

FIGURE 1: Experimental designs of Loop 1 (for the training set) and Loop 2 (for the test set). Each arrow indicates a microarray hybridization experiment. The arrow heads and tails represent samples labeled with Cy5 and Cy3, respectively. The black solid circles stand for the SDP samples and the open circles stand for non-SDP samples. Loop 1 is the experimental design for the training set of 12 individuals. Loop 2 is the experimental design for the test set of the other 12 individuals. The annotations of samples in Loop 1 and Loop 2 are shown below each loop.

the training set. We then used hierarchical clustering to verify whether the gene expression profiles of the 192 biomarker genes could classify the 12 test samples into 2 groups and how well they could distinguish the SDP patients and non-SDP individuals.

2.9. Functional Annotation and Enrichment Analysis. Functional annotation and enrichment analysis were accessed through the database for annotation, visualization, and integrated discovery (DAVID) [19], which performed a modified Fisher's exact test to identify overrepresented functions. DAVID is a widely employed web tool that provides a rapid means to understand the biological meaning of a long list of genes of interest. For any gene list, DAVID can map and convert identifiers (IDs) and accessions among different gene IDs. A long gene list can be reduced into biological theme-related groups of genes, for example, gene ontology (GO) [20] and the Kyoto Encyclopedia of Genes and Genomes (KEGG) pathway [21].

The Entrez gene IDs of 192 biomarker genes were used as the gene ID for bioinformatics analysis. Biological processes of GO terms were used for functional annotation and enrichment analysis of these biomarker genes.

3. Results

3.1. Questionnaires to Obtain a Common Profile for SDP. We distributed questionnaires to 300 senior clinical TCM practitioners, and 43 questionnaires were returned. Our questionnaire listed 41 symptoms related to SDP. In the survey, each senior clinical TCM practitioner assigned a score to each symptom, indicating the correlation between the symptom and SDP, from high to low (5, 4, 3, 2, 1, and 0). Based on the frequency with which participating TCM practitioners assigned a score of 5 to the symptoms, we identified symptoms that collectively constituted a common SDP profile (Figure 2). The frequency threshold was set at higher than 35% of the 43 returned surveys (i.e., symptoms assigned a score of 5 by at least 16 surveys). This process revealed 7 symptoms to form our symptom profile of SDP patients. By grouping related symptoms, we obtained a common profile for SDP as 2 sets of symptoms: (1) pulse feels deep or faint and (2) reversal cold of the extremities. We recruited SDP patients with the 2 sets of symptoms. In this study, 12 SDP patients and 12 non-SDP individuals were recruited from Taipei City Hospital, Linsen Chinese Medicine Branch, Taiwan. All of the participants provided informed consent.

3.2. Identifying Biomarker Genes from the Training Set Microarray Experiment. On the basis of the results for the 4951 genes of Loop 1 (the training set), 192 genes were identified (Table 1) using an F test with null hypothesis H_0: $(\widehat{\lambda_1} + \widehat{\lambda_3} + \widehat{\lambda_5} + \widehat{\lambda_7} + \widehat{\lambda_9} + \widehat{\lambda_{11}}) - (\widehat{\lambda_2} + \widehat{\lambda_4} + \widehat{\lambda_6} + \widehat{\lambda_8} + \widehat{\lambda_{10}} + \widehat{\lambda_{12}}) = 0$, at a Bonferroni-adjusted significance level of 0.05/4951. By applying hierarchical clustering with Spearman distance and average linkage, the 12 training samples were appropriately separated into 2 groups, as shown in Figure 3. In Figure 3,

Table 1: The 192 biomarker genes identified using an F test with null hypothesis H_0: $(\widehat{\lambda_1}+\widehat{\lambda_3}+\widehat{\lambda_5}+\widehat{\lambda_7}+\widehat{\lambda_9}+\widehat{\lambda_{11}})-(\widehat{\lambda_2}+\widehat{\lambda_4}+\widehat{\lambda_6}+\widehat{\lambda_8}+\widehat{\lambda_{10}}+\widehat{\lambda_{12}}) = 0$, at a Bonferroni-adjusted significance level of 0.05/4951.

Gene name				
ABHD3	ABI2	ACSM2B	ACTB	AGFG1
AKAP9	ARG1	ARID5A	ATP1B3	ATP6AP2
ATP6V0B	BLZF1	BPGM	C11orf79	C12orf24
C12orf32	C17orf91	C6orf106	CAPN1	CBARA1
CCL18	CCL5	CD1D	CD24	CD40
CD44	CD83	CD8A	CD93	CDC42
CDC42SE2	CLDN1	COMT	COX10	CP
CREM	CST7	CXCL9	DEFA1	DEFA3
DEFA4	DENND2D	DGCR6L	DLG2	DUSP6
EEF2	EIF3E	EIF3I	EPAS1	EXOSC9
FAM113B	FAM175B	FCER1A	FLNB	FMOD
FOLR3	FOS	FOSB	FYN	GCA
GIMAP1	GLRX	GNG11	GNG2	GNLY
GPR56	GSTA2	GTF2E1	GZMA	H3F3B
HERPUD1	HIST1H2AC	HIST1H2BD	HIST1H2BG	HIST1H2BJ
HIST2H2AA3	HLA-A	HLA-DMA	HLA-DQB1	HLA-DRB1
HLA-G	Hs.282050	Hs.467411	Hs.534061	Hs.586682
Hs.591807	Hs.599359	Hs.655903	Hs.674438	Hs.88605
HSP90B1	HSPA1A	HTATIP2	HTR7P1	ID2
IFIT1	IL10RA	IL15RA	IL1B	IL32
JARID1C	KIF3C	KLF10	KLF6	LCP1
LNP1	LOC400027	LOC729776	LTB	LYRM1
MAPK13	MBP	MCM3AP	MEST	MLH3
MNDA	MRPL3	MRPL49	MTMR6	MYL6
NCRNA00084	NHEDC2	NPY	NUCB1	NUDT16
NUP93	ORM1	PACS1	PCDH8	PDE4B
PEA15	PF4	PLAUR	PNLIPRP2	POLR1C
POLR2D	POU2F2	PPBP	PPP1R12B	PPP1R7
PPP2R2A	PPRC1	PPT1	PRL	PSMC6
RAB4A	RARRES3	RGS18	RGS2	RHOQ
RNF40	RNPEP	RPL41	RPS11	RPS24
RPS27	RPS4X	RPS4Y1	RUNX3	S1PR5
SEC22B	SELL	SERPINE2	SFRS1	SH2B3
SH3D19	SHCBP1	SLC2A3P1	SOD2	SPTY2D1
SRGN	STX8	SYTL2	TADA3L	TARP
THBS1	TIMP1	TMEM176A	TNFAIP8L2	TPCN1
TRA@	TRAPPC1	TRMT11	VIM	VPS13D
WDR42A	WIZ	XPNPEP1	YARS	Unknown*
Unknown*	ZNF286A			

*The sequence of the clone was not yet identified in the BLAST.

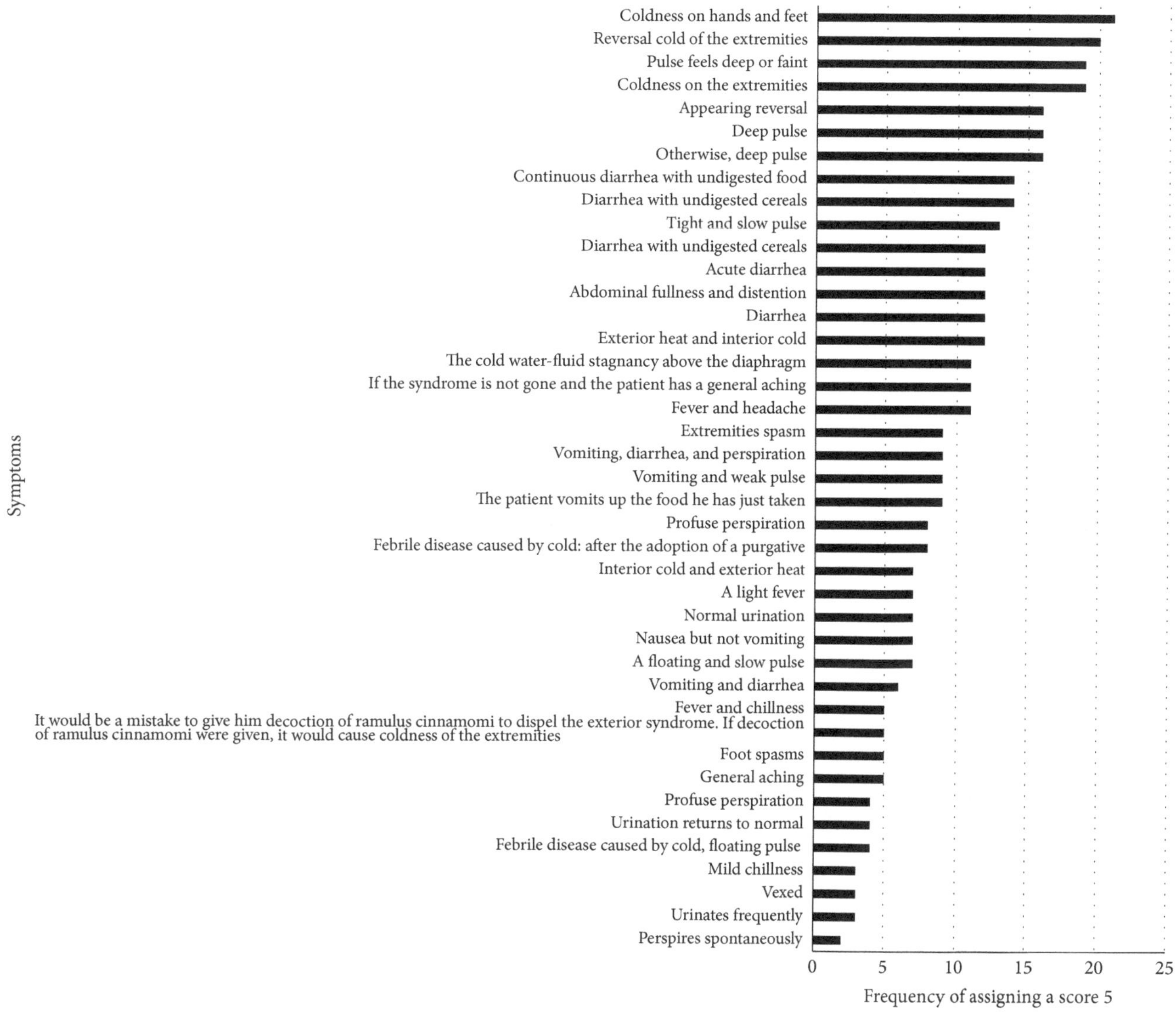

FIGURE 2: Frequency with which survey symptoms were assigned a score of 5 in determining the SDP profile.

the gene expression value used to do the clustering is the relative expressions of the labeled sample.

3.3. Distinguishing Power of the Biomarker Genes to the Test Set Microarray Experiment. The 192 biomarker genes identified in the training set experiments were then used to test the ability to distinguish the SDP patients and non-SDP individuals in the test set. To include additional available genes to be tested, we relaxed the selection criteria of the spot-screening rules for the data of the test set (Loop 2). The logarithm of the ratios for all valid spots on each array was normalized under the same normalization conditions as those for the training set. We then used hierarchical clustering to verify whether the gene expression profiles of the 192 biomarker genes could classify the 12 test samples into 2 groups and how well they could distinguish the SDP patients and non-SDP individuals. Under the same clustering conditions (i.e., hierarchical clustering with Spearman distance and average linkage), Figure 4 showed that the 192 biomarker genes can classify the 12 test samples into 2 groups. One group comprised L2A2, L2A1, L2A3, L2C3, L2C2, and L2D1 samples and the other comprised L2D2, L2B3, L2D3, L2B2, L2C1, and L2B1 samples. Except for L2D1 and L2C1 samples, all of the samples were correctly grouped into SDP and non-SDP groups. In Figure 4, the gene expression value used to do the clustering is the relative expressions of the labeled sample. The microarray data of 4 biomarker genes from 7 samples were confirmed by quantitative PCR (qPCR). The correlation coefficients r between microarray data and qPCR for each gene are 0.73, 0.83, 0.93, and 0.76 (Appendix A).

3.4. Functional Annotation and Enrichment Analysis Results for the 192 Biomarker Genes. The functional annotation and enrichment analysis were accessed using DAVID. Seventy-eight GO terms were enriched with a P value less than 0.05. All enriched GO terms are listed in Appendix B. 78 GO terms

Table 2: The 11 enriched GO terms for 192 biomarker genes (sorted according to P value).

GO term	Description	# gene	P value
GO:0006952	Defense response	24	0.000000
GO:0006955	Immune response	24	0.000002
GO:0009617	Response to bacterium	11	0.000088
GO:0001817	Regulation of cytokine production	11	0.000172
GO:0048534	Hemopoietic or lymphoid organ development	13	0.000562
GO:0030097	Hemopoiesis	12	0.000999
GO:0002520	Immune system development	13	0.001183
GO:0007610	Behavior	14	0.004162
GO:0006412	Translation	12	0.004210
GO:0001775	Cell activation	11	0.008090
GO:0019725	Cellular homeostasis	13	0.009574

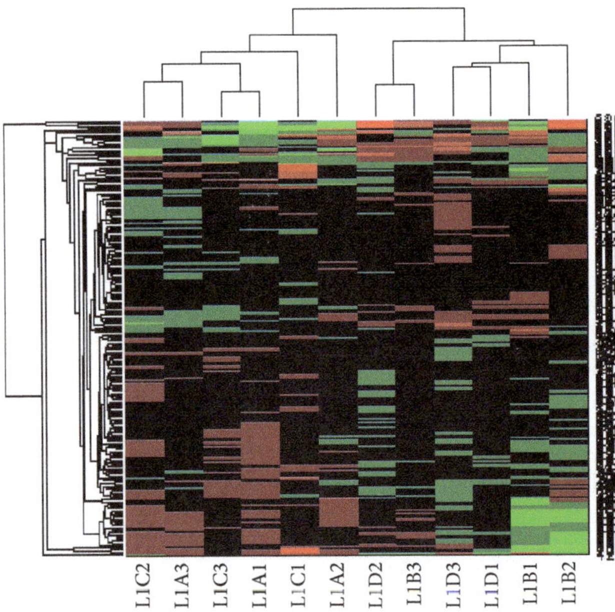

Figure 3: 192 genes, identified using the F test at a Bonferroni-adjusted significance level of 0.05/4951, were clustered into 2 groups. By applying hierarchical clustering with Spearman distance and average linkage, the 12 training samples were appropriately separated into 2 groups according to the 192 marker genes. Samples L1C2, L1A3, L1C3, L1A1, L1C1, and L1A2 comprised the SDP group, and samples L1D2, L1B3, L1D3, L1D1, L1B1, and L1B2 comprised the non-SDP group. In this figure, the gene expression value used to do the clustering is the relative expressions of the labeled sample.

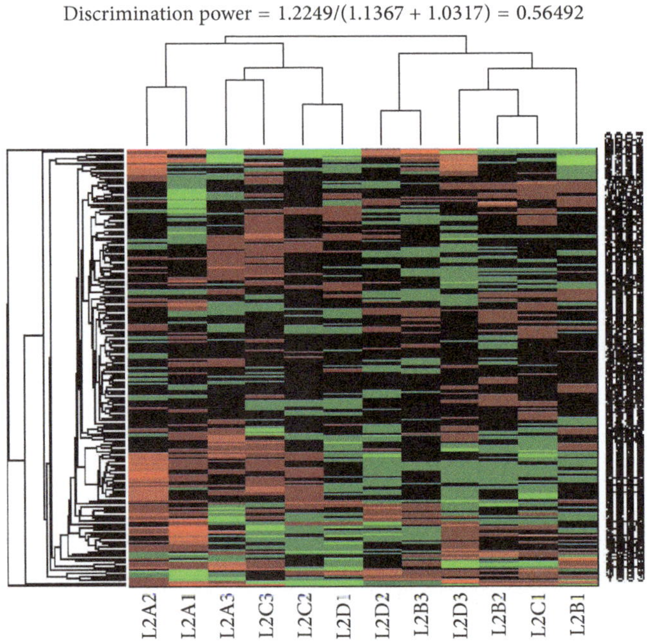

Figure 4: Hierarchical clustering results for the 12 test samples. Under the same clustering conditions (i.e., hierarchical clustering with Spearman distance and average linkage), the gene expression profiles of the 192 marker genes classified the 12 test samples into 2 groups. One group consisted of the L2A2, L2A1, L2A3, L2C3, L2C2, and L2D1 samples and the other consisted of the L2D2, L2B3, L2D3, L2B2, L2C1, and L2B1 samples. Except for the L2D1 and L2C1 samples, all of the samples were correctly grouped into SDP and non-SDP groups. In this figure, the gene expression values that used to do the clustering are the relative expressions of the labeled sample.

were enriched with a P value of less than 0.05. We further applied 2 stringent criteria to filter the high-ranked GO terms: (1) GO terms containing more than 10 genes and (2) a P value of less than 0.01. Consequently, 11 GO terms were identified (Table 2).

Table 2 showed that the 11 GO terms are substantially correlated with immune, inflammation, and hemopoiesis functions. In detail, the immune function includes defense response, immune response, response to bacterium, and immune system development. The inflammation function includes cytokine production regulation, behavior, cell activation, and cellular homeostasis. The hematopoiesis function includes hemopoietic or lymphoid organ development and hemopoiesis.

Table 3: The correlation plots between microarray data and qPCR data.

Genes	Samples	Microarray data: $\log_2$ of microarray relative gene expression data: $\widehat{\lambda}_i$	Microarray data: $\log_2$ ratio of two samples' microarray relative gene expression data: $\widehat{\lambda}_i - \widehat{\lambda}_j$, that is, $(a - b)$	qPCR data: $\log_2$ of qPCR relative gene expression data: ΔCt	qPCR data: $\log_2$ ratio of two samples' qPCR relative gene expression data: −ΔΔCt, that is, $-(a - b)$
GNG2	(a) L2A1 (b) L2B2	0.572 0.097	0.476	−0.35 0.14	0.49
	(a) L2B2 (b) L2A2	0.097 0.235	−0.139	0.14 0.80	0.66
	(a) L2A2 (b) L2D1	0.235 −0.389	0.625	0.80 1.75	0.95
	(a) L2D1 (b) L2C2	−0.389 −0.222	−0.167	1.75 0.50	−1.25
	(a) L2C2 (b) L2D2	−0.222 −0.258	0.035	0.50 1.21	0.71
	(a) L2D2 (b) L2D3	−0.258 0.131	−0.388	1.21 0.67	−0.54
	(a) L2D3 (b) L2A1	0.131 0.572	−0.442	0.67 −0.35	−1.02
RUNX3	(a) L2A1 (b) L2B2	0.835 −0.022	0.858	1.39 2.49	1.10
	(a) L2B2 (b) L2A2	−0.022 −0.042	0.020	2.49 2.81	0.32
	(a) L2A2 (b) L2D1	−0.042 −0.099	0.057	2.81 2.85	0.04
	(a) L2D1 (b) L2C2	−0.099 −0.258	0.159	2.85 2.37	−0.48
	(a) L2C2 (b) L2D2	−0.258 −0.190	−0.068	2.37 2.86	0.49
	(a) L2D2 (b) L2D3	−0.190 0.196	−0.385	2.86 2.37	−0.49
	(a) L2D3 (b) L2A1	0.196 0.835	−0.640	2.37 1.39	−0.98
CST7	(a) L2A1 (b) L2B2	1.301 0.224	1.076	−1.65 −0.90	0.75
	(a) L2B2 (b) L2A2	0.224 0.493	−0.268	−0.90 −0.72	0.18
	(a) L2A2 (b) L2D1	0.493 −0.454	0.946	−0.72 0.04	0.76
	(a) L2D1 (b) L2C2	−0.454 −0.414	−0.039	0.04 −0.01	−0.05
	(a) L2C2 (b) L2D2	−0.414 −0.325	−0.089	−0.01 0.23	0.24
	(a) L2D2 (b) L2D3	−0.325 0.300	−0.626	0.23 −0.62	−0.85
	(a) L2D3 (b) L2A1	0.300 1.301	−1.000	−0.62 −1.65	−1.03
MNDA	(a) L2A1 (b) L2B2	−1.136 0.313	−1.449	2.29 0.76	−1.53
	(a) L2B2 (b) L2A2	0.313 −0.229	0.542	0.76 1.88	1.12
	(a) L2A2 (b) L2D1	−0.229 −0.185	−0.044	1.88 1.31	−0.57

TABLE 3: Continued.

Genes	Samples	Microarray data: $\log_2$ of microarray relative gene expression data: $\widehat{\lambda}_i$	Microarray data: $\log_2$ ratio of two samples' microarray relative gene expression data: $\widehat{\lambda}_i - \widehat{\lambda}_j$, that is, $(a-b)$	qPCR data: $\log_2$ of qPCR relative gene expression data: ΔCt	qPCR data: $\log_2$ ratio of two samples' qPCR relative gene expression data: −ΔΔCt, that is, $-(a-b)$
	(a) L2D1 (b) L2C2	−0.185 −0.015	−0.170	1.31 −0.08	−1.39
	(a) L2C2 (b) L2D2	−0.015 0.349	−0.365	−0.08 0.17	0.25
	(a) L2D2 (b) L2D3	0.349 0.357	−0.008	0.17 1.10	0.93
	(a) L2D3 (b) L2A1	0.357 −1.136	1.493	1.10 2.29	1.19

4. Discussion

Of the 4951 genes of the training set, 192 genes were identified using an F test with null hypothesis. By applying hierarchical clustering with Spearman distance and average linkage, the 12 training samples were appropriately separated into SDP and non-SDP groups. The 192 biomarker genes were then used to distinguish the SDP patients and non-SDP individuals in the test set. Under the same clustering conditions, the 12 test samples were clustered into 2 groups. One group comprised L2A2, L2A1, L2A3, L2C3, L2C2, and L2D1 samples and the other comprised L2D2, L2B3, L2D3, L2B2, L2C1, and L2B1 samples. Except for L2D1 and L2C1 samples, all of the samples were correctly grouped into the SDP and non-SDP groups. Thus, we reviewed the original information of these 2 samples. L2C1 sample (classified as SDP according to TCM but clustered into the non-SDP group by using biomarkers) had a deep, rough, and rapid pulse and reversal cold of the extremities. Among the symptoms of L2C1 sample, reversal cold of the extremities matched the selected symptom of SDP; however, a deep, rough, and rapid pulse was inconsistent with a deep or faint pulse, a selected symptom for SDP. L2D1 sample (categorized as non-SDP according to TCM but clustered into the SDP group by using biomarkers) had a deep and tight pulse, which was particularly deep at the *guan* site (the guan is immediately central to the radial styloid at the wrist, where the tip of the physician's middle finger is placed), and reversal cold of the extremities. Among the symptoms of L2D1 sample, a deep and tight pulse, particularly at the guan site, did not meet the symptom of a deep or faint pulse, and the sample was thus classified as non-SDP according to TCM. However, reversal cold of the extremities matched the selected symptom of SDP. These findings indicate that, in classifying these 2 samples into SDP and non-SDP groups, uncertain areas exist. Nevertheless, determining biomarkers by using the mRNA profiling method can facilitate identifying the SDP group. Therefore, the traditional dialectical method of TCM is quite trustworthy.

The results of the functional annotation and enrichment analysis of 192 biomarker genes revealed that the 11 GO terms were substantially correlated with immune, inflammation, and hemopoiesis functions. Among the symptoms of SDP, a deep or faint pulse implied the insufficiency of *Qi* (in the field of medicine, *Qi* refers both to the refined nutritive substance that flows within the human body and to its functional activities). Insufficiency of *Qi* indicates the body's resistance against disease is weak. Pathogens can invade the human body easily, and viruses and bacteria could then cause inflammation easily.

5. Conclusion

Our results provided the biomarker genes of SDP, which was first mentioned in *Shang Han Za Bing Lun*. The results provide molecular evidence for TCM in the ZHENGs differentiation of SDP. Using mRNA profiling experiments on patients' PBMCs to discover biomarker genes to test an unknown group of individuals can effectively identify a specific ZHENG. We hope that the mRNA profiling method will become a model for TCM physicians in diagnosis and assist TCM practitioners in evaluating the curative effect of the medication.

Appendix

A.

The microarray data of 4 biomarker genes from 7 samples were confirmed by quantitative PCR (qPCR). The correlation plots between microarray data and qPCR data are shown in Table 3. The correlation coefficients r for each gene are 0.73 (GNG2), 0.83 (RUNX3), 0.93 (CST7), and 0.76 (MNDA), shown in Figure 5.

B.

The complete list of all enriched GO terms for 192 biomarker genes (sorted according to P value) is shown in Table 4.

TABLE 4: The complete list of all enriched GO terms for 192 biomarker genes (sorted according to *P* value).

GO term	Description	# gene	*P* value
GO:0006952	Defense response	24	0.000000
GO:0006955	Immune response	24	0.000002
GO:0019882	Antigen processing and presentation	7	0.000073
GO:0009617	Response to bacterium	11	0.000088
GO:0006968	Cellular defense response	7	0.000149
GO:0001817	Regulation of cytokine production	11	0.000172
GO:0048534	Hemopoietic or lymphoid organ development	13	0.000562
GO:0030097	Hemopoiesis	12	0.000999
GO:0002520	Immune system development	13	0.001183
GO:0002696	Positive regulation of leukocyte activation	8	0.001499
GO:0001819	Positive regulation of cytokine production	7	0.001573
GO:0050867	Positive regulation of cell activation	8	0.002053
GO:0007610	Behavior	14	0.004162
GO:0002763	Positive regulation of myeloid leukocyte differentiation	4	0.004167
GO:0006412	Translation	12	0.004210
GO:0002684	Positive regulation of immune system process	10	0.006451
GO:0006414	Translational elongation	7	0.006467
GO:0002822	Regulation of adaptive immune response based on somatic recombination of immune receptors built from immunoglobulin superfamily domains	5	0.007075
GO:0048584	Positive regulation of response to stimulus	10	0.007697
GO:0001775	Cell activation	11	0.008090
GO:0051240	Positive regulation of multicellular organism process	10	0.008151
GO:0002819	Regulation of adaptive immune response	5	0.008161
GO:0030162	Regulation of proteolysis	5	0.008161
GO:0001818	Negative regulation of cytokine production	4	0.008578
GO:0002824	Positive regulation of adaptive immune response based on somatic recombination of immune receptors built from immunoglobulin superfamily domains	4	0.008578
GO:0002544	Chronic inflammatory response	3	0.009217
GO:0010829	Negative regulation of glucose transport	3	0.009217
GO:0050832	Defense response to fungus	3	0.009217
GO:0051043	Regulation of membrane protein ectodomain proteolysis	3	0.009217
GO:0002694	Regulation of leukocyte activation	8	0.009343
GO:0002706	Regulation of lymphocyte mediated immunity	5	0.009351
GO:0019725	Cellular homeostasis	13	0.009574
GO:0002821	Positive regulation of adaptive immune response	4	0.010479
GO:0042742	Defense response to bacterium	5	0.010649
GO:0042592	Homeostatic process	18	0.011731
GO:0006873	Cellular ion homeostasis	11	0.012021
GO:0050865	Regulation of cell activation	8	0.012239
GO:0009611	Response to wounding	15	0.012528
GO:0007267	Cell-cell signaling	15	0.013447
GO:0050778	Positive regulation of immune response	7	0.013518
GO:0031640	Killing of cells of another organism	3	0.013542
GO:0055082	Cellular chemical homeostasis	11	0.013819
GO:0002705	Positive regulation of leukocyte mediated immunity	4	0.014959
GO:0002708	Positive regulation of lymphocyte mediated immunity	4	0.014959
GO:0010827	Regulation of glucose transport	4	0.014959
GO:0034101	Erythrocyte homeostasis	5	0.015220

TABLE 4: Continued.

GO term	Description	# gene	*P* value
GO:0030098	Lymphocyte differentiation	6	0.016523
GO:0051251	Positive regulation of lymphocyte activation	6	0.016523
GO:0050801	Ion homeostasis	11	0.017255
GO:0045639	Positive regulation of myeloid cell differentiation	4	0.017545
GO:0002703	Regulation of leukocyte mediated immunity	5	0.018862
GO:0006935	Chemotaxis	7	0.020473
GO:0042330	Taxis	7	0.020473
GO:0045765	Regulation of angiogenesis	5	0.020868
GO:0006954	Inflammatory response	10	0.021243
GO:0046649	Lymphocyte activation	8	0.024760
GO:0045321	Leukocyte activation	9	0.026088
GO:0002761	Regulation of myeloid leukocyte differentiation	4	0.026706
GO:0050870	Positive regulation of T cell activation	5	0.030175
GO:0048872	Homeostasis of number of cells	6	0.030221
GO:0009620	Response to fungus	3	0.030551
GO:0032655	Regulation of interleukin-12 production	3	0.030551
GO:0031349	Positive regulation of defense response	5	0.032829
GO:0002699	Positive regulation of immune effectors process	4	0.033982
GO:0032103	Positive regulation of response to external stimulus	5	0.035615
GO:0048878	Chemical homeostasis	12	0.036704
GO:0002504	Antigen processing and presentation of peptide or polysaccharide antigen via MHC class II	3	0.037413
GO:0016525	Negative regulation of angiogenesis	3	0.037413
GO:0050850	Positive regulation of calcium-mediated signaling	3	0.037413
GO:0006928	Cell motion	13	0.037784
GO:0006334	Nucleosome assembly	4	0.037967
GO:0031497	Chromatin assembly	4	0.037967
GO:0048002	Antigen processing and presentation of peptide antigen	3	0.044801
GO:0010033	Response to organic substance	18	0.044896
GO:0030218	Erythrocyte differentiation	4	0.046616
GO:0065004	Protein-DNA complex assembly	4	0.046616
GO:0002521	Leukocyte differentiation	6	0.046793
GO:0014070	Response to organic cyclic substance	6	0.049526
GO:0002237	Response to molecule of bacterial origin	5	0.051544
GO:0007626	Locomotory behavior	8	0.052288
GO:0055080	Cation homeostasis	8	0.052288
GO:0050848	Regulation of calcium-mediated signaling	3	0.052676
GO:0051249	Regulation of lymphocyte activation	6	0.055270
GO:0034728	Nucleosome organization	4	0.056149
GO:0045619	Regulation of lymphocyte differentiation	4	0.056149
GO:0002697	Regulation of immune effectors process	5	0.058846
GO:0002712	Regulation of B cell mediated immunity	3	0.060999
GO:0002889	Regulation of immunoglobulin mediated immune response	3	0.060999
GO:0051235	Maintenance of location	4	0.061237
GO:0032914	Positive regulation of transforming growth factor-beta 1 production	2	0.061881
GO:0045651	Positive regulation of macrophage differentiation	2	0.061881
GO:0007611	Learning or memory	5	0.062693
GO:0008285	Negative regulation of cell proliferation	10	0.063328

TABLE 4: Continued.

GO term	Description	# gene	P value
GO:0051241	Negative regulation of multicellular organism process	6	0.064581
GO:0051789	Response to protein stimulus	5	0.066670
GO:0016192	Vesicle-mediated transport	13	0.067653
GO:0042060	Wound healing	7	0.068209
GO:0001906	Cell killing	3	0.069736
GO:0046635	Positive regulation of alpha-beta T cell activation	3	0.069736
GO:0051094	Positive regulation of developmental process	9	0.072195
GO:0050863	Regulation of T cell activation	5	0.075009
GO:0050900	Leukocyte migration	4	0.077725
GO:0009895	Negative regulation of catabolic process	3	0.078852
GO:0046634	Regulation of alpha-beta T cell activation	3	0.078852
GO:0030099	Myeloid cell differentiation	5	0.079368
GO:0055066	Di-, tri-valent inorganic cation homeostasis	7	0.080251
GO:0006323	DNA packaging	4	0.083611
GO:0030217	T cell differentiation	4	0.083611
GO:0043066	Negative regulation of apoptosis	10	0.085435
GO:0046324	Regulation of glucose import	3	0.088316
GO:0002863	Positive regulation of inflammatory response to antigenic stimulus	2	0.091380
GO:0032891	Negative regulation of organic acid transport	2	0.091380
GO:0032908	Regulation of transforming growth factor-beta 1 production	2	0.091380
GO:0051918	Negative regulation of fibrinolysis	2	0.091380
GO:0043069	Negative regulation of programmed cell death	10	0.092873
GO:0060548	Negative regulation of cell death	10	0.095435
GO:0045637	Regulation of myeloid cell differentiation	4	0.095934
GO:0030003	Cellular cation homeostasis	7	0.096877
GO:0045582	Positive regulation of T cell differentiation	3	0.098097

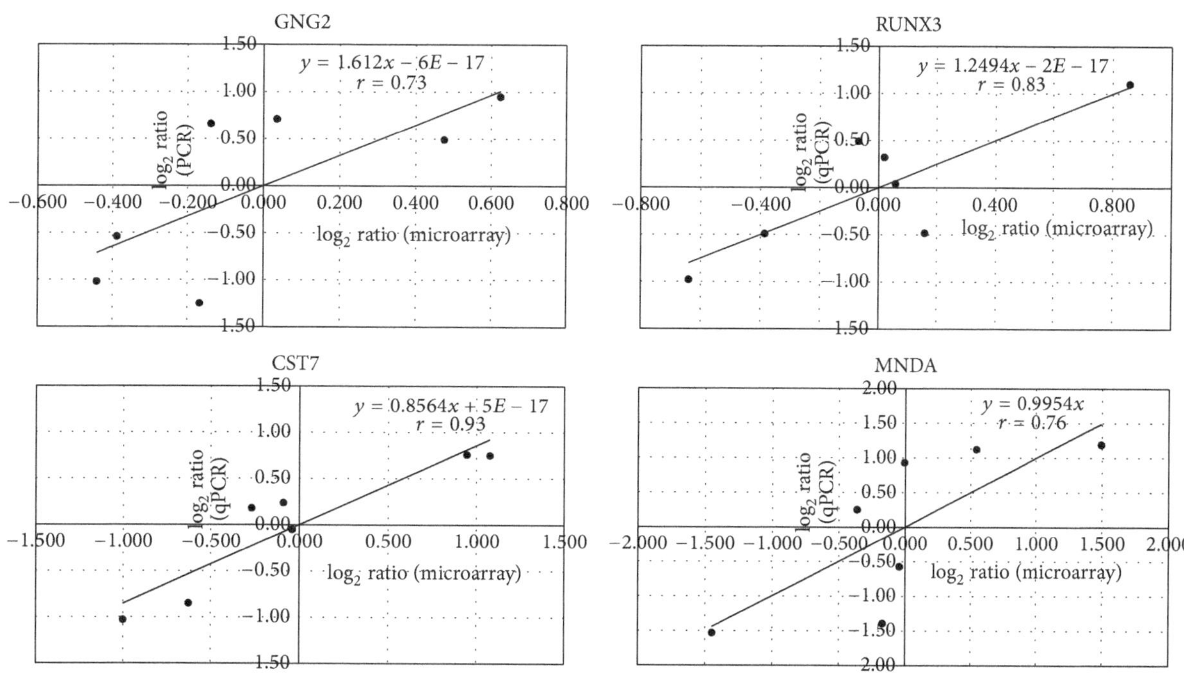

FIGURE 5: The correlation coefficients r for each gene are 0.73 (GNG2), 0.83 (RUNX3), 0.93 (CST7), and 0.76 (MNDA).

Competing Interests

The authors declare that they have no competing interests.

References

[1] P. U. Unschuld, *Huang Di Nei Jing Su Wen*, University of California Press, Los Angeles, Calif, USA, 2003.

[2] K.-H. Lee, S. Morris-Natschke, X. Yang et al., "Recent progress of research on medicinal mushrooms, foods, and other herbal products used in traditional chinese medicine," *Journal of Traditional and Complementary Medicine*, vol. 2, no. 2, pp. 84–95, 2012.

[3] F. Yu, T. Takahashi, J. Moriya et al., "Traditional Chinese medicine and kampo: a review from the distant past for the future," *Journal of International Medical Research*, vol. 34, no. 3, pp. 231–239, 2006.

[4] M. Xue, H. J. Yin, and K. J. Chen, "Some thoughts on studying essence of syndromes based on genomics," *Zhongguo Zhong Xi Yi Jie He Za Zhi*, vol. 26, no. 1, pp. 88–90, 2006.

[5] J. van der Greef, H. van Wietmarschen, J. Schroën, M. Wang, T. Hankemeier, and G. W. Xu, "Systems biology-based diagnostic principles as pillars of the bridge between Chinese and Western medicine," *Planta Medica*, vol. 76, no. 17, pp. 2036–2047, 2010.

[6] W. J. Ding, Y. Z. Zeng, W. H. Li et al., "Identification of linkage disequilibrium SNPs from a kidney-yang deficiency syndrome pedigree," *American Journal of Chinese Medicine*, vol. 37, no. 3, pp. 427–438, 2009.

[7] W. J. Ding, S. L. Yan, Y. Z. Zeng et al., "Insufficient activity of MAPK pathway is a key monitor of Kidney-Yang Deficiency Syndrome," *Journal of Alternative and Complementary Medicine*, vol. 15, no. 6, pp. 653–660, 2009.

[8] L. Yang, M. Wang, W. Wu, and L. Zhang, "Transcriptome analysis of cold syndrome using microarray," *American Journal of Chinese Medicine*, vol. 35, no. 4, pp. 609–620, 2007.

[9] G. Chen, C. Lu, Q. Zha et al., "A network-based analysis of traditional Chinese medicine cold and hot patterns in rheumatoid arthritis," *Complementary Therapies in Medicine*, vol. 20, no. 1-2, pp. 23–30, 2012.

[10] Q. Pan-Hammarström, S. Wen, and L. Hammarström, "Cytokine gene expression profiles in human lymphocytes induced by a formula of traditional Chinese medicine, vigconic VI-28," *Journal of Interferon and Cytokine Research*, vol. 26, no. 9, pp. 628–636, 2006.

[11] C. Lu, C. Xiao, G. Chen et al., "Cold and heat pattern of rheumatoid arthritis in traditional Chinese medicine: distinct molecular signatures indentified by microarray expression profiles in CD4-positive T cell," *Rheumatology International*, vol. 32, no. 1, pp. 61–68, 2012.

[12] J. Liu, K. Peter, D. Shi et al., "Traditional formula, modern application: Chinese medicine formula Sini tang improves early ventricular remodeling and cardiac function after myocardial infarction in rats," *Evidence-Based Complementary and Alternative Medicine*, vol. 2014, Article ID 141938, 10 pages, 2014.

[13] S. M. Sun, *Qian Jin Yi Fang*, People's Medical Publishing House, Beijing, China, 1955.

[14] World Health Organization and Regional Office for the Western Pacific, *WHO International Standard Terminologies on Traditional Medicine in the Western Pacific Region*, World Health Organization Regional Office for the Western Pacific, Manila, Philippines, 2007.

[15] M. K. Kerr and G. A. Churchill, "Experimental design for gene expression microarrays," *Biostatistics*, vol. 2, no. 2, pp. 183–201, 2001.

[16] C.-R. Chen, W.-Y. Shu, M.-L. Tsai, W.-C. Cheng, and I. C. Hsu, "THEME: a web tool for loop-design microarray data analysis," *Computers in Biology and Medicine*, vol. 42, no. 2, pp. 228–234, 2012.

[17] J. Schuchhardt, D. Beule, A. Malik et al., "Normalization strategies for cDNA microarrays," *Nucleic Acids Research*, vol. 28, no. 10, p. E47, 2000.

[18] W.-C. Cheng, W.-Y. Shu, C.-Y. Li et al., "Intra- and inter-individual variance of gene expression in clinical studies," *PLoS ONE*, vol. 7, no. 6, Article ID e38650, 2012.

[19] D. W. da Huang, B. T. Sherman, and R. A. Lempicki, "Bioinformatics enrichment tools: paths toward the comprehensive functional analysis of large gene lists," *Nucleic Acids Research*, vol. 37, no. 1, pp. 1–13, 2009.

[20] M. Ashburner, C. A. Ball, J. A. Blake et al., "Gene ontology: tool for the unification of biology. The Gene Ontology Consortium," *Nature Genetics*, vol. 25, no. 1, pp. 25–29, 2000.

[21] M. Kanehisa and S. Goto, "KEGG: kyoto encyclopedia of genes and genomes," *Nucleic Acids Research*, vol. 28, no. 1, pp. 27–30, 2000.

PERMISSIONS

All chapters in this book were first published in ECAM, by Hindawi Publishing Corporation; hereby published with permission under the Creative Commons Attribution License or equivalent. Every chapter published in this book has been scrutinized by our experts. Their significance has been extensively debated. The topics covered herein carry significant findings which will fuel the growth of the discipline. They may even be implemented as practical applications or may be referred to as a beginning point for another development.

The contributors of this book come from diverse backgrounds, making this book a truly international effort. This book will bring forth new frontiers with its revolutionizing research information and detailed analysis of the nascent developments around the world.

We would like to thank all the contributing authors for lending their expertise to make the book truly unique. They have played a crucial role in the development of this book. Without their invaluable contributions this book wouldn't have been possible. They have made vital efforts to compile up to date information on the varied aspects of this subject to make this book a valuable addition to the collection of many professionals and students.

This book was conceptualized with the vision of imparting up-to-date information and advanced data in this field. To ensure the same, a matchless editorial board was set up. Every individual on the board went through rigorous rounds of assessment to prove their worth. After which they invested a large part of their time researching and compiling the most relevant data for our readers.

The editorial board has been involved in producing this book since its inception. They have spent rigorous hours researching and exploring the diverse topics which have resulted in the successful publishing of this book. They have passed on their knowledge of decades through this book. To expedite this challenging task, the publisher supported the team at every step. A small team of assistant editors was also appointed to further simplify the editing procedure and attain best results for the readers.

Apart from the editorial board, the designing team has also invested a significant amount of their time in understanding the subject and creating the most relevant covers. They scrutinized every image to scout for the most suitable representation of the subject and create an appropriate cover for the book.

The publishing team has been an ardent support to the editorial, designing and production team. Their endless efforts to recruit the best for this project, has resulted in the accomplishment of this book. They are a veteran in the field of academics and their pool of knowledge is as vast as their experience in printing. Their expertise and guidance has proved useful at every step. Their uncompromising quality standards have made this book an exceptional effort. Their encouragement from time to time has been an inspiration for everyone.

The publisher and the editorial board hope that this book will prove to be a valuable piece of knowledge for researchers, students, practitioners and scholars across the globe.

LIST OF CONTRIBUTORS

Imran Khan
Department of Pharmacy, University of Swabi, Khyber Pakhtunkhwa 23340, Pakistan

Nasiara Karim and Waqar Ahmad
Department of Pharmacy, University of Malakand, Khyber Pakhtunkhwa 18800, Pakistan

Abeer Abdelhalim
Faculty of Science, Taibah University, Medina 30001, Saudi Arabia

Mary Chebib
Faculty of Pharmacy, University of Sydney, Sydney, NSW 2006, Australia

L. D. Wang, J. M. Zhao, R. J. Huang, L. Y. Tan, Z. J. Weng, K. Wang, H. G. Wu and H. R. Liu
Key Laboratory of Acupuncture and Immunological Effects, Shanghai Research Institute of Acupuncture and Meridian, 650 South Wanping Road, Shanghai 200030, China

Z. H. Hu
Shanghai TCM-Integrated Hospital, Shanghai University of TCM, Shanghai 200082, China

Mi Mi Ko
KM Fundamental Research Division, Korea Institute of Oriental Medicine, Daejeon 305-811, Republic of Korea

Honggie Kim
Department of Information and Statistics, Chungnam National University, Daejeon 305-764, Republic of Korea

Qin Zheng, Lemin Xia, Yiling Jiang and Meihong Luo
Department of Hematology, Shanghai Baoshan Hospital of Integrated Traditional Chinese andWestern Medicine (Baoshan Branch of Shuguang Hospital Affiliated to Shanghai University of Traditional Chinese Medicine), Shanghai 201999, China

Yu Guan, Xiaofeng Zhang, Jing Xia and GuohuaWang
Department of Central Laboratory Medicine, Shanghai Municipal Hospital of Traditional Chinese Medicine, Shanghai University of Traditional Chinese Medicine, Shanghai 200071, China

Zhicheng Wang
Department of Laboratory Medicine, Huashan Hospital, Shanghai Medical College, Fudan University, Shanghai 200040, China

Jianying Wang and Yiqiong Pu
College of Pharmacy, Shanghai University of Traditional Chinese Medicine, Shanghai 201203, China

Jung-Hoon Kim
1Division of Pharmacology, School of Korean Medicine, Pusan National University, Yangsan 626-870, Republic of Korea

Eui-Jeong Doh
Department of Herbology, College of Korean Medicine, Wonkwang University, Iksan 570-749, Republic of Korea
Center for Metabolic Function Regulation, Wonkwang University, Iksan 570-749, Republic of Korea

Guemsan Lee
Department of Herbology, College of Korean Medicine, Wonkwang University, Iksan 570-749, Republic of Korea

Mohammad Hafiz Abdul Rahim, Zuraini Ahmad and Mohd HijazMohd Sani
Department of Biomedical Science, Faculty of Medicine and Health Science, Universiti Putra Malaysia, 43400 Serdang, Selangor, Malaysia

Zainul Amiruddin Zakaria and Manraj Singh Cheema
Department of Biomedical Science, Faculty of Medicine and Health Science, Universiti Putra Malaysia, 43400 Serdang, Selangor, Malaysia
Integrative Pharmacogenomics Institute (iPROMISE), Faculty of Pharmacy, Universiti Teknologi MARA (UiTM), Puncak Alam Campus, Level 7, FF3, 42300 Bandar Puncak Alam, Selangor, Malaysia

Maizatul Hasyima Omar
PhytochemistryUnit,Herbal Medicine Research Centre, Institute for Medical Research, Jalan Pahang, 50588 Kuala Lumpur, Malaysia

Yusnita Yakob
Molecular Diagnostics and Protein Unit, Specialised Diagnostics Centre, Institute for Medical Research, Jalan Pahang, 50588 Kuala Lumpur, Malaysia

Siew Mooi Ching
Department of Family Medicine, Faculty of Medicine and Health Science, Universiti Putra Malaysia, 43400 Serdang, Selangor, Malaysia

Arifah Abdul Kadir
Department of Veterinary Pre-Clinical Sciences, Faculty of Veterinary Sciences, Universiti Putra Malaysia, 43400 Serdang, Selangor, Malaysia

Jiao Ying Ou
Department of Nephrology, Shuguang Hospital, Shanghai University of Traditional Chinese Medicine, No. 528 Zhang Heng Road, Shanghai 201203, China
TCM Institute of Kidney Disease, Shanghai University of Traditional Chinese Medicine, No. 528 Zhang Heng Road, Shanghai 201203, China
Shanghai Key Laboratory of Traditional Chinese Clinical Medicine, No. 528 Zhang Heng Road, Shanghai 201203, China
Department of Internal Medicine, Shanghai TCM-Integrated Hospital of Shanghai University of Traditional Chinese Medicine, No. 184 Baoding Road, Shanghai 200082, China

Di Huang, Yan Sheng Wu, Lin Xu, Fei He, Hui LingWang, Li Qiang Shi, QiangWan, Li Qun He and Jian Dong Gao
Department of Nephrology, Shuguang Hospital, Shanghai University of Traditional Chinese Medicine, No. 528 Zhang Heng Road, Shanghai 201203, China
TCM Institute of Kidney Disease, Shanghai University of Traditional Chinese Medicine, No. 528 Zhang Heng Road, Shanghai 201203, China
Shanghai Key Laboratory of Traditional Chinese Clinical Medicine, No. 528 Zhang Heng Road, Shanghai 201203, China

Pei-Jing Rong and jing-Jun Zhao
Institute of Acupuncture and Moxibustion, China Academy of Chinese Medical Sciences, Beijing 100700, China

Lei Wang
School of Acupuncture-Moxibustion and Tuina, Beijing University of Chinese Medicine, Beijing 100029, China

Li-Qun Zhou
School of Basic Medical Science, Beijing University of Chinese Medicine, Beijing 100029, China

Xu Sun, Gan-Lin Zhang, Ming-Wei Yu, Yi Zhang, Xiao-Min Wang, Guo-Wang Yang, Lin Yang and Pei-Yu Cheng
Department of Oncology, Beijing Hospital of Traditional Chinese Medicine, Capital Medical University, Beijing 100010, China

Xing Zhang, Jia-Yun Nian and Jiao Guo
Department of Oncology, Beijing Hospital of Traditional Chinese Medicine, Capital Medical University, Beijing 100010, China
Beijing University of Chinese Medicine, Beijing 100029, China

Yi Yin
Department of Oncology,Third Affiliated Hospital of Henan College of Traditional Chinese Medicine, Zhengzhou 450000, China

Jin-Ping Li
Department of Oncology, Beijing Hospital of Traditional Chinese Medicine, Capital Medical University, Beijing 100010, China
Department of Medical Biochemistry and Microbiology, Uppsala University, 75123 Uppsala, Sweden

Najla O. Zarmouh, Samia S.Messeha, FaiselM. Elshami and Karam F. A. Soliman
College of Pharmacy & Pharmaceutical Sciences, Florida A & M University, Tallahassee, FL 32307, USA

Fatai Oladunni Balogun and Anofi Omotayo Tom Ashafa
Phytomedicine and Phytopharmacology Research Group, Department of Plant Sciences, University of the Free State, Qwaqwa Campus, Private Bag X13, Phuthaditjhaba, Free State 9866, South Africa

Peng Wu
Southern Medical University, Guangzhou 510515, China
Beijing Tibetan Hospital, China Tibetology Research Center, Beijing 100029, China

Yuandai Luo, Lifang Zhen, Xianda Hu and Fukai Huang
Beijing Tibetan Hospital, China Tibetology Research Center, Beijing 100029, China

Ying Shang
Beijing Mentougou Hospital of Traditional Chinese Medicine, Beijing 102300, China

Yinuo Liao, Huiyuan Xue and Wei Xiao
Southern Medical University, Guangzhou 510515, China

Chun-Chang Wu
Division of Chinese Medicine, China Medical University Beigang Hospital, Yulin 65152, Taiwan

Tsung-Jung Ho
Division of Chinese Medicine, China Medical University Beigang Hospital, Yulin 65152, Taiwan
Division of Chinese Medicine, An Nan Hospital, China Medical University, Tainan 70965, Taiwan
College of Chinese Medicine, China Medical University, Taichung 40421, Taiwan

Shinn-Jong Jiang and Hao-Ping Chen
Department of Biochemistry, School of Medicine, Tzu Chi University, Hualien 97004, Taiwan

Guang-Huey Lin and Ming-Chuan Hsieh
Department of Microbiology, School of Medicine, Tzu Chi University, Hualien 97004, Taiwan

Tzong Shiun Li
Department of Plastic Surgery, China Medical University Beigang Hospital, Yulin 65152, Taiwan
School of Medicine, China Medical University, Taichung 40421, Taiwan
Department of Plastic Surgery, China Medical University Hospital, Taichung 40447, Taiwan

Lih-Ming Yiin
Department of Public Health, School of Medicine, Tzu Chi University, Hualien 97004, Taiwan

Jai-Sing Yang
Department of Medical Research, China Medical University Hospital, China Medical University, Taichung 40447, Taiwan

Jaung-Geng Lin
Graduate Institute of Chinese Medicine, China Medical University, Taichung 40421, Taiwan

Baoshan Liu, Xiaohong Wang, Hong Wang and Lin Ma
Department of Traditional Chinese Medicine, Tianjin Medical University General Hospital, Tianjin 300052, China

Tong Liu and Xin Zheng
Tianjin Zhongxin Pharmaceutical Group Corporation LTD., Tianjin 300457, China

Ho-Yeol Cha and Jin-Hong Cheon
Department of Korean Pediatrics, Hospital of Korean Medicine, Pusan National University, 20 Geumo-ro, Mulgeum-eup, Yangsan-si, Gyeongsangnam-do 50612, Republic of Korea

Sang-hyun Ahn
Research Institute for Korean Medicine, Pusan National University, 49 Pusandaehak-ro, Mulgeum-eup, Yangsan-si, Gyeongsangnam-do 50612, Republic of Korea

In-Sik Park and Jin-Tack Kim
Department of Anatomy, College of Korean Medicine, Dongguk University, Seokjang-dong, Gyeongju-si, Gyeongsangbuk-do 38066, Republic of Korea

Kibong Kim
Department of Korean Pediatrics, Hospital of Korean Medicine, Pusan National University, 20 Geumo-ro, Mulgeum-eup, Yangsan-si, Gyeongsangnam-do 50612, Republic of Korea
Department of Korean Pediatrics, School of Korean Medicine, Pusan National University, 49 Pusandaehak-ro, Mulgeum-eup, Yangsan-si, Gyeongsangnam-do 50612, Republic of Korea

Hung-Tsu Cheng
Institute of Nano Engineering and Microsystems, National Tsing Hua University, No. 101, Section 2, Kuang-Fu Road, Hsinchu 300, Taiwan
Classics Chinese Medicine Clinic, Taipei 104, Taiwan

Chaang-Ray Chen, Chao-Ying Huang and Ian C. Hsu
Department of Biomedical Engineering and Environmental Sciences, National Tsing Hua University, Hsinchu 300, Taiwan

Chia-Yang Li
Department of Genome Medicine, College of Medicine and Center for Infectious Disease and Cancer Research, Kaohsiung Medical University, Kaohsiung 807, Taiwan

Wun-Yi Shu
Institute of Statistics, National Tsing Hua University, Hsinchu 300, Taiwan

Index